SURGERY OF THE LARYNX, TRACHEA, ESOPHAGUS, AND NECK

SURGERY OF THE LARYNX, TRACHEA, ESOPHAGUS, AND NECK

WILLIAM W. MONTGOMERY, MD

John W. Merriam Professor of Otology and Laryngology

Massachusetts Eye and Ear Infirmary

Harvard Medical School

Boston, Massachusetts

SAUNDERS

An Imprint of Elsevier Science

Philadelphia   London   New York   St. Louis   Sydney   Toronto

Saunders
An Imprint of Elsevier Science

The Curtis Center
Independence Square West
Philadelphia, Pennsylvania 19106

NOTICE

Medicine is an ever-changing field. Standard safety precautions must be followed, but as new research and clinical experience broaden our knowledge, changes in treatment and drug therapy may become necessary or appropriate. Readers are advised to check the most current product information provided by the manufacturer of each drug to be administered to verify the recommended dose, the method and duration of administration, and contraindications. It is the responsibility of the treating physician, relying on experience and knowledge of the patient, to determine dosages and the best treatment for each individual patient. Neither the Publisher nor the Editor assumes any liability for any injury and/or damage to persons or property arising from this publication.

THE PUBLISHER

Library of Congress Cataloging-in-Publication Data

Montgomery, William W., MD
   Surgery of the larynx, trachea, esophagus, and neck / William W. Montgomery.
     p. ; cm.
   ISBN 0–7216–8708–3
    1. Laryngectomy. 2. Larynx—Surgery. 3. Esophagus—Surgery. 4. Neck—Surgery. I. Title.
   [DNLM: 1. Laryngectomy. 2. Esophagus—surgery. 3. Neck—surgery. 4. Trachea—surgery. WV 540 M7879s 2002]
   RF517 .M66 2002
   617.5′3059—dc21   2001–049610

Acquisitions Editor: Stephanie Donley
Publishing Services Manager: Frank Polizzano
Project Manager: Marian A. Bellus
Illustration Specialist: Bob Quinn

SURGERY OF THE LARYNX, TRACHEA, ESOPHAGUS, AND NECK   ISBN 0–7216–8708–3

Printed in the United States of America

Last digit is the print number: 9 8 7 6 5 4 3 2 1

Dedication

We owe much and dedicate this volume to our patients, who have been our life's work. They have contributed themselves with their disorders and support our research and writings.

We thank the nurses in the operating room for their contributions to our medical lives. We have great respect and admiration for these nurses.

Contributors

Mack Lowell Cheney, MD, FACS
Associate Professor of Otolaryngology
Harvard Medical School;
Director of Facial Plastic and Reconstructive Surgery,
Massachusetts Eye and Ear Infirmary,
Boston, Massachusetts

John B. Lazor, MD, MBA, FACS
Instructor in Otology and Laryngology,
Harvard Medical School,
Massachusetts Eye and Ear Infirmary,
Boston, Massachusetts

Stuart K. Montgomery, BS, MBA
President and CEO,
Boston Medical Products, Inc,
Westborough, Massachusetts

William W. Montgomery, MD, FACS
John W. Merriam Professor of Otology and Laryngology,
Harvard Medical School,
Massachusetts Eye and Ear Infirmary,
Boston, Massachusetts

Gregory W. Randolph, MD, FACS
Assistant Professor of Otology and Laryngology,
Harvard Medical School;
Director, General and Thyroid Surgical Service,
Massachusetts Eye and Ear Infirmary,
Boston, Massachusetts

Mark Alex Varvares, MD
Assistant Professor of Otology and Laryngology,
Harvard Medical School;
Associate Surgeon,
Massachusetts Eye and Ear Infirmary,
Boston, Massachusetts

Alfred L. Weber, MD
Professor of Radiology
Harvard Medical School;
Radiologist,
Massachusetts Eye and Ear Infirmary,
Boston, Massachusetts

Preface

The intent of this book is to provide the resident and the practicing otolaryngologist with guidelines for diagnosis and surgical management of diseases of the larynx, trachea, esophagus, and neck.

The first chapter supplies the "tools" necessary for arriving at as exact a diagnosis as possible and for selecting the proper therapeutic measures for the patient who has symptoms referable to this portion of our specialty. Highlighted in the remaining chapters of the book are diagnosis of a cervical mass, blocked neck dissection, pedicle skin flaps, parotid and submandibular gland surgery, facial nerve rehabilitation, laryngeal paralysis, reconstruction of the cervical esophagus, free flap reconstruction, thyroid surgery, snoring and sleep apnea, technique and complications of tracheotomy, and treatment of tracheal and laryngeal stenosis.

We are indebted to the entire resident and visiting staff at the Massachusetts Eye and Ear Infirmary for their direct and indirect contributions to this work. I wish to thank those contributing to this volume: Drs. Mack L. Cheney, Gregory W. Randolph, John B. Lazor, Mark A. Varvares, Alfred L. Weber, and Stuart K. Montgomery.

The modern otolaryngologist must be an accomplished surgeon. A single operation can require the versatility and dexterity needed for handling soft tissues and bone, as well as various macro- and microsurgical procedures and free tissue transfer surgery. The surgeon must have a thorough knowledge of the anatomy and physiology of the involved structures, to enable him to deal efficiently with diseases of the larynx, trachea, esophagus, and neck.

Special recognition goes to Joshua B. Clarke, for his excellent artwork. He possesses a keen intellect, curiosity, thoroughness, and dedication to work. In his artwork he is able to make a complicated problem simple. Joshua Clarke is now retired. The artwork of Robert Galla is also excellent. The manuscript transcription was done by Beverly F. Stone and Candace Thomas.

WILLIAM H. MONTGOMERY, M.D.

Contents

Chapter 1
Anatomy, Examination, and Diagnosis

WILLIAM W. MONTGOMERY   JOHN B. LAZOR   ALFRED L. WEBER

This chapter is intended to provide medical students, residents, and attending physicians with the knowledge and tools that will allow them to arrive at the correct diagnosis and to institute the appropriate treatment. The anatomy, physiology, physical examination, diagnostic procedures, and abnormal findings of the oral cavity, oropharynx, larynx, hypopharynx, cervical esophagus, and neck are discussed.

ORAL CAVITY

The oral cavity extends from the lips to the level of the uvula and the base of tongue (circumvallate papillae). The uvula, palatoglossal fold (anterior tonsillar pillar), and base of the tongue constitute the boundary between the oral cavity and the oropharynx.

Anatomy of the Tongue

The extrinsic muscles of the tongue include the genioglossus, hyoglossus, and styloglossus. Branches of the hypoglossal nerve (Fig. 1–1A) supply the muscles. The palatoglossus muscle is sometimes included in this group; the pharyngeal plexus innervates this muscle. The genioglossus and hyoglossus muscles extend superiorly into the tongue from the sublingual region and make up a large portion of the extrinsic muscular mass. The styloglossus and palatoglossus muscles enter the tongue laterally from above. The intrinsic tongue musculature is made up of complicated interlacing bundles of muscle that are, for the most part, arranged in a vertical or transverse direction. The extrinsic muscles pull the tongue forward, backward, upward, and downward. The intrinsic muscles change the shape of the tongue.

The lingual nerve is distributed to the anterior two thirds of the tongue, or that portion anterior to the circumvallate papillae (Fig. 1–1B). The glossopharyngeal nerve is distributed to the posterior third of the tongue, including the circumvallate papillae. A small portion of the base of the tongue is innervated by a branch of the superior laryngeal (vagus) nerve.

The lingual and glossopharyngeal nerves include fibers for temperature, pain, and touch sensation, as well as some limited taste function. The change in taste function after section of one chorda tympani nerve is much more noticeable to the patient than the change after unilateral section of the glossopharyngeal nerve. Conversely, section of both glossopharyngeal nerves may result in a complete loss of taste.

Anatomy of the Palate

The five paired muscles of the soft palate are important for speech, eustachian tube function, and deglutition. They are shown in Figure 1–1C and Table 1–1.

All muscles of the soft palate are innervated by the pharyngeal plexus (X and IX), with the exception of the trigeminal nerve by way of the otic ganglion.

Anatomy of the Submandibular and Parotid Glands

The submandibular gland occupies most of the submandibular triangle, which is bounded by the anterior and posterior bellies of the digastric muscle and the mandible. The posterior aspect of the submandibular gland is in close proximity to the parotid gland (Fig. 1–2A). The platysma muscle, ramus mandibulae nerve, and anterior facial vein are superficial to the submandibular gland. The facial artery crosses the upper surface of the gland. The anterior portion of the submandibular gland lies directly against the mylohyoid muscle. The lingual nerve is located medial and superior to the submandibular gland; it connects with the submandibular gland by way of the submandibular ganglion. The hypoglossal nerve lies inferior between the submandibular gland and the hyoglossus muscle. The submandibular (Wharton's) duct proceeds forward, above the mylohyoid muscle, where it crosses the descending lingual nerve. The hypoglossal nerve and submandibular duct are closely related until they reach the genioglossus muscle. The submandibular duct lies immediately inferior to the mucous membrane of the floor of the mouth, forming the sublingual fold. It terminates just lateral to the frenulum, in the sublingual papilla.

The parotid gland is located anterior and inferior to the auricle (Fig. 1–2B). Its posterior border is immediately an-

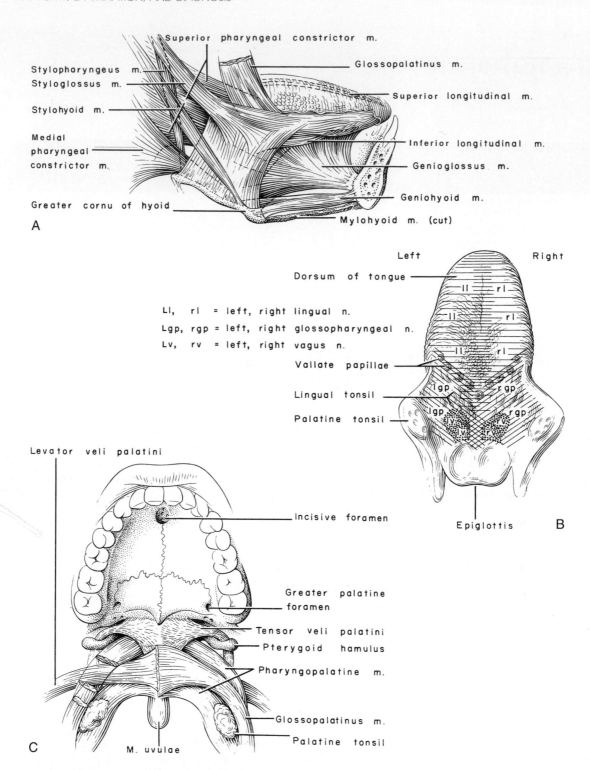

FIGURE 1-1. Anatomy of the tongue and palate. *A,* Tongue musculature. The extrinsic muscles of the tongue include the genioglossus, hyoglossus, styloglossus, and palatoglossus muscles. These muscles are innervated by the hypoglossal nerve, with the exception of the palatoglossus, which is innervated by the pharyngeal plexus. The intrinsic tongue musculature is made up of interlacing vertical and transverse muscle bundles. *B,* Sensory innervation of the tongue. The lingual nerve supplies sensation to the anterior two thirds of the tongue, whereas the facial nerve supplies taste to the anterior two thirds of the tongue. Taste and sensation to the posterior one third of the tongue, including the circumvallate papillae, are by way of the glossopharyngeal nerve. A small portion of the base of the tongue is innervated by the vagus nerve by way of a branch of the superior laryngeal nerve. *C,* Anatomy of the palate. The five-paired muscles of the soft palate include the palatoglossus, palatopharyngeus, levator veli palatini, tensor velipalatini, and uvulae muscles. They are important for speech, eustachian tube function, and deglutition. The incisive foramen is located in the midline, just behind the upper median incisors. The greater palatine foramen can be palpated in the slight depression in the hard palate located just medial to the last molar. Note the relations of the hamulus of the pterygoid and the tendon of the tensor veli palatini muscles.

TABLE 1-1
Anatomy of the Palate

Palatoglossus muscle (anterior pillar)
- Origin: undersurface of soft palate
- Insertion: side of tongue
- Action: lower soft palate

Palatopharyngeus muscle (posterior pillar)
- Origin: inferior surface of soft palate
- Insertion: posterior border of thyroid cartilage
- Action: lowers soft palate

Muscle of uvula
- Origin: posterior nasal spine
- Insertion: aponeurosis of soft palate
- Action: elevates uvula anteriorly and superiorly

Levator muscle of velum palatinum
- Origin: inferior tip of petrous temporal bone and lower cartilaginous eustachian tube
- Insertion: aponeurosis of soft palate
- Action: raises soft palate

Tensor muscle of velum palatinum
- Origin: spine of sphenoid, scaphoid fossa of pterygoid process, and lateral aspect of cartilaginous tube
- Insertion: posterior border of hard palate after passing around the hamular process.
- Action: stretches soft palate and opens eustachian tube

terior to the tragus of the conchal cartilage, mastoid process, and anterior border of the sternocleidomastoid (SCM) muscle. The anterior border of the gland is related to the mid-portion of the masseter muscle and the body of the mandible. The superior border of the gland extends from the tragus to the mid-portion of the masseter muscle. Inferiorly, the gland extends into the neck 2-cm inferoposterior to the angle of the mandible. The outer surface of the gland is found just beneath the subcutaneous layer. The parotid (Stensen's) duct proceeds forward, superficial to the masseter muscle, at the level of a line drawn halfway between the columella and upper lip. At the anterior border of the masseter muscles, the duct is directed medially, where it penetrates the buccinator muscle. It enters the mouth at its papilla, which is located opposite the crown of the second upper molar.

Examination Technique

The oral cavity is the most accessible body orifice; it deserves a thorough examination because it may reveal signs of systemic disease as well as local lesions. Examination of the oral cavity requires a pair of tongue depressors, light source, gauze sponge, glove, and set of lacrimal dilators and probes. The patient is placed in a sitting position with the head resting on a back support.

A systematic examination should include the lips, buccal mucosa, teeth, floor of mouth, tongue, and palate.

Lips
The lips should be examined for symmetry, function, and lesions. Any lesions should be palpated.

Buccal Mucosa
The patient is asked to remove any dentures and to open the mouth slightly. The lips are retracted with a tongue depres-

sor, and the inner aspect of lips, buccal mucosa, and gingivae are carefully inspected. The orifice of the parotid duct enters the mouth through the lateral buccal mucosa at a point opposite the second upper molar (Fig. 1–3A). Saliva can be expressed when the cheek is stroked in an anterior direction along the parotid duct.

Teeth
The teeth are examined for their structure, function, and support of the jaw. Light percussion with the handle of a mirror is useful in locating the source of a painful dental condition. The examiner should look for malocclusion and should observe the excursion of the mandible. At the same time, it is wise to palpate the temporomandibular joint to detect any possible malfunction. The inner aspects of the gingivae are inspected with a mirror.

Floor of the Mouth
The anterior floor of the mouth is examined as the patient places the tip of the tongue against the hard palate (Fig. 1–3B). The sublingual fold (frenulum) is noted. On either side of the frenulum is an elevation known as the sublingual papilla (*arrows*). Saliva can be expressed from the orifice of the duct in a sublingual papilla by massaging the submental and submandibular area. At least 10 sublingual ducts (ducts of Rivinus) empty into the sublingual area on either side of the sublingual fold.

The lateral floor of the mouth is examined by retracting the cheeks laterally with one tongue depressor and displacing the lateral surface of the tongue in a medial direction with another (Fig. 1–3C).

Bimanual palpation of the floor of the mouth is accomplished by inserting an index finger covered with a glove. With this finger in place, the entire floor of the mouth is palpated, while the fingers of the opposite hand palpate, in opposition, the submandibular and submental areas (Fig. 1–3D). Using this bimanual technique, saliva can be expressed from the submandibular papilla by milking the duct forward.

Tongue
The patient is asked to stick out the tongue for inspection of its dorsum. The tongue is then inspected, with the aid of the tongue depressor, for symmetry and muscle coordination. The tongue normally protrudes in the midline. If unilateral paralysis is present, it deviates toward the paralyzed side. The mucous membrane of the tongue is inspected and observed for coating, a black hairy appearance, geographic deformity, tumors, and varicosities.

The lingual and glossopharyngeal nerves distribute sensory fibers to the anterior two thirds and posterior one third of the tongue, respectively. Because the glossopharyngeal nerve mediates the gag reflex, it is best to keep the tongue depressor well forward of the posterior third of the tongue (Fig. 1–4A). Note the circumvallate papillae at the junction of the anterior two thirds and posterior one third of the tongue (arrow). These papillae receive taste fibers from the glossopharyngeal nerve. The facial nerve (chorda tympani) innervates the taste buds on the anterior two thirds of the tongue. If the patient complains of a disturbance in taste, a

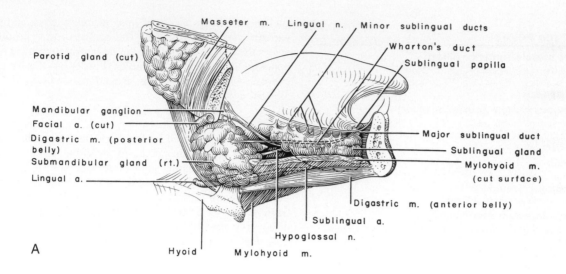

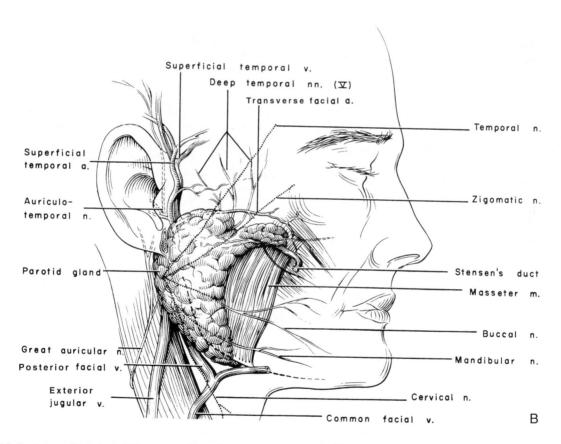

FIGURE 1-2. Submandibular and sublingual glands. *A,* A portion of the mandible has been removed to demonstrate the details of the submandibular triangle. The relationship of the facial artery, lingual nerve, Wharton's duct, and hypoglossal nerve is shown. The relationship of the facial artery to the submandibular gland is variable. Usually it is necessary to retract the mylohyoid muscle anteriorly and the submandibular gland inferiorly to obtain a view of the lingual nerve. The submandibular duct and lingual nerve are near each other in the submandibular triangle. The hypoglossal nerve is found deep and inferior in the triangle. *B,* The parotid gland is shown in relation to the numerous neural and vascular structures in its vicinity. The parotid duct proceeds directly forward, along the external surface of the masseter muscle, until it reaches its anterior border. Here, directed medially, it penetrates the buccinator muscle and enters the mouth, opposite the second upper molar.

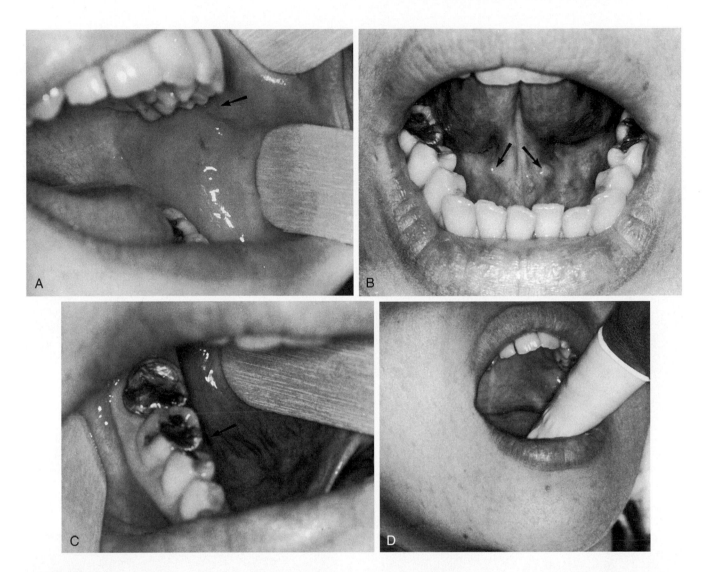

FIGURE 1–3. *A,* The punctum and orifice of the parotid (Stensen's) duct are found on the lateral buccal mucosa at a point opposite the second upper molar (*arrow*). This is best visualized by retracting the lips laterally with a tongue depressor. At times, the orifice is difficult to visualize. Massaging the cheek forward over the parotid duct will express saliva from the duct's orifice, making its location apparent. *B,* The anterior floor of the mouth can be inspected by having the patient place the tip of his or her tongue against the hard palate. The sublingual papillae (*arrows*) can be seen on either side of the frenulum. The orifice of the submandibular duct may be found in the region of the sublingual papillae. Saliva can be expressed from the duct's orifice by massaging the submandibular gland. *C,* Examination of the lateral floor of the mouth (*arrow*) is best accomplished by retracting the cheek laterally with the tongue depressor and by retracting the lateral surface of the tongue medially. *D,* Bimanual palpation of the floor of mouth is valuable for outlining local lesions as well as the contents of the submandibular triangle.

thorough examination of the tongue is performed. The lateral surfaces of the tongue are inspected by pulling the tongue forward and to one side with gauze sponge while retracting the cheek in the opposite direction with a tongue depressor. A referral to a neurologist is ordered for detailed testing. Lesions of the tongue are best evaluated using computed tomography or magnetic resonance imaging (Fig 1–5*A* and *B*).

Palate

The patient is asked to tilt the head back and open the mouth wide. The hard and soft palate can then easily be seen (see Fig. 1–4*B*). The dorsum of the tongue is depressed to observe the function of the soft palate. Elevation of the uvula in the midline is noted as the patient says "ah" (see Fig. 1–4*C*).

The Parotid Gland

In general, one's ability to palpate the medial aspect of the mandibular angle with a finger indicates whether the parotid gland is enlarged (Fig. 1–6).

The signs and symptoms of parotid disease are (1) swelling, (2) pain in the region of the parotid, (3) pain in the ear canal, (4) foul discharge in the mouth, and (5) a mass in the cheek region.

Diagnosis of Parotitis

The upper lip is retracted superiorly, with the teeth in near approximation, to expose the orifice of the parotid duct in the buccal mucosa opposite the second upper molar. The papilla of the parotid duct is often not apparent, and the ori-

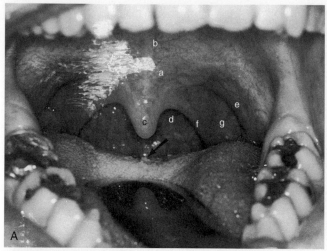

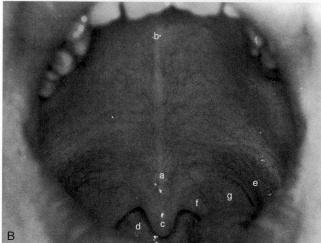

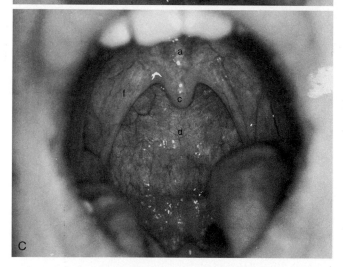

fice is difficult to visualize. It may be necessary to milk the duct several times, wiping away the saliva after each milking, to locate its orifice. Excellent illumination is necessary for the procedure. The parotid duct is palpated by using the bimanual technique. The status of the saliva can be observed by milking forward along the duct.

Topical anesthesia is sprayed on the buccal mucosa opposite the second upper molar. The duct's orifice is dilated with a punctum dilator (Fig. 1–7A). A lacrimal probe is inserted into the orifice. The duct proceeds for a few millimeters in a direction perpendicular to the plane of the cheek, to the level of the external surface of the masseter

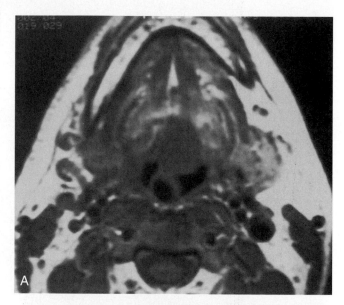

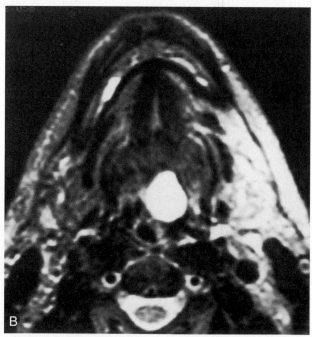

FIGURE 1–4. *A,* The dorsum of the tongue is depressed with the tip of the depressor to view the oropharynx. It is important to place the tip of the tongue depressor anterior to the circumvallate papillae (*arrow*) to avoid stimulating the gag reflex. *B,* The entire palate can be seen by having the patient tilt his or her head back and open the mouth wide. This portion of the examination is often omitted, and obvious lesions are missed. *C,* The functions of the soft palate can be observed and evaluated while depressing the tongue. The soft palate should be elevated symmetrically as the patient says "ah." The uvula should not deviate from the midline. a = soft palate; b = hard palate; c = uvula; d = posterior pharyngeal wall; e = anterior pillar; f = posterior pillar; g = palatine tonsil.

FIGURE 1–5. Thyroglossal duct cyst of posterior tongue. *A,* Axial T1-weighted image of posterior tongue shows a low-intensity cystic lesion in the posterior tongue. *B,* Axial T2-weighted image shows high intensity of the cyst.

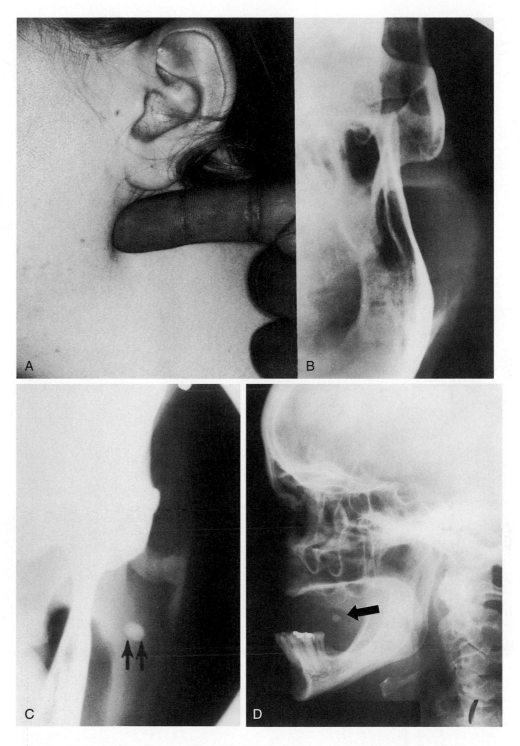

FIGURE 1–6. *A,* Examination of the parotid gland should include external and bimanual palpation of the parotid region and also of the region between the mastoid tip and the angle of the jaw. Often, general enlargement of the gland, which is not obvious by usual methods of palpation, can be determined by attempting to introduce the index finger behind the angle of the mandible. *B,* Radiograph of the parotid duct with patient's cheek "ballooned out." No abnormalities are seen. *C,* An anteroposterior radiograph of the parotid duct taken with the patient's cheek "ballooned out." A large salivary stone (*arrows*) is present in the duct. *D,* Lateral view shows a salivary stone (arrow) in the parotid duct in the region of Stensen's orifice.

muscle (Fig. 1–7*B*). At this point, the duct bends sharply in a posterolateral direction. If the probe does not follow this course, it will puncture the duct. The probe should be inserted gently, to avoid creating unnecessary discomfort or perforating the duct's wall. Stones, strictures, or an abnormal course of the duct can be detected with the lacrimal

probe. After trauma, when transection of the parotid duct is probable, a probe inserted by way of the buccal orifice may appear in the wound.

Stenosis is easily demonstrated by sialography and by delayed emptying time. The stenosis may be in the region of the papilla, especially in patients who wear dentures. Occa-

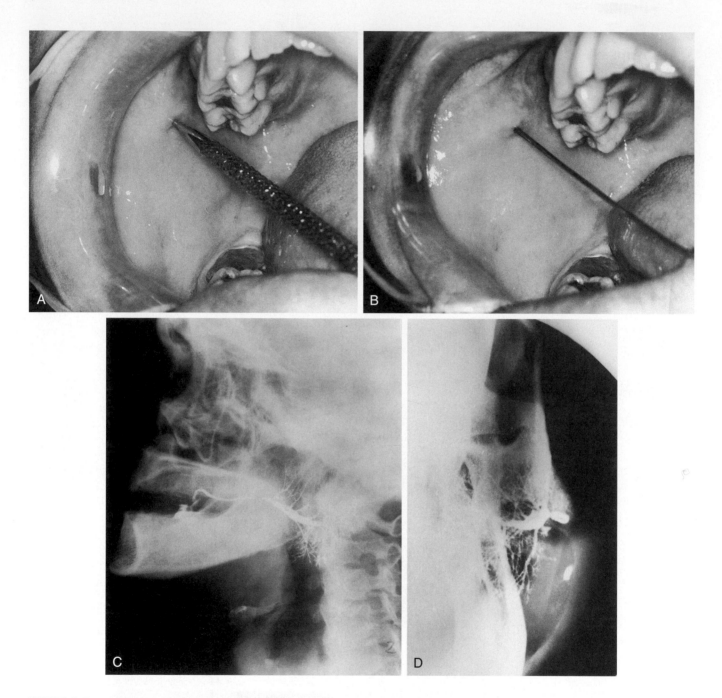

FIGURE 1-7. Parotid sialography. *A,* The parotid duct orifice is gently dilated with a punctum dilator after the application of topical anesthesia to this region. *B,* The lacrimal probe is inserted into the orifice of the parotid duct. It is advanced for a few millimeters, in a direction perpendicular to the plane of the cheek, to the level of the external surface of the masseter muscle. At this point, the duct bends sharply in a posterolateral direction; the probe should be rotated approximately 90 degrees. *C,* An anteroposterior view of the sialogram showing normal filling of the parotid duct and gland. *D,* A sialogram demonstrating a normal parotid duct gland.

sionally, the stenosis occurs at the bifurcation of the main duct. Radiopaque stones are demonstrated in the radiograph taken before sialography, whereas nonradiopaque stones are identified by contrast sialography. Sialectasis is also easily demonstrated by sialography. In general, sialography is not useful in determining the exact site, size, and shape of tumors of the parotid gland, but it may give some indication of their location by compression of the adjacent parotid gland.

Figure 1–8 demonstrates the findings associated with normal parotid and submandibular glands. Contrast computed tomography and magnetic resonance imaging scans have

added much to the diagnostic methods for studying these glands. Figures 1–9 and 1–10 show the typical finding of a pleomorphic adenoma.

The Submandibular Gland

The submandibular gland is palpated directly under the body of the mandible, about halfway between the mental protuberance and the angle. Normally, it has a firm, irregular consistency. It can be palpated with greater accuracy by placing

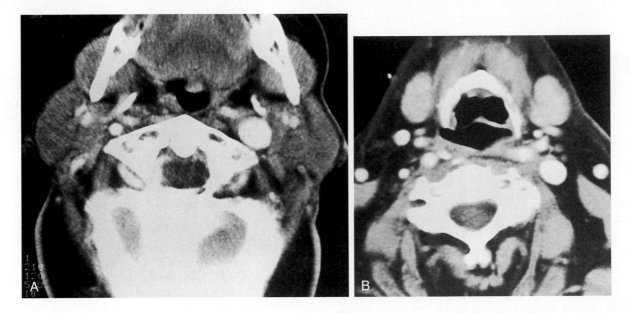

FIGURE 1–8. Normal computed tomography (CT) study of submandibular glands and parotid glands. *A,* Axial CT study shows normal submandibular glands, which are isodense with muscle. *B,* Axial CT study through the parotid gland reveals normal parotid glands. Note retromandibular vein and external carotid artery in the anterior mid-portion of the parotid gland behind the mandible.

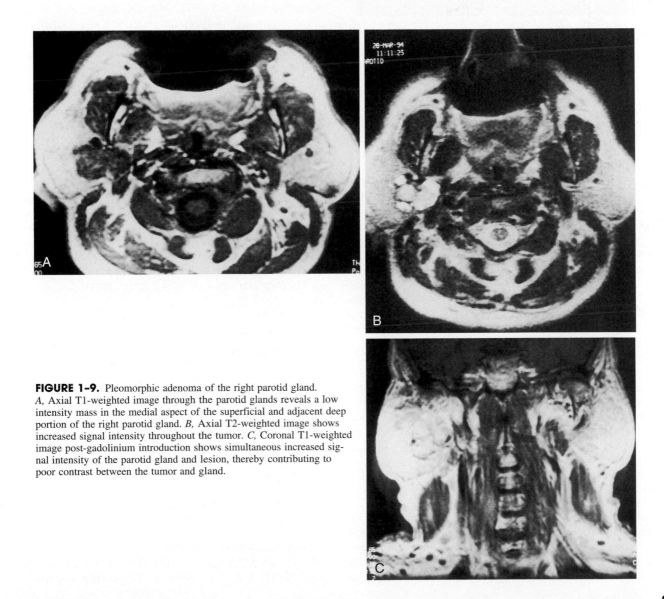

FIGURE 1–9. Pleomorphic adenoma of the right parotid gland. *A,* Axial T1-weighted image through the parotid glands reveals a low intensity mass in the medial aspect of the superficial and adjacent deep portion of the right parotid gland. *B,* Axial T2-weighted image shows increased signal intensity throughout the tumor. *C,* Coronal T1-weighted image post-gadolinium introduction shows simultaneous increased signal intensity of the parotid gland and lesion, thereby contributing to poor contrast between the tumor and gland.

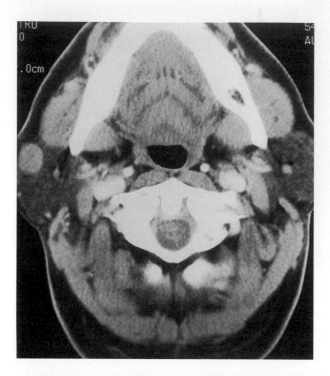

FIGURE 1-10. Pleomorphic adenoma of right parotid gland. Axial CT study demonstrates an oval-shaped, homogeneous sharply defined tumor in the superficial portion of the right parotid gland anteriorly.

the index finger on the lateral floor of the mouth and the fingers of the opposite hand externally over the submandibular triangle. With this technique, the submandibular duct can be carefully palpated for stones or other abnormalities.

Routine radiography of the anterior and lateral floor of the mouth may demonstrate a radiopaque stone in the submandibular duct (Fig. 1–11A and B).

Dilator is in place (Fig. 1–12A). Lacrimal probes of various sizes are inserted into the duct, inferiorly for a few millimeters and then laterally in the horizontal plane, in the direction of the floor of the mouth (Fig. 1–12B). A stone or stricture can be palpated in this fashion. A No. 18 blunt-end needle or No. 90 polyethylene tubing is inserted into the submandibular duct. Approximately 1 mL of contrast material (Diodras or Pantopaque) is slowly injected into the duct. The injection is stopped when the patient reports discomfort in the region of the submandibular gland. The patient should be reassured that the pain is not unusual. Lateral and floor-of-the-mouth radiographs are repeated after injection of the radiopaque substance (Fig. 1–13). Computed tomography scanning has added much in the diagnosis of salivary gland and neck disease (Fig. 1–14).

Congenital Abnormalities of the Oral Cavity

Ankyloglossia (Tongue Tie)

Ankyloglossia is the result of a short lingual frenulum. It interferes with the protrusion of the tongue, and, if marked, may cause lisping during speech and interfere with chewing. The condition is most commonly congenital but may be the result of trauma.

Macroglossia

Congenital enlargement of the tongue is most commonly seen in cretinism and Down's syndrome. It is also seen with angiomatous involvement of the tongue musculature, pituitary tumors, and lesions that interfere with blood circulation or lymphatic drainage of the tongue.

Cleft Lip and Palate

Large congenital clefts of the lip and palate are quite obvious. A small cleft lip may consist of a small notch. A cleft palate may be incomplete. A submucous cleft may be detected by palpation.

Glossitis Rhombica Mediana

This is a congenital defect that is usually oval-shaped and slightly elevated. It is characteristically located in the midline just anterior to the circumvallate papillae. It is of no clinical significance.

Lingual Thyroid

Occasionally the thyroid gland will fail to descend and remains as a mass on the base of the tongue. Although a radioactive iodine study will verify this diagnosis, a computed tomography scan or magnetic resonance imaging should be suggested. Patients with this disorder should be referred to an endocrinologist for evaluation.

Diseases of the Oral Mucosa

Aphthous Stomatitis

This appears first as yellow superficial vesicles that rupture and leave grayish ulcerations surrounded by erythema. They are painful and may recur. They are believed to be of viral origin.

Moniliasis/Thrush

This condition is caused by *Candida albicans* and occurs most commonly as a result of antibiotic therapy or immunosuppression. It usually appears as a glistening, grayish-white membrane on the surface of the mucous membrane that somewhat resembles leukoplakia or lichen planus. Removal of the membrane reveals an angry red mucosa.

Leukoplakia

Leukoplakia appears first as reddish areas on the mucous membrane that gradually become milky-white patches of keratinized epithelium. It usually occurs in patients over 50 years of age who are either heavy smokers or have poor dental hygiene. This condition should be carefully observed because 15% of severe cases undergo malignant degeneration.

Vincent's Stomatitis (Trench Mouth)

Vincent's stomatitis is caused by *Fusiformis dentium* and *Borrelia vincentii;* it usually involves the entire gingiva and buccal mucosa. The gums are swollen and tender, with superficial dirty-green ulcerations of the mucous membrane that bleed easily. Mastication is painful, and there is usually cervical lymphadenopathy.

Streptococcal Stomatitis

Streptococcal stomatitis is caused by beta-hemolytic streptococci. The mucous membrane is markedly reddened, and

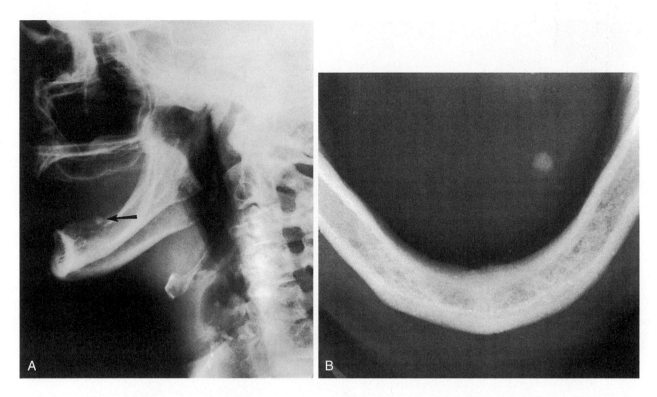

FIGURE 1-11. *A,* Lateral view shows a salivary stone in the submandibular duct (*arrow*). *B,* Radiograph of the floor of the mouth more accurately determines the location of this radiopaque salivary stone.

there may be ulcerations or exudates. The condition is usually associated with streptococcal pharyngitis or tonsillitis.

Toxic Stomatitis

Toxic stomatitis occurs after ingestion of mercury, lead, or bismuth. The characteristic clinical picture is a dark gray or bluish black line on the gingiva.

Stomatitis and Systemic Disease

In patients with diabetes who have stomatitis and systemic disease, the gingivae are dark red and bleed easily. In patients with uremia, the interdental papillae are red, swollen, and ulcerated. In patients with leukemia, the gingivae are red, swollen, and bleed easily. There is usually a foul odor. Approximately 70% of patients with acute

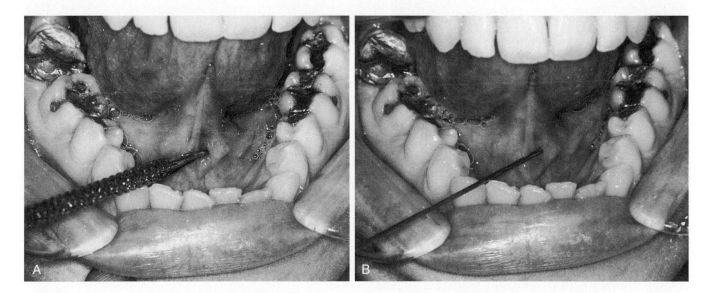

FIGURE 1-12. Submandibular sialography. *A,* After the application of topical anesthesia, the orifice of the submandibular duct is dilated. *B,* The lacrimal probe is inserted in an inferior direction, for a few millimeters, into the submandibular duct, and then laterally in the direction of the plane of the floor of the mouth. When performing submandibular sialography, a blunt No. 18 needle or No. 90 polyethylene tubing is inserted in a similar fashion.

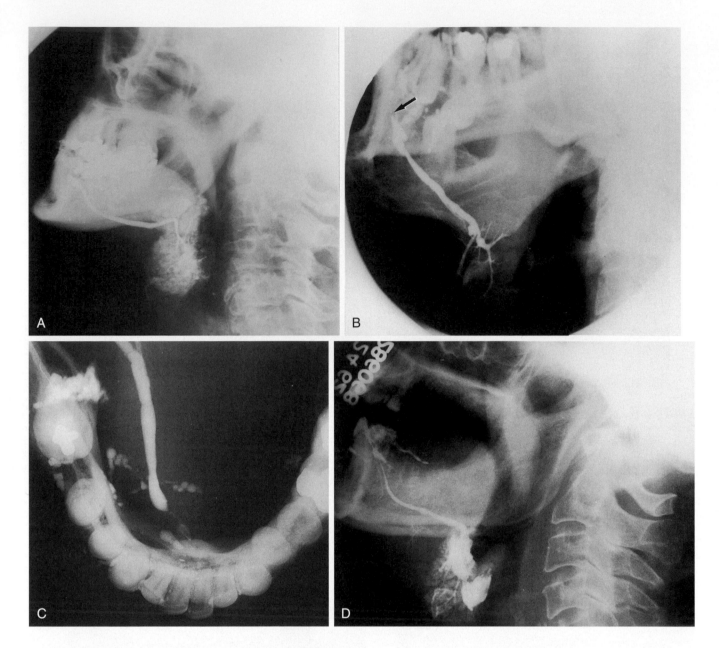

FIGURE 1-13. *A,* Lateral radiograph view of a normal submandibular gland and duct. Globules of radiopaque material are present in the floor of the mouth. *B,* Sialogram demonstrating sialectasia of the submandibular duct to stenosis of the duct at the punctum (*arrow*). *C,* A floor-of-the-mouth view of the same submandibular sialogram as shown in *B*. The dilated submandibular duct and anterior narrowing are obvious. *D,* Submandibular sialogram showing normal filling of the gland and duct. Two cavities, however, are filled with radiopaque substance, indicating sialoangiectasis.

leukemia develop this stomatitis. In patients with anemia, the gums are a pale bluish gray. In patients with polycythemia, the gums are red and hypertrophic and bleed easily. In patients with vitamin C deficiency, the gums are hypertrophic, spongy, and bluish red. They are quite painful and bleed easily.

Fordyce's Disease
Fordyce's disease is characterized by pinhead-sized white or yellowish elevations on the mucous membrane of the gums and lips. It is caused by hypertrophy of aberrant sebaceous glands and usually occurs after puberty.

Diseases of the Tongue

Geographic Tongue
Geographic tongue begins as red, macular spots on the surface of the tongue. As the central portion of the inflammation heals, the periphery spreads in an irregular fashion, producing the characteristic geographic configurations. It is self-limiting and requires no treatment.

Coating of the Tongue
The usual causes for coating of the tongue are smoking, mouth breathing, general debilitation, and dehydration. A

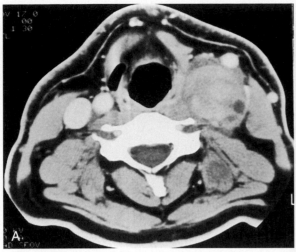
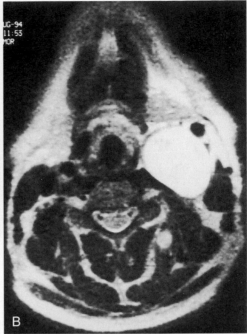
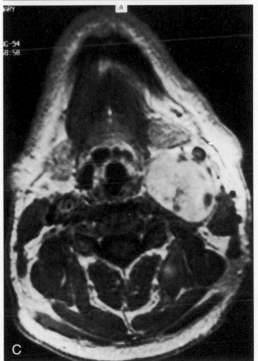

FIGURE 1-14. Malignant schwannoma of the left neck. *A,* Axial contrast CT section shows a fairly well-defined heterogeneous tumor in the left neck at the level of the larynx. *B,* Axial T2-weighted image shows marked increased signal intensity of the lesion. *C,* Axial T1-weighted (post-gadolinium) shows heterogeneous enhancement of the tumor with nonenhancing cystic degenerative areas.

black hairy tongue is the result of elongation of the papillae on the dorsum of the tongue; it frequently follows antibiotic therapy. Yellow hairy tongue can occur. This is also an elongation of the filiform papillae and is most often associated with poor nutrition and vitamin deficiencies. Fungal infection can produce a thick whitish yellow coating of the tongue.

Inflammatory Glossitis

A strawberry appearance of the dorsum of the tongue is seen in cases of scarlet fever and gonorrhea. Tuberculosis of the tongue produces an irregular ulcer without surrounding erythema; the ulceration often resembles a carcinoma with the exception that it has a soft consistency when palpated.

Syphilis

A chancre can occur on the tongue; it has a firm consistency when palpated. If the clinician suspects syphilis, a careful history should be obtained and serologic studies should be conducted. Secondary syphilitic lesions of the tongue often resemble and are associated with carcinoma.

Myxedema

A scalloped tongue is indicative of myxedema; thus, any patient with a scalloped tongue should have a complete thyroid evaluation.

Vitamin Deficiencies

Deficiency of the vitamin B complex is characterized by a reddish or purplish red tongue. The papillae are prominent and edematous. Fissures may occur, and the patients may complain of a burning sensation. In cases of vitamin C deficiency (scurvy), the tongue is smooth and red. The other oral manifestations of this disease are more striking.

Glossodynia (Burning Tongue)

Frequently no local or systemic abnormalities can be found to account for a burning tongue. Glossodynia can occur with systemic diseases such as pernicious anemia, vitamin B complex deficiencies, pellagra, and sprue. Acute or chronic glossitis can produce glossodynia.

Varicosities

Varicosities can occur on the undersurface of the tongue. Local discomfort can occur when thrombosis occurs, and occasionally there is hemorrhage from a glossovaricosity.

Benign Tumors of the Oral Cavity

Hemangiomas can occur in any location in the oral cavity. These lesions should not be treated unless they become bulky and interfere with function. Lymphangiomas of the cavernous or cystic hygroma variety can be quite troublesome when they involve the floor of the mouth and tongue. Papilloma is a common lesion found anywhere in the oral cavity. These tumors are removed by simple excision as are numerous other benign tumors that can occur in the oral cavity.

Malignant Lesions of the Oral Cavity

Malignant lesions of the oral cavity vary widely. They can be exophytic, ulcerative, or infiltrative lesions. An immediate biopsy of any suspicious lesion is required.

Contrast-enhanced computed tomography or magnetic resonance imaging is essential to outline the extent of a lesion of the oral cavity as well as its local extension and any cervical metastasis (Fig. 1–15).

THE OROPHARYNX

Anatomy

The oropharynx is that portion of the pharynx directly behind the oral cavity. It should be regarded as a space surrounded by muscles serving as an area of communication between the oral cavity, nasopharynx, and laryngopharynx. It is limited above by the inferior border of the soft palate and below by the lingual surface of the epiglottis. The superior aspect of the oropharynx includes the posterior soft palate, uvula, and opening into the nasopharynx. On the lateral wall are the palatine tonsil and its fossa. The anterior pillar of the tonsillar fossa is formed by muscle. The lymphoid tissue of the palatine tonsil is arranged around crypts or small pockets, in contrast to the ridges or folds found in the pharyngeal tonsil (adenoids); the portion of the lateral wall posterior to the palatine tonsil is formed by mucous membrane covering the middle constrictor muscle. The posterior wall is composed of mucous membrane covering the middle constrictor muscle, which in turn is directly anterior to the prevertebral fascia.

Pharyngeal Musculature

1. Superior constrictor
   Origin: (1) hamulus of medial pterygoid; (2) pterygo-

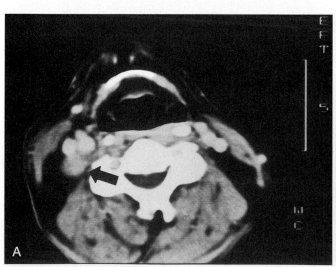
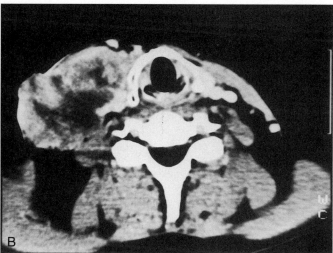

FIGURE 1-15. *A,* Contrast-enhanced axial CT scan of the neck at the level of the upper epiglottis reveals an enlarged lymph node posterior to the internal carotid artery and internal jugular vein on the right (*arrow*). The laryngeal structures are normal. *B,* Contrast-enhanced axial CT scan of the neck at the level of the mid-larynx reveals an irregular necrotic mass in the right neck that is secondary to metastatic lymph nodes. Note normal left side for comparison.

mandibular ligament; (3) mylohyoid line of the mandible.

Insertion: (1) medial raphe; (2) pharyngeal tubercle of occipital bone. The fossa of Rosenmüller is formed by an absence of muscle between the median raphe and the pharyngeal tubercle. The eustachian tube and the levator velopalatini pass through the defect.

2. Middle constrictor

   Origin: (1) hyoid bone; (2) stylohyoid ligament.

   Insertion: median raphe.

   The upper border of the inferior constrictor overlaps the inferior border of the superior constrictor.

3. Inferior constrictor muscle

   Origin: (1) oblique line of thyroid cartilage; (2) cricoid cartilage.

   Insertion: median raphe.

   The lower portion of this muscle is referred to as the cricopharyngeal muscle.

4. Palatopharyngeus muscle

   Origin: from the hard palate passing between tensor and levator palatini muscles.

   Insertion: (1) pharyngeal aponeurosis; (2) posterior border of thyroid cartilage.

   Forms the posterior pillar of the tonsillar fossa.

5. Palatoglossal muscle

   Origin: soft palate.

   Insertion: dorsum of tongue.

   This muscle forms the anterior pillar of the tonsillar fossa.

6. Salpingopharyngeal muscle

   Origin: lower cartilage of the eustachian tube.

   Insertion: lateral wall of the pharynx, adjacent to the palatopharyngeus muscle.

7. Stylopharyngeus muscle

   Origin: medial base of the styloid.

   Insertion: posterior surface of middle constrictor.

Pharyngeal Innervation

Sensory innervation of the pharyngeal plexus occurs through the glossopharyngeal nerve; motor innervation occurs through the pharyngeal branches of the vagus nerve. Both the motor and sensory components of the pharyngeal plexus follow the course of the stylopharyngeal muscle. The motor fibers are distributed to all muscles of the pharynx and soft palate, with the exception of the tensor veli palatini (V) and the stylopharyngeus (IX). The sensory component of the pharyngeal plexus supplies the entire pharynx.

Pharyngeal Tonsil

The pharyngeal tonsil is situated in a fossa created by the palatoglossal and palatopharyngeal muscles. Its arterial supply consists of branches to the lower pole from the dorsal lingual artery anteriorly, the ascending pharyngeal artery posteriorly, and the facial artery between the dorsal lingual and ascending palatine arteries. The branches to the upper pole are from the ascending pharyngeal artery posteriorly and the lesser palatine artery anteriorly.

Veins from the pharyngeal tonsil are distributed to the lingual vein and the pharyngeal plexus of veins.

Sensory innervation to the upper pole is by way of branches from the palatine nerve (V). Innervation to the lower pole is by way of a branch from the glossopharyngeal nerve.

Lymphatic drainage is accomplished by (1) the upper deep cervical nodes (especially a lymph node below the angle of the mandible, known as the tonsillar node), (2) the submandibular nodes, and (3) the superficial cervical lymph nodes.

Physiology

The oropharynx serves as a respiratory passage and as a drainage passage from the nasopharynx. It also assists with articulation and deglutition. During deglutition, as the pharynx receives the food bolus, the soft palate is elevated against the posterior pharyngeal wall, at which point a transverse elevation occurs to assist the sphincteric action of Passavant's fold. This elevation is the result of contractions of the palatopharyngeal and superior constrictor muscles. The palatopharyngeal and stylopharyngeal muscles draw the pharynx superiorly as the bolus begins to descend into the hypopharynx. The remaining musculature of the pharynx then contracts, in a peristaltic fashion, to force the bolus into the entrance of the esophagus. The tongue rises against the palate, and the palatoglossus muscle contracts, preventing return of the bolus into the oral cavity. The sphincters of the larynx contract and simultaneously open the pyriform sinuses and upper esophageal sphincter. A fraction of a second later the inferior constrictor muscle is stimulated, so that the cervical esophagus becomes widely patent. The inferior constrictor muscle contracts to close the esophagus after the food bolus passes through it.

Examination Technique

The examination of the oropharynx is conducted immediately after the examination of the oral cavity. The only additional equipment required is a laryngeal mirror, which is necessary to examine the lingual tonsils and vallecula. The various walls of the pharynx described above are carefully inspected for physical and functional disorders. Many patients can voluntarily depress the base of their tongue and thus simplify this examination. Before insertion of the tongue depressor, note the V-shaped row of circumvallate papillae at the junction of the anterior two thirds and posterior one third of the tongue. The tongue is depressed by exerting pressure with the tip of the tongue depressor placed well anterior to the circumvallate papillae (Fig. 1–16A). This affords a view of the entire oropharynx with the exception of the base of the tongue. The tonsillar pillars are accentuated as the tongue is depressed (Fig. 1–16B). The tonsils are inspected carefully. Any portion of the oropharynx can be palpated with the index finger if necessary. The lingual tonsils are located on each side of the midline at the extreme base of the tongue. In some patients, the lingual tonsils can be viewed as the tongue is pulled forward. As a rule, a laryngeal mirror is necessary for proper evaluation of these structures. The space between the base of the tongue and the lingual surface of the epiglottis known as the vallecula should be inspected carefully with the laryngeal mirror.

Abnormalities

Because the oropharynx includes the base of the tongue and is a continuation of the oral cavity, the pathologic findings are not unlike those described in the preceding section.

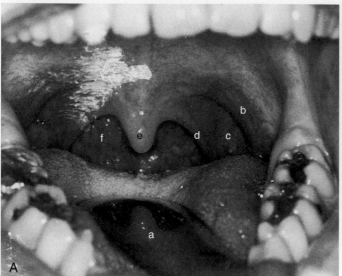
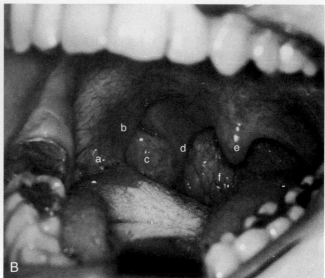

FIGURE 1-16. *A,* View of the oropharynx obtained by depressing the dorsum of the tongue anterior to the circumvallate papillae. The posterior dorsum of the tongue, pharyngeal tonsils, lateral and posterior pharyngeal walls, and soft palate are inspected. *B,* The right side of the tongue is depressed, giving the examiner a view of the retromolar trigone. The tonsillar fossa and posterolateral floor of the mouth are better visualized: a = posterolateral floor of the mouth; b = anterior pillar; c = palatine tonsil; d = posterior pillar; e = uvula; f = posterior pharyngeal wall.

THE LARYNGOPHARYNX

The laryngopharynx extends from the upper margins of the epiglottis to the subglottic larynx and cervical esophagus.

Anatomy

The portion of the laryngopharynx that extends from the tip of the epiglottis to the introitus of the esophagus is called the hypopharynx. It includes the pyriform sinuses on each side of the larynx but does not include the larynx. When the sphincters of the larynx are contracted, the hypopharynx and the cervical esophagus are adjusted into direct continuity. The lateral and posterior walls of the hypopharynx are formed by the middle and inferior constrictor muscles and the stylopharyngeus muscle (pharyngeal constrictors).

The thyroid, cricoid, and arytenoid cartilages make up the framework for the larynx (Fig. 1–17*A*). The thyroid cartilage sits on top of the signet ring–shaped cricoid cartilage and is anchored to it by the cricothyroid membrane (anteriorly) and the lateral and posterior cricothyroid ligaments. The lateral and posterior cricothyroid ligaments support the cricothyroid joint, which is formed by the inferior horn of the thyroid cartilage and the lamina of the cricoid cartilage. The upper border of the thyroid cartilage is attached superiorly to the hyoid bone by the thyrohyoid membrane.

The arytenoids form a joint on each side of the superior border of the posterior cricoid lamina. The cricoarytenoid joint is arthrodial in type, possessing a joint cavity and synovial lining. It is supported by the cricoarytenoid ligament. The joint movements are gliding and rotatory.

The intrinsic ligaments of the larynx make up a sheet of elastic membrane that connects the cartilaginous framework of the larynx to the laryngeal mucosa. The upper portion of this membrane extends from each side of the epiglottis to the arytenoids. It thus forms the framework for the aryepiglottic folds and the wall between the pyriform sinus and the intrinsic larynx. The lower portion of the intrinsic ligament of the larynx is a layer of elastic tissue arising from the upper border of the cricoid cartilage laterally and the inner aspect of the thyroid cartilage anteriorly. It sweeps upward and medially to the true vocal cord and is often referred to as the conus elasticus. The anterior aspect of the vocal cords, where the conus elasticus attaches to the inner aspect of the thyroid cartilage, is known as the anterior commissure.

The intrinsic muscles of the larynx (Fig. 1–17*B*) are:

1. Cricothyroid muscle
   Origin: the arch of the cricoid.
   Insertion: the inferior horn and the inferior border and inner surface of the thyroid cartilage.
   Innervation: external branch of the superior laryngeal nerve.
   Action: tilts the thyroid forward and the cricoid backward through the cricothyroid joint, thus lengthening or stretching the vocal cord.
2. Posterior cricoarytenoid muscle
   Origin: posterior surface of the cricoid lamina.
   Insertion: the muscular process of the arytenoid.
   Innervation: recurrent laryngeal nerve.
   Action: only true abductor of the vocal cords; it swings the muscular process medially and posteriorly, displacing the vocal process laterally.
3. Arytenoid muscle
   Origin: has an oblique and transverse portion, from one arytenoid to the other; the oblique portion continues on as the aryepiglottic muscle.
   Innervation: recurrent laryngeal nerve.
   Action: adducts the arytenoid; the aryepiglottic muscle pulls the epiglottis posteriorly and accomplishes the sphincteric action of the aryepiglottic folds during the act of swallowing.

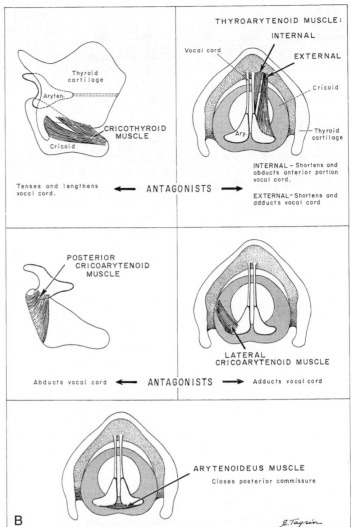

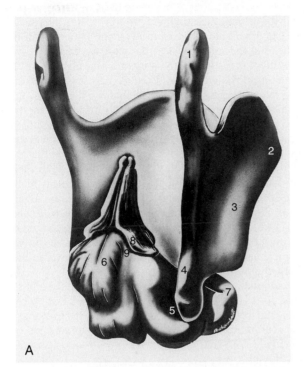

FIGURE 1-17. *A* and *B*, the laryngeal cartilages. 1. Superior cornu thyroid cartilage; 2. Thyroid notch (not seen); 3. Thyroid lamina; 4. Inferior cornu thyroid cartilage; 5. Cricothyroid joint; 6. Posterior cricoid lamina; 7. Cricoid arch; 8. Arytenoid cartilage—corniculate process, superior; muscular process, lateral; vocal process, anterior; 9. Cricoarytenoid joint.

4. Thyroarytenoid muscle

　Origin: the anterior inner aspect of the thyroid cartilage.

　Insertion: the arytenoid cartilage and vocal cord.

　Innervation: recurrent laryngeal nerve.

　Action: draws the arytenoids forward and rotates them medially, thus relaxing and adducting the vocal cords; when the arytenoids are fixed in the midline, a portion of this muscle can adduct or bow the vocal cords.

The recurrent laryngeal nerve innervates all intrinsic muscles of the larynx, with the exception of the cricothyroid, which is innervated by the external branch of the superior laryngeal nerve.

The interarytenoid muscle is supplied bilaterally by both recurrent laryngeal nerves. When these nerves are sectioned, the vocal cords assume the median or paramedian position. They do not assume the cadaveric position because the effect of cricothyroid muscles, which are sup-

plied by the superior laryngeal nerve, produces a degree of adduction. The adductor muscles of the larynx are supplied by the larger, more heavily myelin-coated fibers in the recurrent laryngeal nerve. The stimulus is required to produce a response in the abductor muscles of the larynx. The stimulus required to produce a response in these adductor muscles is approximately one tenth of that required to produce the response in the abductor muscles of the larynx.

Sensory innervation of the larynx is by way of the internal branch of the superior laryngeal nerve. This innervation extends from the supraglottic area to the lower border of the true vocal cord. Sensory innervation of the subglottic area is by way of the recurrent laryngeal nerve.

Sympathetic and parasympathetic innervation of the larynx is by way of the superior laryngeal nerve, the superior cervical ganglion, and the recurrent laryngeal nerves. This innervation regulates the vascular flow in the larynx and its secretory functions.

Physiology

Respiration

An adequate airway through the larynx is provided by contraction of the posterior cricoarytenoid muscles, which abduct the vocal cords. The larynx remains in this position except during deglutition and phonation.

Sphincteric Function

The sphincteric action of the larynx not only prevents the passage of food into the trachea but also opens the mouth of the esophagus. Three layers of sphincters guard the larynx. The aryepiglottic muscles pull the epiglottis posteriorly and the aryepiglottic folds medially. The epiglottis does not completely cover the larynx during swallowing. Adduction of the false and true vocal cords forms the second and third level of sphincteric protection.

Phonation

The current accepted definition of phonation is the passive vibration of the vocal cords by subglottic air pressure. The sound is monitored by the degree of tension of various laryngeal muscles. The theory that the laryngeal muscles oscillate at high frequencies to produce sound has been discredited, as the discharge of recorded motor units has been found not to exceed 40 to 50 per second, a frequency range too small to be of any great importance in tone production.

The vocal intensity is thus a production of the aerodynamic force of expiration and the glottal resistance. Various levels of intensity are achieved either by a change in the rate of airflow or by a change in the rate of the stimulation intensity of the laryngeal motor nerves.

The suprahyoid and extralaryngeal muscles play an important part in phonation. An increased pitch is accomplished by use of these muscles, which narrow and decrease the diameter of the phonatory tract above the larynx. The larynx is displaced inferiorly, increasing the length of the phonatory tract during the production of low-pitched tones. These muscles also stabilize the thyroid cartilage during contraction of the cricothyroid muscles as it tilts the cricoid lamina posteriorly, lengthening and tensing the vocal cords. This has been demonstrated by the close correlation between the electrical activity in the cricothyroid muscle and glottal muscle resistance. The electrical activity in the cricothyroid muscles increases with rise in the vocal pitch when the loudness of the voice is maintained at a constant level. There is marked decrease in the electrical activity of the cricothyroid muscle when phonation is changed from the chest registrar to falsetto. In this situation, there is segmental tensing of the true vocal cord by selective fibers in the vocal muscle.

Increased activity in the cricothyroid muscle is necessary for a rise in pitch. The vocal arch becomes thinner and longer as the pitch rises.

Vocal pitch and intensity are closely related. It is not possible to change the pitch without changing the intensity. Pitch does not rise because of increased airflow alone but is strongly influenced by the tension of the vocal cords (cricothyroid and thyroarytenoid muscle activity). Conversely, the expiratory effort of subglottic pressure and airflow bear a direct relation to vocal intensity or loudness.

The thyroarytenoid muscle affects minor regulation of vocal pitch and intensity. This muscle has great versatility. It can regulate the tension of the vocal cord anterior to the vocal process and both abduct and adduct this portion of the vocal cord.

The activity of the lateral cricoarytenoid muscle is not certain. Most likely, this muscle serves as a rapid adductor for sphincteric function.

Examination Technique

Indirect Laryngoscopy (Mirror Examination)

A No. 4 to No. 6 laryngeal mirror is used. Fogging is prevented by warming the mirror.

The examiner should sit in front of the patient with his or her head at the same level as the patient's head.

The patient is instructed to sit up straight, far back in the chair. The head should be projected slightly forward so that the tongue can be grasped between folder gauze pads. It is important that the examiner's thumb be on top of the patient's tongue and his or her second finger underneath the tip of the tongue. The index finger is used to elevate the upper lip. (Fig. 1–18A)

After testing the mirror on the back of the hand to make certain that it is not too hot, the clinician places it in the oropharynx in such a manner that it elevates the uvula. Touching the lateral walls or back of the tongue will cause gagging. If the patient has a sensitive gag reflex, the examination must be interrupted and the pharynx must be sprayed with topical anesthesia. The indirect laryngoscopy can then be resumed after 4 or 5 minutes.

The examiner asks the patient to breathe quietly and not hold his or her breath and then to say "a-a-a-a" or "e-e-e-e." This will bring the larynx up and backward so that it may be seen more easily. The following structures are observed (Fig. 1–18B and C):

1. Base of the tongue—lingual tonsils
2. Lingual surface and margins of the epiglottis
3. Arytenoids

Direct Laryngoscopy

Direct laryngoscopy can be performed with either local or general anesthesia. For internal administration of anesthesia (Fig. 1–19), the lips, gingivobuccal sulcus, floor of the mouth, and pharynx are sprayed with 4% cocaine or lidocaine (Xylocaine) solution. The hypopharynx and larynx are anesthetized with a ball of cotton, approximately 1 cm in diameter, that has been saturated with a topical anesthetic agent and placed at the end of a laryngeal applicator. The applicator is inserted down along the lateral hypopharyngeal wall into the pyriform sinus. The examiner should palpate the tip of the applicator externally, with the fingers of his or her free hand over the lateral aspect of the patient's larynx, to make certain that the applicator is in the pyriform sinus. The cotton should remain in the pyriform sinus for 1 to 2 minutes and then be transferred quickly to the opposite sinus.

The patient's tongue is pulled forward, either by the assistant or by the patient. The larynx is viewed with the laryngeal mirror held in the left hand, and 1 to 2 mL of topical anesthetic agent is injected subglottically between the

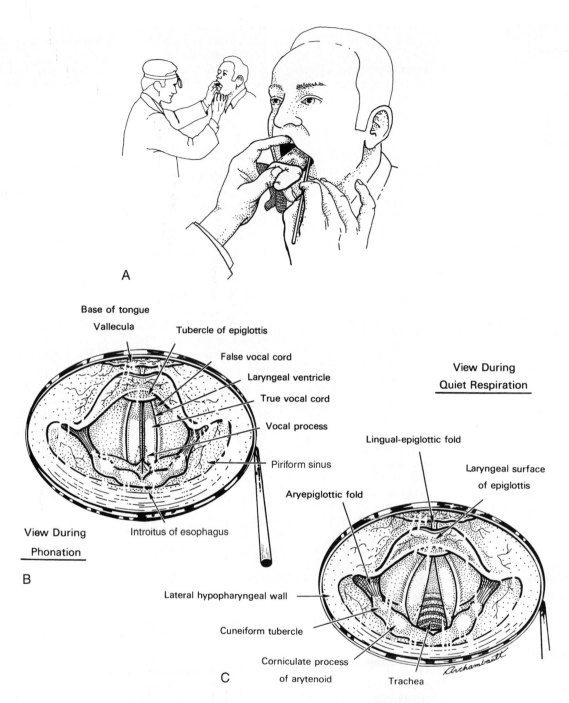

Base of tongue

Vallecula

Tubercle of epiglottis

False vocal cord

Laryngeal ventricle

True vocal cord

Vocal process

Piriform sinus

View During

Quiet Respiration

Lingual-epiglottic fold

Laryngeal surface

of epiglottis

Aryepiglottic fold

Introitus of esophagus

View During

Phonation

B

Lateral hypopharyngeal wall

Cuneiform tubercle

Corniculate process

of arytenoid

Trachea

C

FIGURE 1-18. Indirect laryngoscopy. *A,* The technique for indirect laryngoscopy (mirror examination of the larynx). The examiner should sit directly in front of, and at the same level as, the patient. The patient sits far back in his chair with the chest and head slightly forward. The patient projects the chin forward as the tongue is grasped, with folded gauze square, by the examiner. The examiner's index finger elevates the upper lip, while his thumb is placed on the dorsal surface of the tongue and the second finger underneath it. The laryngeal mirror is heated. The stem of the mirror should touch the lip as it is introduced in a posterior direction to elevate uvula. Any contact of the mirror with the lateral pharyngeal wall or base of the tongue will stimulate gagging. With the mirror in place, the patient is asked first to breathe quietly and not hold his breath. Often, at this point, the entire larynx can be viewed in partial abduction, including the subglottic region and cervical trachea. The glottis is evaluated as the patient attempts to say "A-a-a-a" and then "E-e-e-." *B and C,* The laryngeal structures as seen with the laryngeal mirror during phonation and respiration, the aryepiglottic folds, false and true vocal cords, trachea, walls of the hypopharynx, pyriform sinuses, and introitus of the esophagus.

vocal cords at the end of an expiration. The patient should be warned that a cough will be initiated when the solution enters the trachea.

In the external method for injection of local anesthesia, the mouth and pharynx are sprayed as described above. The superior laryngeal nerves are anesthetized by making a skin wheal immediately inferior and anterior to the tip of the hyoid bone on each side. One milliliter of 2% lidocaine (Xylocaine) solution is injected into the thyrohyoid membrane at the wheal, on each side. Another skin wheal is made in the anterior midline just below the cricoid cartilage over the trachea. A No. 20 needle is inserted into the lumen of the

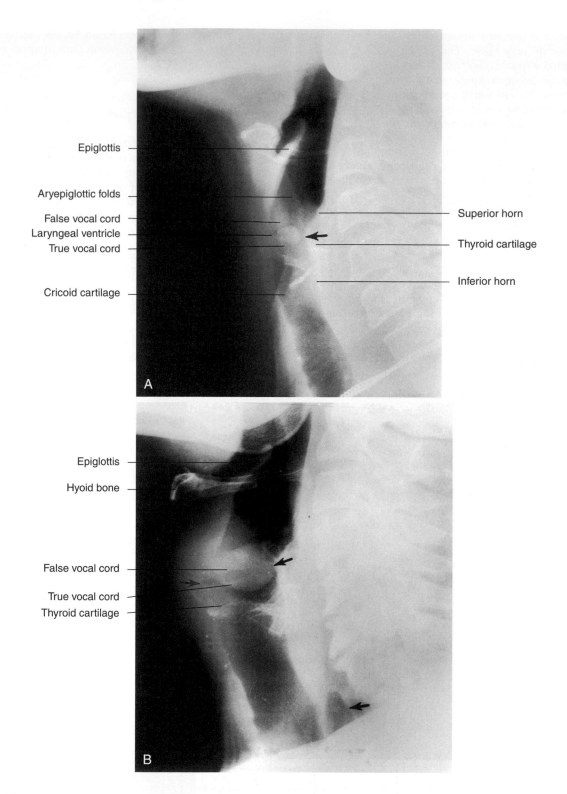

FIGURE 1–21. *A* and *B,* the *arrows* point to a moderate-sized polypoid mass attached to the anterior aspect of a vocal cord or the anterior commissure. This polypoid mass obscures the usual radiolucency representing the laryngeal ventricles. A large polyp is attached to the region of the anterior commissure. The horizontal translucency representing the laryngeal ventricles can be seen. The polyp extends above and below the glottis. This patient was admitted to the hospital with acute airway obstruction and a history of 1-year hoarseness and with months of recurrent bouts of intermittent respiratory obstruction.

ities, which extends into the nasopharynx, can be viewed. A foreign body may be present and easily seen, or an air column may be obliterated by a tumor mass or by atresia.

2. *Nasopharynx:* A good view of the nasopharynx is often obtained. The vault of the nasopharynx, posterior surface of the hard and soft palates, posterior wall of the nasopharynx, tori, and orifice of the eustachian tube can be viewed.

3. *Oropharynx:* The mandible obscures much of the oropharynx. The dorsal surface of the tongue, the uvula, the posterior pharyngeal wall, and density of the palatine tonsils can usually be seen.

4. *Hypopharynx:* The air column of the hypopharynx is translucent. It is crossed horizontally by the greater horns of the hyoid bone. Often it is also crossed obliquely by calcified stylohyoid ligaments. The base of the tongue, vallecula, epiglottis, and posterior hypopharyngeal wall are readily apparent. The irregular outline at the posterior third of the base of the tongue may represent the cobblestone effect of the lingual tonsil. The first three cervical vertebrae lie behind the posterior wall of the hypopharynx. The thickness of the soft tissue of the posterior wall of the hypopharynx should be noted. Normally this is approximately one third the width of the fourth cervical vertebra. The earlobe may create a false shadow here. Widening of the soft tissue in this area may represent an inflammatory process, edema, or tumor. In the event of abscess formation, air may be present in the soft tissues.

5. *Epiglottis:* The slightly S-shaped density behind the base of the tongue represents the epiglottis. The tip and anterior and posterior surfaces should be smooth. Normally, the epiglottis is quite thin. An air shadow anterior to the epiglottis represents the vallecula. The base of the tongue, represented by the anterior border of the air shadow, is usually smooth but may be irregular because of the lingual tonsil. Hypertrophy of the lingual tonsils, lingual thyroid, or a tumor mass may obliterate the vallecula. The base of the epiglottis extends to the anterior aspect of the thyroid of the thyroid cartilage in the region of the anterior aspect of the horizontal radiolucency, representing the laryngeal ventricle. This point also represents the anterior commissure and the anterior aspect of the true vocal cords. Air shadow represents the inferior surface of the false vocal cords, whereas the inferior surface represents the superior aspect of the true vocal cords. The area of the cricoarytenoid joint is located posterior to the true vocal cords.

6. *Laryngeal inlet:* The aryepiglottic fold can be seen extending from the posterior surface of the epiglottis to the density that represents the corniculate processes of the arytenoid cartilages. The air column of the laryngeal inlet or vestibule can be seen between the aryepiglottic folds and the posterior surface of the base of the epiglottis.

7. *Glottis:* The most striking landmark in the glottic region is the horizontal radiotranslucency representing the laryngeal ventricle. This is most often seen as the shape of a cross-section of an airplane wing. The superior surface of this air shadow represents the inferior surface of the false vocal cords, whereas the inferior surface represents the superior aspect of the true vocal cords. The area of the cricoarytenoid joint is located posterior to the true vocal cord.

8. *Laryngeal cartilages:* The densities of the laryngeal cartilages are often difficult to interpret because of irregular or partial calcification. The epiglottis and the corniculate and cuneiform cartilages are fibroelastic and, as a rule, contain no calcium. The thyroid cartilage is visualized best. All margins can usually be identified along with the superior and inferior horns. The arytenoid cartilages are often obscured by the superimposed thyroid cartilage. On occasion, they are clearly visible along with the mass of the corniculated cartilages. The signet-ring shadow of the cricoid cartilage can often be seen. Portions of the cricoid cartilage, however, are often obscured by the overlying thyroid cartilage.

9. *Hyoid bone:* The body and greater cornus of the hyoid bone are easily seen at the level of the third cervical vertebra. The lesser horn is often indistinct, even when the stylohyoid ligament is calcified. The greater horns of the hyoid bone are at right angles with the middle of the epiglottis.

10. *Subglottic region:* The contour of the subglottic region is clearly outlined by the air shadow. Any abnormalities in this area can be clearly seen.

11. *Cervical esophagus:* The width of the soft-tissue shadow of the cervical esophagus behind the larynx is usually two thirds the width of the fourth cervical vertebra. Increased thickness in this region usually represents infection, edema, injury, or tumor. Osteophytic changes are often noted in the anterior cervical vertebrae. Most foreign bodies in the cervical esophagus are found at the level of the cricopharyngeal muscle. The soft-tissue thickness of the cervical esophagus behind the trachea is somewhat narrower than the retrolaryngeal cervical esophagus. An air column, usually in the shape of a bullet (*arrow*), may be a normal finding inferiorly. Below this level, however, it is commonly associated with obstruction of the esophagus.

12. *Anterior soft tissue:* Any swelling, which may represent a solid or cystic tumor, is readily apparent. An air pocket may represent an abscess or subcutaneous emphysema and is readily seen in this area.

The most common sites for foreign bodies seen in a lateral neck radiograph view are (1) nasal cavity, (2) nasopharynx, (3) palatine tonsils, (4) vallecula epiglottica, (5) pyriform sinus, and (6) cervical esophagus (Fig. 1–22). Some radiodensities may be misinterpreted as being caused by foreign bodies. Partial calcification of the posterior aspect of the thyroid or cricoid cartilages is often misinterpreted as a foreign body in the upper cervical esophagus. The thyrohyoid ligament (cartilago triticea) may be calcified. The superior and inferior horns of the thyroid cartilage often project posteriorly. The stylohyoid ligament may be calcified. The earlobe may cast a shadow on the hypopharynx or pharynx. Calcium deposits in the carotid artery, salivary glands, lymph nodes, or a thyroid adenoma may also be misinterpreted as foreign bodies.

Laminagraphy

Laminagraphy of the larynx (Fig. 1–23) is valuable for demonstrating defects of the laryngopharynx and outlining tumor masses more accurately than lateral neck radiography. The lower hypopharynx, laryngeal inlet, false vocal cords, laryngeal ventricle, true vocal cords, pyriform sinuses, and subglottic region are clearly outlined in this technique.

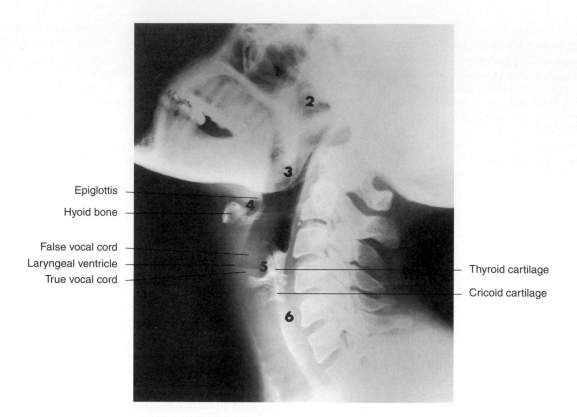

Epiglottis
Hyoid bone

False vocal cord
Laryngeal ventricle
True vocal cord

Thyroid cartilage
Cricoid cartilage

FIGURE 1-22. The most common sites for a foreign body to lodge in the upper respiratory system are as follows: 1, nasal cavity; 2, nasopharynx; 3, palatine tonsils; 4, vallecula, 5, pyriform sinus; and 6, cervical esophagus.

The best views are obtained as the patient phonates softly during both inspiration and expiration. The structures above the vocal cords can be more clearly outlined by increasing the supraglottic pressure with the Valsalva's maneuver. The subglottic structures are better seen in a view projected as the patient attempts forced expiration against adducted vocal cords.

Laryngograms
Laryngograms are often valuable for outlining the surface anatomy of tumors involving the larynx (Figs. 1–24 and 1–25). They should supplement the lateral neck radiograph and the laminagraph. They provide an outline of the hypopharynx, laryngeal inlet, and pyriform sinuses. In the anteroposterior and lateral views, the true vocal cords, false vocal cords, laryngeal ventricles, vallecula, epiglottis, laryngeal inlet, and subglottic region can be outlined accurately. The surface anatomy of tumors also can be delineated accurately to aid in determining the extent of disease and the relationship between the tumor and surrounding normal structures.

Computed Tomographic Scanning of the Larynx
Computed tomographic scanning of the larynx has been used for a number of years. It is an accurate method for assessing the extent of disease; in the future, it may well change our current TNM classification of laryngeal carcinoma (Fig. 1–26). At the present state of the art, however, the authors prefer a soft-tissue series of the larynx and trachea along with polytomography, in addition to computed tomographic and magnetic resonance imaging.

Abnormalities

Hoarseness. Hoarseness is abnormal phonation in which the voice is husky and raspy. Pitch is lower than normal, and the volume is decreased.

Hoarseness may be caused by inflammatory edema of the vocal cords as part of the common cold. The laryngeal mucosa is red and edematous. The true vocal cords remain pale at first, but they may become fiery red. Secretions may be seen on the cords. Ecchymotic spots on the cords are caused by coughing.

Inflammatory edema of the vocal cords may also be caused by acute specific laryngitis associated with measles, pertussis, scarlet fever, infectious mononucleosis, influenza, Vincent's angina, diphtheria, or croup.

Acute laryngotracheal bronchitis (croup) is accompanied by inflammatory edema of the vocal cords. The mucosa of the larynx is a deep red, except for the mucosa of the true vocal cords, which is somewhat paler and edematous. Subglottic edema and redness can be seen through the cords. Croup is common in children, and a hereditary factor is involved. Sudden onset and cough are characteristic, and stridor and suprasternal retractions soon develop.

Hoarseness may also be caused by chronic laryngitis. Nonspecific chronic laryngitis is probably caused by a number of factors, such as repeated infections, voice abuse, smoking, or poor nasal respiration. The laryngeal mucosa is dull red. The true vocal cords lose their nearly white appearance and are boggy. Engorged capillaries may be present on the cords, and thick stringy secretions are also seen.

Laryngeal tuberculosis is always secondary to pulmonary

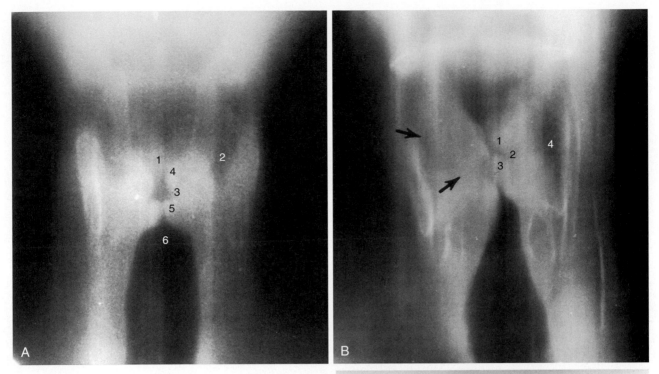

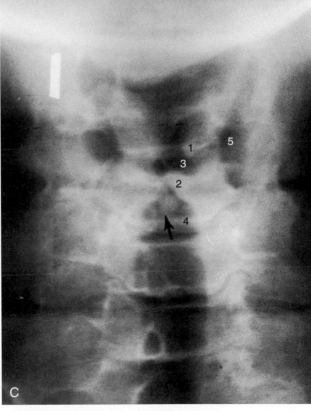

FIGURE 1-23. *A,* Laminagram of the normal larynx. The laryngeal inlet, pyriform sinuses, false vocal cords, laryngeal ventricles, true vocal cords, and subglottic region are clearly seen. The symmetry of the air column is normal. 1 = laryngeal inlet; 2 = pyriform sinus; 3 = laryngeal ventricle; 4 = false vocal cord; 5 = truce vocal cord; 6 = subglottic region. *B,* A large tumor is present, distorting the normal anatomy of the right larynx. This mass extends into the supraglottic region and 2.5 cm subglottically. The upper arrow points to a partially obliterated right pyriform sinus. The lower arrow indicates the tumor mass. 1 = false vocal cord; 2 = laryngeal ventricle; 3 = true vocal cord; 4 = pyriform sinus. *C,* A laminagram showing a small tumor mass (*black arrow*) attached to, and extending downward from, the right true vocal cord. This film was taken during expiration against a closed glottis. 1 = false vocal cord; 2 = true vocal cord; 3 = laryngeal ventricle; 4 = subglottic region; 5 = pyriform sinus.

involvement and is not frequently seen today. It usually involves the posterior aspect of the larynx. Early in the disease, the arytenoids and cords are red and edematous. Nodules are common in the interarytenoid space. Late in the disease, pale edema and ulceration of the mucous membrane become apparent.

Arthritis. In arthritis of the cricoarytenoid joints, a bright red swelling occurs over the arytenoid during both the acute stage and exacerbations. The arytenoids are fixed or have decreased motion. Speaking and swallowing are painful, and pain may radiate to the ears. The true vocal cords may be normal. Hoarseness is not an outstanding symptom of this

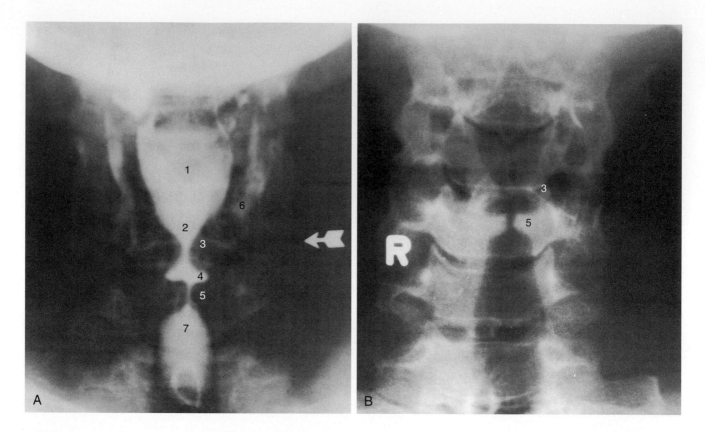

FIGURE 1-24. *A,* A laryngogram of the normal larynx. This clinical study is regarded as supplemental to lateral neck radiograph and laminagraphy. The surface anatomy of defects can be accurately outlined by the technique. The patient was phonating softly as this radiograph was taken. 1 = hypopharynx; 2 = laryngeal inlet; 3 = false vocal cord; 4 = laryngeal ventricle; 5 = true vocal cord; 6 = pyriform sinus; 7 = subglottic region. *B,* This radiograph demonstrates the excellent view obtained of the laryngeal structures and the minimal amount of radiopaque substance necessary when performing a laryngogram. The walls of the hypopharynx, laryngeal inlet, and pyriform sinuses are outlined. The false vocal cords, laryngeal ventricle, true vocal cords, and subglottic region are also clearly seen. 1 = hypopharynx; 2 = laryngeal inlet; 3 = false vocal cords; 4 = laryngeal ventricle; 5 = true vocal cord; 6 = pyriform sinuses; 7 = subglottic region.

disease. The mucosa over the arytenoids is roughened and thickened in the chronic stage. The symptoms depend on the degree of joint fixation; inspiratory stridor occurs when the arytenoids are fixed in the midline. Cricoarytenoid arthritis is often misdiagnosed as pulmonary disease.

Congenital Abnormalities. Laryngomalacia is characterized by hoarseness, noisy respiration, and stridor in infants from birth to $1^{1}/_{2}$ years of age. Symptoms improve when the child lies on his or her stomach. The diagnosis is based on the presence of a small, lax, and curled epiglottis. The arytenoids are lax and flutter with respiration.

Congenital web of the larynx is usually found anteriorly.

A laryngocele is an enlargement of the laryngeal ventricle. It may be present internally and cause hoarseness, or it may penetrate the thyrohyoid membrane and appear as an external laryngocele.

Neoplasms

The most common benign tumor of the larynx is papilloma. It occurs in all age groups, usually as a mole. It tends to recur after removal.

Varix (organized varicosity) of the larynx is usually caused by voice strain.

Polyps are common and may become large and even obstructive.

Vocal nodules are found at the junction of the middle and anterior thirds of the vocal cords.

Amyloid tumors of the larynx are rare.

Intrinsic carcinoma of the larynx produces hoarseness early in the course of the disease. Stridor, dysphagia, severe pain (local or radiating to one or both ears), halitosis, widening of the thyroid cartilage, hemoptysis, and cervical adenopathy are signs of advanced disease.

Extrinsic carcinoma of the larynx involved the epiglottis, aryepiglottic folds, pyriform sinuses, or hypopharynx. Hoarseness is not an early symptom. A feeling of having a lump in the throat, discomfort, painful swallowing, (odynophagia), pain radiating to one ear, and cervical adenopathy are the first symptoms.

Speech Defects. Most dysphonias are caused by voice abuse and misuse. The false cords may take over phonation (dysphonia plicae ventricularis). Psychic shock can cause aphonia.

Paralysis. Paralysis of the vocal cords can be unilateral, bilateral, complete, or incomplete. The cause may be trauma, inflammation, neoplastic disease, aortic aneurysm, or a central nervous system disorder. Paralysis may result from cervical or thoracic trauma to the recurrent laryngeal nerve(s) (especially thyroidectomy), direct trauma to the larynx, or

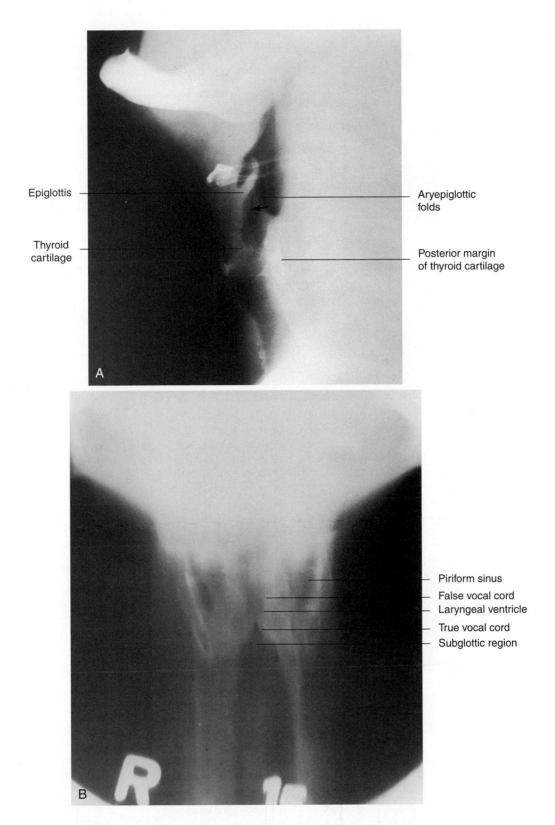

Epiglottis

Thyroid
cartilage

Aryepiglottic
folds

Posterior margin
of thyroid cartilage

Piriform sinus

False vocal cord
Laryngeal ventricle

True vocal cord

Subglottic region

FIGURE 1–25. The patient, a 56-year-old woman, when first examined had a history of increasing hoarseness, slight odynophagia without radiation of the pain, and odynophonia for 3 months. She had no other symptoms. With indirect laryngoscopy, a lesion was seen, beginning at the middle third of the laryngeal surface of the epiglottis and extending in the midline to the region of the anterior commissure and the anterior aspect of the right false vocal cord. The anterior third of the true vocal cords could not be seen clearly. The cervical lymph nodes are not enlarged. The lower limit of the lesion could not be accurately determined by indirect laryngoscopy. This case was presented to demonstrate the value of laminagraphy of the larynx and laryngograms. *A,* The lateral neck radiograph shows no abnormality except for a radiodensity (*arrow*) involving the inferior half of the laryngeal surface of the epiglottis. The horizontal translucency representing the laryngeal ventricles is not seen because of the degree of calcification of the thyroid cartilages. *B,* A laminagram of the larynx shows symmetry and no abnormality except for an apparent obliteration of the laryngeal ventricles. The true vocal cords and false vocal cords do not appear to be abnormal.

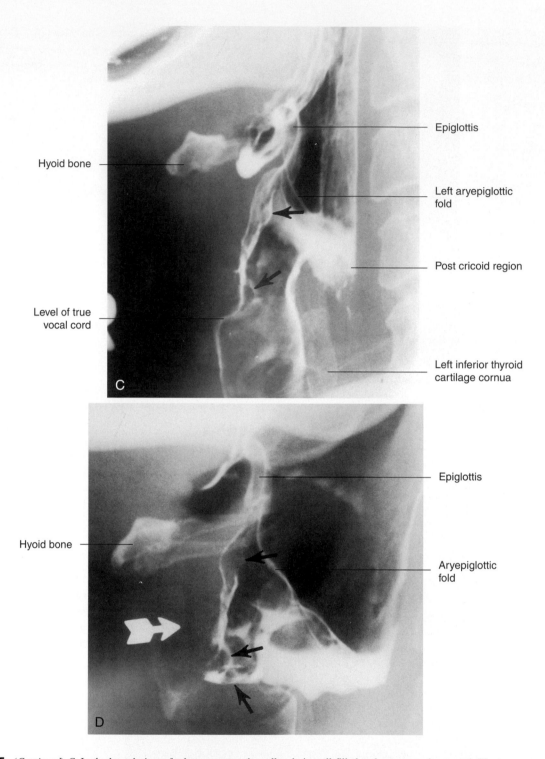

FIGURE 1-25. (*Continued*) *C,* In the lateral view of a laryngogram, the vallecula is well filled and appears to be normal. The tumor mass involving the laryngeal surface of the epiglottis is clearly outlined (*upper arrow*). The lower arrow designates an area that may represent an extension of the tumor to the region of the anterior commissure and anterior aspect of the false vocal cord. *D,* The *upper arrow* points to the tumor mass attached to the laryngeal surface of the epiglottis. The *middle arrow* designates an extension of the tumor to the region of the anterior commissure and the anterior aspect of the false vocal cords. The *lower arrow* indicates the upper surface of the true vocal cords.

complications of a fractured skull. Inflammatory disease, such as thyroiditis or mediastinitis, may result in vocal cord paralysis. Pulmonary, mediastinal, or cervical neoplasms cause paralysis of the vocal cords. Central nervous system disorders that may cause laryngeal paralysis include bulbar paralysis, tabes, multiple sclerosis, and cerebrovascular accidents.

Laryngeal Stridor. The following must be considered in the differential diagnosis of laryngeal stridor.

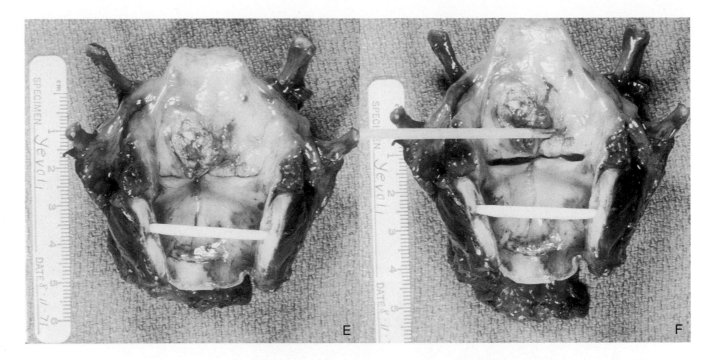

FIGURE 1-25. (*Continued*) *E,* A direct laryngoscopy was performed, and a biopsy specimen was obtained from the laryngeal surface of the epiglottis. The lesion was found to be squamous cell carcinoma. The true vocal cords and anterior commissure were free of disease. The tumor, however, extended into the anterior aspect of the false vocal cords and also involved their undersurface. Because of the close proximity of the tumor to the right true vocal cord, a total laryngectomy rather than a conservation procedure was elected. The lesion appears to extend into the anterior commissure, as well as into the false vocal cords. *F,* The tumor mass is elevated, demonstrating that it does not involve the anterior commissure. The involvement of the right false vocal cord and ventricle are apparent (*arrow*).

1. Edema due to infection, allergy, instrumentation, or myxedema;
2. Tumors such as neonatal subglottic hemangioma;
3. Bilateral paralysis of the larynx in the midline position;
4. Foreign bodies;
5. Congenital malformation;
6. Ankylosis of the cricoarytenoid joint (usually rheumatoid arthritis); and
7. Laryngeal spasms.

THE CERVICAL ESOPHAGUS

Anatomy

The cervical esophagus is situated directly behind the larynx and cervical trachea. Its introitus includes both pyriform sinuses and the postcricoid region. The true esophagus begins at the inferior border of the cricoid cartilage, or the inferior margin of the cricopharyngeal muscle, which is its narrowest portion. The cervical portion of the esophagus is slightly convex to the left, thereby projecting to the left of the trachea. This may be one reason why one usually finds a hypopharyngeal diverticulum on the left side and why the surgical approach to the cervical esophagus is best made on that side.

The anterior surface of the cervical esophagus is directly posterior to the cervical trachea and the posterior cricoarytenoid muscles. The recurrent laryngeal nerves are located on the anterolateral surface of the esophagus. The left recurrent laryngeal nerve tends to lie more medially because of the left lateral curvature of the cervical esophagus. The lateral lobes of the thyroid gland are in an anterolateral relation to the cervical esophagus. Posteriorly, the cervical esophagus lies directly over the prevertebral fascia.

The musculature of the esophagus is arranged in inner circular and outer longitudinal layers. The circular layer is continuous with the inferior fibers of the inferior constrictor muscle. This portion is referred to as the cricopharyngeal muscle.

The cervical esophagus receives its innervation from the recurrent laryngeal nerves. The inferior constrictor and cricopharyngeal muscles are supplied by the pharyngeal plexus (X) and the recurrent laryngeal nerves. The blood supply is from the inferior thyroid arteries.

The function of the cervical esophagus is described in the section on physiology of the oropharynx.

Examination Technique

Radiographic Study

Radiographic examination of the cervical esophagus includes a lateral neck radiograph and fluoroscopy with a contrast material. The consistency of the contrast material should vary to stimulate a semi-solid or liquid bolus.

The lateral neck radiograph is most valuable in outlining abnormalities. The thickness of the soft-tissue shadow of the retrolaryngeal portion of the cervical esophagus is usually two thirds the width of the fourth cervical vertebra. The thickness of the soft tissue of the posterior wall of the hypopharynx is one third the width of the fourth cervical ver-

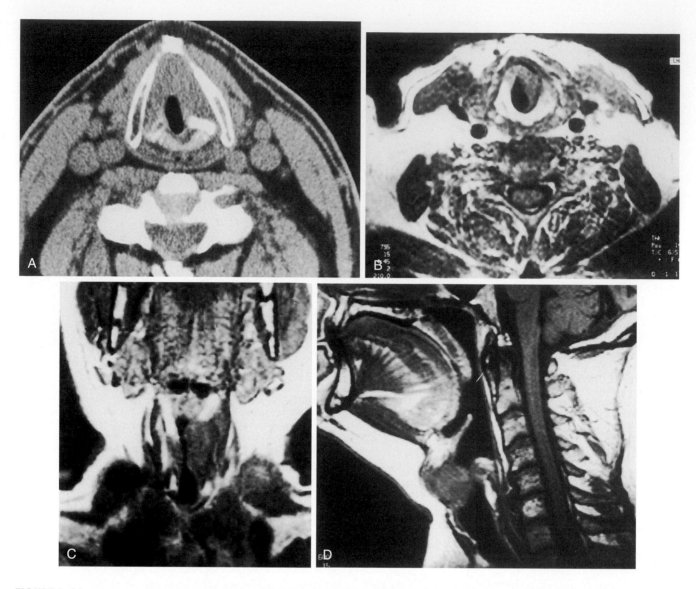

FIGURE 1-26. Carcinoma of the left vocal cord. *A,* Axial CT section through the level of the vocal cords shows diffuse thickening of the left vocal cord with extension into a thickened anterior commissure. *B,* Axial MRI T1-weighted image through the vocal cords shows hypointensity with thickening of the left cord. *C,* Coronal MRI T1-weighted image through the larynx shows a markedly thickened hypointense left vocal cord, obliteration of left laryngeal ventricle and a thickened false cord. *D,* Sagittal MRI T1-weighted image through the larynx shows a mass in the central and anterior portion of the larynx within the vocal cords and anterior commissure with extension to the false cords and subglottic space.

tebra. The width of the retrotracheal cervical esophagus is somewhat less than the portion posterior to the larynx. On occasion, an air column is present in the lower cervical esophagus below the cervical region.

Foreign bodies in the cervical esophagus are best viewed on the lateral neck radiograph film (Figs. 1–27 and 1–28). The most common site is at the level of the cricopharyngeal muscle (Fig. 1–29). A nonopaque foreign body can often be seen during fluoroscopy with a contrast material. Another technique is to have the patient swallow a small piece of cotton impregnated with a radiopaque substance. The cotton will become lodged with the nonopaque foreign body.

The function of the cervical esophagus can be observed during contrast fluoroscopy (Fig. 1–30), and the presence of aspiration into the larynx during deglutition can be noted. Defects, such as a hyopharyngeal diverticulum (see Chap-

ter 4) or a cervical esophageal web, are clearly outlined using this diagnostic procedure.

Esophagoscopy

Endoscopic examination of the cervical esophagus is conducted as outlined in the section on direct laryngoscopy using either local or general anesthesia. A hypopharyngoscope or cervical esophagoscope can be used. As a rule, the introitus of the esophagus is approached in the midline behind the cricoid lamina. If this is not possible, the tip of the scope is inserted into a pyriform sinus and then gradually slid toward the midline in the postcricoid region. During this procedure, the esophagus should be observed for (1) the status of the mucous membrane, (2) the diameter of the lumen, (3) defects in the esophageal wall, (4) areas of stricture, (5) webs, and (6) lesions.

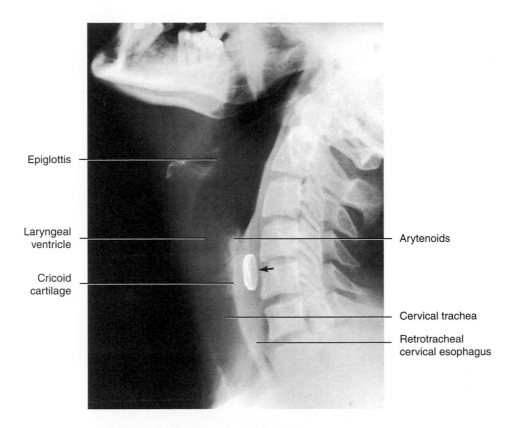

Epiglottis

Laryngeal
ventricle

Cricoid
cartilage

Arytenoids

Cervical trachea

Retrotracheal
cervical esophagus

FIGURE 1–27. A metallic foreign body (*top arrow*) is seen lodged in the upper cervical esophagus (retrolaryngeal) at the level of the cricoid cartilage. It had been present for only a short time, thus accounting for the minimal soft-tissue swelling. Note that the retrolaryngeal soft-tissue width exceeds that of the retrotracheal soft-tissue width. There is an air column (bullet) in the lower cervical esophagus (*bottom arrow*).

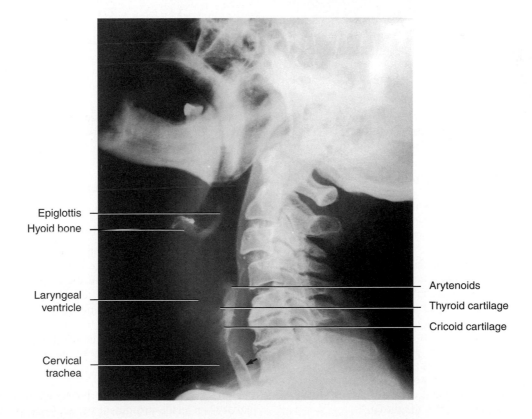

Epiglottis
Hyoid bone

Laryngeal
ventricle

Cervical
trachea

Arytenoids

Thyroid cartilage

Cricoid cartilage

FIGURE 1–28. A linear foreign body is present in the lower cervical esophagus (*arrow*). There is more of an increase in soft-tissue swelling in this region compared with that shown in Figure 1–29.

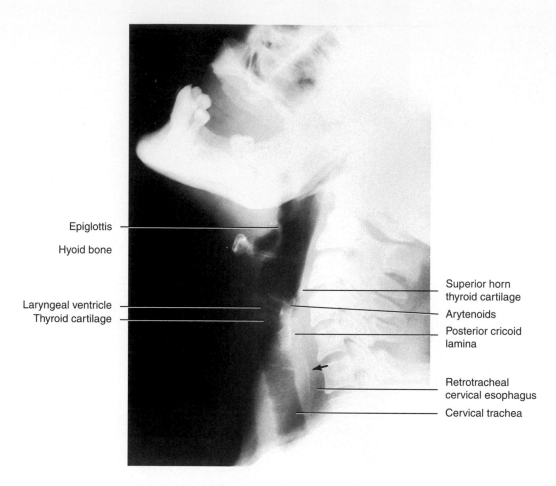

Epiglottis

Hyoid bone

Superior horn
thyroid cartilage

Laryngeal ventricle

Arytenoids

Thyroid cartilage

Posterior cricoid
lamina

Retrotracheal
cervical esophagus

Cervical trachea

FIGURE 1-29. The linear vertical foreign body (*arrow*) in the mid- or upper retrotracheal cervical esophagus of a chicken bone. Moderate soft-tissue swelling is present at this level.

Abnormalities

Foreign bodies in the esophagus are a common cause of dysphagia. A detailed case history and lateral neck radiograph usually provide the diagnosis.

Carcinoma of the esophagus is the most common cause of dysphagia (Fig. 1–31). The diagnosis often is not made until complications such as weight loss, odynophagia, pain radiating to the ear(s), bleeding, and metastasis are evident.

A history of swallowing a caustic substance provides the diagnosis for cicatricial stenosis. Esophageal web is more common in older women than in other persons and may be accompanied by anemia, achlorhydria, glossitis, or splenomegaly. Cardiospasm (achalasia) is a spasmodic condition of the cardiac sphincter at the junction of the esophagus and stomach.

A hypopharyngeal diverticulum is an outpouching of the upper cervical esophagus through the inferior constrictor muscle. It is usually found on the left side. Symptoms include dysphagia, retrosternal discomfort while eating, regurgitation of food, choking and coughing spells after eating or at night, and "gurgling in the throat."

Odynophagia (painful swallowing) results from any insult to the glossopharyngeal or vagal sensory distribution to the hypopharynx, larynx, or cervical esophagus. The pain may be referred to the ear(s).

THE NECK

Applied Anatomy

Triangles of the Neck

The fundamental oblong for the formation of the triangles of the neck is bounded by the anterior vertical midline of the neck, the anterior border of the trapezius muscle posteriorly, the clavicle inferiorly, and the lower border of the mandible superiorly. This oblong is divided into the anterior and posterior triangles by the sternocleidomastoid muscle. The various triangles of the neck (Fig. 1–32 and Table 1–2) are covered superficially by the platysma muscle.

Important Landmarks

The greater cornu (tip end) of the hyoid bone is easily palpated when made prominent by applying pressure against the opposite greater cornu of the hyoid. The tip of the hyoid is in close relationship to most important structures of

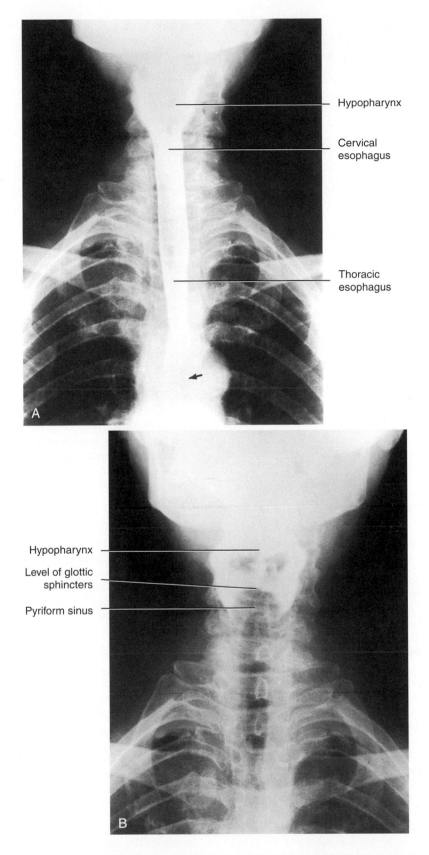

FIGURE 1-30. *A,* An anteroposterior view showing a normal cervical esophagus. The *arrow* indicates the deviation created by the aortic arch. *B,* A radiograph taken before the contrast medium entered the cervical esophagus; the hypopharynx and pyriform sinuses are clearly outlined. The glottic sphincteric action is normal, and there is no aspiration into the layer.

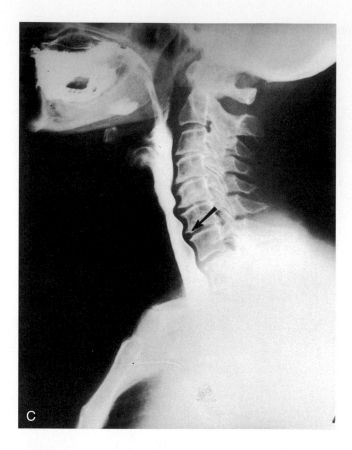

FIGURE 1-30. (*Continued*) *C*, A lateral view of the barium-swallow examination in the same patient. Posterior irregularities can be accounted for by the osteophytic changes on the anterior aspect of the cervical vertebrae (*arrows*). In this patient, they did not produce any disturbance in deglutition.

the neck (see Fig. 1–33 and Table 1–2). These include the following:

1. The carotid bulb and its bifurcation into the external and internal carotid arteries, which is directly behind the tip of the hyoid.

2. The internal jugular vein, which is slightly posterior and more superficial to the carotid artery.

3. The vagus nerve, which lies between the carotid bulb and the internal jugular vein.

4. The hypoglossal nerve, which passes lateral to the internal and external carotid arteries, just above the level of the tip of the hyoid.

5. The lingual vein, which is immediately superior to the level of the hyoid tip.

6. The superior thyroid and facial veins, which enter the internal jugular vein at the level of the tip of the hyoid.

7. The superior thyroid artery and the superior laryngeal nerve and artery, which are at a level slightly inferior to the tip of the hyoid bone.

The superior thyroid artery has its origin from the external carotid artery, just below the level of the tip of the hyoid. The superior laryngeal artery leaves the superior thyroid artery at about the same level and is directed anteriorly along with the internal branch of the superior laryngeal nerve (Fig. 1–34A).

8. The external branch separates from the superior laryngeal nerve at the tip of the hyoid, as it appears from behind the internal and external carotid arteries. This branch descends in close relationship to the superior thyroid artery on the surface of the inferior constrictor muscle to supply the cricothyroid muscle.

The internal branch of the superior laryngeal nerve follows the upper border of the interior constrictor muscle and then pieces the thyrohyoid membrane at the lateral border of the thyrohyoid muscle (Fig. 1–34B).

The transverse process of the atlas (Fig. 1–35) is an excellent guide to the superior aspect of the internal jugular vein; cranial nerves IX, X, XI, and XII; and the internal carotid artery. When palpating the neck, the transverse process of the atlas can be located just anterior and inferior to the tip of the mastoid process. During neck dissection, after the inferior portion of the parotid gland has been resected and the upper end of the sternocleidomastoid muscle has been transected and reflected inferiorly, the prominence of the transverse process of the atlas can easily be palpated a finger breadth anterior and inferior to the mastoid process. Blunt dissection over the anterior aspect of the transverse process of the atlas will lead directly to the internal jugular vein. The glossopharyngeal, vagus, spinal accessory, and hypoglossal nerves enter the neck anterior to the internal jugular vein. The vagus nerve is the only one of these four nerves that takes a direct inferior course. The spinal accessory nerve is the only one of the four that progresses in a posterior direction. It usually crosses superficial to the internal jugular vein. The glossopharyngeal and hypoglossal nerves descend in a forward direction. Superiorly, all four nerves lie between the internal jugular vein and the carotid artery.

This approach to the superior aspect of the internal jugular vein is particularly important when a high ligation is anticipated and for positive identification of the last four cranial nerves.

The transverse process of the sixth cervical vertebra (carotid tubercle) is found at the level of the arch of the cricoid cartilage. It lies just posterior to the common carotid artery, which can be compressed against the carotid tubercle as an emergency procedure. An incision along the anterior border of the sternocleidomastoid muscle at this point is used for rapid exposure of the common carotid artery. The vertebral artery enters the foramen at this level.

The fascia of the neck is shown in Figure 1–36.

Examination Technique

General Inspection
The neck is viewed anteriorly, posteriorly, and laterally for symmetry and posture. Its mobility is checked during rotation, flexion, and extension. The trapezius and sternocleidomastoid muscles are carefully observed for physical and functional disorders.

A detailed examination of the neck is conducted by palpation from the anterior, lateral, and posterior position.

Examination of the Anterior Neck
The submental area is the first to be examined. If this area is under suspicion, a bimanual examination, with the index finger of one hand in the anterior floor of the patient's mouth palpating against fingers of the opposite hand placed in the submental region, should be performed (Fig. 1–37A). The hyoid bone and the entire laryngeal skeleton, with particular reference to the precricoid area, should be carefully pal-

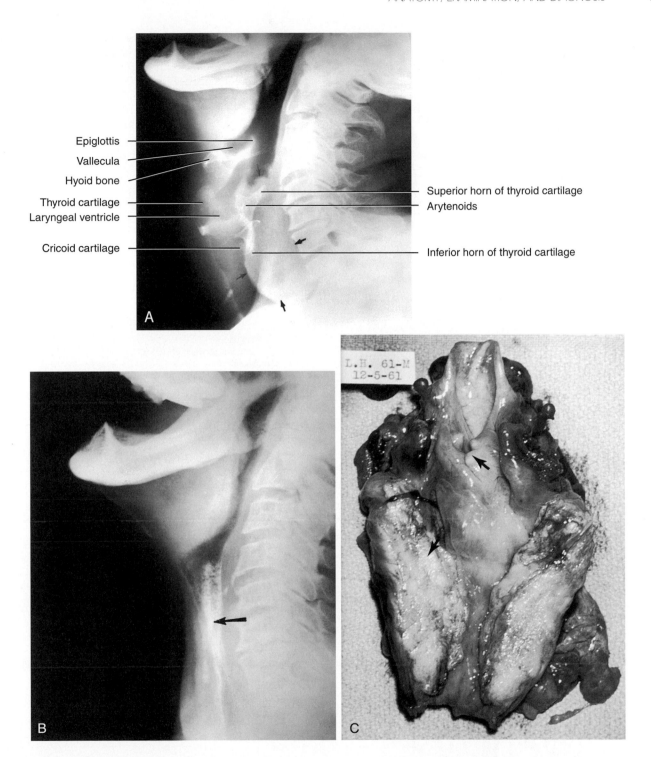

FIGURE 1-31. *A,* A 65-year-old man entered the hospital with a 1-week history of inability to swallow. Gradual increasing dysphagia had been present for 2^1/$_2$ months. A lateral neck radiograph study demonstrated a large soft-tissue mass (*arrows*) involving the entire cervical esophagus and extending to the thoracic inlet. A barium-swallow examination demonstrated complete obstruction of the cervical esophagus. At endoscopy, the larynx and hypopharynx were found to be normal; a mass obstructing the cervical esophagus was found just below the level of the esophageal inlet. The remainder of the cervical esophagus could not be examined by endoscopy, nor could a nasogastric feeding tube be inserted. Laryngoesophagectomy and thyroidectomy were performed. A 2-cm margin of normal esophagus was resected with the lower margin of the tumor, and a first-stage reconstruction of the cervical esophagus was accomplished at this time. The second stage of the cervical esophagectomy reconstruction was accomplished 6 weeks later. The patient has remained well and without recurrent carcinoma for 9 years. *B,* A barium-swallow examination after reconstruction of the cervical esophagus (*arrow*). The lumen is adequate for a normal diet. This patient remained well and free from disease for 9 years. *C,* Carcinoma of the cervical esophagus. The *top arrow* points to the postarytenoid area. The *lower arrows* indicate the right and left halves of the carcinoma.

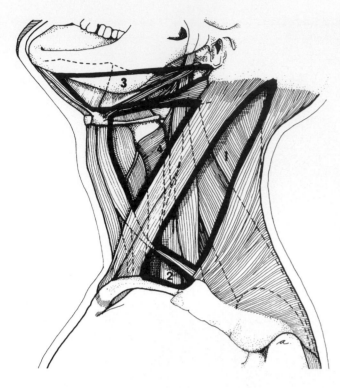

FIGURE 1–32. Triangles of the neck. (see Table 1–2)

pated. The entire length of the cervical trachea is palpated for motility, position, and structure. The thyroid gland can be palpated either from behind or from in front of the patient. The information gained from this examination should include the gland's position, size, shape, consistency, sensitivity, and movability. The patient should be sitting erect with hands relaxed in the lap. The examiner should sit in front of, and at the same level as, the patient. When the right

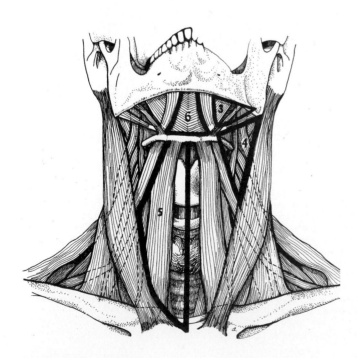

FIGURE 1–33. Triangles of the neck. (see Table 1–2)

thyroid gland is being examined, the patient is asked to turn the head to the left. The examiner's right thumb is placed over the cricoid cartilage with fingers extended around the side of the patient's neck (Fig. 1–37B). The cricoid and trachea are pressed to the left. The index finger of the examiner's left hand palpates posterior to the tensed right sternocleidomastoid muscle, pushing the thyroid forward. The right thyroid gland is then palpated between the index finger and thumb of the left hand. It may help if the patient

TABLE 1–2
Triangles of the Neck

1. Occipital triangle
   Posterior
      Trapezius
   Anterior
      Sternocleidomastoid
   Inferior
      Posterior omohyoid
   Floor
      Splenius
      Levator scapulae
      Scalenus anterior, medius, posterior
2. Subclavian triangle
   Superior
      Posterior omohyoid
   Anterior
      Sternocleidomastoid
   Inferior
      Clavicle
   Floor
      Scalenus medius and anterior
3. Digastric triangle
   Superior
      Mandible
   Infero-anterior
      Anterior belly of the digastric
   Inferoposterior
      Posterior belly of the digastric
   Floor
      Mylohyoid muscle
      Hyoglossus muscle
4. Carotid triangle
   Superior
      Posterior belly of the digastric
   Anterior
      Omohyoid
   Posterior
      Sternocleidomastoid
   Floor
      Thyrohyoid
      Inferior constrictor
5. Muscular triangle
   Posterosuperior
      Anterior belly of the omohyoid
   Anterior
      Midline of the neck
   Posteroinferior
      Sternocleidomastoid
   Floor
      Sternohyoid
      Sternothyroid
6. Submental triangle
   Laterally
      Two anterior bellies of the digastric
   Inferior
      Hyoid bone
   Floor
      Mylohyoid

Numbers coincide with numbers in Figures 1–32 and 1–33.

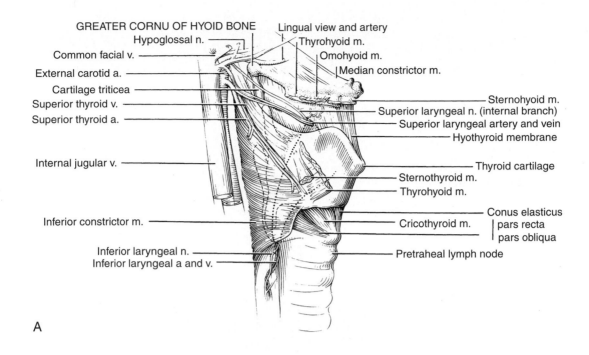

GREATER CORNU OF HYOID BONE
Hypoglossal n.
Common facial v.
External carotid a.
Cartilage triticea
Superior thyroid v.
Superior thyroid a.
Internal jugular v.
Inferior constrictor m.
Inferior laryngeal n.
Inferior laryngeal a and v.

Lingual view and artery
Thyrohyoid m.
Omohyoid m.
Median constrictor m.
Sternohyoid m.
Superior laryngeal n. (internal branch)
Superior laryngeal artery and vein
Hyothyroid membrane
Thyroid cartilage
Sternothyroid m.
Thyrohyoid m.
Conus elasticus
Cricothyroid m.   pars recta
                  pars obliqua
Pretraheal lymph node

A

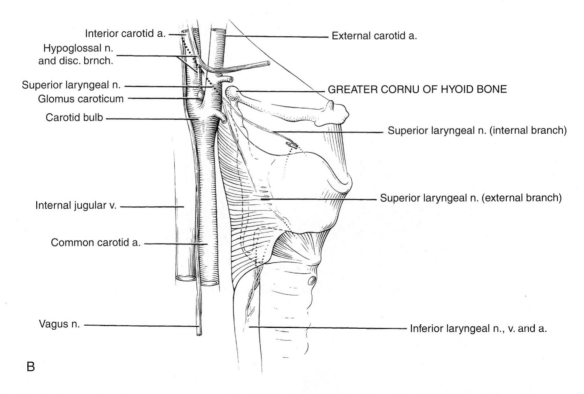

Interior carotid a.
Hypoglossal n. and disc. brnch.
Superior laryngeal n.
Glomus caroticum
Carotid bulb
Internal jugular v.
Common carotid a.
Vagus n.

External carotid a.
GREATER CORNU OF HYOID BONE
Superior laryngeal n. (internal branch)
Superior laryngeal n. (external branch)
Inferior laryngeal n., v. and a.

B

FIGURE 1-34. Deep anatomy of the neck. The tip or end of the greater cornus of the hyoid bone is near a number of important structures in the neck. The carotid bulb and its bifurcation into the external and internal carotid arteries are located directly behind the tip of the hyoid. The internal jugular vein is found slightly posterior and more superficial compared with the carotid artery system. The vagus nerve descends vertically between the carotid artery and internal jugular vein. The hypoglossal nerve crosses external to both the internal and external carotid arteries; it begins its anterior course just above the tip of the hyoid bone. The lingual vein is immediately superior to he level of the hyoid tip. The superior thyroid and facial veins enter the internal jugular vein at the level of the tip of the hyoid bone. The superior thyroid artery and the superior laryngeal nerve and artery are found just below the level of the tip of the hyoid. The superior laryngeal artery branches from the superior thyroid artery soon after it leaves the external carotid artery. The superior laryngeal nerve descends from the vagus nerve and passes behind both the internal and external carotid arteries, at about the same level that the hypoglossal passes external to both of these arteries. It divides into the internal and external branches, just behind and inferior to the tip of the hyoid bone. The internal branch follows the upper borders of the inferior constrictor and pieces the thyrohyoid membrane at the lateral border of the thyrohyoid muscle. The external branch descends in close proximity to the superior thyroid artery on the surface of the inferior constrictor muscle, on its way to supply the cricothyroid muscle.

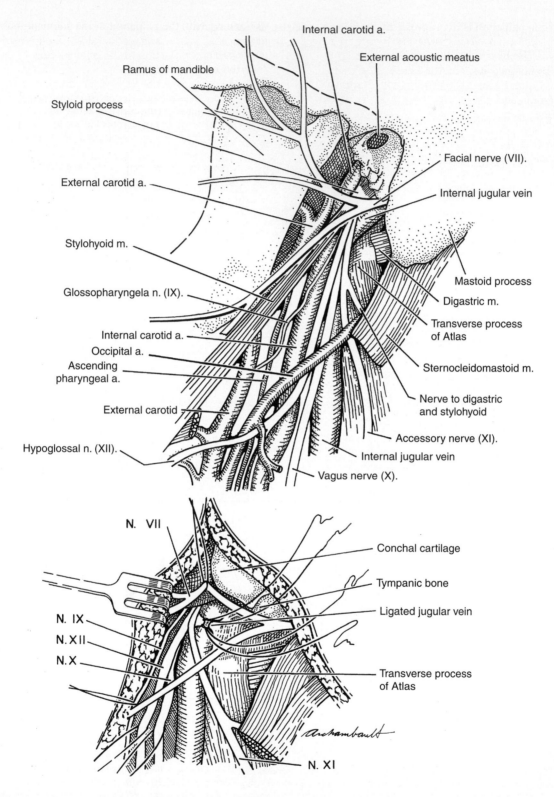

FIGURE 1–35. The transverse process of the atlas is one of the most valuable landmarks in the neck and an excellent guide to the internal jugular vein; glossopharyngeal, vagus, spinal accessory, and hypoglossal nerves; and internal carotid artery. The transverse process of the atlas is palpated just anterior and inferior to the tip of the mastoid bone. This landmark can be more easily palpated during a radical neck dissection, after the inferior pole of the parotid gland and the upper end of the sternocleidomastoid muscle have been transected and reflected inferiorly. The internal jugular vein is identified by retracting the posterior belly of the digastric muscle anteriorly and dissecting bluntly immediately anterior to the transverse process of the atlas. The facial nerve can be identified by dissecting superiorly. The glossopharyngeal, vagus, spinal accessory, and hypoglossal nerves are seen as they enter the neck anterior to the internal jugular vein. Each of these nerves can also be identified at this level. The vagus nerve is the only one of the four that takes a direct inferior course. The spinal accessory nerve is the only one of the four that descends posteriorly. This nerve crosses superficial to the internal jugular vein. The glossopharyngeal and hypoglossal nerves descend in a forward direction. The former is smaller and superior to the hypoglossal nerve. Identification of the internal jugular vein at the level of the transverse process of the atlas during a radical neck dissection is important when a high ligation of the vein is anticipated. In such instances, a high ligation can be easily accomplished without danger to the adjacent four cranial nerves.

swallows while palpation is in progress. If the trachea is deviated to one side a substernal goiter may be present. Coughing may raise a substernal goiter into the neck. If the thyroid gland is enlarged, it should be ascertained whether it is smooth or nodular. Firmness, fixation, or tenderness may indicate a thyroid cancer.

The space immediately above the manubrium, the suprasternal notch, is best examined with the patient's neck in extension (Fig. 1–37C). Normally, only adipose tissue is palpated subcutaneously. In a very thin neck, the inferior aspect of the cervical trachea can be palpated. An enlarged lymph node or abnormal pulsation may be found in this area.

Examination of the Lateral Neck
The examination is continued with the patient sitting down while the examiner stands facing the side to be examined.

Beginning with the palpation of the submandibular triangle, the patient's neck is placed in slight flexion and rotated to the left for examination of the right submandibular triangle. The fingers of the examiner's left hand are inserted deeply underneath the mandible, moving the contents of the submandibular triangle inferiorly (Fig. 1–37D). The entire contents of the submandibular triangle can be palpated between the fingers of the left hand and the right index finger, which has been inserted into the lateral floor of the patient's mouth (Fig. 1–37E). Bimanual palpation may be useful to detect deep lymph nodes. Pseudohypertrophy of the submandibular gland occurs in middle-aged or elderly patients and merely represents submandibular gland ptosis.

When examining the right carotid chain of lymph nodes, the examiner can stand on either side of the patient. The patient's head is rotated slightly to the left and flexed, to al-

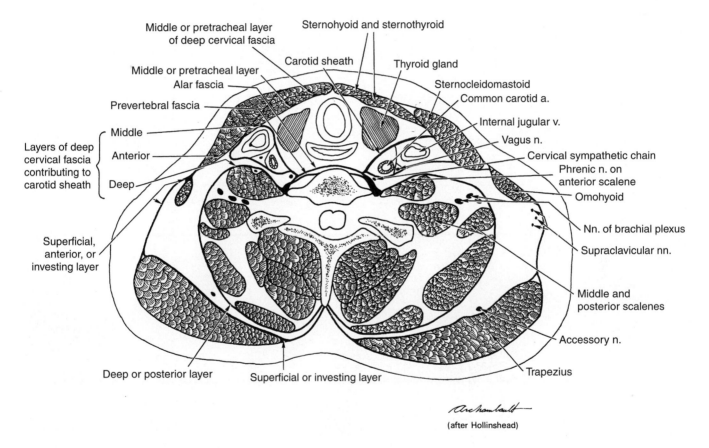

Middle or pretracheal layer of deep cervical fascia
Sternohyoid and sternothyroid
Middle or pretracheal layer
Carotid sheath
Thyroid gland
Alar fascia
Sternocleidomastoid
Common carotid a.
Prevertebral fascia
Internal jugular v.
Layers of deep cervical fascia contributing to carotid sheath
Middle
Vagus n.
Anterior
Cervical sympathetic chain
Phrenic n. on anterior scalene
Deep
Omohyoid
Nn. of brachial plexus
Supraclavicular nn.
Superficial, anterior, or investing layer
Middle and posterior scalenes
Accessory n.
Deep or posterior layer
Superficial or investing layer
Trapezius

(after Hollinshead)

FIGURE 1-36. Fascia of the neck. The superficial cervical fascia consists of the subcutaneous tissue of the neck. The platysma muscle is embedded in this fascial layer. The fascia on the undersurface of the platysma lies against the superficial layer of deep cervical fascia; it allows for the free movement of the platysma. A superficial layer of deep cervical fascia lies deep to the superficial cervical fascia. It is attached to the nuchal ligament and the spines of the cervical vertebrae. It completely invests the neck like a sleeve. This layer is attached to the base of the skull, the mandible, clavicle, sternum, and hyoid bone; it splits to enclose the trapezius, sternocleidomastoid, and omohyoid muscles. Superiorly, it splits to surround the submandibular and parotid glands. Anteroinferiorly, between the sternal heads of the sternocleidomastoid muscle, it splits into two layers, one attaching to the anterior and the other to the posterior surface of the sternum. The space thus created is known as the suprasternal space of the Burns; it contains the inferior aspect of the anterior jugular veins, their transverse connecting branch, and one or two lymph nodes. The middle layer of deep cervical fascia is merely a deeper reflection of the anterior aspect of the superficial layer and contributes to the anterolateral wall of the carotid sheath. It extends forward, anterior to the thyroid gland and trachea. This layer is deep to the sternothyroid and sternohyoid muscles and is commonly referred to as the deep pretracheal fascia. The deep layer of deep cervical fascia arises from the nuchal ligaments and covers the muscles attached to the vertebral column. This fascia thus covers the splenius capitis, splenius cervicis, and levator scapulae muscles. As it progresses anteriorly, it covers the outer surface of the posterior, middle, and anterior scalenes. This portion of the deep layer of fascia is often referred to as the "fascial carpet." All three layers of deep cervical fascia contribute to surround the carotid artery, the carotid sheath, the internal jugular vein, and the vagus nerve. After passing anteriorly over the anterior scalene muscle, the deep layer of the fascia becomes attached to the anterior tubercles of the cervical transverse processes. The fascia then extends across the vertebral column. This fascia is quite thick and consists of two layers. The phrenic nerve is found deep to this fascia on the anterior scalene muscle. The brachial plexus also is found deep to the fascia, between the anterior and middle scalene muscles.

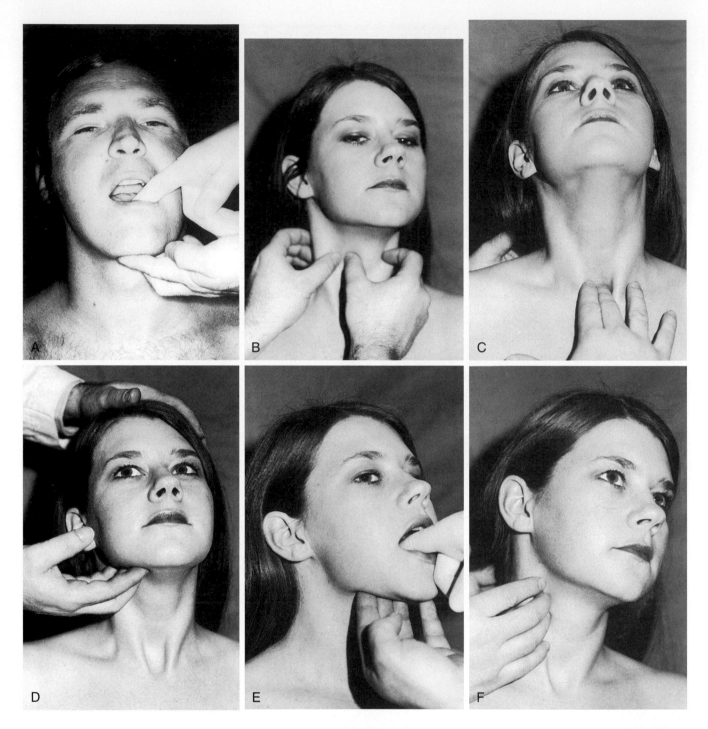

FIGURE 1-37. Examination of the neck. *A,* Submental region. This region is examined by bimanual palpation in addition to the routine external palpation. The index finger of one hand is placed on the anterior floor of the patient's mouth to palpate against the fingers of the opposite hand, which have been placed in the submental region. After this, the laryngeal skeleton and trachea are examined for motility, position, and structures. *B,* Thyroid gland. To examine the thyroid gland, the examiner sits in front of, and at the same level as, the patient. The patient's neck is rotated slightly to the left when the right lobe is examined. The examiner's right thumb is placed over the lateral cricoid cartilage arch with the fingers extending around the left side of the neck. The cricoid is pressed to the left. The right index finger is placed posterior to the tensed right sternocleidomastoid muscle, pushing the thyroid anteriorly. The right thyroid is then palpated between the index finger and the thumb of the left hand. *C,* Suprasternal notch. This area is palpated with the patient's neck in extension. The inferior aspect of the cervical trachea can be palpated, unless excessive adipose tissue is present. Enlarged lymph nodes or pulsations in this region are considered abnormal until proven otherwise. *D,* Submandibular triangle. To examine the right submandibular region, the patient's neck is slightly flexed and rotated to the left. The examiner's fingers are inserted deep underneath the mandible and its contents are palpated. *E,* Bimanual palpation of submandibular triangle. This is performed in a manner similar to, and usually at the same time as, bimanual examination of the submental region. *F,* Examination of the right carotid chain of lymph nodes.

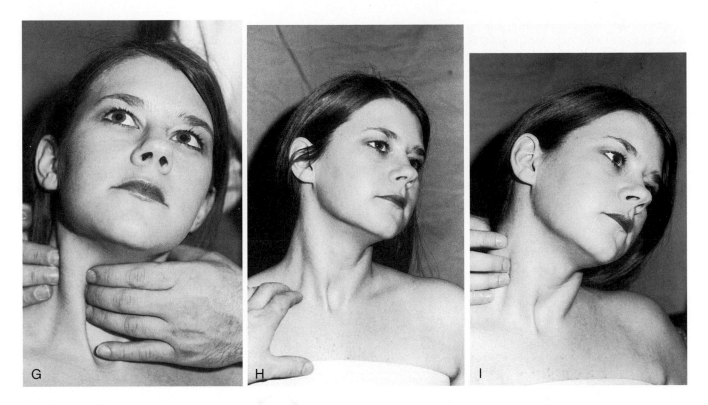

FIGURE 1–37. (*Continued*) *G*, Examination of the right lateral neck from the opposite side. The technique is similar to that mentioned above (*F*). The background for palpating the lateral neck is the transverse processes of the cervical vertebrae. The carotid bulb can be palpated at the level of the thyroid cartilage notch. *H*, Supraclavicular region. This often-neglected region is palpated with the flat surfaces of the fingers. This is accomplished with the patient's neck in flexion and extension. Abnormal masses and pulsations may be detected. *I*, Posterolateral neck. The patient's neck is slightly flexed to the right side as the right posterolateral region is examined with the flat surfaces of the examiner's fingers. The examiner stands behind the patient. The function of the trapezius muscle is evaluated as the patient elevates her shoulder.

low relaxation of the right sternocleidomastoid muscle. The fingers of the examiner's right hand are placed in front of the sternocleidomastoid muscle while the examiner's fingers of the left hand are placed behind this muscle when examining from the same side (Fig. 1.35*F*). The hands are, of course, reversed when examining from the opposite side (Fig. 1–35*G*). A careful search for lymph nodes is conducted anterior and posterior to the carotid artery, along its entire course in the neck. The background for this palpation is the transverse processes of the cervical vertebrae. Pulsations of the carotid bulb are easily palpated anterior and deep to the sternocleidomastoid muscle at about the level of the thyroid cartilage notch. The common artery can be palpated below this level, especially in the region of the carotid tubercle (transverse process of the sixth cervical vertebra).

The supraclavicular triangle is examined with the flat surfaces of the fingers while the patient's neck is in slight extension and then flexion (Fig. 1–37*H*). This is often neglected in a routine examination of the neck. Abnormal masses and pulsations in this area should be carefully evaluated.

Examination of the Posterolateral Neck

The posterior triangle of the neck is examined by palpating with the flat surfaces of the fingers, while the patient's neck is slightly flexed to the side being examined (Fig. 1–37*I*). The function of the trapezius muscle is easily tested by placing a hand on the patient's shoulder and asking him or her

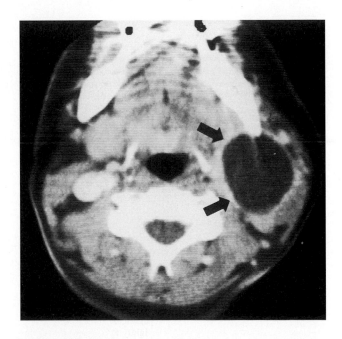

FIGURE 1–38. Axial CT section through the neck at the level of the oropharynx shows a water-density sharply defined mass posterior to the mandible and medial to the sternocleidomastoid muscle. There is a slight enhancement of the medial wall of this mass (*arrows*). Note slight skin bulge laterally, secondary to the underlying mass.

to elevate the arm. The posterior triangle of the neck (the space anterior to the trapezius muscle) is carefully palpated for enlarged lymph nodes or other tumor masses.

Computed Tomography

The advent of computed tomography gives a new dimension to the diagnosis and treatment of neck disease. Computed tomography scanning has become extremely valuable in assessing cervical metastatic disease and cervical abscesses (Fig. 1–36). Solid, cartilaginous, and bony lesions can be differentiated. Extension to the base of the skull and thorax can be determined, as can the extent of the tumor in relation to the larynx, esophagus, thyroid gland, carotid sheath, cervical spine, and brachial plexus.

Chapter 2
Surgery of the Neck

WILLIAM W. MONTGOMERY   MARK A. VARVARES

DIAGNOSIS OF A CERVICAL MASS

Neoplastic Disease

Benign Tumors
In general, benign lesions in the cervical region are discreet, moveable, and nontender. They constitute approximately 20% of all masses occurring in the neck.

Salivary Gland Tumors
Benign tumors that are most commonly associated with the parotid and submandibular glands are mixed tumors, Warthin's tumors (papillary cystadenoma lymphomatosum), adenomas, reactive intraparotid lymph nodes, HIV-associated lymphoepithelial cysts, and sebaceous cysts.

Mixed tumors of the parotid gland may arise from that part of the gland that projects into the cervical region, but they are most commonly found in the main portion of the gland or in the angle between the mandible and the mastoid. A tumor may be palpated as a cystic or solid lesion. Tumors of the submandibular gland are much less common (4:1) and are more likely to be malignant than tumors of the parotid gland.

Thyroid Gland Lesions
In general, a goiter is not difficult to diagnose. It is evident by diffuse or nodular swelling in the region of the thyroid gland or thyroid isthmus. The mass moves up and down as the patient swallows. Subacute thyroiditis (Hashimoto disease) is characterized by painful and tender swelling over one or both thyroid lobes. The protein-bound iodine and radioactive iodine uptake tests are useful in establishing the diagnosis. In both tests the values are below normal when the disease is present (see Chapter 18).

Carotid Body Tumor
This tumor is located at the bifurcation of the common carotid artery. Often, a bruit can be heard over it. The lesion tends to be fixed to the arteries and may increase the separation between the internal and external carotids. Arteriography of a carotid body tumor shows a vascular mass with displacement of the internal and external carotid arteries, the "lyre" sign.

Neurofibromas and Schwannomas
These tumors are most commonly associated with the cervical sympathetic trunk. They produce signs and symptoms of Horner's syndrome. They also may be associated with the glossopharyngeal nerve and taste disturbance, the vagus nerve and vocal cord paralysis, the spinal accessory nerve and shoulder drop, or the hypoglossal nerve and tongue paralysis. A neurofibroma occurring with von Recklinghausen disease is more apt to be associated with the trigeminal and facial nerves and to be accompanied by multiple skin lesions.

Fibroma
Fibromas occur in the cervical region. They are usually not diagnosed until they are removed.

Lipoma
Lipomas are usually superficial, soft, and typical.

Lymphangioma (Cystic Hygroma)
These lesions occur in infants and young children. They are often large, soft, and nontender, tending to be more common in the submandibular and supraclavicular regions than in other locations. They feel somewhat fluctuant, and they transilluminate. The lesion may present as a small mass with a large underlying tumor. Surgical excision is a treatment of choice, although in many instances, only a partial removal is possible.

Chondrosarcoma of the Cricoid
This usually presents as an intralaryngeal mass but may be first palpated externally. The mass is typically bony, hard, smooth, and globular when palpated. Lateral neck radiographs and laminography as well as computerized tomography scanning confirm the diagnosis.

Cystic Lesions
The dermoid cyst is usually a single enlargement and is most often found in the midline. The thyroglossal duct cyst is most often found in the midline, anywhere from the suprahyoid region to the suprasternal notch. This cyst is superficial compared with the dermoid cyst. First, second, and third branchial cleft cysts occur in the lateral cervical region. The

location of these cysts is usually indicative of the diagnosis. Occasionally, however, a thyroglossal duct cyst may be laterally placed and may mimic a second branchial cleft cyst.

The laryngocele, esophageal diverticulum, and carotid aneurysm can be confused with a true cyst of the neck. The laryngocele is soft and increases in size as intralaryngeal pressure increases. It is common among glassblowers and wind instrument musicians. Its close association with thyrohyoid membrane and its radiographic appearance may suggest the diagnosis. The esophageal diverticulum may present as a big mass in the cervical region anterior to the sternocleidomastoid muscle. The typical history of dysphagia and aspiration, along with contrast radiography, establishes this diagnosis. The carotid aneurysm is rare. Palpating the pulsating mass indicates the diagnosis, which is confirmed by angiography.

Malignant Tumors

A mass in the lateral neck of an adult should be considered a metastasis from a primary carcinoma of the head and neck until proven otherwise. An enlarged cervical lymph node, suspected of being involved with malignant disease, should be carefully considered to be due to primary lesion of the head and neck (85%), a distant primary lesion (9%), an occult (hidden) primary lesion (5%), or a constitutional neoplasm (1%).

Primary Lesions of the Head and Neck

The incidence of metastasis to cervical nodes from a primary lesion of the head and neck varies considerably. Lindberg reviewed the records of 2,044 patients with squamous cell carcinoma of the upper aerodigestive tract who were previously untreated. The incidence of metastatic squamous cell carcinoma based on anatomic location of the primary tumor is shown in Table 2–1.

Usually, when a patient has a neck mass presumed to be an enlarged cervical lymph node, he will have other signs and symptoms directing the examining physician to the site of the primary lesion. Occasionally, however, the site of the primary lesion is completely asymptomatic. In such cases, the surgeon's experience with tumor diagnosis and his or her knowledge of the usual site of cervical lymph node metastasis from a given primary lesion become invaluable.

Shah reviewed a series of 1,081 patients who underwent radical neck dissection, of these 776 with clinically positive nodal disease. The oral cavity was the most common source of metastatic disease with nearly 50% of patients presenting with an oral cavity primary. The oropharynx was a source in 20%, the larynx in 25%, and the hypopharynx in 12%. Levels I, II, and III were at highest risk for metastasis from carcinoma of the oral cavity, and levels II, III, and IV were at highest risk for metastasis from carcinomas of the oropharynx, hypopharynx, and larynx.

Some primary lesions of the head and neck are difficult to diagnose because certain areas such as the posterior nares, nasopharynx, and larynx are occasionally inaccessible for inspection. The rough and irregular surfaces of the tonsils, adenoids, and tongue can obscure a small lesion. Lesions can remain asymptomatic in areas with a sparse sensory nerve supply. Tumors in the nasopharynx, pharynx, hypopharynx, and pyriform sinuses can become large before they interfere with function. A good rule of thumb is that masses in the superior and middle jugular groups arise more commonly from the tonsil, oropharynx, nasopharynx, and supraglottic larynx than from other sites. Masses in the middle and inferior jugular group usually arise from the larynx. Masses in the supraclavicular region most frequently originate from primary lesions below the clavicle, in the stomach, intestinal tract, lungs, or breast. Posterior neck masses usually arise from the nasopharynx or paranasal sinuses or are primary lymphomas.

Neoplastic disease is responsible for 80% of lateral cervical neck masses, and 85% of these masses are derived from primary lesions of the head and neck. The most common site of primary disease is of the nasopharynx, tonsils, base of tongue, supraglottic region, thyroid gland, pharynx, floor of mouth, and palate.

If the primary lesion is not apparent after a careful search, the examiner should consider the possibility of an occult (hidden) primary lesion. When a neck mass is present, it is imperative that the examiner realizes never to use an incisional biopsy. Fine needle aspiration is very useful in differentiating a mass that is malignant from that which is benign. It is also very useful in differentiating metastatic squamous cell carcinoma from lymphoma. It should be liberally used in patients who present with a neck mass without an obvious primary tumor. The sensitivity and specificity of fine needle aspirate biopsy may be as high as 97% and 98%, respectively. The work-up of the occult head and neck primary tumor is discussed later in this chapter.

Distant Primary Lesions

The patient should be questioned carefully regarding any symptoms or history of disorder in any portion of the body to direct attention toward a distant primary lesion in the stomach, lungs, kidneys, pancreas, breast, bowels, lymphatic system, or circulatory system. Unless there is an obvious focus, it is best at this point to refer the patient to an internist.

Constitutional Neoplasm

Certain constitutional neoplasms may be first manifest as a single node in the neck. These include Hodgkin's disease, lymphosarcoma, reticulum cell carcinoma, and leukemia. Fine needle aspiration will often be helpful in establishing a diagnosis. A thorough search of the axilla, groin, and abdomen for other enlarged nodes is usually fruitful when any of these diseases is present. A blood count and biopsy excision of an enlarged node will confirm the diagnosis if the fine needle biopsy is not diagnostic.

TABLE 2–1
Incidence of Metastatic Squamous Cell Carcinoma Based on Anatomic Location of the Primary Tumor

Anatomical Area	Percent
Oral tongue	35%
Floor of mouth	30.5%
Retromolar trigone and anterior faucial pillar	45%
Soft palate	44%
Tonsillar fossa	76%
Base of tongue	78%
Oropharyngeal walls	59%
Supraglottic larynx	55%
Hypopharynx	75%
Nasopharynx	87%

Occult (Hidden) Primary Lesions

Approximately 5% of malignant lesions of the cervical lymph nodes are considered to be so-called occult primary lesions. This diagnosis is made only after a thorough search for a primary lesion in the head and neck region or a metastasis from a distant site has been conducted. The patient should be questioned carefully concerning any abnormal symptoms pertaining to the ear, nose, nasopharynx, pharynx, larynx, or esophagus that he or she may have experienced. The work-up should include a panendoscopy that includes nasopharyngoscopy, laryngoscopy, rigid esophagoscopy, and bilateral tonsillectomy. Computerized tomography scanning or magnetic resonance imaging scanning of the head and neck as well as chest radiograph is also indicated. Positron emission tomography scanning has been found to be ineffective in isolating an occult primary tumor in the head and neck. Lesions located in the supraclavicular fossa have a much higher incidence of being metastatic from a lesion located below the clavicle.

After the diagnosis of an occult primary lesion has been made by exclusion of other possibilities, a biopsy of the lesion is indicated. Open excisional biopsy should be used only when needle biopsy does not yield a definitive diagnosis. In general, an open incisional biopsy of any suspected squamous cell carcinoma metastatic to the neck is to be avoided.

The fine needle technique is preferred in most instances. Fine needle biopsy is recommended because its cutting edge provides a sample of tissue that allows cytologic evaluation. The dissemination of malignant tumor cells is virtually unreported in the use of fine needle aspirate biopsy. If the fine needle aspirate biopsy does not provide a definitive diagnosis, the next step is open biopsy with frozen section. An excisional biopsy is preferred. The specimen should be secured in the operating room with the patient prepared for a comprehensive neck dissection. The skin incision is made as small as possible and within the boundaries of a neck dissection. A frozen section diagnosis of thyroid carcinoma, adenocarcinoma, or undifferentiated squamous cell carcinoma may indicate the inadvisability of neck dissection. If the diagnosis is undifferentiated carcinoma, no additional surgery should be performed and the nasopharynx should be very carefully scrutinized for the possibility of an occult lesion. If the frozen section diagnosis is not definitive, further treatment should be postponed pending the examination of permanent tissue sections.

A primary lesion will ultimately become apparent approximately in 50% of occult primary tumors. Thus, the search for a primary lesion should continue even after definitive management (especially during radiation therapy) of the cervical lesion. The other 50% of primary lesions will not be evident even at autopsy. When an occult primary is treated with radiation to both necks and to all of Waldeyer's ring, a complete search for the primary site should be conducted after 2,000 centigray (cGy) has been administered. At this point, there is maximal difference between normal and cancerous tissue, and inconspicuous primary lesion may become apparent and be identified.

The staging of metastatic squamous cell carcinoma is an important part of the comprehensive care of the head and neck cancer patient. The patient's primary tumor, cervical lymph node metastasis, and distant disease status are all addressed in the staging system. The most recent staging system developed by the American Joint Commission of Cancer (AJCC) is listed in Table 2–2.

When patients present with bilateral neck disease, the neck should be individually staged with respect to multiplicity of nodes and node size.

TABLE 2-2
Staging System Developed by the American Joint Commission of Cancer (AJCC)

Stage	Parameters
N_x:	Regional nodes cannot be assessed.
N_0:	No regional lymph node metastasis.
N_1:	Metastasis in a single ipsilateral lymph node, less than or equal to 3 cm in greatest dimension.
N_2:	Metastasis in a single ipsilateral node or multiple ipsilateral nodes, greater than 3 cm, but less than 6 cm; bilateral or contralateral nodes none greater than 6 cm.
N_{2a}:	Metastasis in a single ipsilateral node, greater than 3 cm, but less than 6 cm.
N_{2b}:	Metastasis to multiple ipsilateral nodes, none greater than 6 cm.
N_{2c}:	Bilateral or contralateral nodes, none greater than 6 cm.
N_3:	Any node greater than 6 cm in greatest dimension.

DEVELOPMENTAL ABNORMALITIES

Developmental abnormalities include branchial cleft cyst, cystic hygromas, thyroglossal duct cyst, and, uncommonly, dermoid cyst.

Branchial Cleft Cyst

The first branchial cleft cyst is characterized by an opening into the external auditory canal anteriorly. The sinus extends anteroinferiorly and is closely related to the parotid gland and facial nerve. The patient rarely has otorrhea. The sinus progresses roughly in the direction of the eustachian tube to the submandibular triangle of the neck. It may course through the parotid gland, in close proximity to the facial nerve. Pressure on the mass, whether it is anterior or inferior to the auricle, may express mucopurulent discharge into the external auditory canal.

The cyst of the second arch (second cleft cyst) is located anterior to the sternocleidomastoid muscle. It courses over the 9th and 12th cranial nerves and between the external and internal carotid arteries into the pharynx, in the tonsillar fossa or nasopharynx.

The third cleft cyst in its complete form is a rare lesion. The sinus extends over the 12th and under the 9th cranial nerve. It runs behind both the external and internal carotid arteries and finally into the hypopharynx through the thyrohyoid membrane. The occurrence of a fourth cleft cyst has not been reported. The external opening should be along the anterior border of the sternocleidomastoid muscle. Internally the sinus tract should descend, passing inferior to the aortic arch on the left or the subclavian artery on the right (arteries of the fourth branchial arch), before ascending along the common carotid artery to pass superior to the 12th nerve to enter the upper esophagus.

Cystic Hygroma (Lymphangioma)

The cystic hygroma is an ill-defined doughy mass formed by failure of the lymph channels to develop. It occurs at the root of the neck, in the angle of the jaw (where it may involve the parotid gland), and in the midline (where it may involve the tongue, floor of mouth, and larynx).

Cystic hygromas transilluminate; they feel somewhat like lipomas, which do not transilluminate. The margins of the lipomas are much better defined than those of a cystic hygroma. Aspiration of cystic hygromas will produce straw-colored fluid. These lesions may get confused with angiomas, which are compressible, pneumatoceles from the apex of the lung, and aneurysms. An arteriogram will differentiate a hygroma from a vascular lesion. It is usually impossible to remove a cystic hygroma completely. If it is unsightly or if it interferes with function, subtotal removal is indicated.

Thyroglossal Duct Cyst

These account for approximately 70% of congenital abnormalities of the neck. They may be situated anywhere from the region of the foramen cecum at the base of tongue to the level of the suprasternal notch. A thyroglossal duct cyst may be present in the form of a cyst alone, a cyst in the sinus tract, or a solid core of thyroid tissue. Its size varies from a very small, barely perceptible lesion to one the size of a grapefruit.

The thyroglossal duct cyst is usually located in the midline at or below the level of the hyoid bone. It will move up and down when the patient swallows. Sometimes the tract can be palpated as the cyst is displaced inferiorly. A radioactive iodide scan or thyroid ultrasound is indicated if the thyroid gland is not definitely palpated in its normal position. The thyroid ultrasound will demonstrate absence of the thyroid gland in its normal position, and a thyroid scan will demonstrate a lingual thyroid and will help differentiate the cyst from a thyroid adenoma. A dermoid cyst should not be confused with a thyroglossal duct cyst because a dermoid cyst is deep in the floor mouth and is more solid than the thyroglossal duct cyst. A ranula is located very superficially in the floor of the mouth and is usually off to one side of midline; it is not at all like the thyroglossal duct cyst or dermoid cyst.

The thyroglossal duct cyst may rupture, resulting in a thyroglossal fistula that discharges a milky mucus. The discharge is purulent when an infection is present.

Inflammatory Cervical Masses

Acute infection of the neck, or cervical adenitis, is most commonly the result of infections of dental origin, tonsillitis, or pharyngitis. A constitutional reaction, tenderness of the cervical mass, and an obvious site for an infectious source confirm the diagnosis. Infections of the fascial spaces of the neck can present real diagnostic problems, especially when the signs and symptoms are masked by antibiotic therapy.

Probably the most common acute infection of the neck is the parapharyngeal abscess with extensions into the cervical region. Extensions into the various cervical fascial compartments can result in a variety of symptoms. Horner syndrome, such as ptosis, myosis, and anhidrosis, associated with involvement of the cervical sympathetic nerve and vocal cord paralysis from vagus nerve involvement, is a classic example. Abscesses in the submandibular and submental spaces are usually associated with an abscessed tooth.

LYMPH NODES OF THE HEAD AND NECK

The lymph nodes of the head and neck (Fig. 2–1 and Fig. 2–2) may be grouped as follows:

1. Occipital
2. Postauricular
3. Parotid
4. Submandibular
5. Submental
6. Facial
7. Sublingual
8. Retropharyngeal
9. Lateral cervical
10. Anterior cervical

The first six groups form a collar situated at the junction of the head and neck. The sublingual and retropharyngeal groups lie inside this collar near the site where the tongue touches the pharyngeal wall; these are not palpated during a routine examination for lymph nodes of the head and neck. The remaining nodes form a chain along the front and side of the neck.

Occipital Nodes

The occipital nodes are suprafascial, subfascial, and submuscular nodes. The one or two suprafascial nodes are rarely absent. They are intimately related to the external branch of the occipital artery and greater occipital nerve in the uppermost part of the occipital triangle.

Usually only one subfascial node lies beneath the deep fascia. Occasionally no subfascial node is present.

Usually one to three submuscular nodes lie near the occipital vessels.

Afferent vessels are located in the occipital region.

Efferent vessels are primarily part of the deep lateral accessory nerve chain.

Postauricular Nodes

The postauricular nodes usually appear as one or two nodes.

Afferent vessels are located in the parietal region and a portion of the auricular chain.

Efferent vessels are found in the infra-auricular parotid nodes and substernomastoid nodes in the superior internal jugular chain.

Parotid Nodes

The parotid nodes include the suprafascial, subfascial extraglandular, and deep intraglandular nodes.

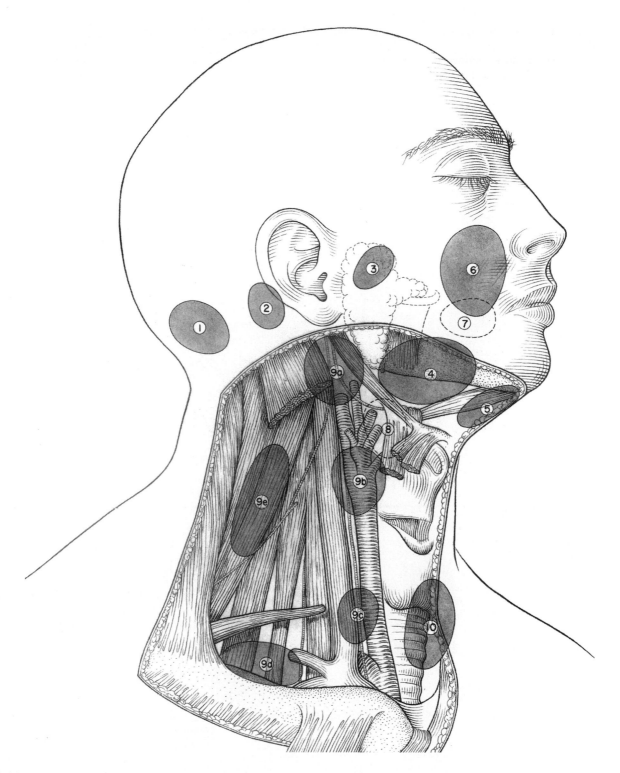

FIGURE 2–1. Lymph nodes of the head and neck, general grouping. (1), Occipital; (2), mastoid; (3), parotid; (4), submandibular; (5), submental; (6), facial; (7), sublingual; (8), retropharyngeal; (9), lateral cervical (a, upper jugular; b, midjugular; c, inferior jugular; d, supraclavicular; e, posterior triangle); (10), anterior cervical.

The suprafascial nodes consist of one or two superficial preauricular nodes lying near the tragus.

The subfascial extraglandular nodes form a small group of nodes lying beneath the parotid sheath (fascia parotideomasseterica). Some of them are preglandular, whereas others are infra-auricular at the lower pole of the parotid gland. (The latter are routinely removed in a block dissection when the inferior extremity of the parotid gland is excised.)

The 4 to 10 deep intraglandular nodes are located near the isthmus that unite the superficial and deep lobes of the parotid gland.

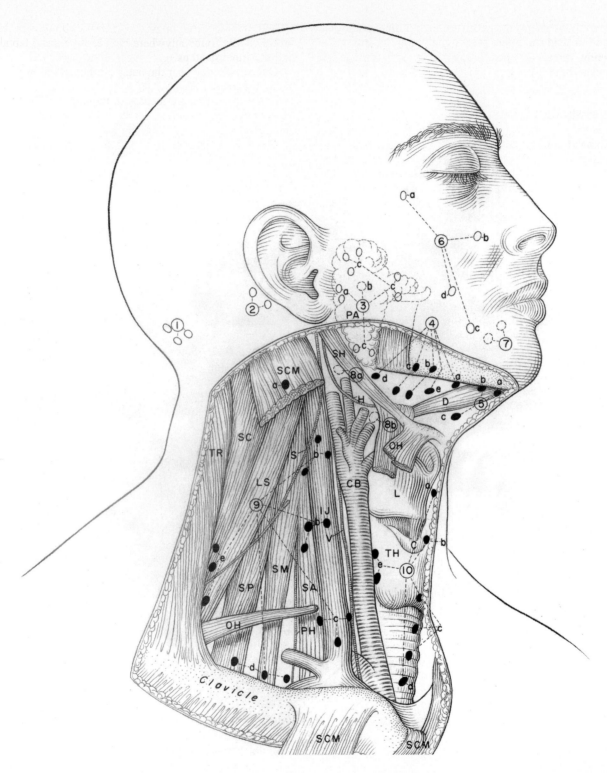

FIGURE 2-2. Lymph nodes of the head and neck, detailed grouping. (1), Occipital; (2), mastoid; (3), parotid (a, suprafacial; b, deep intraglandular; c, subfacial extraglandular); (4), submandibular (a, preglandular; b, prevascular; c, retrovascular; d, retroglandular; e, intracapsular); (5), submental (a, anterior; b, middle; c, posterior); (6), facial (a, malar; b, infraorbital; c, inferior maxillary; d, buccinator); (7), sublingual; (8), retropharyngeal (a, medial; b, lateral); (9) lateral cervical (a, superior jugular; b, midjugular; c, inferior jugular; d, transverse cervical (supraclavicular); e, spinal accessory (posterior triangle); (10), Anterior cervical (a, superficial anterior jugular chain; b, prelaryngeal; c, pretracheal). TR, trapezius; SC, scalenus capitus; SCM, sternocleidomastoid; SH, stylohyoid; D, anterior belly of digastric; L, larynx; OH, anterior border of omohyoid muscle; CB, carotid bulb; C, cricothyroid membrane; TH, thyroid; PH, phrenic nerve; OH, posterior belly digastric; SP, splenius posticus muscle; SM, splenius medius muscle; SA, splenius anticus muscle; V, vagus nerve; IJ, internal jugular vein; S, spinal accessory nerve; LS, levator scapulae muscle.

Afferent vessels are located from the midline, anteriorly over the forehead and upper face to the postauricular region.

Efferent vessels are positioned directly or indirectly to the jugular chain.

Submandibular Nodes

The submandibular nodes include the preglandular, prevascular, retrovascular, retroglandular, and intracapsular nodes.

One or two preglandular nodes are located anterior to the submandibular gland and lie on the submental vessels.

Usually only one large prevascular node is present, located in front of the anterior facial vein and on the external maxillary artery.

One or two retrovascular nodes are situated behind the anterior facial vein.

The retroglandular nodes are found medial to or below the angle of the mandible (uncommon).

One or more intracapsular nodes lie within the capsular or substance of the submandibular gland.

Afferent vessels are located on the lateral chin, lower lip, cheeks, nose, mucosa of the anterior part of the nasal fossa, gums, teeth, lids, soft and hard palate, tongue anterior to the lingual vein, submandibular gland, sublingual gland, and floor of mouth.

Efferent vessels are in the internal jugular chain.

Occasionally, an efferent vessel from a preglandular or prevascular node extends to a lateral submental node and may drain into the internal jugular vein on the opposite side.

Submental Nodes

The submental nodes may be classified as the anterior, middle, and posterior nodes.

One or two anterior nodes are found in the anterior part of the submental triangle.

The middle nodes are found midway between the hyoid bone and the mandible and are medially or laterally situated in the submental triangle.

One or two posterior nodes are located near the hyoid bone in the posterior part of the submental triangle.

Afferent vessels are located in the chin, middle lower lip, cheeks, incisor region of the gums, anterior floor of the mouth, and tip of the tongue.

Efferent vessels are in the submaxillary nodes and the internal jugular vein; these may cross to the opposite side.

Facial Nodes

The facial nodes are found along the anterior facial vein and external maxillary artery. They consist of the inferior maxillary node, and the buccinator, infraorbital, and malar groups.

There is usually only on inferior maxillary (midmandibular) node on the external surface of the mandible and masseter muscle.

The buccinator group consists of one or two nodes approximately 2.5 cm posterior to the angle of the mouth, near Stensen's duct.

One small node belonging to the infraorbital (nasal labial) group can be found anywhere between the nasal labial fold and the inner canthus.

One small node near the outer canthus of the eye belongs to the malar group.

Afferent vessels are located in the upper and lower lids, nose, upper and lower lips, entire cheek, and rarely, the gums and palate.

Efferent vessels are in the submaxillary nodes.

Retropharyngeal Nodes

The retropharyngeal nodes may be divided into the medial and lateral groups.

The medial nodes are intercalated (interrupting nodules) in the lymphatics from one pharyngeal wall draining into the lateral nodes. They may be found anywhere on the posterior pharyngeal wall from the base of the skull to the level of the hyoid bone.

The lateral nodes consist of one or two nodes lying between the prevertebral fascia and the lateral pharyngeal wall at the level of the atlas near the carotid as it enters the carotid canal, and adjacent to the upper pole of the superior cervical ganglion.

Afferent vessels are located in the nasal fossae, sinuses, nasopharynx, oropharynx, palate, and mid-middle ear.

Efferent vessels are found in the internal jugular chain.

Lateral Cervical Nodes

Lateral cervical nodes are both superficial and deep. In the external jugular chain, one to four superficial nodes occur over the upper half of the sternocleidomastoid muscle in relation to the external jugular vein. They are usually found in close relation to the lower pole of the parotid gland.

The deep lateral cervical nodes consist of three chains: the internal jugular, the spinal accessory, and the transverse cervical.

The internal jugular chain lies along the anterolateral aspect of the internal jugular vein and spirals laterally to the posterior aspect of the vein in the lower neck. In relation to the posterior belly of the digastric muscle are the subdigastric nodes; in relation to the carotid bifurcation are the carotid nodes; and in relation to the superior belly of the omohyoid muscle are the omohyoid nodes. The nodes near the clavicle are called the supraclavicular nodes. At the lower end of the chain, the lymph collects into the jugular lymphatic trunk, which empties on the left side into the arch of the thoracic duct and on the right into the right lymphatic duct. An anteriorly located jugular node near the lower border of the posterior belly of the omohyoid muscle is called a principle node of Kuttner because of its clinical importance in cancer metastasis.

The spinal accessory chain consists of 5 to 10 nodes that extend along the course of the spinal accessory nerve. Lymph from these nodes flows into the transverse cervical chain.

The transverse cervical (supraclavicular) chain consists of 1 to 10 lymph nodes lying between the spinal accessory chain and the jugulo-subclavian junction. These nodes accompany the transverse cervical artery and vein. The most medial node in this chain is the node of Troisier, to which carcinoma of the stomach may metastasize. Lymph from this group of nodes flows on the right side into the right lymphatic duct.

Anterior Cervical Nodes

The anterior cervical nodes lie between the two carotid sheaths below the level of the hyoid bone. They consist of the superficial anterior jugular chain and the deep anterior cervical nodes.

The nodes of the superficial anterior jugular chain lie in relation to the anterior jugular chain and usually drain into the lower internal jugular nodes. There are three groups of deep anterior cervical nodes: the prelaryngeal nodes, the pretracheal nodes, and the nodes of the recurrent nerve chain.

The prelaryngeal nodes are one or two intercricothyroid nodes on the cricothyroid infraglottic larynx and pyriform sinuses. Occasionally, they include small lymphoid nodules in front of the thyrohyoid membrane and thyroid cartilage.

The pretracheal nodes accompany the thyroid veins behind the pretracheal fascia. They receive lymph from the thyroid gland. Their efferent vessels extend to the recurrent nerve nodes, internal jugular nodes, and anterior mediastinal nodes.

The recurrent nerve chain nodes consist of 4 to 10 nodes on each side. They receive lymph from the posterior part of the infraglottic larynx as well as from the pretracheal nodes and thyroid gland. Their efferent vessels extend to the internal jugular chain.

Cervical lymph node groups may be grouped simply as clinical levels I to VI.

Level I includes the submental and submandibular nodes.

Levels II to IV are the jugular nodes that are found lateral to the jugular vein. The anterior and posterior limits of levels II to IV are the anterior and posterior borders of the sternocleidomastoid muscle, respectively. Level II includes the upper jugular nodes in the region extending from the base of skull to the hyoid bone or carotid bifurcation.

Level III includes the jugular nodes found between the hyoid bone superiorly and the omohyoid muscle inferiorly.

Level IV includes lymph nodes of the lower jugular group in the region that extends from the omohyoid muscle superiorly to the clavicle inferiorly.

Level V is composed of the lymph nodes of the posterior triangle that include the accessory nodes that are found near cranial nerve XI and the supraclavicular fossa. The boundaries are the trapezius posteriorly, the clavicle inferiorly, and the sternocleidomastoid muscle anteriorly.

Level VI describes the anterior compartment nodes. Included are the pretracheal, paratracheal, precricoid (Delphian), and perithyroidal nodes. The lateral boundaries are the common carotid arteries, the superior boundary is the hyoid bone, and the inferior boundary is the sternal notch.

BLOCK DISSECTION OF THE NECK

Indications

A block neck dissection is elective when no enlarged cervical lymph nodes are palpable; definitive or therapeutic when enlarged cervical nodes are present; and functional when the sternocleidomastoid muscle, internal jugular vein, and cranial nerve XI are preserved.

A neck dissection is indicated when the overall plan for care of the patient includes surgical management of the neck. This may be in conjunction with radiation, either administered before or after neck dissection.

A neck dissection is contraindicated in large fixed nodes, which are inoperable, and when it is believed that there is no hope of controlling the primary tumor.

Elective neck dissections are performed in the clinically N_0 neck. Most surgeons now agree that in this setting, at the very least, cranial nerve XI should be preserved. Many would agree that a functional neck dissection that preserves the spinal accessory nerve, sternocleidomastoid muscle, and jugular vein may be performed in this setting. With increased frequency, surgeons are performing elective neck dissection for the clinically N_0 neck. The type of selective neck dissection and the region they encompass are noted in Table 2–3. Essentially the elective neck dissection includes some components of a functional neck dissection, again which preserves the sternocleidomastoid muscle, cranial nerve XI, and the internal jugular vein.

To help clarify the classification of comprehensive neck dissections, terminology has been devised to describe the modified radical neck dissection as a comprehensive dissection of levels I to V. The subcategories define the type of dissection depending on which of the nonlymphatic structures, that is the sternocleidomastoid muscle, jugular vein,

TABLE 2–3
Types of Selective Neck Dissection and the Regions They Encompass

Selective Neck Dissections	Regions Dissected	Usually Primary Site Involved
Supraomohyoid	I–II	Oral cavity and oropharynx, excluding tongue
Extended supraomohyoid neck dissection	I–IV	Tongue
Posterolateral	II–V, including retroauricular and suboccipital nodes	Scalp and postauricular skin
Lateral neck dissection	II–IV	Larynx, hypopharynx, and oropharynx
Anterior compartment	VI	Thyroid

or accessory nerve, are preserved. In a Type I modified radical neck dissection, only cranial nerve XI is spared. In a Type II modified radical neck dissection, two of the three nonlymphatic structures are spared. In a Type III modified radical neck dissection, all three nonlymphatic structures are spared. This is identical to a functional neck dissection.

A therapeutic neck dissection is performed when there is clinically manifest cervical metastasis. In most therapeutic neck dissections, the jugular vein and sternocleidomastoid are sacrificed. It has been demonstrated that in many cases of N(+) neck disease, a cranial nerve XI sparing neck dissection (modified radical neck dissection Type I) may be used without an increased risk of cervical recurrence when compared with a standard radical neck dissection. In cases of large fixed nodes in region 2 when cranial nerve XI is intimately associated with metastatic disease, it is advisable to sacrifice this nerve. It may be grafted to decrease the associated morbidity of trapezius muscle denervation.

Preoperative Preparation

The patient's neck and upper chest are shaved to prepare for the operation. The patient is placed on the operating room table with a pillow or inflatable rubber bag under his shoulders. His head should be extended so that the occiput rests against the upper end of the table. The upper half of the operating room table is elevated to approximately 30 degrees. This will decrease the amount of bleeding during the procedure. The patient's lower face, ears, neck, shoulders, and upper chest are prepared with solutions of the surgeon's choice.

Proper draping of the patient for a block neck dissection is important. A towel placed over a half sheet is slid under the patient's head. This is then draped around the head to exclude the anesthesia tubing from the field. The towel is secured with a towel clip just above the patient's chin. The lower lip is left partially exposed to visualize lip movement should the marginal mandibular nerve be stimulated with a nerve stimulator. The lobule of the ear on the side on which the operation is to be performed remains uncovered. Four towels are then placed and sutured to the skin: (1) from the chin to the mastoid over the body of the mandible; (2) horizontally across the upper chest from midline to the shoulder; (3) from the mastoid tip to the shoulder; and (4) in the midline vertically. A half sheet is placed across the patient's chest. A thyroid sheet covers the entire patient and table except for the field of operation. The Mayo stand is draped. Suction tubing and the cautery cord are secured in place.

Incisions and Flaps

The double Y incision (Fig. 2–3A) was formerly the most popular for block neck dissection. The upper incision extends from the mid-submental area, running posteroinferiorly to a point just below the submandibular gland. From here it extends posterosuperiorly to the tip of the mastoid process. The lower incision extends from the suprasternal notch, running posterosuperiorly to approximately 4 cm above the clavicle and the mid-clavicular region. It then runs

posteroinferiorly to the junction of the trapezius muscle and the clavicle. The vertical arm of the incision, which connects with the upper and lower incisions, should be placed posterior to the carotid vessels. If a laryngectomy has already been performed, the carotid artery is found in the more anterior position. The cosmetic result is improved by giving the vertical or connecting incisions a slightly S-shaped curve.

Some surgeons prefer the single Y incision (Fig. 2–3B). Use of this incision can make dissection of the lateral subclavian triangle difficult. Extensions and modifications of this incision to include surgery of the larynx, mandible, mouth, and pharynx are presented as alternatives.

Many surgeons use the apron flap incision (Fig. 2–3C) when a block neck dissection is to be combined with a total laryngectomy. This incision begins at the tip of the hyoid on the contralateral side, extending inferiorly along the anterior border of the sternocleidomastoid muscle to a level just below the cricoid arch. From this point, it is extended posterosuperiorly along the posterior aspect of the sternocleidomastoid muscle to the mastoid process. Another extension is made to the lateral aspect of the subclavian triangle.

The Schobinger flap (Fig. 2–3D) is designed to protect the carotid artery, especially when the block neck dissection follows radiation therapy to the neck. A large anteriorly based pedicled skin flap is elevated.

The H incision (Fig. 2–3E) provides inferiorly and superiorly based flaps. The blood supply to both flaps is good, affording good protection for the carotid artery in the postradiation therapy neck. The flaps give excellent exposure and may be best in certain situations, although the cosmetic result is not good.

Most head and neck surgeons now use the Conley modification of the Schobinger flap (Fig. 2–3F) for block neck dissections. It brings the posterosuperior aspect of the flap a little further anteriorly than does the Schobinger incision. This area occasionally becomes devitalized when the Schobinger flap is used. The vertical portion of the incision extends in a more posterior direction than the Schobinger. It crosses over the clavicle at its lateral one third.

A block dissection can also be accomplished with parallel transverse incisions (Fig. 2–3G). The bipedicled flap (the "MacFee") thus elevated enjoys an excellent blood supply and therefore is advocated by many for surgery after radiation therapy. This approach can be used with or without primary resection of the lesion. The cosmetic and functional results are excellent. It is not practical for simultaneous bilateral neck dissections or for patients with large metastatic lesions of the neck. It has been said that the parallel transverse incisions allow sufficient coverage to the carotid artery in patients who have had radiation therapy. This is not true. Carotid artery protection with a levator muscle, dermal graft, or fascia lata graft is still necessary. Block neck dissection using parallel transverse incision is a more tedious procedure and is attended by somewhat greater difficulty in control of the blood vessels than with other incisions.

The authors prefer a further modification of the Conley and Schobinger incisions. This incision (Fig. 2–4A) begins in the submental region and extends posteriorly about two finger breadths inferior to the mandible at the level of the mandibular notch. It then extends posterosuperiorly and is

Text continued on page 54

rounded off just below the tip of the mastoid process. At this point, the incision is directed inferiorly along the posterior border of the sternocleidomastoid muscle and then onto the chest, across from the clavicle at the junction of its anterior middle thirds. Flaps are elevated in all directions and shown in Figure 2–4B. In the authors' experience, this incision gives excellent exposure with a little extra retraction and will almost invariably heal without complications, even after a full course of radiation therapy.

The chosen incision is carried through the skin, subcutaneous tissue, and platysmal muscle. It is best to either ligate or cauterize all bleeders as they are encountered so that hemostats, which interfere with the elevation of the skin flaps, will not be required. The platysmal muscle is included with the skin flaps because it provides additional blood supply that assists in the healing process. The lymphatics associated with the platysma are seldom involved with metastatic disease. The external jugular vein is not included with the skin flap. The skin flaps are elevated in four directions to expose (1) the mandibular ramus, superiorly, (2) the midline or strap muscles, anteriorly, (3) the clavicle, inferiorly, and (4) the anterior border of the trapezius muscle, posteriorly (see Fig. 2–4).

If one suspects that the metastatic disease might involve the subcutaneous or dermal layers, a wide area of skin must be excised in continuity with the block neck dissection. A small skin defect is covered with a split-thickness skin graft or by rotating a pedicled skin flap. In patients in whom a wide area of skin has been excised, as well as all of those who have received radiation therapy, the carotid artery should be covered with either a muscle pedicle or a dermal and fascial graft. A pectoralis myocutaneous flap may be necessary.

It is functionally and cosmetically important to preserve the mandibular branch of the facial nerve. The ramus mandibulae nerve crosses just deep to the superficial layer of deep cervical fascia, but superficial to both the anterior facial vein and the external maxillary artery. This nerve is identified after the superior flap is elevated over the submandibular gland, exposing the superficial layer of deep cervical fascia. Occasionally it can be detected easily through the fascia; in most instances, however, a nerve stimulator is required to make the identification. This technique is tedious and requires extra equipment.

An almost foolproof technique for preserving the mandibular nerve is to locate the notch on the inferior border of the mandible made by the external maxillary vessels. Following this point inferiorly, the anterior facial vein is located over the inferior aspect of the submandibular gland by incising the superficial layer of deep cervical fascia. This fascia is then incised along the inferior aspect of the submandibular gland. The anterior facial vein is divided and ligated at this level. The superior ligature on the anterior facial vein is left long and reflected superiorly with a hemostat (see Fig. 2–4). The superficial layer of deep cervical fascia is then undermined and incised both anteriorly and posteriorly at the horizontal level closely approximating the upper skin incision. The anterior facial vein and superficial layer of deep cervical fascia are reflected superiorly with the skin flap, exposing the submaxillary gland, the tail of the parotid gland, the anterior body of the digastric muscle, and the inferior margin of the mandible. Although the ramus mandibularis may not be seen, it is automatically reflected superiorly and not injured.

Inferior Aspect of the Sternocleidomastoid Muscle

An incision is made over the fascia covering the sternocleidomastoid muscle (Fig. 2–5A). The sternal and clavicular head to this muscle is delineated using sharp dissection (Fig. 2–5B). With curved dissecting scissors or a heavy curved hemostat, the undersurface of the muscle is separated from the carotid sheath (Fig. 2–5C). Injury to the carotid artery, vagus nerve, or internal jugular vein is avoided if this dissection is performed just external to the fascia surrounding the muscle and the muscle retracted laterally as it is transected (Fig. 2–5D).

The bellies of the sternocleidomastoid muscle are retracted posterosuperiorly, exposing the carotid sheath and the omohyoid muscle, which overlies the great vessels (Fig. 2–6A). The internal jugular vein, carotid artery, and vagus nerves are identified. The omohyoid muscle is then divided above the clavicle. Its upper portion can be mobilized medially to the hyoid bone to define the anteromedial aspect of the neck dissection.

The inferior aspect of the internal jugular vein is skeletonized using curved scissors or a hemostat and broad fixation or vein forceps. There is much less chance of injuring the vein if the dissection is performed close to the adventitial layer of the vein. When dissecting on the medial surface of the vein, the dissection should proceed in a horizontal direction rather than vertical to prevent avulsion of small branches off the jugular vein. Both anterior and posterior branches may be encountered entering the vein at this level. These usually come from the transverse cervical, transverse scapular, and anterior jugular veins. At least 2 cm of the internal jugular vein is isolated before clamping. It is important to visualize the common carotid artery and vagus nerve before clamping the jugular vein. Two Kelly clamps are placed on the vein, 1 cm apart, with both handles in the same direction. It is best to place the clamps so that their tips are facing laterally and away from the vagus nerve. The vein is transected between these clamps. A 2-0 silk ligature is placed around the vein below the lower clamp. This clamp is loosened as the first knot is tied and then reapplied. A 2-0 black silk suture ligature is placed through the vein above the first tie. It is tied around the vein, and the clamp is removed. The upper cut end of the vein is secured in a similar fashion. Another, possibly simpler, method to transect and suture ligate the internal jugular vein is to pass a loop of 2 black silk suture posterior to the vein, as shown in Figure 2–6B. A loop is then cut to create two ligatures posterior to the internal jugular vein. The superior ligature is tied first (Fig. 2–6C). The vein is transected after the inferior ligature is tied (Fig. 2–6D). Each end of the vein is then grasped with a hemostat and suture ligature applied as illustrated in Figure 2–6E.

The carotid sheath is opened, exposing the common carotid artery and vagus nerve. The thoracic duct usually enters the posterolateral aspect of the left internal jugular vein just above

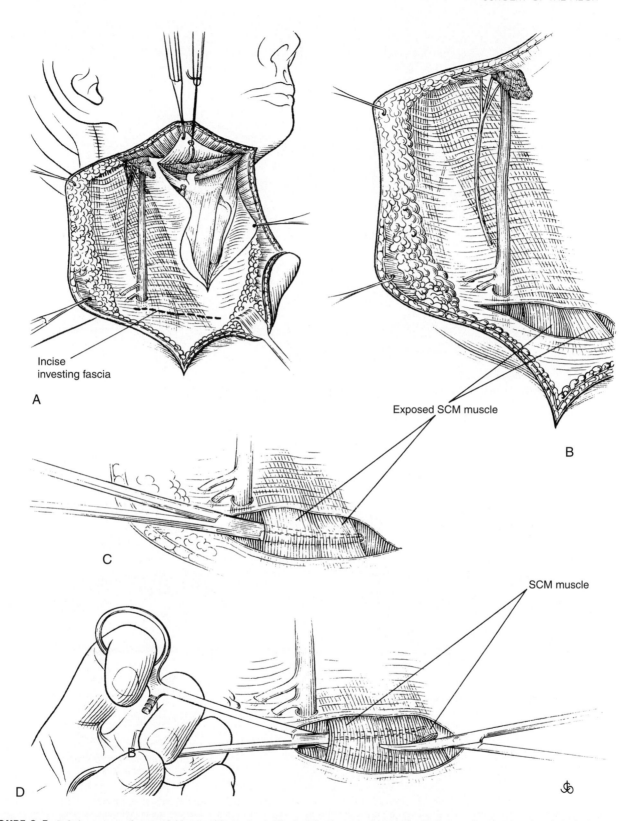

Incise
investing fascia

A

B

Exposed SCM muscle

C

SCM muscle

D

FIGURE 2–5. Inferior aspect of sternocleidomastoid muscle. *A,* The incision is made through the fascia covering the sternal and clavicular heads of the sternocleidomastoid (SCM) muscle just above the clavicle. *B,* Both heads of the sternocleidomastoid muscle are dissected so that the anterior and posterior borders of this muscle complex are clearly delineated. Using blunt dissection, the plane is established posteriorly between the heads of the sternocleidomastoid muscle and the carotid sheath. *C,* A large blunt-end hemostat serves best for this dissection. *D,* With the hemostat in place between the sternocleidomastoid muscle and the carotid sheath, the muscle is transected as it is resected laterally.

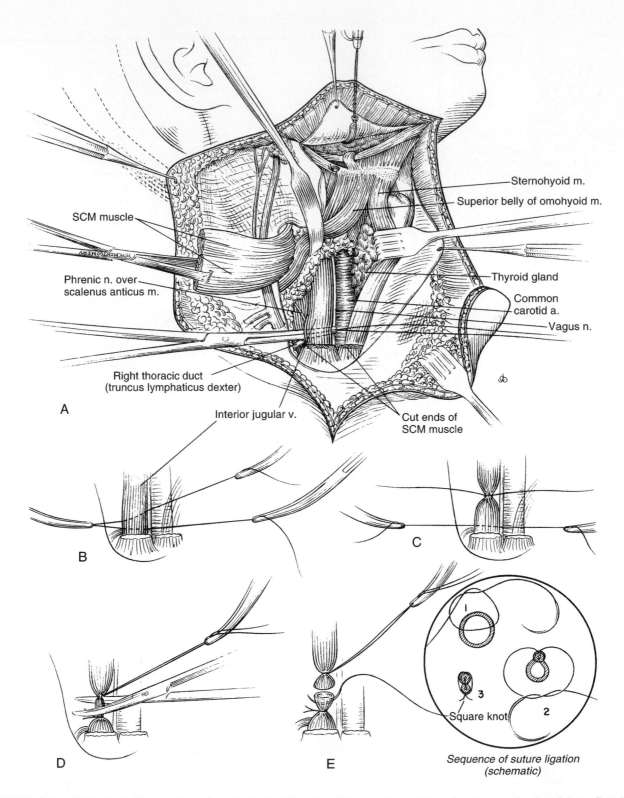

Sternohyoid m.

Superior belly of omohyoid m.

SCM muscle

Thyroid gland

Phrenic n. over scalenus anticus m.

Common carotid a.

Vagus n.

Right thoracic duct (truncus lymphaticus dexter)

Interior jugular v.

Cut ends of SCM muscle

A

B

C

D

E

Square knot

Sequence of suture ligation (schematic)

FIGURE 2–6. Carotid sheath. *A,* The sternal and clavicular heads of the sternocleidomastoid muscle have been transected and are being reflected posterosuperiorly along with the anterior belly of the omohyoid muscle. The carotid sheath is dissected to identify the internal jugular vein, carotid artery, and vagus nerve. The internal jugular vein is dissected free from its surrounding tissue using fixation forceps and blunt dissection. During this dissection it is essential not to injure the accessory thoracic duct (*right side*), which enters the posterolateral aspect of the internal jugular vein just above its junction with the subclavian vein. The duct is not injured if the dissection is carried out above this level. *B–E,* A loop of 2-0 silk suture material is passed behind the internal jugular vein. The loop is cut and the upper ligature tied. The lower ligature is tied and the internal jugular vein transected. The cut end of the internal jugular vein is grasped with a hemostat and is ligated with sutures as illustrated.

its junction with the subclavian vein. The accessory thoracic duct empties into the venous system at about the same point on the right side. If the internal jugular vein has been transected at too low a level, or if the thoracic duct enters at a high level, it may be injured or transected. Injury to the duct is easily recognized, for when it occurs chyle flows freely into the operating field. It is best to identify the point of leakage at once and to ligate it with sutures to prevent formation of a postoperative chyloma. The fascia of the carotid sheath is then stripped from the common carotid artery and vagus nerve so that it may be removed with the specimen.

Thyroid Gland

In some cases, it may be desirable to include the ipsilateral thyroid lobe with the neck dissection. The thyroid isthmus and gland on the side of the neck dissection may be removed with the specimen if there is any question of their involvement. This step is especially indicated when there is subglottic extension of a transglottic lesion, or if the cricothyroid lymph node is involved.

The thyroid gland is exposed by transecting the sternohyoid and sternothyroid muscles on the side of the neck dissection. These muscles, along with the internal jugular vein, are retracted superiorly. A neat dissection can be accomplished by isolating and ligating the superior thyroid artery and vein, the middle thyroid vein, and the inferior thyroid artery and vein. The thyroid isthmus is transected between clamps and ligated with sutures (Fig. 2–7A).

If the larynx is not to be removed with the radical neck dissection, the recurrent laryngeal nerve must be identified and preserved. As the thyroid gland is dissected, the recurrent laryngeal nerve can be identified as it runs medial to the inferior pole of the gland. A further guide is the inferior thyroid artery, which intertwines with the nerve in its terminal position (Fig. 2–7B and C). The authors prefer to begin dissection of the thyroid gland inferiorly and then use a nerve stimulator for positive identification of the recurrent laryngeal nerve.

Dissection of the Subclavian Triangle

After transecting the sternocleidomastoid muscle and the internal jugular vein, dissection of the fascia from the common carotid artery and vagus nerve, and freeing the thyroid gland, elevation of the specimen can begin. With blunt dissection lateral to the carotid artery, the fascia over the anterior scalene muscle (fascial carpet) is identified (Fig. 2–8). This is an important landmark because it is the deep limit of the neck dissection and should not be disturbed. The phrenic nerve can be seen beneath this fascia, descending in a lateral to medial direction across the anterior scalene muscle. Its location and identification can be confirmed with a nerve stimulator. At this point, the surgeon should begin watching for an abnormally high apical pleura or subclavian vein.

The transverse scapular and transverse cervical arteries are identified and ligated as they branch from the thyrocervical trunk at the medial border of the anterior scalene muscle. They are again ligated adjacent to the anterior border of the trapezius muscle.

The inferior aspect of the external jugular vein reaches the posterior margin of the sternocleidomastoid muscle approximately 2 cm above the clavicle, where it pierces the deep cervical fascia, enters the posterior triangle of the neck, and communicates with the subclavian vein. Just before entering the subclavian vein, the external jugular vein receives branches that include the transverse cervical, transverse scapular, and the anterior and posterior jugular veins. The external jugular vein, with these branches, is carefully ligated.

Having identified the fascial carpet, the dissection is carried laterally to the anterior border of the trapezius muscle. The transverse scapula and transverse cervical arteries are again encountered at this time.

Any dissection deep to the layer of deep cervical fascia covering the anterior scalene muscle may result in injury to the phrenic nerve and the brachial plexus.

Anterior Border of the Trapezius Muscle

Elevation of the posteroinferior aspect of the specimen commences as soon as the subclavian triangle dissection reaches the anterior border of the trapezius muscle (Fig. 2–9). The middle scalene, posterior scalene, levator scapula, and splenius capitus muscles are identified as the dissection is carried superiorly.

The nodes of the spinal accessory group are much less likely to be involved with metastatic disease from carcinoma of the head and neck than are the nodes of the internal jugular group. Many authors note that the spinal accessory area is still a possible site of metastasis and that the spinal accessory nerve should be included routinely in a block neck dissection. The controversy concerning the preservation of this nerve stems from patients' complaints of persistent shoulder pain and shoulder droop when it has been removed. One seemingly logical approach to this problem would be to include the nerve with the block dissection if there is any question of the presence of palpably enlarged nodes and to preserve the nerve when the prophylactic neck dissection is performed. If the spinal accessory nerve is to be preserved, it is identified as it approaches the anterior border of the trapezius muscle at the junction of the lower one third and upper two thirds of the distance between the mastoid tip and the clavicle. This nerve is usually associated with the posterior border of the levator scapulae muscle. It follows this border superiorly and disappears underneath the posterior belly of the digastric muscle. After its identification, the nerve is mobilized out of the posterior triangle contents. Dissection and division of the muscle continue until the nerve is noted on the anterior and deep aspect of the upper portion of the sternocleidomastoid muscle.

The spinal accessory nerve is usually crossed by a cutaneous sensory branch at the point where it enters the posterior aspect of the sternocleidomastoid muscle. Caution must be used not to confuse this nerve with the spinal accessory nerve. During dissection, the nerve must be handled with care because excessive retraction will result in a traction injury to the nerve. This may cause a severe neuropraxia or even nerve degeneration, resulting in trapezius muscle weakness and shoulder pain, although the nerve is "anatomically intact." In some cases, such a nerve may never recover functionally. The branch of the spinal accessory nerve to the ster-

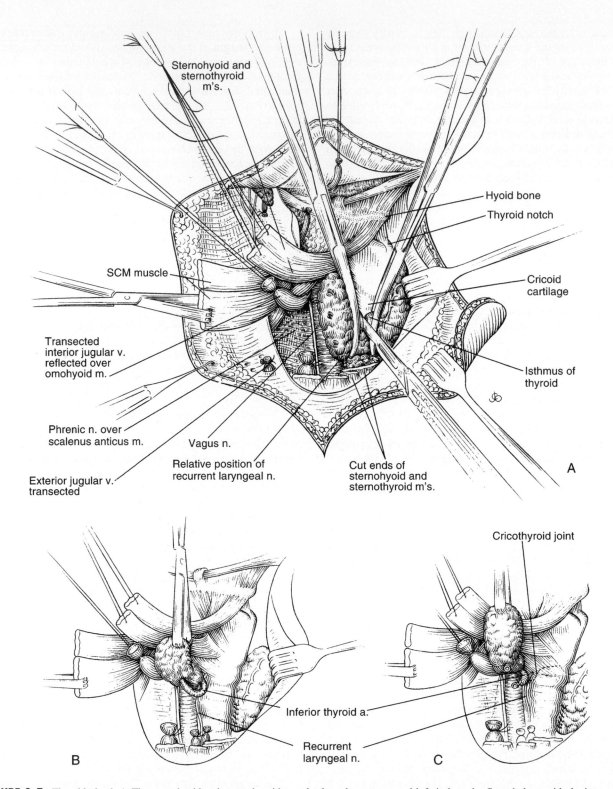

FIGURE 2-7. Thyroid gland. *A,* The sternohyoid and sternothyroid muscles have been transected inferiorly and reflected along with the internal jugular vein in a posterosuperior direction. A lobe of the thyroid gland to be resected along with the block neck dissection and thyroid isthmus is thus exposed. The place of cleavage is established between the trachea and thyroid isthmus using hemostat dissection. The thyroid isthmus is transected between clamps and ligated using 2-0 chromic catgut suture material. *B,* The inferior pole of the thyroid gland is elevated and separated from the trachea. The recurrent laryngeal nerve can be identified as it runs medial to the inferior pole of the gland. As the dissection progresses the inferior thyroid artery is identified. *C,* The inferior thyroid artery, which intertwines with the recurrent laryngeal nerve, is ligated as the thyroid gland is dissected superiorly. A nerve is valuable during this portion of the dissection if there is any difficulty locating the recurrent laryngeal nerve.

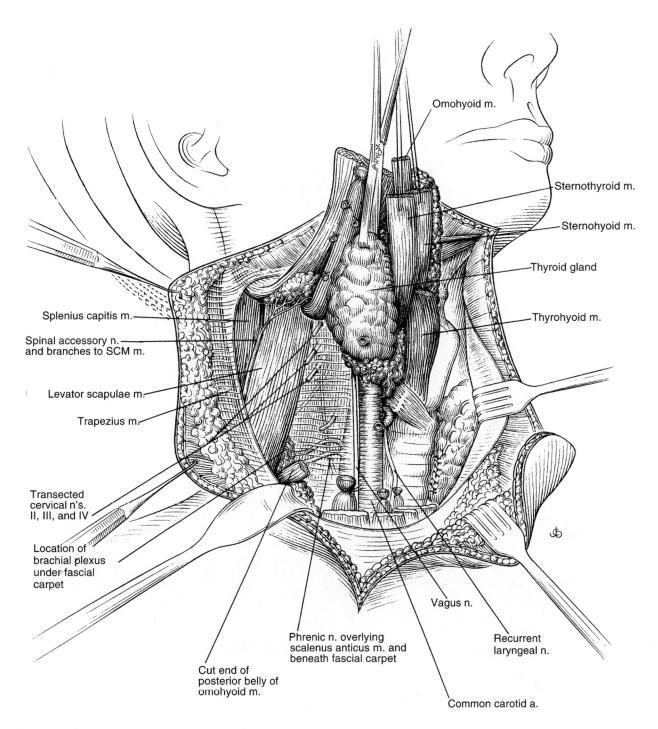

Omohyoid m.

Sternothyroid m.

Sternohyoid m.

Thyroid gland

Thyrohyoid m.

Splenius capitis m.

Spinal accessory n. and branches to SCM m.

Levator scapulae m.

Trapezius m.

Transected cervical n's. II, III, and IV

Location of brachial plexus under fascial carpet

Vagus n.

Phrenic n. overlying scalenus anticus m. and beneath fascial carpet

Recurrent laryngeal n.

Cut end of posterior belly of omohyoid m.

Common carotid a.

FIGURE 2-8. Dissection of the subclavian triangle. The thyroid gland has been dissected superiorly, exposing a good portion of the common carotid artery. The thyroid gland has been dissected superiorly, exposing a good portion of the common carotid artery. The recurrent laryngeal nerve remains intact. The vagus nerve is freed from surrounding structures so that it is not injured. The deep cervical fascia covering the scalenus muscles is identified, establishing the plane of the so-called fascial carpet. This represents the deep, or posterior, extent of the radical neck dissection. The phrenic nerve can be visualized through this fascia and on the surface of the muscle inferiorly, just above the level of the clavicle. All veins and arteries are identified and transected as the dissection progresses. The posterior belly of the omohyoid muscle is transected as far posterosuperiorly as possible. The posterior aspect of the transverse scapular and transverse cervical arteries are encountered in this region.

nocleidomastoid muscle is usually transected. In cases where the sternocleidomastoid muscle is preserved, its motor branch may be preserved as well.

The most common complaint after a block neck dissection is the discomfort of shoulder droop. The pain is often severe and overshadows deglutitory and phonatory disabil-

ities resulting from resection of the primary lesion. If at all possible, the spinal accessory nerve should be grafted when resected during a block neck dissection. Successful results have been reported after the replacement of the resected portion of the nerve with a great auricular nerve graft. To accomplish this, the great auricular nerve, which is closely as-

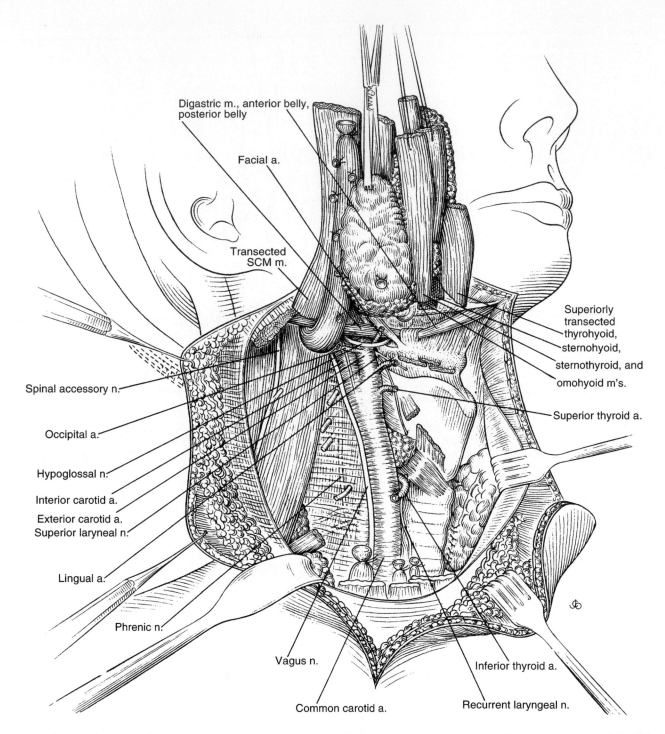

Digastric m., anterior belly, posterior belly

Facial a.

Transected SCM m.

Spinal accessory n.

Occipital a.

Hypoglossal n.

Interior carotid a.

Exterior carotid a.
Superior laryneal n.

Lingual a.

Phrenic n.

Vagus n.

Common carotid a.

Superiorly transected thyrohyoid, sternohyoid, sternothyroid, and omohyoid m's.

Superior thyroid a.

Inferior thyroid a.

Recurrent laryngeal n.

FIGURE 2-9. Anterior border of the trapezius muscle. The dissection is carried up along the anterior border of the trapezius muscle. The spinal accessory nerve has been preserved. The branch to the sternocleidomastoid muscle is to be cut. The spinal accessory nerve is shown descending along the posterior aspect of the levator scapulae muscle. The locations of the recurrent laryngeal, vagus, phrenic, and brachial plexus nerves are shown. Both the phrenic nerve and the brachial plexus nerves are deep through the fascial carpet. Injury to the subclavian vessels and pleura is avoided by remaining above the level of the clavicle.

The sensory cervical nerves are transected as the specimen is elevated superficial to the fascial carpet; this is another area where dissection can become too deep.

The upper end of the sternocleidomastoid muscle is transected, exposing the posterior belly of the digastric muscle, which remains intact until the superior dissection has been completed, thus protecting the upper end of the jugular vein. The block dissection has been further elevated. The insertions of the superior omohyoid, sternothyroid, and sternohyoid muscles are transected. Additional branches of the cervical plexus of nerves are transected as the dissection continues superiorly. The carotid bulb and internal and external carotid arteries are exposed. The hypoglossal nerve can be seen crossing external to both these arteries approximately 2 cm above the carotid bulb. At this same level the superior laryngeal nerve extends behind both carotid vessels. The facial and occipital arteries have been ligated, whereas the lingual artery has been preserved. The anterior and posterior bellies of the digastric muscle are dissected free.

sociated with the external jugular vein on the surface of the sternocleidomastoid muscle, is transected at the superior aspect of the dissection and inferiorly as it stems from the superficial branches of the cervical nerves. It is then placed in saline solution until the block dissection has been completed. It is sutured to the upper and lower transected ends of the spinal accessory nerve after all nerve endings have been freshly cut with a new blade. The use of the surgical microscope and a 9-0 nylon suture facilitates this repair. The repair is performed using an epineurial suture technique.

After dealing with the spinal accessory nerve, the block dissection is carried superiorly along the anterior border of the trapezius muscle to a point where this muscle meets the posterior upper margin of the sternocleidomastoid muscle.

At this point, the upper end (insertion) of the sternocleidomastoid muscle is transected, exposing the posterior belly of the digastric muscle. The posterior belly of the digastric muscle is not transected at this time, for it is a landmark to, and protection for, the upper end of the internal jugular vein.

Anterior of Dissection

Anteriorly, the dissection is carried upward along the lateral margin of the sternohyoid muscle (see Fig. 2–9) if the thyroid gland has not been included in the block dissection. If the thyroid gland has been included, it is best to also include the sternohyoid and sternothyroid muscles. The internal jugular vein is easily dissected from the common carotid artery and vagus nerve. The fascia is carefully dissected from the common carotid artery, taking care not to injure its adventitia. Both the common carotid artery and the vagus nerve are brought into clear view, facilitating the ascending dissection and preventing injury to these structures. The numerous branches of the cervical plexus of nerves are transected. Many of these nerves are quite large, and it is often disturbing to cut them, especially because some of them stem from the same cervical roots as the phrenic nerve. Consequently, this dissection is greatly simplified by identifying the entire length of the phrenic nerve. The various branches of the internal jugular vein are divided and ligated as they are encountered. The insertion of the anterior belly of the omohyoid muscle is transected at the level of the hyoid bone.

The carotid bulb and superior thyroid artery are identified. It is wise to inject the fascia over the carotid bulb with 2% lidocaine without epinephrine to prevent the reflex hypotension that can occur with manipulation of the carotid bulb. Many surgeons do not inject lidocaine unless the anesthesiologist reports a change in the blood pressure or pulse rate.

Next, the hypoglossal nerve is identified as it crosses superficial to both the internal and external carotid arteries, approximately 1.5 cm above the carotid bifurcation. The ranine vein, which descends from the tip of the tongue and empties into the common facial vein, accompanies the hypoglossal nerve. This vein also makes dissection of the nerve quite troublesome.

The superior laryngeal nerve passes deep to internal and external carotid arteries and can be seen as it emerges anteriorly from beneath the external carotid artery. It then divides into the internal branch superiorly, which then penetrates the thyrohyoid membrane for its sensory distribution to the larynx, and into the external branch, which descends to supply (motor) to the cricothyroid muscle. Injury to the superior laryngeal nerve can result in considerable deglutitive dysfunction. This may be avoided by keeping the plane of dissection superficial, not deep or medial, to the carotid artery.

Submandibular and Submental Triangles
(FIGURE 2-10)

The tendon of the digastric muscle is identified just above the insertion of the omohyoid muscle to the hyoid bone. The anterior border of the digastric muscle is followed superiorly to a point just below its insertion to the mandible. Using cautery dissection, the contralateral anterior belly of the digastric muscle is identified. All of the fascia and fat is mobilized from the contralateral anterior digastric belly to the ipsilateral submandibular triangle. The plane of dissection is the fascia of the suprahyoid musculature. The attachment of the deep cervical fascia to the entire lower border of the mandible is detached by sharp dissection. A portion of this fascia may have been detached previously during the maneuver to preserve the marginal mandibular nerve.

The upper end of the external jugular vein is transected before dealing with the parotid gland. After the deep cervical fascia has been detached from the lower pole of the mandible, the dissection is carried posteriorly across the lower pole of the parotid gland, which is removed primarily to facilitate visualization of the upper end of the internal jugular vein as a termination of the procedure. This also eliminates the infraparotid group of lymph nodes, which are occasionally involved with metastatic disease.

The thickened portion of he deep cervical fascia, which is in essence the stylomandibular ligament, is also divided when performing this dissection across the superior aspect of the submandibular triangle and the lower pole of the parotid gland. The mylohyoid muscle is identified beneath the anterior belly of the digastric muscle. Its fibers run at right angles to those of the digastric muscle. Its posterior border is delineated and retracted anteriorly. By simultaneously retracting the submaxillary gland in the posterior inferior direction, the lingual nerve and submaxillary duct are identified. The former is carefully preserved. The latter is transected and ligated. The superior aspect of the submandibular gland is then dissected. If not previously ligated, the fascial artery is transected and ligated just below the mandible. This vessel will be ligated again where it enters the deep and posterior surface of the gland after crossing over the posterior belly of the digastric muscle.

Posterosuperior Dissection

The block dissection specimen is retracted anteriorly (Fig. 2–11). The posterior belly of the digastric muscle and the stylohyoid muscles are identified. In the situation where disease is located very high in the neck along the jugular chain, these muscles may be divided to give extra cephalad exposure of the jugular vein. The facial artery and occipital ar-

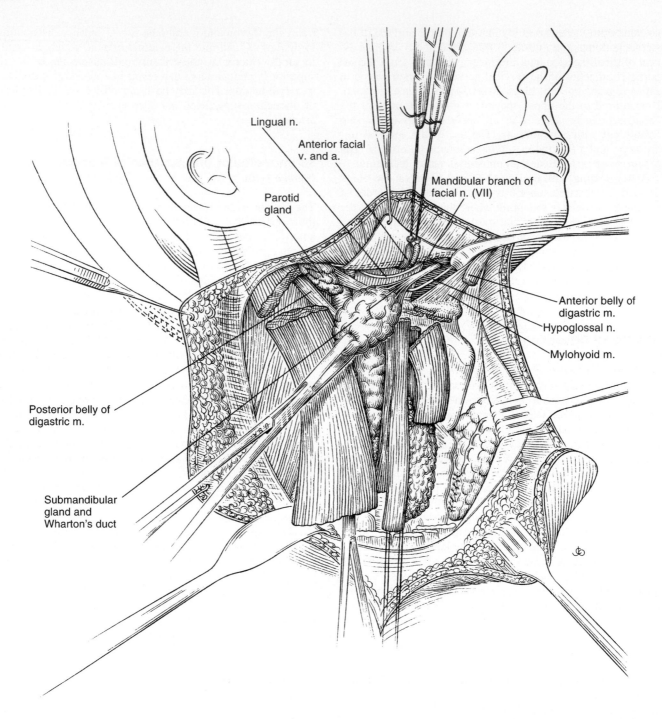

Lingual n.

Anterior facial
v. and a.

Parotid
gland

Mandibular branch of
facial n. (VII)

Anterior belly of
digastric m.

Hypoglossal n.

Mylohyoid m.

Posterior belly of
digastric m.

Submandibular
gland and
Wharton's duct

FIGURE 2–10. Submandibular triangle. The specimen of the radical neck dissection is reflected inferiorly to expose the contents of the submandibular triangle. There are three nerves to be preserved in this area: the mandibular branch of the facial nerve, the lingual nerve, and the hypoglossal nerve. To avoid injury to the lingual nerve during the block neck dissection, the posterior border of the mylohyoid muscle is retracted anteriorly and the submandibular gland is pulled in a posteroinferior direction. This maneuver pulls this lingual nerve inferiorly, where it can be readily identified using hemostat dissection. The submandibular (Wharton's) duct is found near the lingual nerve anteriorly. The anterior belly of the digastric muscle is transected and reflected beneath the specimen in this illustration. Some surgeons prefer to leave this muscle intact. The submandibular duct is transected and reflected inferiorly with the specimen. At this point the hypoglossal nerve can be visualized as shown in the illustration. As the dissection in the submandibular triangle continues posteriorly, the tail of the parotid gland is transected.

teries are identified and ligated. At this point, the block dissection is complete except for the transection of the upper end of the internal jugular vein. In most patients, the vein can be transected in a manner similar to that described for the lower end. However, occasionally, a high metastatic node makes this orderly transection impossible without violating a safe margin around the tumor bearing area. In such instances, moderate inferior tension is placed on the vein. The vein is grasped with a heavy hemostat just below the jugular foramen and transected. It may be impossible to place a satisfactory ligature around the vein at this level in which case the clamp is released and the jugular foramen is packed with surgical gauze. This procedure controls the hemorrhage, eliminates a necessity for a tie, and causes no postoperative complications.

Closure

Careful hemostasis is time-consuming but rewarding. The entire field should be thoroughly irrigated with normal saline and bacitracin solutions. If the patient received a full course of radiation therapy before the radical neck dissection, then the carotid artery is covered with a dermal graft (Fig. 2–12A).

Another option to cover the carotid artery is to use the levator scapulae muscle (Fig. 2–13). The levator scapulae muscle should not be used for carotid coverage in patients who have had cranial nerve XI sacrificed, as this muscle is important for shoulder stabilization after the loss of trapezius muscle innervation.

Dermal and fascia lata grafts have also proved satisfactory for covering the carotid artery. The autogenous dermal graft is preferable because it is readily available, it has great strength and stability, it quickly revascularizes from both sides in 2 to 5 days, and it is relatively resistant to purulent and salivary secretions.

The thigh is the usual donor site for dermal graft. The dermatome is adjusted to the width and thickness (0.012 to 0.014 inches) of the split-thickness graft, which is to be elevated and remain attached at one end. The flap of the split-thickness graft is deflected forward after detaching it from the dermatome. A dermal graft of the same thickness (or thicker) is obtained after slightly reducing the width adjustment of the dermatome. The dermatome is again withdrawn, and the dermal graft is attached. The split-thickness flap is returned to its original position and sutured with 4-0 chromic catgut. The graft is pie-crusted, and a pressure dressing is applied.

Before closing the skin flaps, it is wise to review certain structures to detect any disturbance in their normal continuity. These structures include (1) the lingual nerve, (2) the hypoglossal nerve, (3) the ligatures on the branches of the external carotid artery, (4) the vagus nerve, (5) the superior laryngeal nerve, (6) the phrenic nerve, (7) the brachial plexus, (8) the spinal accessory nerve, and (9) the recurrent laryngeal nerve if a thyroidectomy has been performed. It is important to close the incisions in two layers (Fig. 2–12B). The platysma is sutured with buried catgut sutures, and the skin is sutured with either silk or nylon sutures or skin clips. The use of constant suction, provided by multi-perforated plastic tubing inserted beneath the flaps, seems far superior to the ordinary Penrose drains and a bulky-type dressing. The tubes are inserted and placed anterior and posterior to the carotid artery and secured in place with silk suture before closure of the incisions.

TECHNIQUE OF MODIFICATION OF THE RADICAL NECK DISSECTION

When indicated, a modified radical neck dissection may be performed sparing one or more of the nonlymphatic structures in the neck. These structures include the sternocleidomastoid muscle, spinal accessory nerve, and the jugular vein.

When sparing all three structures, the dissection is also described as a "functional" neck dissection or a modified radical neck dissection with preservation of cranial nerve XI, the sternocleidomastoid muscle, and the jugular vein. The preparation, positioning, and exposure necessary to perform a modified radical neck dissection is no different than the standard radical neck dissection. The flap elevation proceeds in a similar fashion. Once the flaps have been elevated and the borders of the dissection have been delineated, the dissection has begun. There are varying techniques for performing this dissection, and what will be illustrated is the technique used by the authors.

The first step is to incise the fascia overlying the sternocleidomastoid muscle. This is the investing layer of deep cervical fascia that splits to envelop this muscle. The fascia is incised along the anterior border of the sternocleidomastoid muscle where it is thickest. The initial incision parallels the anterior border. Horizontal incisions are made at the superior- and inferior-most areas of muscle exposure. This fascia is sharply dissected off the anterior and lateral aspect of the muscle, and it is pedicled at its posterior border. The dissection proceeds along the medial aspect of the muscle peeling the fascia off the muscle completely. The spinal accessory nerve is identified in the upper most aspect of the dissection as it passes lateral to the jugular vein to enter the superior medial aspect of the sternocleidomastoid muscle. The nerve is found again at the posterior border of the sternocleidomastoid muscle at Erb's point. It is protected there. This allows the muscle to be completely elevated out of the neck dissection specimen but maintain its mastoid and sternoclavicular attachments.

The next step is to follow the eleventh cranial nerve from its point of exit on the posterior aspect of the sternocleidomastoid muscle to the trapezius muscle. The nerve is identified, followed from superior and anterior to posterior and inferior. Once the muscle has been completely uncovered in the posterior triangle soft tissues, it is elevated from the soft tissues by sharp dissection and preserved.

Once the sternocleidomastoid muscle and the eleventh cranial nerve have been identified, freed, and preserved, attention is then turned toward the jugular vein. At its supraclavicular insertion, the sternocleidomastoid muscle is retracted laterally. The omohyoid muscle is identified, divided, and mobilized anteriorly and medially to demarcate the anteromedial limits of the dissection. The jugular vein is identified, and the carotid sheath fascia overlying the vein is divided from inferior to superiorly, exposing the vein. The jugular vein is then carefully dissected out of the fascia of the carotid sheath in a plane of 360 degrees. Once the vein is completely immobilized off the tissues that surrounded it, the neck dissection can be performed as would a standard radical neck dissection, only with preservation of the three structures that have just been identified, mobilized, and preserved. At this point in a modified radical neck dissection, dissection begins posteriorly to the jugular vein with identification of the fascial carpet. The standard dissection is performed from this point lateral to the trapezius and then along the anterior border of the trapezius muscle in the layer of the deep cervical fascia (fascial carpet) to the junction of the sternocleidomastoid muscle and trapezius muscles. The entire dissection is taken from inferior to superior, the entire width of the neck dissection until the carotid bifurcation is

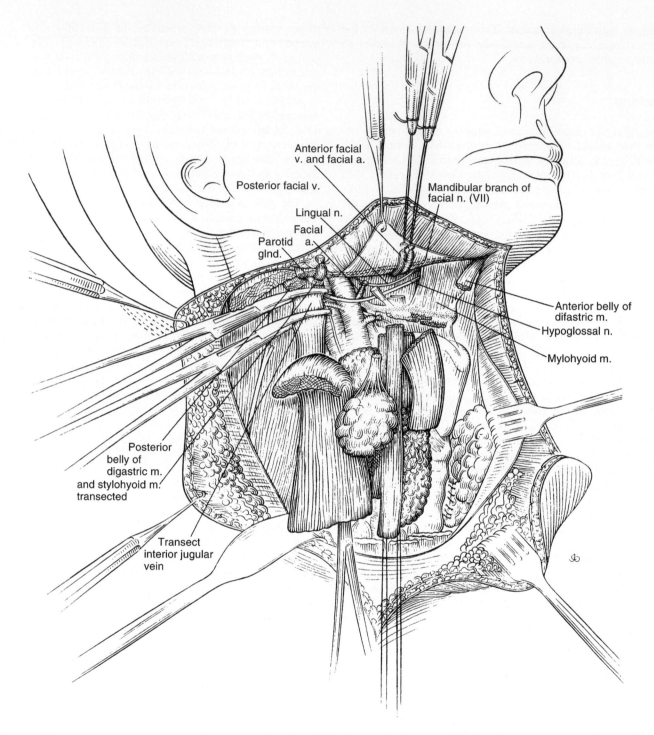

Anterior facial
v. and facial a.

Posterior facial v.

Mandibular branch of
facial n. (VII)

Lingual n.

Facial
a.

Parotid
glnd.

Anterior belly of
difastric m.

Hypoglossal n.

Mylohyoid m.

Posterior
belly of
digastric m.
and stylohyoid m.
transected

Transect
interior jugular
vein

FIGURE 2–11. Superior dissection. The inferior pole of the parotid gland has been transected as well as the posterior bellies of the digastric and sty-lohyoid muscles. This dissection should be completed below the level of the mandibular branch of the facial nerve. The upper end of the internal jugu-lar vein has been clamped in readiness for transection and removal of the block neck dissection. The upper end of the internal jugular vein is ligated with sutures.

encountered. The dissection of the submental and sub-mandibular triangles proceeds as described above in the rad-ical neck dissection technique. The specimen is delivered from the wound.

A somewhat difficult portion of the dissection is the up-per most aspect of the posterior triangle that lies deep to the upper sternocleidomastoid muscle. This portion of the dis-section may be tedious. The fascia on the deep surface of

the sternocleidomastoid muscle must be taken down sharply, and often this can result in troublesome bleeding. Care must be taken to carefully cauterize each individual vessel as it is encountered. The floor of the posterior triangle deep to the sternocleidomastoid muscle may be difficult to dissect, again, because of inferior exposure compared with that of a radical neck dissection. With careful retraction, and as not to stretch the spinal accessory nerve, this dissection can be

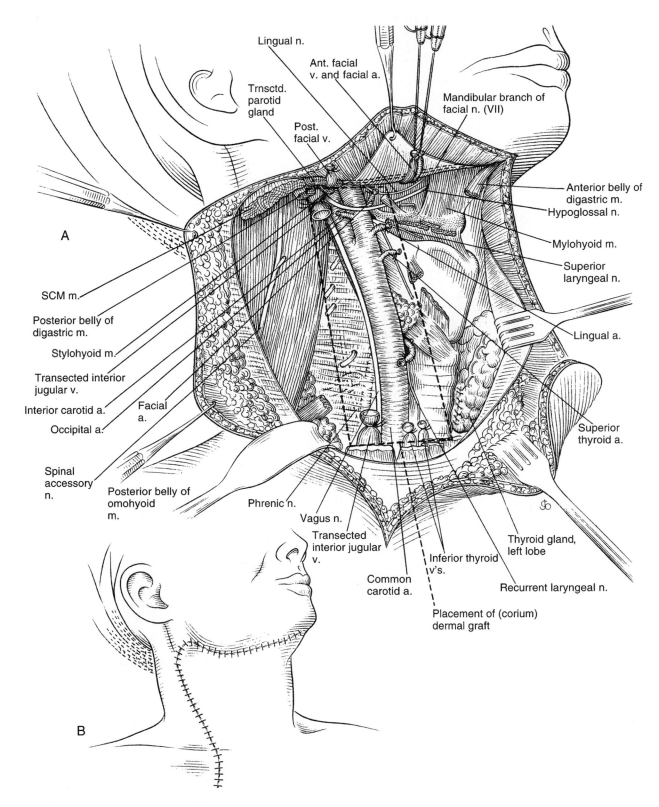

FIGURE 2-12. Completed dissection and closure. The incisions have been closed in two layers. The skin is closed using sutures or skin clips. A multiperforated plastic suction drainage tube is inserted beneath the flaps both anterior and posterior to the common carotid artery. This tubing exits and is secured in place below the clavicle.

A, The radical neck dissection is completed as the upper end of the jugular vein is suture-ligated. The specimen has been removed. It is essential to identify certain structures before closing, including the lingual nerve, the mandibular branch of the facial nerve, the hypoglossal nerve, ligatures of all branches of the external carotid artery, the vagus nerve, the superior laryngeal nerve, the phrenic nerve, the brachial plexus, the spinal accessory nerve, and the recurrent laryngeal nerve. The broken line indicates the size, shape, and placement of the dermal graft that is to cover the entire carotid artery system in the cervical region.

B, A two-layer closure is important. The platysma is sutured with buried catgut sutures and the skin approximated with dermal sutures or clips. Closed suction drainage is an important part of the closure.

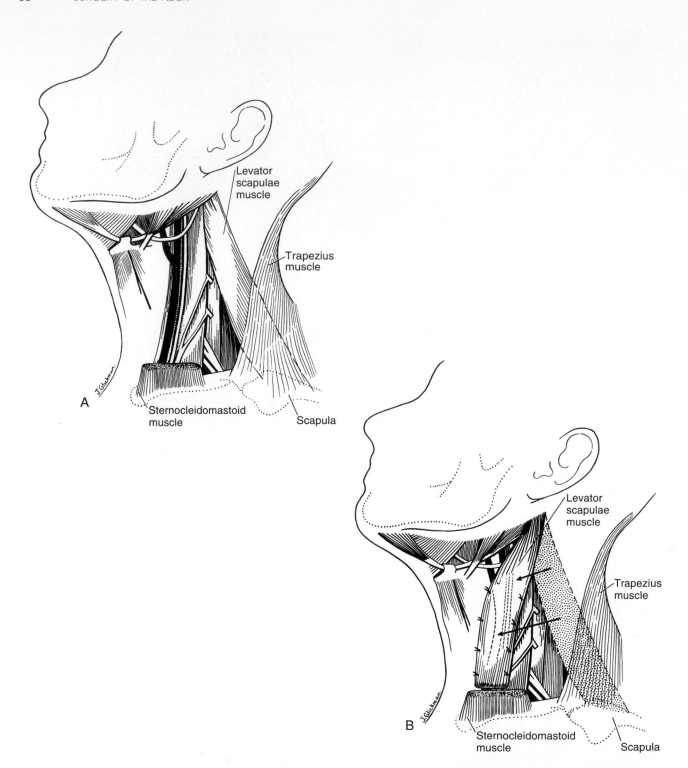

FIGURE 2-13. Carotid artery protection with the levator scapulae muscle. *A,* After completion of the block neck dissection, the levator scapulae muscle is found posterior to the scalenus medius and posterior muscles. The levator scapulae originates from the transverse processes of the first four cervical vertebrae and descends in a posterolateral direction to the vertebrae and descends in a posterolateral direction to the vertebral border of the scapula. To cover the carotid artery sufficiently the levator scapulae muscle should be transected inferiorly and dissected free, with the exception for its superior attachment. Sufficient length of muscle can be obtained to cover the entire carotid artery by dissecting beneath the trapezius and transecting the levator scapulae muscle just above its scapular attachment.

B, The levator scapula has been advanced forward to cover the common carotid artery, carotid bulb, and beginning of the internal and external carotid arteries. The margins of the muscle are anchored and placed anterior and posterior to the carotid artery system with a few interrupted catgut sutures. (*From* Gacek RR, Zonis R: Carotid artery protection with levator scapulae muscle, Arch Otolaryngol 1966; 84(2):198–200; with permission.)

completed with the specimen remaining in continuity with the remaining portion of the functional neck dissection.

SELECTIVE NECK DISSECTIONS

The Supraomohyoid Neck Dissection

The supraomohyoid neck dissection is a more limited version of the functional neck dissection. The confines of the dissection include posteriorly the rootlets to the cervical plexus, inferiorly the upper border of the omohyoid muscle, and superiorly the lower border of the mandible.

The preparation and exposure for the supraomohyoid neck dissection should be no different than that afforded a standard radical neck dissection. However, the incision may be more limited and can often be accomplished with an apron flap incision that does not pass inferior to the mid-horizontal plane of the neck. The flaps are elevated in a subplatysmal plane, and the marginal mandibular nerve is preserved as outlined in the section on radical neck dissection.

The authors' usual technique is to begin this dissection anteriorly and pass posteriorly. Dissection is begun in the submental and submandibular triangles, which proceeds as described in the radical neck dissection. Once reaching the posterior aspect of the submandibular triangle, regions II and III are encountered. The dissection passes posteriorly first overlying the carotid artery and vagus nerve. Once the vagus nerve has been identified along the entire length of the exposure of the neck dissection and freed, the jugular vein is encountered. The anterior aspect of the jugular vein is exposed by incising the fascia overlying it. The vein is circumferentially freed from the specimen, and the specimen is further mobilized posteriorly. Posterior to the vessels, then the plane of the fascial carpet is identified, and dissection proceeds posteriorly until the rootlets of the cervical plexus are encountered. Once the cervical plexus rootlets are encountered, the specimen may be transected starting posteriorly and inferiorly and working superiorly until the specimen is pedicled up in the area of the superior aspect of the posterior triangle. This represents the soft tissues of the posterior triangle superior and posterior to the spinal accessory nerve. The specimen can then be sharply dissected as was discussed for a functional neck dissection, and the specimen may then be delivered from the wound.

Lateral Neck Dissection

The preparation and draping for a lateral neck dissection is usually encompassed in the standard draping for a laryngectomy. The most common scenario in which a lateral neck dissection is performed is during laryngectomy and laryngopharyngectomy.

The confines of the dissection are the clavicle inferiorly, the transverse process of C1 superiorly, the posterior border of the sternocleidomastoid posteriorly, and the larynx medially.

The anterior aspect of the sternocleidomastoid muscle is mobilized away from its investing fascia, exposing the carotid sheath and its contents. The authors' technique is to usually begin this dissection inferiorly where the jugular vein is identified just above the clavicle. The fascia overlying the jugular vein is incised vertically as is the omohyoid muscle. The vein is circumferentially mobilized out of the fascia that surrounds it. The plane of the posterior triangle fascia is identified just posterior and lateral to the inferior aspect of the jugular vein, and this plane of dissection is followed from inferior to superior. The specimen is mobilized from posterior to anterior, encountering next the vagus nerve and the carotid artery. It may be further mobilized with sharp dissection and left pedicled medially onto the larynx or the laryngopharyngectomy specimen, or it may be transected as a separate specimen.

Postoperative Care

When a block neck dissection is combined with a tracheotomy or tracheostomy, special nursing care is necessary for at least 3 days postoperatively. This care ensures continuous high humidity, adequate airway, early ambulation, and adequate attention to the closed suction drainage. Deep breathing exercises or positive pressure breathing ensures against alveolar collapse and pneumonitis. Intravenous antibiotic therapy is begun before surgery and is continued 2 days postoperatively. This is essential in all patients in whom the block neck dissection has been combined with an opening in the upper respiratory system and regardless of whether the patients have received radiation therapy. In patients in whom the upper respiratory system has not been violated, 24 hours of antibiotic therapy is adequate.

Nausea is controlled by such medications as Zofran, administered orally or intravenously, and prochlorperazine (Compazine), administered intramuscularly. A nasogastric tube, inserted when the block neck dissection has been combined with a laryngectomy, should remain open while nausea is present. Water and dilute feedings are given in small amounts on the first day. As soon as the patient's intake is adequate, either orally or by nasogastric feeding tube, the use of intravenous fluids is discontinued. Closed suction drainage is discontinued 48 hours after surgery unless there is an unusually large amount of serous or bloody drainage.

The skin sutures or clips can be removed in the sixth or seventh postoperative day, unless the patient has received radiation therapy. When radiation therapy has been given, the skin sutures should remain in place for at least 10 days after surgery.

COMPLICATIONS OF UNILATERAL OR BILATERAL NECK DISSECTION

Hemorrhage at the Time of Operation

Excessive blood loss can be prevented by meticulous hemostasis during surgery. Too many hemostats left in place are probably the most common cause of unnecessary blood loss. A hemostat can be pulled away from a blood vessel inadvertently, and considerable loss of blood can remain undetected until the situation is serious. Tie as you go.

It is unusual for a patient who had a normal hematocrit preoperatively to require a blood transfusion postoperatively. Patients who are having a concomitant primary tumor ablation or a bilateral neck dissection should be typed and crossed for two units of packed red blood cells preoperatively.

Hemorrhage from either the upper or lower end of the jugular vein, from the subclavian vein, or from the carotid artery can be a serious problem. Occasionally the subclavian vein may be incised or a large vessel may be retracted beneath the clavicle. The surgeon should not hesitate to transect the clavicle so that proper exposure may be obtained. When the tumor involves the carotid artery and it is necessary to ligate and remove this vessel, there is approximately a 40% chance of hemiparesis and the patient may die. It is crucial at this time to have the patient's pulse and blood pressure at normal levels when the carotid artery is ligated. The anesthesiologist should be alerted as soon as the decision to ligate the carotid artery has been made. When the carotid is ligated, a bolus of heparin should be administered. The anesthesiologist may wish to lighten the anesthesia and to increase the rate of flow of intravenous fluids or to administer an artificial stimulus to raise the blood pressure. In most cases, the need to resect the carotid artery is predictable and may be managed safely. Further discussion appears later in this chapter.

Delayed Bleeding

Hematoma can be a serious postoperative complication. It is prevented by careful ligation of all vessels and the placement of suction-type drainage systems. Suction drainage seems to be superior to all other drainage methods. If a hematoma forms, it should be evacuated. Pressure is then applied so that it does not reform. If active bleeding occurs in the postoperative period, the patient should be returned to the operating room, and under sterile technique, the flaps opened, the clots expressed, and the vessels ligated.

Often, no serious bleeding point can be identified after a large hematoma has been evacuated, and hemorrhage continues from multiple small areas. When this occurs, the authors routinely administer high doses of steroids intravenously. This therapy is continued for at least 48 hours.

Shock

Shock can be a complication during or after a unilateral or bilateral neck dissection. However, with modern anesthesia and proper replacement therapy, shock can usually be avoided.

Airway Obstruction

During the operation, an obstruction is usually caused by a kink in the endotracheal tube or a blood clot in the tracheobronchial tree. Pneumothorax may be a cause of respiratory embarrassment.

Postoperative laryngeal edema may develop, especially after a bilateral neck dissection. It can be of rapid onset and produce asphyxia during the postoperative period. A tracheotomy should be performed immediately after the appearance of laryngeal edema. When performing bilateral radical neck dissection, a prophylactic tracheotomy is advised, particularly in the patient who has undergone irradiation. The airway obstruction may be caused by extrinsic pressures such as hemorrhage or a dressing that is too tight. Other causes of destruction in the postoperative period are aspiration of blood clots, vomitus, mucus, or occlusion of the upper respiratory tract.

Carotid Sinus Reflux

The incidence of a decrease in blood pressure when an operation is being performed in the region of the carotid bulb is high. This decrease in blood pressure can be avoided by injecting about 1 mL of 1% or 2% lidocaine (Xylocaine) without epinephrine into the adventitial layer of the carotid bulb, making certain that some of the anesthetic agent diffuses to the region between the bifurcation of the carotid artery. Many surgeons carry out this injection routinely as soon as the carotid bulb is exposed. The signs of carotid sinus reflux are hypotension, bradycardia, and cardiac irregularities.

Pneumothorax

Pneumothorax is a rare complication of neck surgery. It is usually caused by air entering the mediastinum and rupturing through the thin mediastinal pleura rather than direct injury to the pleura. The treatment consists of immediate tube thoracostomy, a suction, and water seal system. If the leak is detected in the subclavian triangle at the time of the operation, the area is temporarily packed. The anesthesiologist inflates the lungs to obliterate the trapped air, after which the area of leakage is suture ligated. The anesthesiologist may notice a pneumothorax developing by change in the respiratory pattern or signs of circulatory failure. An air-sucking wound may be a tip off. Postoperative chest radiographs are, of course, indicated.

Air Embolism

Air embolism occurs rarely. When it does, the leak should be located immediately and ligated. The head of the operating room table is immediately lowered and the patient is turned on his left side to allow air to arise and settle in the apex of the right ventricle. An air embolism is serious; advanced cardiac life-support may be necessary to resuscitate the patient.

Nerve Damage

The section of one superior laryngeal nerve produces some interference with normal swallowing. The patient usually adjusts to the situation within 1 month. Section of both nerves can leave the patient with a functionless larynx; a laryngectomy may be necessary.

Paralysis of the facial nerve is not common and is usually temporary and caused by stretching, blunt trauma, or hematoma rather than to transsection. Although this is a temporary problem, it is disturbing because recovery may take several months. The marginal mandibular branch of the facial nerve is often sectioned during a blocked neck dissection when there is metastatic disease in the submandibular triangle. The resulting paralysis is troublesome to the patient, resulting in drooling, especially if combined with an inferior alveolar nerve deficit. This paralysis is difficult to correct.

Unilateral sacrifice of the vagus nerve results in ipsilateral laryngeal paralysis, which is of no serious consequence unless the paralyzed side of the larynx remains in the position of abduction. The manifestation of abduction is poor voice, frequent aspirations, and the inability to produce an effective cough. This may be corrected by medialization thyroplasty (see Chapter 13). Gastrointestinal and cardiac manifestations are not severe unless both vagus nerves are sectioned. Bilateral paralysis usually requires an immediate tracheotomy.

If only one phrenic nerve is sectioned, the respiratory embarrassment is mild. If both are sectioned, there can be severe respiratory difficulty requiring use of a respirator.

Unilateral sectioning of the hypoglossal nerve will cause only moderate speech and masticatory difficulties. If the hypoglossal nerve is near a metastatic lesion, it should be sacrificed. Bilateral section results in complete immobilization of the tongue, severely interfering with both speech and deglutition.

Section of the cervical sympathetics or injury thereof results in only minor symptoms, most notably, upper lid ptosis. Horner's syndrome can sometimes be detected after a radical neck dissection.

Probably the most troublesome complication of radical neck dissection is the shoulder syndrome, resulting from denervation of the trapezius muscle after resection of the spinal accessory nerve in the posterior triangle of the neck. This is especially true for patients who earn their livelihood by manual labor. The shoulder syndrome is characterized by weakened, deformed, and painful shoulder.

The shoulder syndrome can be prevented by preserving the spinal accessory nerve. The ability to preserve the spinal accessory nerve in therapeutic neck dissection has been controversial. Researchers have presented evidence that the spinal accessory nerve should not be preserved during either therapeutic or an elective radical neck dissection. They found that cancerous lymph node metastasis from head and neck primary cancers occurs almost as frequently among the spinal accessory nerve as in any other area of the radical neck dissection. They analyzed 50 radical neck dissections. All of the specimens contained spinal accessory lymph nodes; the average number was 11 for each neck. Twenty-eight of the 50 radical neck dissection specimens (elective, 5; therapeutic, 23) contained cancerous lymph nodes. Seven of the 28 contained positive jugular lymph nodes and negative spinal accessory lymph nodes. Twenty-one contained a positive spinal accessory lymph node and a negative internal jugular lymph node. Fourteen specimens contained positive lymph nodes in the both the spinal accessory and internal jugular areas.

Brandenburg evaluated a total of 370 cases of neck dissection comparing both classic radical neck dissection and radical dissection with preservation of cranial nerve XI. The overall rate of recurrent tumor in the neck with the classic neck dissection was 12%, whereas the rate of recurrence when the spinal accessory nerve was spared was 6%. Based on his observations, it was felt that the classical radical neck dissection could be modified to preserve the spinal accessory nerve without jeopardizing the chances for cure in elective neck dissection and some selected therapeutic neck dissections.

The authors prefer to preserve cranial nerve XI in all cases where it is believed to be possible. Contraindication to preserving cranial nerve XI is significant lymphadenopathy along the route of cranial nerve XI that shows any degree of adherence of the nerve to the lymphadenopathy. This is particularly true in patients who have had previous radiation therapy. If the nerve is near an involved lymph node, but easily freed from the surrounding areolar tissue and not adherent, the nerve is preserved.

Grafting a segment of the great auricular nerve between the proximal and distal ends of the spinal accessory nerve that is transected during radical neck dissection is too infrequently performed by head and neck surgeons. At least 75% of such grafts have been reported to be successful in preventing the painful shoulder syndrome.

Exercise has a definite roll in the management of the shoulder syndrome. A series of exercises can be used as physiotherapy rehabilitation in patients with disabled and deformed shoulders. These exercises should be offered to every patient with a post-radical neck dissection shoulder syndrome. The exercises include (1) strengthening the scapular retractors and elevators using regressive resistance technique, (2) range of motion exercises to increase scapular-humeral joint motion, and (3) active stretch of the shortened scapular protractor (serratus anterior).

It is usually not necessary to sacrifice the lingual nerve. When it is necessary, however, the resulting anesthesia of the tongue is not of serious consequence. Because there are fairly consistent landmarks in the vicinity of this nerve to facilitate its identification, there is no need for its inadvertent sacrifice.

Injury to the brachial plexus is a disastrous and unnecessary complication of a block neck dissection. The sectioned nerve should be carefully approximated with 8-0 nylon sutures.

Chylous Fistula

If the thoracic duct is inadvertently transected during the procedure, it should be ligated immediately. After ligation, the anesthesiologist should administer a positive breath and hold it for several seconds. This will test the repair and look for a residual fistula. If a chylous fistula is noted postoperatively, the drain should continue on closed suction, a pressure dressing should be applied, and the patient should be placed on a medium triglyceride diet. The leakage of lymph usually stops after 7 to 10 days. If the leakage of lymph is profuse and prolonged, the electrolyte balance may be disturbed and the patient may become malnourished. Patients in whom the leak is profuse should either be explored and the duct ligated, or the neck sclerosed using a doxycycline solution on a Gelfoam sponge. When these techniques are not successful, a transthoracic ligation may be performed.

Subcutaneous Emphysema

Subcutaneous emphysema can occur even with a small perforation of the upper respiratory tract. It may follow a tracheotomy. Medication is administered to suppress the cough reflex. It may be necessary to locate and eliminate the point of air leakage. If a cuffed tracheotomy tube is in place, the cuff should remain inflated until the condition improves.

Wound Infection

Meticulous aseptic techniques should be adhered to preoperatively, intraoperatively, and postoperatively. Tissue is handled with care because necrosis breeds infection. Tissues should not be allowed to become dry during the procedure. Antibiotics are used routinely, especially when the block neck dissection is combined with total or partial laryngectomy. Preoperative evaluation of oral hygiene as well as postoperative mouth care is very important. There has been a marked decrease in the occurrence of postoperative wound infection since beginning the practice of irrigating the operative field with bacitracin solution several times during the operation.

If a wound infection does occur, materials are taken for culture, sensitivity tests are performed, and the proper antibiotics are administered. Adequate drainage and obliteration of dead space are still necessary and very important in treating patients with a postoperative wound infection. If the area of wound infection is large, the wound should be packed with antibiotic impregnated iodoform gauze. The surgeon must be alert for diabetes or poor liver function when faced with postoperative infection because they may lead to delayed wound healing.

Gangrene of Flap Tissue

Gangrene of flap tissue occurs more commonly when surgery follows radiation therapy. The tissue necrosis may be apparent during the immediate postoperative period or may not develop until the 10th postoperative day. At times, the gangrenous process is progressive and disastrous, especially when the result is an exposed carotid artery. Thus, when operating on a patient who has had radiation therapy, prophylactic coverage of the carotid artery with adjacent muscle tissue or dermal graft is excellent insurance. There are a number of intraoperative ways to reduce the incidence of this disheartening complication, including (1) judicious atraumatic handling of tissues, (2) the prevention of tissue drying, (3) periodic irrigation of the operative field with bacitracin solution, and (4) the use of closed suction drainage.

Fluid and Electrolarynx Imbalance

Careful postoperative management and nursing care will avoid fluid and electrolarynx imbalance.

Increased Intracranial Pressure After Removal of Both Internal Jugular Veins in a Bilateral Neck Dissection

Some surgeons who perform simultaneous bilateral neck dissections leave one internal jugular vein intact. Most surgeons stage the procedures, performing the second operation 4 to 6 weeks after the first. This gives time for collateral venous outflow to develop. In a situation where bilateral simultaneous jugular sacrifice must be done, preservation of the external jugular veins may decrease cerebral venous engorgement.

If edema of the head develops during the operation, the head should be elevated. The patient should remain in a semi-sitting position at all times postoperatively. No tight ties should be placed around the neck, and no pressure should be placed against the back of the neck, as both will decrease venous flow in the vertebral venous plexus. Some physicians advocate the use of diuretics and a low-salt diet for the reduction of lymph edema. It is known that patients develop a syndrome of inappropriate antidiuretic hormone secretion when they undergo bilateral simultaneous jugular vein sacrifice. Perioperative steroids may help with the situation of cerebral edema and facial edema following bilateral simultaneous jugular vein sacrifice.

Complications Involving the Parotid Gland

Two complications involving the parotid gland may result from block neck surgery. The first is a persistent swelling of the inferior aspect of the gland, probably due to the trauma of surgery. The second is a persistent salivary leak from the gland. These complications are not common, and the manifestations subside spontaneously.

Injury to the Cervical Vertebrae

Extremes in positioning of the head during the operation may produce varying degrees of injury to the cervical vertebrae. A dislocation requires reduction by traction.

Salivary Fistula

Salivary fistula is a complication that occurs when the radical neck dissection is combined with total laryngectomy or laryngopharyngectomy. Aseptic technique, careful suturing of the gullet, and proper handling of tissues will markedly reduce this incidence. Treatment consists of the reinsertion of the nasogastric feeding tube, packing of the fistulous tract with iodoform gauze, use of a salivary bypass tube, and application of a pressure dressing. A large fistula may require secondary surgical repair.

Pulmonary Complications

Possible pulmonary complications are bronchopneumonia, atelectasis, and lung abscess. Early ambulation, adequate bronchopulmonary toilet, and the use of antibiotics can usually prevent these complications. Respiratory obstructions have been discussed.

Feeding Tube Syndrome

Dehydration, hypernatremia, hyperchloremia, and azotemia may result as complications of nasogastric tube feedings. Early clinical signs are lacking because the dehydration is initially intracellular. There may be weight loss, increased hematocrit values, and serum osmolarity. Mental confusion and disorientation, fever, increased urinary output, and tachycardia are signs of disease progression.

This syndrome is caused by high protein content in the feedings to elderly patients with cerebral-centered dysfunction with respect to sodium metabolism, renal tubule function, and primary deficit in body water.

Regarding treatment, early recognition is imperative because 150 mEq/L can be fatal within a few days.

Withdrawal or reduction of the feeding tube diet and administration of 3 to 4 L of 5% dextrose and water per day are necessary. Sodium or potassium depletion should be avoided during this treatment.

This syndrome can be prevented by a diet consisting of less than 70 g/L of protein. Milk contains 35 g/L of protein. In addition, a concentrated diet can easily exceed 70 g/L and thus provide an excessively solute load to elderly patients.

Hyponatremia from excessive free water administration is another common complication of tube feedings. Patients on tube feedings should have regular evaluation of their serum electrolytes.

Carotid Artery Replacement and Ligation

The word "carotid" is derived from the Greek word *karos*, which means to sleep. The carotid artery was initially described by Aristotle, who wrote of people lapsing into sleep when their carotid artery was incised. We now call this phenomenon carotid artery reflex. Carotid artery ligation was performed as early as 1652, when Ambroise Paré ligated this vessel while repairing an extensive sword wound in the neck. The patient developed aphasia and hemiplegia. In 1803, Flemming ligated both common carotid arteries without sequela in a patient who had attempted suicide. The first emergency ligation to be reported in this country was performed in 1807 in Keene, New Hampshire, also without sequela. Mott, in 1857, described bilateral carotid ligations for the treatment of head tumors and reported that the tumors "melted away" after this therapy.

In 1863, during the Civil War, bilateral carotid ligation was performed on a man who had received gunshot wounds; the patient did not survive. A century later, Catlin described bilateral staged carotid ligations in treatment of a patient with large supraglottic lesions with metastasis. The carotids were ligated because of imminent rupture. After the procedure, subclavian arteriograms were obtained that showed well-functioning vertebral vasculature providing adequate cerebral flow. The patient was asymptomatic.

Watson and Silverstone reported a series of 20 consecutive carotid artery ligations performed because of tumor; the mortality rate in this group of patients was 55%. In a series of carotid artery ligations for vascular lesions, atrioventricular malformations, and intracranial aneurysms, Dandy reported a mortality rate of 10% and Matas only 5%.

De'Fourmestraux reported the following mortality figures: ligation for hemorrhage (blow-out), 54%; ligation for tumors, 46%; ligation for aneurysms, 13.5%; and ligation for aneurysms with pulsing exophthalmos, 7%.

More and Baker contributed a classic article on carotid artery ligation and outlined the necessary criteria for optimum results from the procedure. In a series of 88 patients (78 with cancer), 40 developed cerebral complications following ligation and 30% of these patients died. Of the 40 with cerebral complications, the onset immediately followed ligation in only 21. The period of delayed onset ranged from 8 hours to 5 days in the remaining 19 patients. Only 4 of the 28 who survived had complete regression of symptoms. The most noteworthy fact in this study was that among the last 35 consecutive patients the mortality rate was 11.5%, and in the last 15 it was 0, with none of the latter group having complications. These increasingly favorable results were obviously owing to improved preoperative management, emphasis on the maintenance of adequate blood volume, and prevention of hypotension at the time of ligation.

The early literature on carotid artery ligation is limited to reports and discussions of ligation without anastomosis of the external or internal arteries. Subsequent literature on the subject embraces vessel anastomosis, transpositions, and autogenous or synthetic grafts. Connolly and Pack advocated anastomosing the external carotid to the internal carotid; they believed that the retrograde flow from the external carotid system would contribute to the intracranial flow by way of this anastomosis. Sweet, Sarnoff, and Bakay had already contradicted this theory, demonstrating by main of metrics that there was equally as great a chance for retrograde flow from the internal to the external carotid systems. Hardesty and associates found that, after occlusion of the common carotid artery in 15 patients, the flow of the internal carotid continued forward in 8, and the other 7 this direction became retrograde. They also showed that occlusion of one carotid vessel increased the flow in the opposite vessel.

Conley reported the use of autogenous vein grafts that was successful in the transport of blood in an otherwise unresectable lesion. Attention was directed to the need for a receptive field (free from infection and tumor) if success was to be expected. Rella, Rongetti, and Bisi reported a successful prosthetic grafting procedure with normal function at the end of 3 months. Lore contributed much to the current concept of carotid artery replacement using both autogenous vein grafts and woven Dacron as prosthetic replacement material.

McCoy and Barsocchini presented a comprehensive article concerning carotid artery ligation at which they pointed out that the prognosis for success with carotid artery ligation can be predicted fairly accurately. They discuss several evaluation measures to be used preoperatively, provided that no emergency situation exists. The Matas test, consisting of digital compression of the carotid artery, when combined with simultaneous electroencephalography indicates the response to ischemia. Angiograms are exceedingly important and should include both carotid and vertebral systems as well as intracranial vasculature. An assessment of the collateral flow can be made.

The management of metastatic squamous cell carcinoma to the neck with potential carotid involvement remains controversial. Many surgeons believe that carotid involvement defines an unresectable tumor. Brennan and coworkers found that patients who underwent carotid resection and who were proven histologically to have invasion of the carotid fascia had no improvement in long-term survival and that the potential morbidity and mortality do not justify carotid sacrifice.

Snyderman and colleagues performed a meta-analysis of all published cases of carotid resection that involved squamous cell carcinoma of the neck. They found that 2-year disease-free survival was 22% and that survival rate compared favorably with a similarly staged control group. They concluded that carotid involvement is not a poor prognostic factor when compared with patients with matched tumor stage without carotid involvement.

The determination of carotid involvement ultimately is made intraoperatively. A good sense, however, can be achieved preoperatively. A large mass that directly overlies the carotid artery and that is fixed will most likely have carotid sheath, fascia, or vessel wall involvement. An associated vocal cord paralysis or Horner syndrome is also indicative of carotid involvement.

Ultrasound and magnetic resonance imaging (MRI) may be the most sensitive studies to determine carotid wall involvement. Ultrasound evaluation will show a step-off in the echo dense signal in any plane and discontinuity of the signal in transverse and longitudinal planes. Vessel lumen invasion may also be seen. Ultrasound has 100% sensitivity and 75% specificity in predicting carotid involvement. Magnetic resonance imaging scan will demonstrate a loss of fascial plane around the carotid when it is involved. The sensitivity and specificity of MRI in predicting carotid involvement is 100% and 87%, respectively.

The computed tomography (CT) criterion for carotid artery invasion is greater than 25% effacement of the circumference of the artery. A CT will accurately exclude patients without carotid involvement but has a false-positive rate of 94%.

Multiple preoperative studies have been advocated to predict the patient's ability to tolerate carotid resection with or without reconstruction. These include the Matas test, oculoplethysmography, arterial stump pressures, progressive vascular clamps, and temporary balloon occlusion (TBO) of the carotid artery with or without xenon-enhanced CT scan.

At the authors' institution, TBO of the carotid artery with electroencephalogram (EEG) monitoring and induced hypotension is an excellent predictor of the ability of patients to tolerate carotid sacrifice. In patients with a high likelihood of carotid involvement who pass TBO and in whom a carotid reconstruction is not planned, at angiography permanent balloons will be placed in the proximal common artery and distal internal carotid artery just proximal to the ophthalmic artery. This has the advantage of eliminating the distal carotid stump that is present after ligation alone and that may be a source of platelet emboli.

At this institution, carotid sacrifice and reconstruction are performed in conjunction with a vascular surgeon. These are usually reserved as the last portion of the neck dissection and are performed when the specimen is pedicled at the carotid involvement. Early on in the neck dissection if extensive soft tissue disease is found involving the paraspinous musculature, the patient is deemed unresectable and the procedure is terminated. Once the carotid is clamped and resected, the segment is reconstructed either with direct end-to-end anastomosis, saphenous vein graft, or synthetic vascular prosthesis. When a segment needs to be replaced, the saphenous vein is the graft of choice. After resection and reconstruction of the artery, it is imperative that vascularized tissue covers the reconstructed segment. If there is no communication with mouth or pharynx and no potential for salivary contamination and if the skin flaps appear healthy, no tissue transfer may be needed. In such a case, planning a neck incision so that there is no trifurcation overlying the vessel is critical. If there is a connection with the upper aerodigestive tract and a potential for salivary contamination, a myocutaneous flap must be mobilized to cover the reconstructive segment of the carotid. In such a case, it may be advisable to create a controlled pharyngostome.

Carotid sacrifice with or without reconstruction is a high-risk procedure. The perioperative mortality ranges from 0 to 31%. The neurologic morbidity ranges from 0 to 45%, with most series reporting a rate of less than 25%.

CONGENITAL CYSTS AND SINUSES

Thyroglossal Duct Cyst and Lingual Thyroid

The thyroid gland originates in the tuberculum impar, which is the point of the foramen cecum at the medial aspect of the sulcus terminalis. In the 3-mm embryo, it appears as an outpocketing in the floor of the foregut between the first and second pharyngeal pouches. Normally, it descends anteriorly and inferiorly in the neck through the area that is to become the hyoid bone. From there, it descends anteriorly to the laryngeal structures and divides into two pouches that form its lateral lobes. These lobes are connected, anterior to the trachea and below the cricoid cartilage, by the thyroid isthmus. A third lobe, the pyramidal lobe, arises from the superior aspect of the isthmus or from an adjacent portion of a lateral lobe. A pyramidal lobe may ascend as far as the hyoid bone.

Congenital abnormalities concerned with the formation and descent of the thyroid gland can occur anywhere from the foreman cecum to the pyramidal lobe of the gland. These may be present in the form of (1) solid thyroid tissue, (2) cyst, or (3) sinus tracts (Fig. 2–14A). Occasionally, the thyroglossal duct (from the foramen cecum to the pyramidal lobe of the thyroid gland) fails to become obliterated and persists to the sinus tract lined by columnar epithelium. As a rule, it descends behind the hyoid bone; however, it may pass through or anterior to this structure.

The thyroglossal duct cyst occurs as a dilated portion of the thyroglossal duct. In 90% of patients, it is present in the midline. It is most frequently found below the level of the hyoid bone (85%). It may occur above the hyoid (8%), at the base of the tongue (1.2%), or low in the neck (5%) (Fig. 2–14B). A thyroglossal fistula is a sinus tract or cyst that has been involved with secondary infection and ruptured through the skin or is a result of incomplete surgical removal of a sinus tract or cyst.

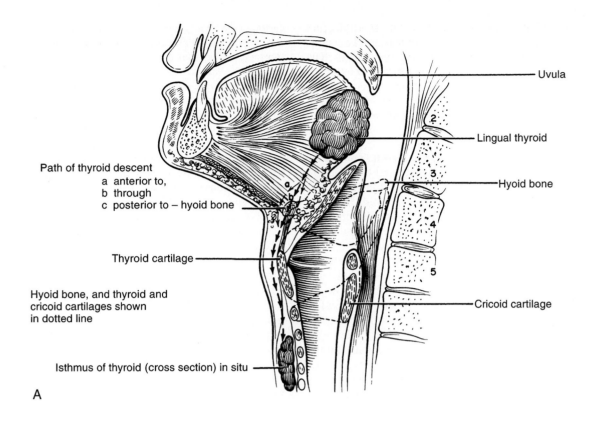

Uvula

Lingual thyroid

Path of thyroid descent
  a anterior to,
  b through
  c posterior to – hyoid bone

Hyoid bone

Thyroid cartilage

Hyoid bone, and thyroid and
cricoid cartilages shown
in dotted line

Cricoid cartilage

Isthmus of thyroid (cross section) in situ

A

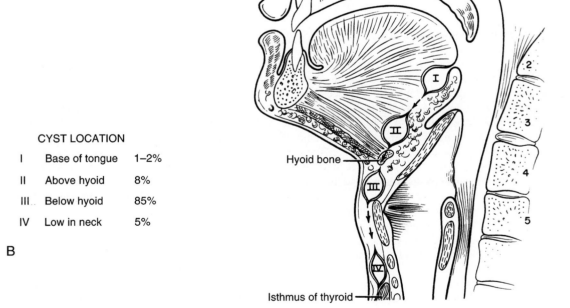

CYST LOCATION

I	Base of tongue	1–2%
II	Above hyoid	8%
III	Below hyoid	85%
IV	Low in neck	5%

Hyoid bone

Isthmus of thyroid

B

FIGURE 2–14. *A,* A midsagittal sketch showing the position of the lingual thyroid and partway for descent of the thyroid gland and position of the thyroglossal duct. Theoretically, the duct passes either anterior to or through the hyoid bone and not behind it. Clinical reports, however, indicate that the duct is often found passing posterior to the hyoid body.

B, The various locations of the thyroglossal cyst, which most commonly occurs in the infrahyoid region over the thyrohyoid membrane. These positions can be classified as intralingual, suprahyoid, infrahyoid (thyrohyoid), and suprasternal.

On occasion, either a portion or the entire thyroid gland will fail to descend and persist as thyroid tissue, known as a lingual thyroid, in the region of the foramen cecum. The lingual thyroid is usually not symptomatic until puberty, when it increases in size. It may also enlarge during pregnancy or in association with infection. In 70% of cases having lingual thyroid, there is no thyroid tissue in the neck.

Diagnosis

A thyroglossal duct cyst at the foreman cecum is easily diagnosed as a soft cystic midline mass covered by stratified squamous epithelium. Its surface is pink or bluish in contrast to the dark red and vascular lingual thyroid. It is usually found in the midline below the level of the hyoid bone, over the thyrohyoid membrane. A thyroglossal duct cyst may also appear above the hyoid bone or low in the neck. Occasionally, the thyroglossal cyst may deviate sufficiently from the midline to be confused with lateral neck cysts such as those of branchial origin. There may be a history of the cyst varying in size. The patient may mention a peculiar taste associated with a decrease in the size of the cyst. The cyst may be tender to palpation even without evidence of infection. In fact, secondary infection in, or trauma to, the cyst can cause enlargement and symptoms. A few patients have a history of repeated infection. The presence of a sinocutaneous fistula represents either rupture of an infected thyroglossal duct cyst or incomplete resection of the sinus tract. Instances of thyroglossal sinus tracts that are sufficiently patent for ingested liquids to appear in the external opening have been reported. The patient may complain of dysphagia, odynophagia, or hoarseness, especially when the thyroglossal sinus or cyst is infected.

In general, the diagnosis of lingual thyroid is not difficult. The mass is in midline, in contrast to the laterally situated lingual tonsils. It is dark red, and its epithelial surface is vascular. These characteristics are not apparent when the patient is examined during an inflammatory process or after hemorrhage in the region due to trauma. A patient presenting with a midline mass at the base of tongue at the time of puberty or during pregnancy should arouse suspicion of the presence of a lingual thyroid. The symptoms associated with lingual thyroid include the sensation of a mass in the throat, dysphagia, an occasionally, dyspnea. Tests with radioactive iodide I 131 will indicate the presence of thyroid tissue at the base of tongue and also whether thyroid tissue is present in the neck. An MRI scan would be useful and a better study than a contrast-enhanced CT scan, which would preclude a radioactive iodide scan for several weeks.

Differential Diagnosis

An adenoma of the pyramidal lobe of the thyroid gland may simulate a thyroglossal duct cyst. Often the two can be differentiated by palpation. Needle aspiration is valuable for a differentiation. The diagnosis may not be made until the time of operation. A suprahyoid thyroglossal cyst may be confused with a dermal cyst from the floor of mouth. However, the thyroglossal cyst is superficial to the mylohyoid muscle, which is invariably external to the dermoid cyst. A laterally placed thyroglossal duct cyst may be confused with an external laryngocele or a cyst of branchial origin. Anterior, posterior, and lateral radiographs with and without Valsalva's maneuver will usually establish a diagnosis of a laryngocele. An infected lymph node in the anterior cervical region may be confused with an infected thyroglossal duct cyst. The two can usually be differentiated after antibiotic therapy.

Other benign, solid, and cystic tumors of the extralaryngeal region can be confused with a thyroglossal cyst. The diagnosis in these instances may not be established until the time of operation, when the relation between the cyst and thyrohyoid membrane has been determined.

The differential diagnosis between a lingual thyroglossal duct cyst and a lingual thyroid is not difficult. The characteristics of each have been described previously. If a diagnosis cannot be established after visualization and palpation, the radioactive iodide test should be used. This test will indicate the presence of thyroid tissue at the level of the base of tongue.

Treatment

The lingual thyroid should not be resected unless symptoms of cough, odynophagia, dysphagia, dyspnea, or hemorrhage persist. This is especially true when normal thyroid tissue is not present in the neck. A subtotal or complete resection of the lingual thyroid is indicated when uncontrolled hyperthyroidism is present or if malignant change is suspected.

The lingual thyroidectomy is conducted with the patient under endotracheal anesthesia administered with a cuffed tube in place. If possible, the patient is placed in a semisitting position. The tongue is pulled forward with stay sutures, and the hypopharynx is packed with gauze. The incisions are made immediately anterior and lateral to the mass. The lingual thyroid is then dissected from the tongue musculature by means of sharp scissors dissection. Bleeding is controlled with No. 00 chromic catgut sutures. A tracheotomy should be performed if the lingual thyroid is sizable. Fluids are administered intravenously for several days until a soft diet can be tolerated. Some surgeons advocate leaving a small portion of the lingual thyroid if there is no evidence of normal thyroid tissue elsewhere. The administration of thyroid extract to prevent hypothyroidism is indicated after total removal. Other surgeons will use a suprahyoid pharyngotomy approach to resection of a lingual thyroid.

The treatment for a thyroglossal sinus, fistula, or cyst is surgical excision. A horizontal anterior cervical incision is used in the infrahyoid region directly over the thyroglossal duct cyst. If the cyst occurs above the hyoid bone (Fig. 2–15A), the horizontal incision can be made in the immediate suprahyoid region. A transverse elliptical incision is made to encompass the fistula of a thyroglossal sinus tract (Fig. 2–15B). Occasionally, the thyroglossal duct cyst will be found low in the neck. In these instances, the so-called "step ladder" incisions (Fig. 2–15C) are necessary for resection of the cyst and the sinus tract.

Adequate exposure and careful dissection are essential because unless the entire epithelium is removed, recurrence is inevitable. Some surgeons prefer to inject methylene blue into the cyst or sinus tract before preparation for surgical treatment. To be effective, this should be done at least 15 minutes before the onset of the operation. If the cyst is tense, fluid should be aspirated before methylene blue is injected.

It is essential to remove the body of the hyoid bone along with sinus tract (Fig. 2–16). As mentioned previously, this tract may pass anterosuperior to or through the hyoid bone

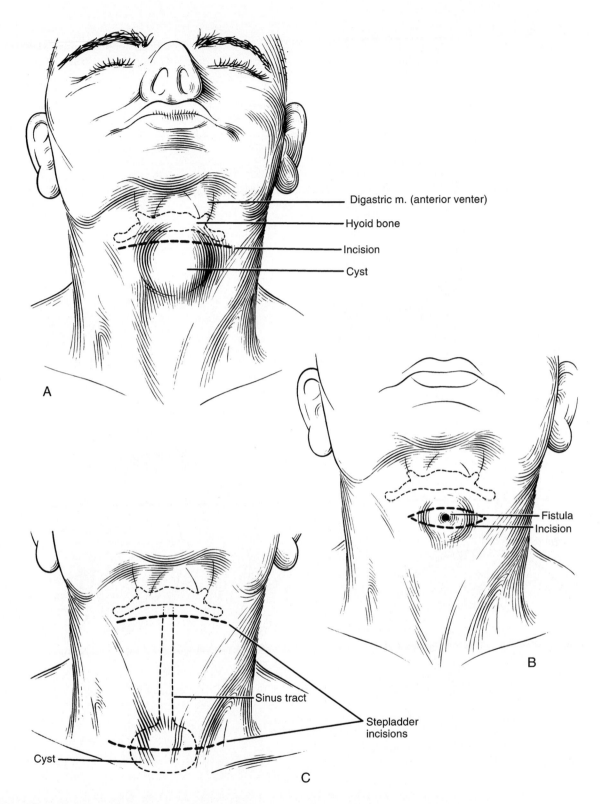

Digastric m. (anterior venter)

Hyoid bone

Incision

Cyst

A

Fistula

Incision

B

Sinus tract

Stepladder
incisions

Cyst

C

FIGURE 2-15. *A,* The usual incision for exposure of a thyroglossal cyst is made horizontally in the infrahyoid region over the thyrohyoid membrane. *B,* A horizontal eliptical incision is made to encompass the fistulous opening of the thyroglossal sinus tract. *C,* Occasionally, the thyroglossal cyst or fistulous opening is found low in the neck in relation to the pyramidal lobe of the thyroid gland. Stepladder incisions are necessary for complete resection in such instances.

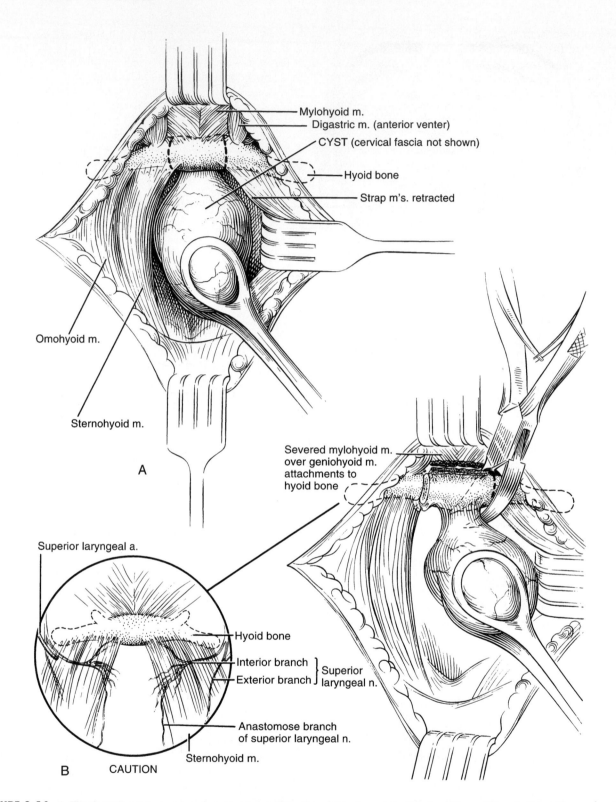

Mylohyoid m.

Digastric m. (anterior venter)

CYST (cervical fascia not shown)

Hyoid bone

Strap m's. retracted

Omohyoid m.

Sternohyoid m.

A

Severed mylohyoid m.
over geniohyoid m.
attachments to
hyoid bone

Superior laryngeal a.

Hyoid bone

Interior branch ⎫ Superior
Exterior branch ⎬ laryngeal n.

Anastomose branch
of superior laryngeal n.

Sternohyoid m.

B   CAUTION

FIGURE 2-16. *A,* The thyroglossal duct cyst or sinus tract is carefully dissected to the region of the hyoid bone. When dealing with a cyst or fistula in the lower anterior neck, the surgeon should be on the lookout for an extension of the tract inferior to the cyst or fistula. If these extensions are not resected, a troublesome recurrence will develop.

The infrahyoid and suprahyoid musculatures are carefully dissected from the body of the hyoid bone. The dotted lines indicate the portion of the body of the hyoid bone that is to be resected in continuity with the sinus tract.

B, The body of the hyoid bone is being transected on each side with bone-cutting forceps. The dissection in this region should not be carried too far laterally for fear of injury to the superior laryngeal nerve.

on its way to the foramen cecum. After the central portion of the body of the hyoid bone has been resected in continuity with the sinus tract, the latter is carefully dissected toward the base of the tongue (Fig. 2–17A). As this dissection approaches the base of the tongue, the surgeon's index finger is inserted into the patient's mouth to the region of the foramen cecum to ensure complete removal of the tract (Fig. 2–17B). The tract is ligated with No. 00 chromic catgut sutures (Fig. 2–18A). A rubber or closed suction drain is inserted into the region of the base of the tongue (Fig. 2–18B), and the wound is carefully closed in layers (Fig. 2–18C and D). If there is any history of recent or past infection, the antibiotic therapy should be continued for several days after the operation. The drain is removed on the second or third postoperative day.

The postoperative discomfort is usually minimal. Occasionally a patient may complain of discomfort in his upper neck while swallowing. This sensation lasts for only 1 or 2 weeks.

Branchial Cysts

A branchial cyst may be discovered as a lateral mass in the neck in a person of any age, from birth to old age. There is no predominance in sex or side of neck incidence. Branchial cysts are usually discovered as painless swellings in the neck, along the anterior border of the sternocleidomastoid muscle and in the region of the mandibular angle. *Bailey* divides them into four types, according to their anatomic location (Fig. 2–19).

An exact diagnosis is difficult to make preoperatively. Aspiration of the cysts' contents will reveal the presence of cholesterol crystals. Computed tomography scanning is useful to differentiate branchial cysts from cystic lymphadenopathy.

The branchial cyst may increase in size during an upper respiratory infection. However, its contents may not become infected. The swelling is usually caused by the lymphoid tissue of the cystic wall.

Cervical adenitis should be considered in a differential diagnosis. Usually the distinction between it and a branchial cyst can be made on the basis that, in cervical adenitis, more than one lymph node is enlarged. An abscessed cervical lymph node may be indistinguishable from an infected branchial cyst before surgery. A lymph node involved with metastatic cancer and having undergone cystic degeneration is also difficult to distinguish from a branchial cyst. A cystic hygroma tends to be less spherical than a branchial cyst, and it is lobulated and translucent. Also, it is usually present in the lower neck. Other lesions that can be confused with a branchial cyst are solid tumors (such as neurofibroma, lipoma, lymphoma, carotid body tumor, and hemangioma), dermoid cysts, and rarely, laterally displaced thyroglossal duct cysts.

Treatment

An infected branchial cyst should be vigorously treated with antibiotics before resorting to incision and drainage. Repeated aspiration of the cyst may prove successful. Branchial cysts are usually removed by way of an upper horizontal cervical incision unless they are unusually large, in which case it is best to make the incision along the anterior border of the sternocleidomastoid muscle. Every effort should

be made to resect the cyst intact. In some instances, a portion of the cyst's contents can be aspirated to reduce its size. If this is not successful, the contents of the cyst are evacuated and a small incision is made in the lateral aspect of the cyst. The surgeon introduces a finger through this incision, which he keeps in place within the cyst during dissection. Care is used to avoid injury to the various cranial nerves in this area, with particular attention paid to the vagus, hypoglossal, and spinal accessory nerves. A pedicle may extend from the cyst to the pharynx. This, of course, should also be carefully excised.

Branchial Sinus Tracts and Fistulas

Congenital sinus tracts of branchial origin may be either complete or incomplete. The incomplete variety may have an external or an internal fistula. The external fistulas are found near the external auditory canal and at any point along the skin over the anterior margin of the sternocleidomastoid muscle. The position of the internal opening of the sinus tract varies from the nasopharynx to the hypopharynx.

The first branchial cleft sinus tract arises from the first branchial groove and thus may contain mesodermal cartilage as well as ectodermal structures. This tract extends from the submandibular region, continuing superficially to the mandible, and on to the external auditory canal (Fig. 2–20A). During its course, it is usually closely associated with the parotid gland and the facial nerve, passing to the former. The superior portion of the first branchial sinus tract is near the junction of the cartilaginous and bony external auditory canal. The tract may be found internal, external, or between the branches of the facial nerve.

It is often difficult to diagnose the first branchial sinus tract. Repeated incision and drainage, as well as subtotal resection, on many of these tracts are performed before the diagnosis is correctly established. The external opening, or cystic end, of the tract is usually in the submaxillary triangle. Discharge from the upper end of the sinus tract by way of the external auditory canal is unusual. On rare occasions, the entire sinus tract can be outlined after injection of radiopaque material.

The incision required for the removal of a first branchial sinus tract is similar to that for a parotidectomy (Fig. 2–20B). The facial nerve and its branches are identified before any attempted dissection is made. The external lobe of the parotid gland is dissected forward; it is usually necessary to remove a portion of the structure to obtain an adequate exposure. Dissection of the tract begins in the submaxillary region. The skin surrounding the external opening is included with the specimen to be removed. Dissections continue to the tract's attachment at the junction of the cartilaginous and bony external auditory canal (Fig. 2–20C).

Whereas the first branchial sinus tract is located entirely above the hyoid bone, the second, third, and fourth branchial sinus tracts are located below this level. The external openings of the second, third, and fourth tracts may be found in the skin at any level along the anterior border of the sternocleidomastoid muscle (usually the lower third). The internal openings vary in location from the nasopharynx to the hypopharynx. Cysts may occur at any level along the course of these sinus tracts. The second branchial sinus tract pen-

Text continued on page 82

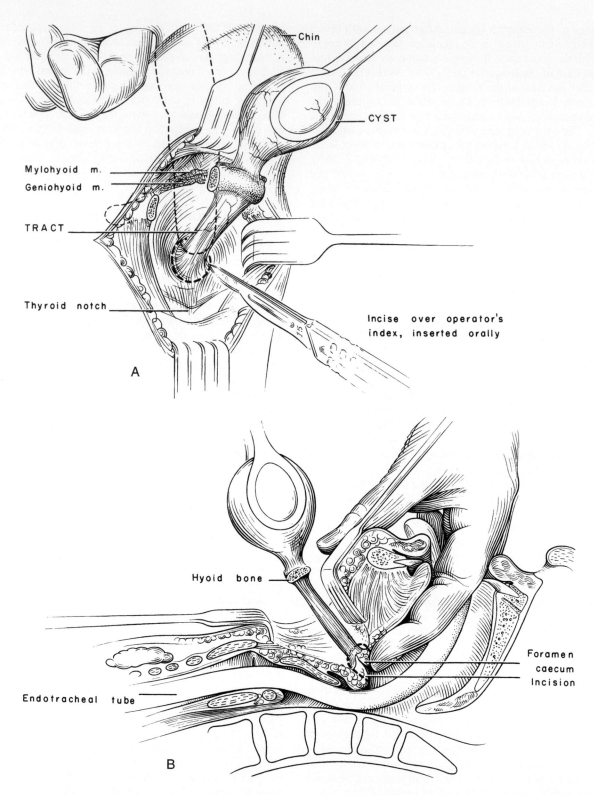

Chin

CYST

Mylohyoid m.

Geniohyoid m.

TRACT

Thyroid notch

Incise over operator's
index, inserted orally

A

Hyoid bone

Foramen
caecum
Incision

Endotracheal tube

B

FIGURE 2-17. *A,* The thyroglossal cyst, sinus tract, and body of the hyoid bone are elevated as dissection is continued towards the base of the tongue. Careful dissection in this region will ensure against recurrence. In most series, there is less than 1% incidence of recurrence, providing the sinus tract is dissected to the submucosal region. *B,* When dissection of the sinus tract, approaches the base of the tongue, the index finger of the surgeon's left hand may be inserted into the patient's mouth to the region of the foramen cecum for bimanual palpation and to facilitate the dissection.

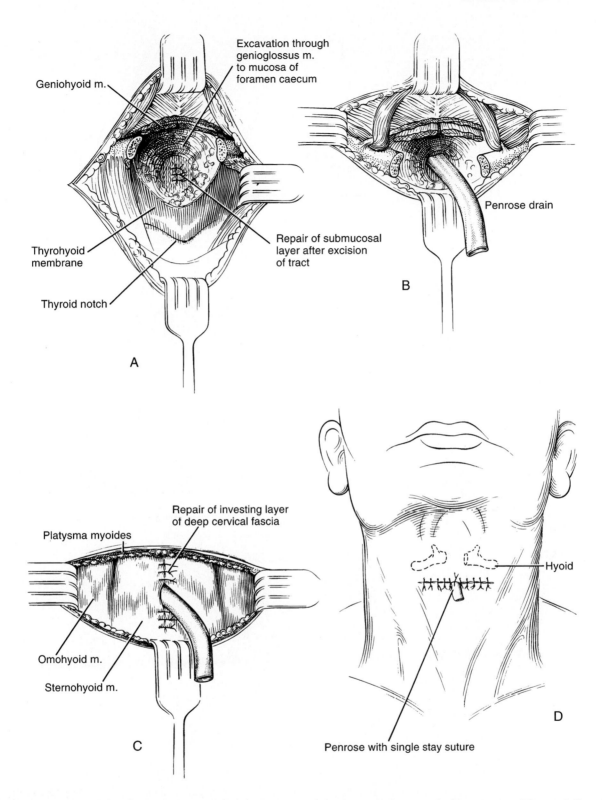

FIGURE 2–18. *A,* The thyroglossal sinus tract has been transected in the submucosal region adjacent to the foramen cecum. The tract is ligated with No. 00 catgut before it is transected. The submucosal layer is repaired with chromic catgut sutures. *B,* A rubber drain is inserted in to the depths of the dissection and secured in place. *C,* Muscles are approximated with chromic catgut suture material to obliterate the defect resulting from the dissection. The sternohyoid muscles are shown approximated in the midline. *D,* The subcutaneous and dermal sutures are in place and the Penrose drain is secured in the center of the incision. Both incisions of the stepladder approach should be drained. The drain can be removed on the first or second postoperative day.

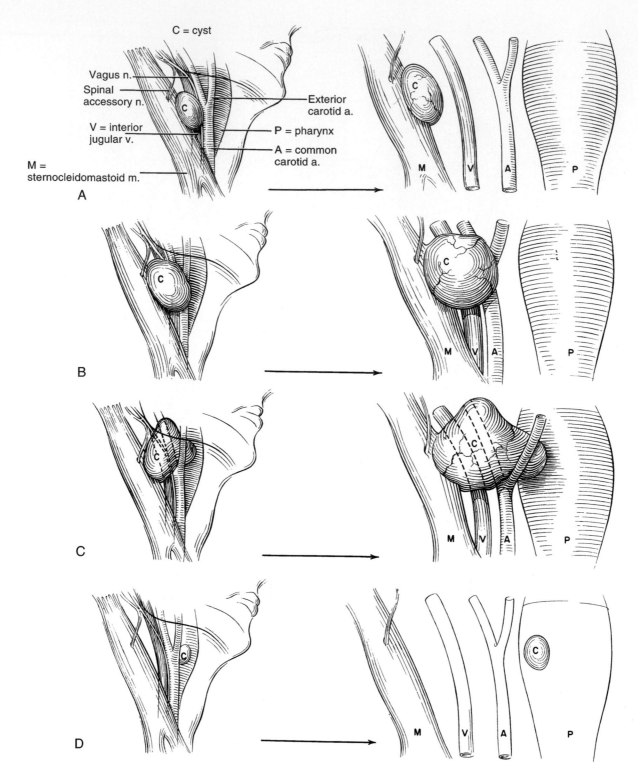

FIGURE 2-19. Bailey (1922) divides the branchial cleft cysts into four types based on their anatomic location. *A,* Type I is found superficially on the anterior border of the sternocleidomastoid muscle beneath the cervical fascia. It probably has its origin from a remnant of the external tract connecting the cervical sinus to the external surface. *B,* Type II, the most common type, lies deep to the investing fascia, is in contact with the great vessels, and may be adherent to the jugular vein. It probably originates from a persistend cervical sinus. *C,* Type III is similar to Type II except that it passes between the internal and external carotid arteries and extends to the pharyngeal wall. It probably originates from a dilated second external pharyngeal duct. *D,* Type IV is found adjacent to the pharyngeal wall medial to the great vessels. It probably has its origins from a remnant of the internal pharyngeal duct.

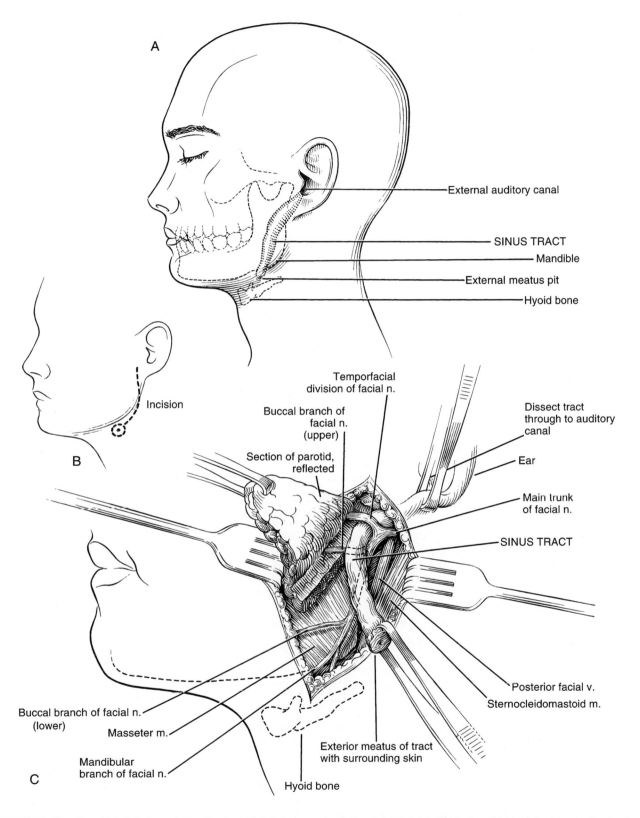

A

External auditory canal

SINUS TRACT

Mandible

External meatus pit

Hyoid bone

B

Incision

Temporfacial
division of facial n.

Buccal branch of
facial n.
(upper)

Section of parotid,
reflected

Dissect tract
through to auditory
canal

Ear

Main trunk
of facial n.

SINUS TRACT

Posterior facial v.

Sternocleidomastoid m.

Buccal branch of facial n.
(lower)

Masseter m.

Mandibular
branch of facial n.

Exterior meatus of tract
with surrounding skin

C

Hyoid bone

FIGURE 2–20. First branchial cleft sinus. *A,* The first branchial cleft sinus extends from an external fistula in the submandibular triangle. It extends superficial to the angle of the mandible to the external auditory canal and is near the parotid gland and facial nerve. *B,* The incision for removal is similar to that for parotidectomy. The facial nerve must be identified before the sinus tract is dissected. *C,* The external lobe of the parotid gland is dissected forward for exposure. It may be necessary to remove a portion of the parotid gland. The skin around the external opening in the submandibular triangle is included with the specimen. It may also be necessary to remove a fistulous opening at the junction of the cartilaginous and bony external auditory canal. In this instance the sinus passes between the division of the facial nerve. It can pass deep or superficial to the facial nerve.

etrates the platysmal muscle at the level of the external fistulous opening. There is a definite relationship between this sinus tract, the internal and external carotid arteries, and the hypoglossal and glossopharyngeal nerves.

Second branchial sinus tracts are reported to be the most common (Fig. 2–21A). A complete fistula of the second branchial sinus tract has an external opening in the skin at the anterior border of the sternocleidomastoid muscle in the lower third of the neck. The tract penetrates the platysmal muscle and ascends along the carotid sheath. It passes deep to the external carotid artery and superficial to the internal carotid artery. It remains superficial to the hypoglossal nerve, stylopharyngeus muscle, and glossopharyngeal nerve. The internal opening is usually found in the region of the tonsillar fossa.

The external fistula of the third branchial sinus tract is found in approximately the same location as that of the second branchial sinus tract (Fig. 2–21B). It also ascends in close relationship to the common carotid artery until it reaches the region of the carotid bifurcation. At this point, it passes behind both the internal and external carotid arteries. It remains superficial to the vagus and hypoglossal nerves. It descends into the lower hypopharynx and penetrates the thyrohyoid membrane and, therefore, is not found in close relationship to the glossopharyngeal nerve and stylopharyngeus muscle. Patients with third branchial sinus tracts may present initially with thyroiditis related to the proximity of the tract to the thyroid lobe.

A fourth branchial sinus tract has not yet been reported (Fig. 2–21C). Theoretically, the external opening would be situated like that of the second and third branchial sinus tracts. After piercing the platysma, the tract would descend into the mediastinum and would pass under the right subclavian artery or the arch of the aorta. From this point, it would ascend along the common carotid artery, hook over the hypoglossal nerve, and pass behind both the internal and external carotid arteries, from whence it would again descend. The internal opening would be in the upper esophagus or pyriform sinus.

Treatment
Occasionally, the outline of the sinus tract can be determined after injecting radiopaque material. To facilitate the dissection, methylene blue can be injected by using a blunt needle and applying minimal pressure immediately before the operation. Stepladder incisions are necessary for adequate exposure. The lower horizontal incision should include the skin surrounding the external opening of the sinus tract (Fig. 2–22A). As the sinus tract is resected during its ascent, deep to the platysma and along the carotid sheath, superior traction is necessary for adequate exposure. Dissection is continued to the level of the carotid bifurcation. It is imperative to identify the hypoglossal nerve and determine the relationships of the sinus tract to the internal and external carotid arteries (Fig. 2–22B). Because the second branchial sinus tract is the most common, it usually passes between the external and internal carotid arteries. Care should be used to avoid injury to the hypoglossal and glossopharyngeal nerves. When dealing with a third branchial sinus tract cyst, which passes behind both the internal and external carotid arteries, care should be used to avoid injury to the vagus, hypoglossal, and superior laryngeal nerves.

PEDICLED SKIN FLAPS

Classification

Local or Distant
A local pedicled skin flap is advanced to rotate to cover an adjacent area denuded of epithelium. An example of this type of flap is that used with a Z-plasty. A distant pedicled skin flap is one that is transferred to an area not adjacent to the operative field. An example of this type of flap is a chest pedicled skin flap that is transferred to resurface an area in the cervical region.

Single Pedicled or Bipedicled
In most instances, a single pedicled skin flap will effect a necessary repair. Occasionally, a bipedicled skin flap is used to provide additional length to augment the blood supply. It is especially useful when the recipient area has a poor blood supply, as is often the case after radiation therapy.

Open or Closed (Tubed)
In most instances, an open flap can be used for resurfacing. Tubing increases the chance for survival of the flap. It eliminates the denuded subcutaneous layer between the base of the flap and the recipient area. Both single and bipedicled skin flaps can be tubed.

Delayed or Nondelayed
Most pedicled skin flaps can be supplied with an adequate arterial supply and venous return without any need for delay. The main indications for a delayed pedicled skin flap are (1) poor circulation in the recipient site after infection, (2) radiation therapy, (3) diabetes, and (4) arteriosclerosis. Occasionally, healing will be delayed without any apparent cause, in which case the delayed flap is the first choice. The number of blood vessels supplying the pedicled flap from the base increases with each delay. Delay allows the recruitment of vascular supply from an angiosome once removed by opening the "choke" area between two neighboring angiosomes. As a rule, a pedicled skin flap is elevated in its entirety as a delayed flap and sutured into its anatomic position. Sometimes a partial delay, consisting of only the skin incision, is necessary. The pedicled flap can be elevated and rotated to the recipient site 10 days to 3 weeks after either a first or second delay. Some evidence indicates that a prolonged delay (in excess of 3 weeks) is undesirable, as the circulation from the periphery increases while that from the base decreases.

Simple or Compound
A simple pedicled skin flap consists of skin, subcutaneous tissue, and occasionally, underlying fascia.

A compound pedicled skin flap is lined with a split-thickness skin graft, cartilage, or bone. It is important that these grafts be placed accurately and not exceed the desired amount of tissue.

Local Pedicled Skin Flaps

Advancement Flap. The straight advancement flap can be used to close small adjacent areas denuded of epithelium (Fig. 2–23A). The flap is constructed, elevated, and stretched to cover the defect (Fig. 2–23B). The elasticity of the skin per-

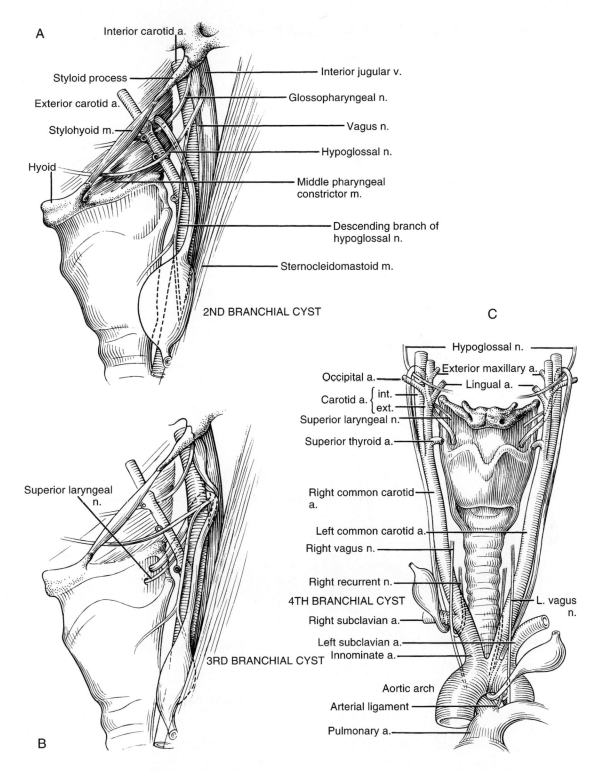

A
Interior carotid a.
Styloid process
Exterior carotid a.
Stylohyoid m.
Hyoid
Interior jugular v.
Glossopharyngeal n.
Vagus n.
Hypoglossal n.
Middle pharyngeal constrictor m.
Descending branch of hypoglossal n.
Sternocleidomastoid m.
2ND BRANCHIAL CYST

B
Superior laryngeal n.
3RD BRANCHIAL CYST

C
Hypoglossal n.
Exterior maxillary a.
Occipital a.
Lingual a.
Carotid a. { int. ext.
Superior laryngeal n.
Superior thyroid a.
Right common carotid a.
Left common carotid a.
Right vagus n.
Right recurrent n.
4TH BRANCHIAL CYST
Right subclavian a.
Left subclavian a.
Innominate a.
L. vagus n.
Aortic arch
Arterial ligament
Pulmonary a.

FIGURE 2-21. Second, third, and fourth branchial-cleft sinus tracts. *A,* Second branchial cleft sinus. The internal opening is in the region of the tonsillar fossa. The external opening is in the skin along the anterior border of the sternocleidomastoid muscle (usually the lower third). The tract passes deep to the external carotid artery and superficial to the internal carotid artery. It remains superficial to the hypoglossal nerve, stylopharyngeus muscle, and glossopharyngeal nerve. *B,* Third branchial-cleft sinus. The internal opening is in the lower lateral hypopharynx. The external opening is the same as that of the second branchial cleft sinus. The tract passes behind both the internal and external carotid arteries. It remains superficial to the vagus and hypoglossal nerve. *C,* Fourth branchial-cleft sinus (not reported—theoretical). The internal opening is in the pyriform sinus or cervical esophagus. The external opening is the same as that of the second branchial cleft sinus. The tract passes into the mediastinum and under the subclavian artery or arch of the aorta. It ascends along the common carotid artery, hooks over the hypoglossal nerve, and passes behind both the internal and external carotid arteries.

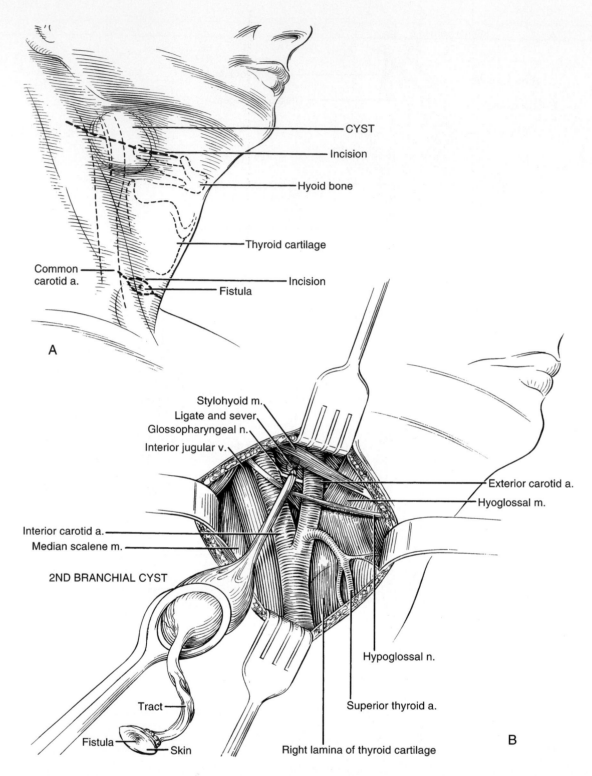

CYST

Incision

Hyoid bone

Thyroid cartilage

Common carotid a.

Incision

Fistula

A

Stylohyoid m.

Ligate and sever

Glossopharyngeal n.

Interior jugular v.

Exterior carotid a.

Hyoglossal m.

Interior carotid a.

Median scalene m.

2ND BRANCHIAL CYST

Hypoglossal n.

Tract

Superior thyroid a.

Fistula

Skin

B

Right lamina of thyroid cartilage

FIGURE 2–22. Resection of second and third branchial-cleft sinuses. *A,* Upper and lower horizontal (stepladder) cervical incisions are necessary for this resection. The skin around the external opening is included with the lower incision. The upper incision is made at the level of the carotid bulb. *B,* It is imperative to determine the relationship between the sinus tract and the internal and external carotid arteries and the hypoglossal nerve. Care should be taken to avoid the glossopharyngeal nerve with a second branchial-cleft sinus tract, and the vagus and superior laryngeal nerve with a third branchial-cleft sinus tract.

Advancement flaps

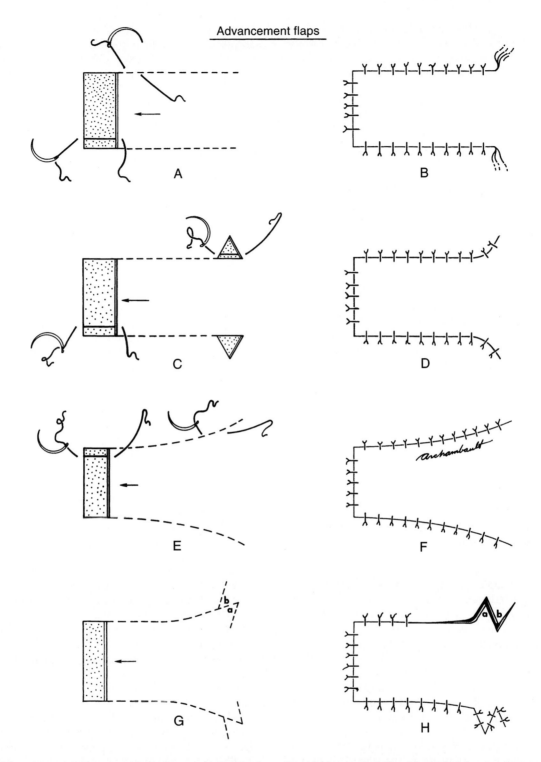

FIGURE 2-23. Advancement flap. *A,* A single advancement flap has been elevated. The sutures indicate the method for advancement. Skin folds will be formed adjacent to each side of the base of the flap if this advancement is excessive. *B,* A sketch illustrating the placement of sutures and completed repair. Skin folds are present on each side of the base. *C,* The skin folds adjacent to the base formed by the advancement of the pedicled skip flap can be avoided by removing two triangular pieces of skin, as shown. The triangles should be equilateral. The sutures indicate the method for closing the triangles and advancement of the pedicled flap. *D,* The suture line at the base is directed laterally, as the triangular defects are closed. The cosmetic result from this type of repair is usually excellent. *E,* Another technique for advancement of a local pedicled skin flap, which enjoys an excellent blood supply and does not create skin folds at its base, is constructed as shown. The slightly curved incisions and broadened base allow for advancement without creating skin folds. *F,* The sketch shows the completed repair and placement of sutures. *G,* A Z-plasty on each side of the base of an advancement flap can be used to facilitate the advancement and effect better cosmesis at its base. *H,* The flaps (a and b) of the Z-plasty have been transposed, and the pedicled flap advanced to cover the defect.

mits this stretching and advancement. If the adjacent area denuded of epithelium is large, two skin folds will be performed adjacent to the base of the flap as it is advanced. If these folds are small they will eventually disappear. They can, however, be avoided by removing a triangular section of skin lateral to the base of each side (Fig. 2–23C and D). They can also be avoided by gradually increasing the width of the flap towards its base (Fig. 2–23E and F). A Z-plasty, performed on each side of the base, will allow for greater advancement and eliminate the skin folds (Fig. 2–23G and H).

Rotation Flaps. Rotation flaps are of particular value in closing defects to the lateral cheek and infraorbital region. The gradual curve of this incision allows for easy advancement and a greater degree of mobility. The skin is rotated without any stretching, and the flap enjoys a wide base, which ensures an ample blood supply. A triangular section of skin can be resected at the end of the incision to facilitate closure (Fig. 2–24A and B). Greater mobility is obtained by directing the end of the incision into the base of the flap (Fig. 2–24C to E). The length of this extension is directly proportional to the degree of release. In addition to effecting a release, this incision, which extends into the base of the flap, facilitates closure and provides a better cosmetic result.

Another technique for resurfacing this type of defect is that of rotating a rectangular pedicled skin flap (Fig. 2–24F). A triangular defect is created as the flap is rotated, and this may close as shown in Figure 2–24G and H.

VY Advancement. Structures such as the palate, portions of the tongue, or columella of the nose can be lengthened or shortened by the VY triangular advancement flap technique. Advancement is accomplished by transforming a V incision into a Y closure (Fig. 2–25A to C). Shortening is accomplished by transforming a Y incision into a V closure (Fig. 2–25D to F).

Z-plasty. The principle use for the Z-plasty, which consists of transposing two triangular skin flaps, is to release linear scar contractures or break up a linear scar. The Z-plasty repair is used for cosmesis and to improve the mobility and function of the involved area. It redistributes tension by dispersing it in a number of directions. A classic example of its lengthening effect is that accomplished in the repair of a contracture scar of the upper lip. The Z-plasty releases the contracture, breaks up the scar, and transposes a portion of it to correspond with the nasolabial fold.

Technique. When planning a Z-plasty, it is best to draw an equilateral triangle on each side of the scar. This results in a parallelogram. The next task is to select the more suitable of the two sets of limbs (Fig. 2–26). If possible, the limb should correspond with the lines of minimal tension. One set may offer a better blood supply than the other.

The angle of the outer limbs to the line of the scar can be varied. As the angles increase, so does the amount of lengthening. For example, with angles of 45 degrees, there will be a 50% lengthening of the contracture. With angles of 60 degrees, there will be a 75% increase. When the angles approach 30 degrees, the base is too narrow, and the

blood supply is rather poor. Any tension release of the flap transposition would be minimal, thus defeating the object of the Z-plasty. If, conversely, the angle exceeds 60 degrees, the flaps lack sufficient mobility for easy transposition. Flaps designed with an 80-degree angle would produce unsightly "dog ears." Therefore, except in unusual circumstances, the 60-degree angles are preferable for the Z-plasty repair.

After the Z-plasty has been carefully designed, the scar or central limb is excised first. Subcutaneous scar tissue must be included with this elevation. The outer limbs of the Z-plasty are then incised, and the triangular flaps elevate in a subcutaneous plane (Fig. 2–26B). The thickness varies with the area of the problem at hand. The adjacent skin is also undermined, as needed. The two triangular flaps are transposed (Fig. 2–26C). Skin hooks rather than forceps should be used to avoid injury to the flaps. Each flap is advanced by applying No. 4-0 chromic catgut suture material. The skin is approximated with fine dermal sutures (Fig. 2–26D).

The ideal situation for a Z-plasty occurs when the scar is narrow and not too long and the surrounding tissue is sufficiently lax to permit mobilization to the skin and ease a flap transposition. Often, the scar is long and the surrounding tissues lack the necessary mobility. Attempts to transpose large flaps can produce undesired tension and the formation of "dog ears." In such instances, it is best to construct a four-flap Z-plasty (Fig. 2–26E and F) or a series of Z-plasties to break up the contracture. These may be made in parallel or skew formation (Fig. 2–26G to K). The W-plasty can also be used to repair a long scar (Fig. 2–26L to N).

Tetrahedral Z-plasty. The tetrahedral Z-plasty can be used to convert a peak (web) into a valley (cleft) or vice versa. Usually the 60-degree angled flaps produce the best symmetry. The techniques for this repair are described and illustrated in Figure 2–27.

T-plasty. Certain lesions of the face (Fig. 2–28A) can be resected with T-plasty excision, which results in minimal scarring and minimal loss of normal tissue as compared with the usual elliptical excision, with or without a Z-plasty closure. The method is especially desirable when the long axis of a tumor is at right angles to the skin lines. The base of the T-plasty corresponds to a skin line, crease, or fold. Although considerable tension exists on the vertical limb of the closure, contractions of hypertrophic scars generally do not occur.

The incisions that form the vertical limb of the T-plasty are identical to those making up half an elliptical excision (Fig. 2–28B). The horizontal incision is made along the skin line. Extensive subcutaneous undermining is necessary in all directions (Fig. 2–28C). The subcutaneous closure of the vertical limb should be carefully executed with multiple sutures (Fig. 2–28D). If the skin is approximated, a slight buckling occurs below the horizontal closure. This flattens out in a week or two (Fig. 2–28E).

Fat Flip Flap (Millard's Tongue-Twister). Often after transposing tissue to close the defect by means of a pedicle skin flap, the repaired area is elevated in comparison with the surrounding skin. This is especially apt to occur in

Text continued on page 92

Rotation flaps

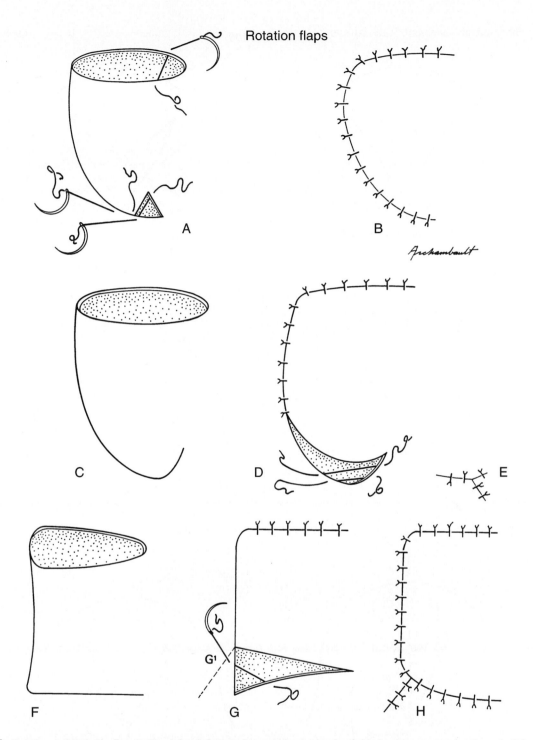

Archambault

FIGURE 2–24. Rotation pedicled skin flap. *A,* The defect is indicated superiorly. A triangle of skin has been removed at the end of the curved incision. The suture indicates the method for closure of the triangular defect and advancement of the rotational flap. *B,* The superior and triangular defects are closed as the rotational flap is advanced superiorly. *C,* The curved incision for construction of the rotational flap has been extended at a right angle into the base of the flap. The amount of release is directly proportional to the length of this incision. *D,* The rotational flap has been advanced to close the superior defect. In so doing, a defect occurs inferiorly. The sutures indicate the method for repair of the defect. *E,* This sketch illustrates the completed repair of the inferior defect. *F,* Larger defects, especially triangular- or oval-shaped ones, are repaired by constructing a rectangular pedicled skin flap as shown. *G,* A triangular-shaped defect is created inferiorly as the flap is rotated superiorly. The inferior defect is closed as shown. If this is not possible, a triangular flap is constructed (*broken line*). *H,* The completed repair.

Local flaps

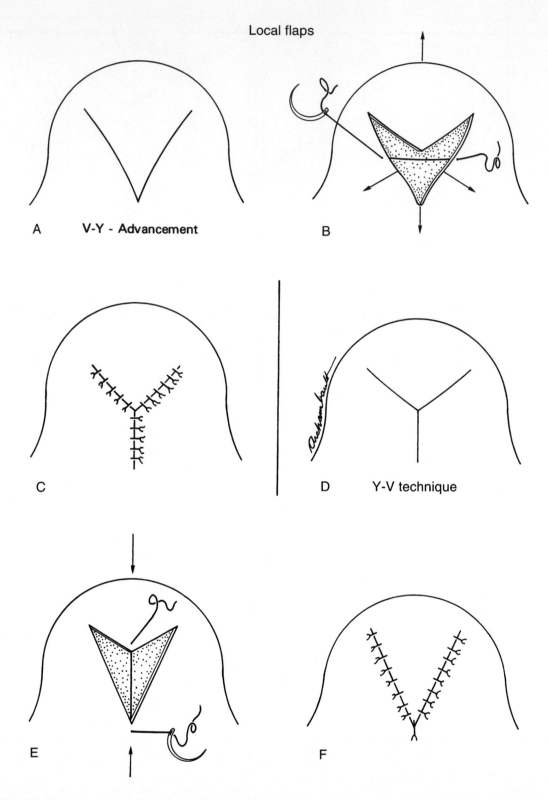

FIGURE 2-25. V-Y advancement flap. *A,* A V incision is made, and the surrounding tissue is undermined. *B,* The superiorly based triangular flap is advanced superiorly as the surrounding skin or mucous membrane is undermined. The Y closure is commenced as illustrated. *C,* The complete Y closure. *D,* The Y incision is made for shortening. *E,* The surrounding mucous membrane or skin has been undermined. The superiorly based triangular flap is advanced inferiorly. *F,* Shortening has been accomplished by the V closure.

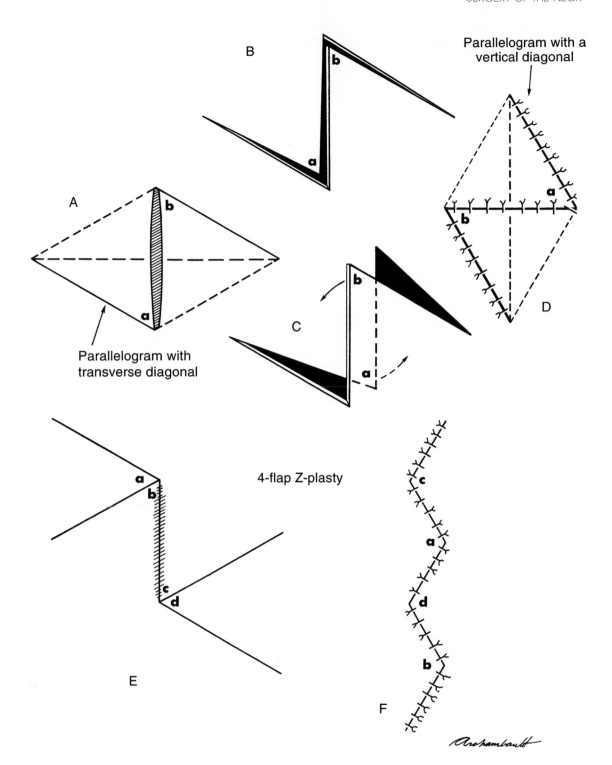

FIGURE 2-26. Z-plasty. *A,* A vertical scar line is indicated. Equilateral triangles are constructed on each side of the scar, using the 60-degree angle for the outer limbs of the Z-plasty. In so doing, a parallelogram with a transverse diagonal is constructed. *B,* The vertical scar has been excised, and the lateral limbs of the Z-plasty incised. Both flaps are elevated, and the surrounding skin is undermined. *C,* This figure illustrates the direction of transposition for the two triangular flaps of the Z-plasty. *D,* The Z-plasty has been completed, and lengthening has been accomplished by producing a parallelogram with a vertical diagonal. *E,* A four-flap Z-plasty can be used when the scar is long and the surrounding tissues lack mobility, in order to avoid undesired tension and the formation of "dog ears." *F,* The four flaps have been transposed and the repair is complete.

Illustration continued on following page

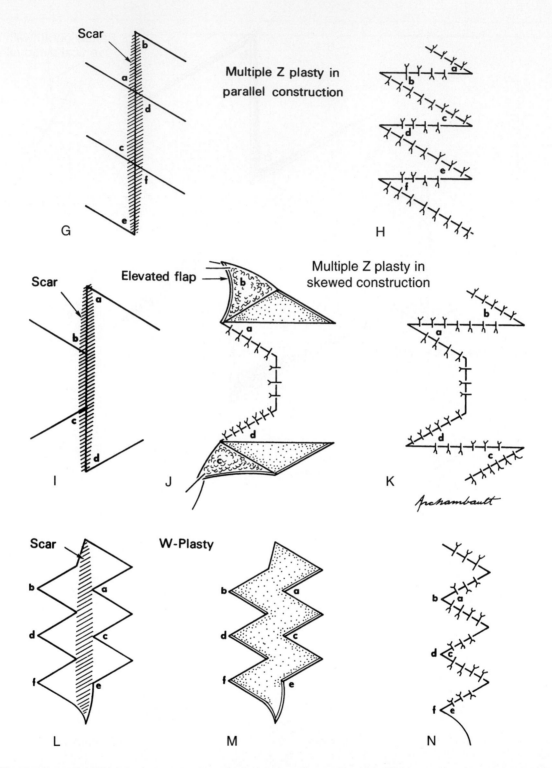

Scar

Multiple Z plasty in parallel construction

G

H

Scar

Elevated flap

Multiple Z plasty in skewed construction

I

J

K

Archambault

Scar

W-Plasty

L

M

N

FIGURE 2–26. (*Continued*) *G,* Multiple Z-plasties in parallel construction can be used to spread the lateral tension over several transverse diagonals. This type of repair is essential when there is sufficient mobility in the surrounding tissues. *H,* This illustrates the repair with multiple Z-plasties in parallel construction. *I,* Multiple Z-plasties in skewed construction can also be used to correct the contracture of a long linear scar. *J,* The flaps are elevated and the surrounding tissues widely undermined. The central portion of the repair is first accomplished. *K,* The final repair made with the skewed Z-plasty technique. *L,* The W-plasty technique can be used to break up a straight-line scar; this is particularly useful when the scar is depressed and does not require lengthening. *M,* The scar and triangles of the skin have been resected. Undermining is accomplished on each side. *N,* The triangular flaps have been advanced and sutured in position.

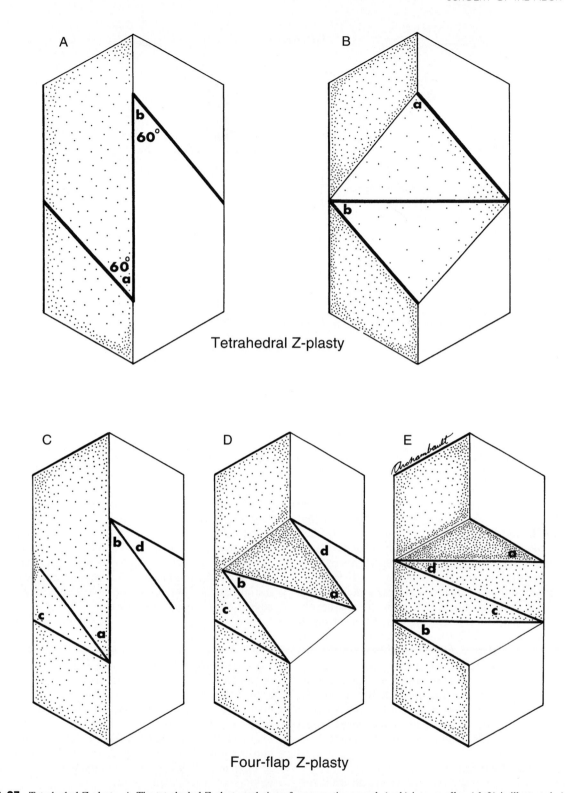

Tetrahedral Z-plasty

Four-flap Z-plasty

FIGURE 2–27. Tetrahedral Z-plasty. *A,* The tetrahedral Z-plasty technique for converting a peak (web) into a valley (cleft) is illustrated. Angles of 60 degrees are usually used because the result is symmetrical. *B,* The flaps of the tetrahedral Z-plasty have been transported, creating a valley. The process can be reversed, transforming a cleft (valley) into a peak. *C* and *D,* The four-flap tetrahedral Z-plasty is used to create a U-shaped rather than a V-shaped cleft. Flaps 1 and 2 are first transposed. Flaps 1 and 4 and flaps 3 and 2 are transposed to complete the repair. *E,* The completed four-flap tetrahedral Z-plasty repair.

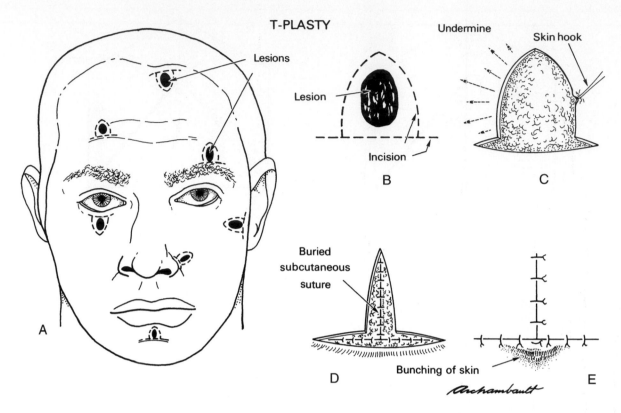

FIGURE 2–28. T-plasty. *A,* Areas on the face that are amenable to the T-plasty excision and repair are shown. The outline for the T-plasty excision is approximately one half of an "elliptical" excision. *B,* The incisions for the T-plasty are shown. The margin of normal tissue around the tumor is at least equal to that of the "elliptical" excision, and yet less normal tissue is excised. *C,* Extensive subcutaneous undermining is necessary in all directions. *D,* The subcutaneous layer is closed with fine chromic catgut sutures. *E,* The T-closure is completed. The bunching of skin adjacent to the horizontal closure spontaneously smoothes out in a week or two.

the face when the surrounding area is scarred or rendered atrophic by radiation therapy. *Millard and associates* had described a unique method to transfer subcutaneous tissue from the "donor" tissue to the surrounding recipient area. They refer to it as the fat flip flap.

Up to one half of the circumferential scar is excised (Fig. 2–29*A*). The skin is elevated over half of the flap tissue, exposing the excess adipose tissue. The skin of the surrounding area is elevated (Fig. 2–29*B*). A layer of excess adipose tissue is elevated as a flap, which is based towards the surrounding tissue. The fat flap is then turned like a page of a book to the surrounding area (Fig. 2–29*C*). The free edge of the flap is sutured as far as possible underneath the surrounding skin that has been elevated. The margins are then closed (Fig. 2–29*D*). The second half of the raised defect can be repaired in a similar fashion in about 1 month.

Pedicled and Distant Flaps

In the last 30 years, the ability for the head and neck surgeon to do more aggressive and complete resections has been dependent on the development of viable tissue transfer for reconstruction of head and neck defects. With the advent of the deltopectoral flap and more importantly the pectoralis major myocutaneous flap, surgeons became able to more reliably resect with wider margins and be able to reconstruct the defect in the upper aerodigestive system. The development of the pectoralis major myocutaneous flap, however, still had as a major drawback the inability to transfer composite tissue for reconstruction of bony as well as

mucosal and cutaneous defects. With the introduction and increased use of free tissue transfer, surgeons are now able to transfer composite flaps that more appropriately meet the demands of the defects. These reconstructive advances have allowed improved patient function and improved quality of life in patients that could not have been offered before the advent of free tissue transfer.

Pedicled Flaps

Cervicothoracic Pedicled Skin Flap *(FIGURE 2–30).* The open pedicle skin flap may be single or bipedicled, delayed or nondelayed. The portion of the open flap, between the donor and recipient sites, may be tubed at the time of transfer to avoid the denuded undersurface. The flap is used to resurface the entire anterior cervical region. It is simple to construct, need not be delayed, and, before the introduction of the pectoralis major myocutaneous flap, was the one the authors most frequently used.

Cervicothoracic flap enjoys a rich blood supply from the branches of the thyrocervical trunk and an excellent venous return.

Technique of Harvest. The medial vertical incision extends inferiorly in the lateral neck to the level of the sternoclavicular joint or is represented by the lateral margin of the anterior cervical defect (Fig. 2–30*A*). The medial vertical incision is extended directly inferiorly over the anterior chest. The lateral vertical incision begins in the mid-cervical region of the

FAT FLIP FLAP (Millard)

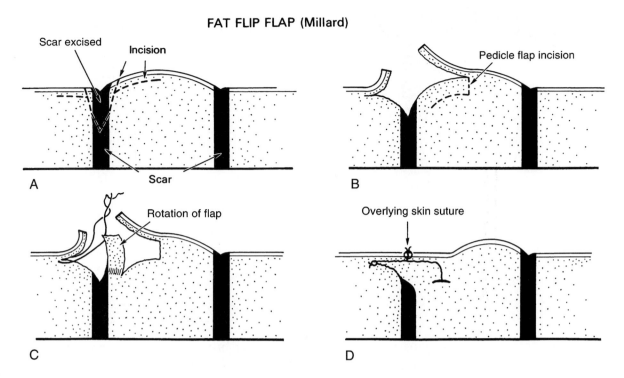

FIGURE 2–29. Fat flip flap. *A,* A cross section of the raised donor tissue (*center section*) compared with the surrounding recipient tissue. The irregular contour results from a difference in the amount of adipose tissue. Incisions are shown for excision of the scar tissue and elevation of the adjacent skin over the recipient and donor tissues. *B,* The skin has been elevated and the subcutaneous fat layers on both sides of the scar are exposed. The broken line indicates a cross section of the incisions to be used to elevate the pedicled fat flap. *C,* The fat flap is turned like the page of a book to the adjacent subcutaneous space. *D,* The fat flap has been reduced and secured in place. The overlying skin is sutured, completing the operation.

anterior border of the trapezius muscle. It extends slightly in the medial direction to the clavicle and then directly inferior. The level of the inferior horizontal incision determines the length of the pedicle flap. The flap is rotated 90 degrees to cover the anterior cervical defect (Fig. 2–30*B*). The resulting dog ear should not be disturbed lest the blood supply be impaired. It will disappear in time. The chest defect can be partially closed by advancing its margins. The remaining defect is covered with a split-thickness skin graft (Fig. 2–30*C*).

The Pectoralis Major Myocutaneous Flap.
The pectoralis major myocutaneous flap has added much to our technique for repair of head and neck defects after extirpative surgery. The technique for the pectoralis major myocutaneous flap was first published by Ariyan in 1979. This flap has the advantage of a constant blood supply from the pectoralis branch of the thoracoacromial artery (Fig. 2–31). The pectoral branch of the thoracoacromial artery is a branch of the axillary artery. The artery runs inferomedially along the posterior surface of the pectoralis muscle within an adipose layer that is surfaced medially with fascia between it and the pectoralis minor muscle. It is thus important to separate the pectoralis major muscle from the pectoralis minor muscle as the former is elevated. The myocutaneous flap does not need to be delayed as do many pedicled flaps, since the blood supply is derived directly from those branches of the pectoralis artery in the underlying pectoralis major muscle.

Design of the Skin Flap *(FIGURE 2–32A).*
The usual size of the flap varies from 100 to 200 cm². Ariyan reports is-

land flaps as large as 12×18 cm with good survival and primary closure of the donor site in the chest. Begin the procedure by drawing the line from the shoulder to the xiphoid process (xiphoid-acromial line). The vascular pedicle can be drawn coming down at a right angle from the midclavicular region, meeting the xiphoid-acromial line at a right angle. At approximately this point, the artery is directed medially and inferiorly along the xiphoid-acromial line. The skin paddle is then outlined over the vascular pedicle between the nipple and the midline. A length of up to 12 cm can be used when surfacing large areas in the neck or reconstructing the cervical esophagus. The distal one quarter of the flap can extend onto the rectus sheath, especially when the distance to the recipient site is long. The flap can be used even with full-breasted women by elevating the breast from the pectoralis major muscle and fashioning the skin paddle inferior and medial to the mammary region.

The skin is incised around the designed skin island. The dissection is continued into the pectoralis major muscle as identified.

Incision From the Island Skin Flap to the Deltopectoral Groove.
A vertical incision (Fig. 2–32*B*) is made from the superior lateral aspect of the skin island in line of the acromial xiphoid axis. The dissection is continued until the pectoralis major muscle is exposed. An alternative incision that spares the deltopectoral flap on that side can be created by an incision that runs from the superior lateral aspect of the skin island to the axilla. Another incision is made near the clavicle to allow full elevation of the intervening deltopectoral skin

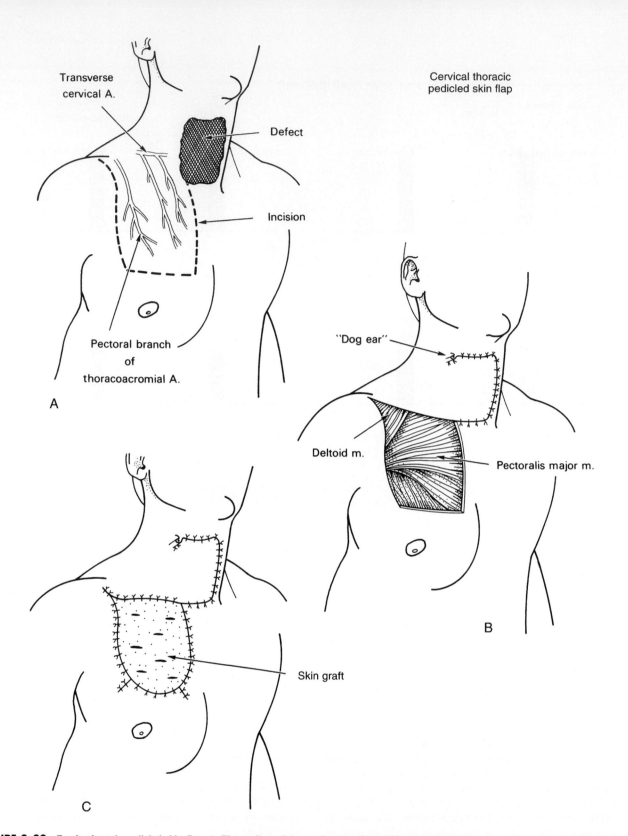

FIGURE 2–30. Cervicothoracic pedicled skin flap. *A,* The outline of the cervicothoracic pedicles skin flap, its blood supply and an anterior cervical defect are shown. The medial vertical incision extends inferiorly in the lateral neck to the sternoclavicular joint or is represented by the lateral margin of the cervical defect. It is then extended inferiorly over the anterior chest to the required length.

The lateral vertical incision begins in the lower lateral cervical region at the anterior border of the trapezius muscle. It extends slightly in a medial direction to the level of the clavicle and then directly inferior to match the length of the medial incision. The lateral and medial vertical incisions are connected inferiorly by a horizontal incision.

B, The flap is elevated with the fascia covering the pectoralis major muscle. Dissection of the flap to the level of the clavicle can be rapidly accomplished. Dissection above this level is carried out with care to avoid disturbing its blood supply. A "dog ear" is created on the flap and is rotated 90 degrees to cover the anterior cervical defect. This should not be altered and will flatten with time. A delay of this flap is not necessary. Carefully applied subcutaneous sutures ensure against any tension of the skin sutures.

C, The cervicothoracic pedicled skin flap has been sutured in place. The chest defect is partially repaired by closing the corners. The remainder is covered with split-thickness skin graft. "Pie-crusting" of the skin graft prevents loss by underlying collection of serum.

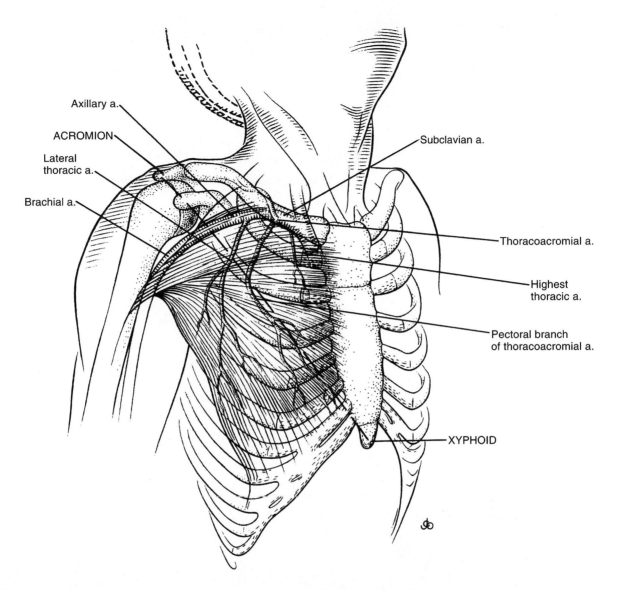

Axillary a.

ACROMION

Lateral
thoracic a.

Brachial a.

Subclavian a.

Thoracoacromial a.

Highest
thoracic a.

Pectoral branch
of thoracoacromial a.

XYPHOID

FIGURE 2-31. The pectoral branch of the thoracoacromial artery, which supplies the pectoralis major myocutaneous flap, is illustrated. A line from the shoulder to the xyphoid process (xyphoacromial line) is drawn on the skin surface. The location of the vascular pedicle can then be drawn coming down at a right angle from the midclavicular region, meeting the xyphoacromial line at a right angle.

from both inferior and superior. The major perforators to the deltopectoral flap in the internal mammary chain are left undisturbed. The pectoralis muscle is then transposed underneath the skin bridge connecting the parasternal to the deltoid region. This also serves as a primary delay for the deltopectoral flap if it is needed to be used later.

Elevation of Flaps. The flaps are elevated (Fig. 2–32C) by exposing the pectoral major muscle and making certain not to disturb the skin island, which would create a sheering effect that would disturb its blood supply from the underlying pectoralis major muscle. The flap is also elevated superiorly to the cervical wounds superior to the clavicle.

Tacking of the Skin Island to Pectoralis Major Muscle. Using No. 3-0 chromic catgut, sutures are passed through the pectoralis major muscle, subcutaneous tissue, and the subcutaneous layer. If these sutures are placed through the skin, the blood supply to the margin of the island flap could

be jeopardized. If the island extends below the level of the pectoralis major muscle and onto the rectus fascia, it is important that the sutures tack the subcutaneous layer to the rectus fascia. This fascia is, of course, incised and elevated with the skin island.

Dissection of the Pectoralis Major Muscle. The lateral aspect of the pectoralis major muscle is dissected free (Fig. 2–33A), leaving its attachment to the humerus. The clavicular and costal fibers of the pectoralis major muscle are identified and separated by blunt dissection. Once this is accomplished, the pectoralis major muscle can be cut from its medial origin.

Elevation of the Pectoralis Major Muscle and Identification of the Pectoralis Artery. This dissection is begun inferiorly, noting that the rectus fascia must be included if the flap extends inferior to it. The pectoralis major muscle is elevated (Fig. 2–33B) by sharp dissection from its origins

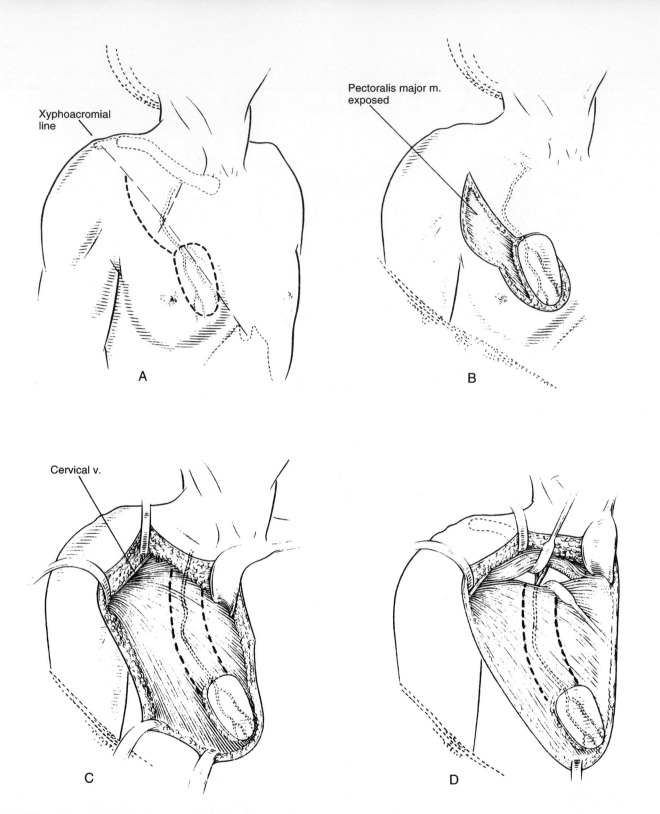

FIGURE 2-32. *A,* The approximate location of the pectoral branch of the thoracoacromial artery. The xyphoacromial line is again illustrated. The outline of the myocutaneous island flap is demonstrated. A flap as large as 12 × 18 cm can be harvested. An incision extending in a superior direction lateral to the xyphoacromial line is demonstrated. This is used to expose the pectoralis major muscle superiorly.

B, The vertical incision has been completed and the flaps elevated medially and laterally to expose the pectoralis major muscle. An incision is made through the skin, fat, and muscle around the island flap. Interrupted sutures through the muscle, subcutaneous tissue, and subcutaneous layer secure the underlying muscle and skin flap together, thus avoiding their separation by a shearing effect.

C, The lateral aspect of the pectoralis major muscle is dissected free, leaving it attached superiorly. The outline of the pectoralis major myocutaneous flap is shown with broken lines. The clavicular and costal fibers of the pectoralis major muscle are identified and dissected by blunt dissection. The medial aspect of the pectoralis major muscle is then incised by sharp dissection.

D, The pedicled skip flap and the pectoralis major muscle are elevated by sharp dissection. Perforating branches of the internal mammary artery are identified, clamped, and ligated. As this dissection is carried superiorly, it is important to make certain that the pectoralis major muscle is being dissected from the pectoralis minor muscle. As soon as the flap is elevated superiorly, the pectoral branch of the thoracoacromial artery becomes visible through the deep fascia.

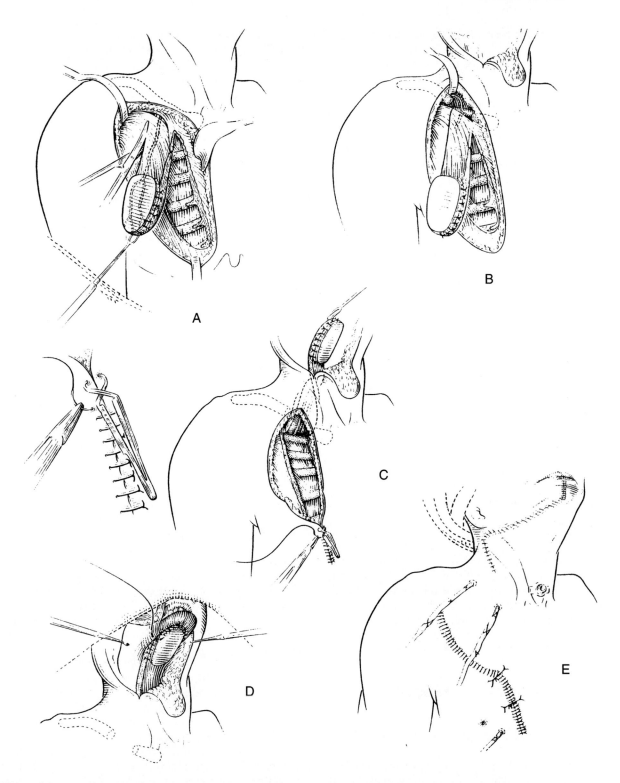

FIGURE 2–33. *A,* Beginning inferiorly and laterally, the insertion of the pectoralis major muscle is dissected with a hemostat. Before each progression of dissection, the flap is elevated to make certain that the pectoral branch of the thoracoacromial artery is not included.

B, A generous tunnel is accomplished in the cervical region so that the pectoralis major myocutaneous flap can be rotated 180 degrees and directed superiorly. The central portion of the clavicle can be resected. This provides greater length to the flap and also eliminates pressure on the flap between the skin and the clavicle.

C and *D,* The skin island is elevated into the defect. It can be trimmed and designed to repair the defect accurately.

E, Primary closure of the chest flap can be accomplished by elevating flaps widely medially and laterally. The repair can be simplified by bringing the skin edges together using towel clips (see part C). The repair is accomplished using No. 2-0 Dexon and skin sutures of clips. Closed-suction drainage is necessary.

from the ribs. Perforating branches of the internal mammary artery are identified, clamped, and ligated. As the dissection is carried superiorly, it is important to separate the pectoralis major muscle from the pectoralis minor muscle. About half way up toward the clavicle, the pectoralis artery becomes visible through the fascia (see Fig. 2–33B).

Transection of the Insertion of the Pectoralis Major Muscle. Beginning laterally, portions of the insertion of the pectoralis major muscle are dissected with a hemostat. Before they are sectioned, the flap is elevated to make certain that the pectoralis artery is not included. The muscle dissection is carefully continued until a narrow pedicle or completely transected, leaving the artery free with its surrounding fascia.

The motor nerve supply of the pectoralis major muscle can be easily identified using a stimulator. The nerves can be left intact if muscle bulk is desired. If not, the resections of the muscle will gradually atrophy.

As the insertion of the pectoralis major muscle is dissected, smaller pectoralis arterial branches are encountered. Once they are identified, they are divided and ligated. They are not necessary for nourishment of the island flap.

Subcutaneous Tunneling. A generous tunnel (Fig. 2–33C) is accomplished in the cervical region so that the pectoralis muscle island flap can be rotated 180 degrees and directed superiorly. Fabian has gained extra length by resecting the central portion of the clavicle. His technique adds little to the morbidity following the operation and also prevents pressure on the flap between the skin and underlying clavicle, which, at times, may reduce the blood supply to the skin paddle. The skin island is elevated into the defect. It can be trimmed and designed to repair the defect accurately.

Closure of the Chest Defect. A primary closure of the chest defect can almost invariably be accomplished (Fig. 2–33C to E). The flaps are elevated widely, medially, and laterally. This repair can be simplified by bringing the skin edges together with towel clips. These remain in place during the closure to prevent tension on the suture line. No. 2-0 Vicryl suture material is suitable for this subcutaneous repair. Either sutures or skin clips can be used. Closed suctioned drainage is a necessity.

MEDIAL BASED HORIZONTAL PEDICLED SKIN FLAP (FIGURE 2-34)

Sternocleidomastoid Myocutaneous Flap

Anatomy. The sternocleidomastoid muscles arise by two tendonous portions. The sternal head arises from the anterolateral aspect of the sternum just below the suprasternal notch. The clavicular portion arises from the medial third of the clavicle.

Blood Supply (FIGURE 2–35). *Superior:* The sternomastoid artery has its origin from the occipital artery. It arises just superior to the hypoglossal nerve and passes superficial to the hypoglossal nerve at the point where the descending hypoglossal nerve has its origin. Several branches of this artery can enter the upper third of the sternocleidomastoid muscle.

Middle: Branches of the superior thyroid artery supply the mid-portion of the sternocleidomastoid muscle.

Inferior: Branches of the thyrocervical trunk supply the sternocleidomastoid muscle, usually by way of the transverse cervical artery. The muscle may also receive blood from the inferior thyroid artery, which is a branch of the thyrocervical trunk.

Technique. The sternocleidomastoid myocutaneous flap can be used at the time of a functional neck dissection or as a separate operation.

The skin island is attached to the inferior aspect of the sternocleidomastoid muscle (Fig. 2–36A). The entire length of the sternocleidomastoid muscle is exposed after the skin paddle has been incised. The skin island or paddle is secured to the underlying sternocleidomastoid muscle with interrupted 3-0 chromic sutures, which pass through the muscle and subcutaneous layers (Fig. 2–36B). The sternocleidomastoid muscle is sectioned just above the sternum and clavicle (Fig. 2–36C and D). The muscle is elevated carefully, to preserve its superior arterial and venous blood supply (inferiorly based flap) or its inferior blood supply (superiorly based flap). The blood supply from the superior thyroid artery is preserved whether the sternocleidomastoid flap is based inferiorly or superiorly.

The size of the skin paddle or island should not exceed 5 to 6 cm. The superiorly based flap enjoys a better blood supply, and the skin in the supraclavicular region is almost invariably free of hair.

The sternocleidomastoid myocutaneous flap is rotated into the recipient site, and the donor is closed (Fig. 2–37). Skin grafting to the donor area is not necessary.

The sternocleidomastoid myocutaneous flap can be used to repair defects of the lip, chin, and face resulting from tumor removal or trauma and defects of the anterior and lateral floor mouth, base of tongue, and retromolar trigone (Fig. 2–38).

Temporoparietal Fascial Flap

The temporoparietal fascial flap (TPFF) (Fig. 2–39) has been used extensively for reconstruction of defects of the extremities, ear, nose, and scalp. The flap was first described in 1898 for use in eyelid reconstruction and has, in the last decade, been rediscovered as useful tissue transfer technique, either pedicled or free, for repair of a variety of defects. In particular, this flap lends itself to the reconstruction of cervical defects in which tissue coverage must be thin, durable, conforming, vascular, and capable of accepting a split-thickness skin graft. This flap can be designed as a large flap, transferring essentially the entire temporoparietal fascia overlying temporalis fascia and extending up into the galeal tissues superior to the superior temporal line. The authors have transferred this flap with extensions all the way to midline with excellent viability. An additional feature may be the use of this flap as a hair-bearing scalp flap. A major advantage to this flap is the invisible donor site, well camouflaged in the patient's hair-bearing scalp in the temporal region, and the minimal contour deformity with harvest of this thin layer of fascia.

Vascular Anatomy. The temporoparietal fascial flap is given a robust blood supply from the superficial temporal artery. Its venous outflow is provided through the superficial temporal vein. These vessels branch in the temporal area

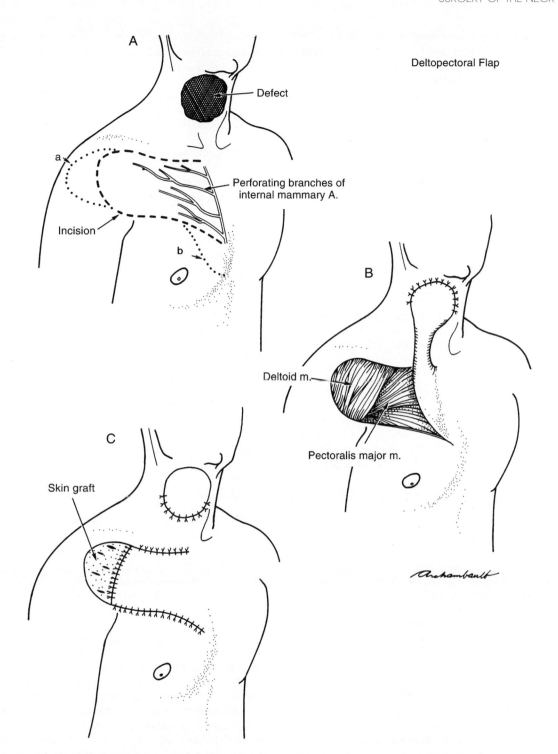

Deltopectoral Flap

A

Defect

a

Perforating branches of
internal mammary A.

Incision

b

B

Deltoid m.

Pectoralis major m.

C

Skin graft

Archambault

FIGURE 2–34. Medially based horizontally pedicled chest skin flap. *A,* The usual incisions for the medially based horizontal pedicled chest skin flap are indicated by interrupted lines.

The superior horizontal incision is extended from the level of the sternoclavicular joint, at a level just below the clavicle, to the superior deltoid region.

The inferior horizontal incision extends from the lower deltoid region across the chest, a few centimeters above the nipple. The lateral incision is made according to the length of flap necessary. The flap may be extended over the deltoid as indicated by *dotted line a.*

The medial aspect of the inferior horizontal incision can be extended inferiorly to widen the base as indicated by *dotted line, b.*

B, This flap is elevated in a plane that includes the fascia overlying the pectoralis major and deltoid muscles. The medially based horizontal chest flap may be delayed, nondelayed, or tubed. Usually, it is not necessary to delay this flap.

C, The denuded area over the deltoid muscle is covered with split-thickness skin graft following return of the unused portion of pedicled skin flap to its anatomic position. *D,* The inferior aspect of the cervical repair is sutured following section of the pedicled skin flap.

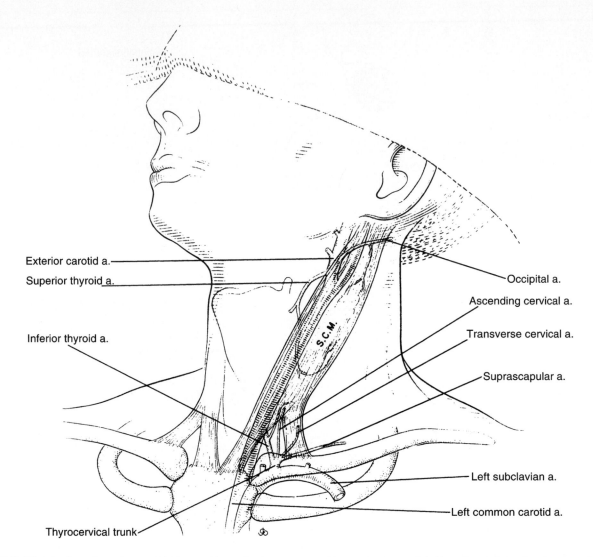

Exterior carotid a.

Superior thyroid a.

Inferior thyroid a.

S.C.M.

Occipital a.

Ascending cervical a.

Transverse cervical a.

Suprascapular a.

Left subclavian a.

Left common carotid a.

Thyrocervical trunk

FIGURE 2–35. Blood supply to the sternocleidomastoid muscle: the sternomastoid artery leaving occipital branches and entering the sternocleidomastoid muscle; branches of superior thyroid artery to sternocleidomastoid muscle; branches from thyrocervical trunk inferiorly by way of the transverse cervical artery and inferior thyroid artery.

into an anterior and posterior branch. The flap is usually elevated with care to transfer at least one of these two branches.

Flap Harvest and Donor Site Closure. The TPFF can usually be harvested without shaving the hair. The superficial temporal artery is outlined preoperatively using a Doppler ultrasound. The standard approach is an extension of a facelift incision from the preauricular area. This is terminated superiorly in a Y-shaped incision to allow greater exposure of the superior most aspect of the temporoparietal fascia. The initial skin incision is made to the level of the subcutaneous tissue. The flap is elevated anteriorly, superiorly, and posteriorly in a plane immediately below the hair follicles. It is the elevation of the scalp flaps that is the tedious portion of this procedure. The dissection must be in a plane immediately below the hair follicles. Elevation too superficially will cause damage to the hair follicles, which would result in hair loss. Dissection too deeply can cause disruption of the superficial temporal vessels and risk flap

viability. When dissecting anteriorly, care must be used to not injure the frontal branch of the facial nerve. The structure can usually be located along the line between a point that is 0.5 cm below the tragus to a point 2 cm above the lateral brow. Both the anterior and posterior branches of the superficial temporal artery are identified and captured in the flap. Once the skin flaps are elevated, mobilization of the temporoparietal fascial flap then begins at the level of the superior temporal line. The medial plane of dissection is in the avascular plane of loose areolar tissue just lateral to the true muscular fascia of the temporalis muscle. Dissection is done from distal or superior to proximal or inferior. Care must be used as the flap is dissected inferiorly, particularly around the helical attachment as the vein can sometimes run more posteriorly than the artery and can be injured at this point of dissection. The flap elevation can be taken as far as the tragus, but usually not beyond.

Donor site closure is rather simple. A large suction drain is placed, and then a single layer closure is performed of the scalp.

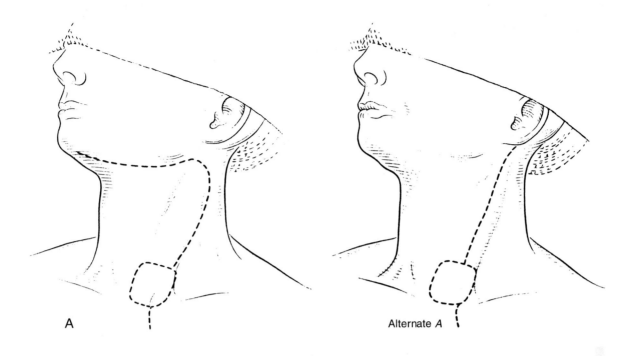

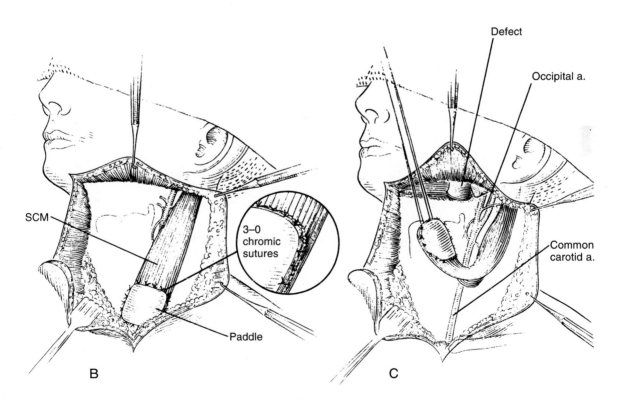

FIGURE 2-36. *A,* The incision for a functional neck dissection is indicated. The size of the supraclavicular skin paddle should not exceed 5 to 6 cm. *Alternate A,* The incision for the sternocleidomastoid myocutaneous flap when a radical neck dissection is not performed.

B, The skin paddle is secured to the inferior aspect of the sternocleidomastoid muscle using No. 3-0 chromic catgut sutures. The sutures pass through the muscle and subcutaneous layers.

C, The sternocleidomastoid muscle has been sectioned just above the sternum and clavicle and is being elevated to close a defect in the posterior tongue and floor of mouth.

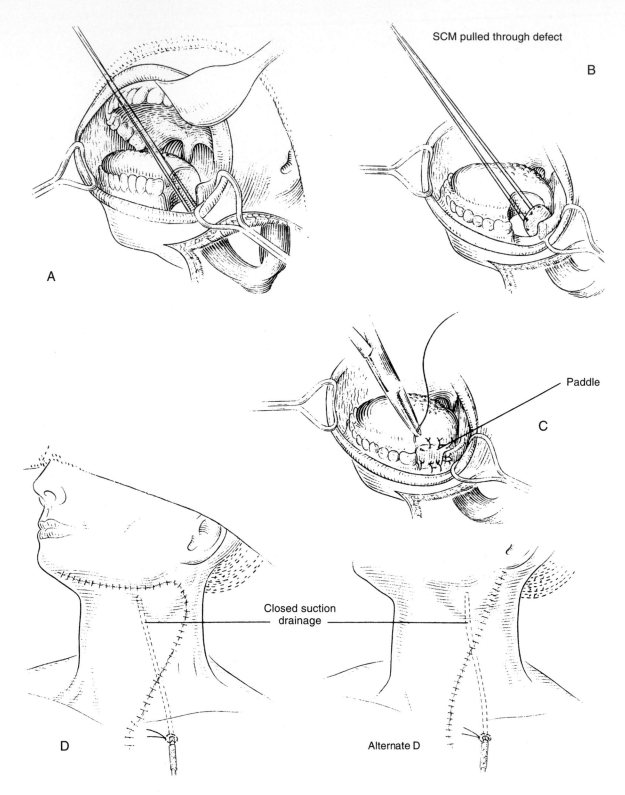

FIGURE 2–37. *A* and *B,* The sternocleidomastoid muscle and skin paddle are elevated to repair a defect in the posterior tongue and floor of mouth. *C,* The skin paddle is secured in place. *D,* The subcutaneous layers and skin have been repaired and closed-suction drainage applied.

The authors find this flap extremely versatile in the reconstruction of a variety of head and neck defects. It is used for reconstruction of the external ear and defects of the scalp and orbit and is particularly useful in obliteration of the mastoid after revision surgery for chronic otitis media.

A major limitation of the temporoparietal fascial flap is that it is pedicled and has a limited arc of rotation. When vascular pedicle length is a problem, it can be transferred as free tissue transfer. The vessels, although small, can be successfully anastomosed to vessels elsewhere in the head and

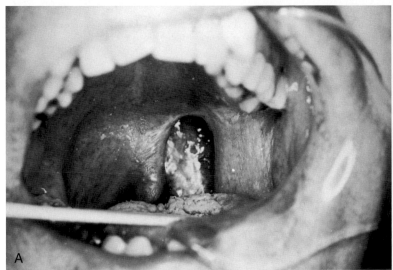

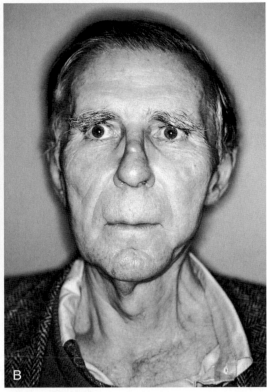

FIGURE 2–38. *A,* Photograph of sternocleidomastoid muscle myocutaneous flap in place 1 year postoperatively. The patient underwent removal of persistent tumor of the base of the tongue and retromolar trigone 8 months following 6500 rads of radiation therapy. *B,* Photograph of the patient from the front side 1 year after sternocleidomastoid repair, following resection of left base of tongue and retromolar trigone.

neck. Alopecia is a possible disadvantage; again, this is related to inappropriate scalp flap elevation. Although the frontal branch of the facial nerve is at risk for injury, careful adherence to the anatomic location of the frontal branch at the lateral eyebrow should avoid this problem.

Pericranial Flap

The pericranial flap is a reliable flap for repair of defects of the anterior cranial fossa following craniofacial resection (Fig. 2–40 *A–D*).

The pericranium consists of two layers of soft tissue, the periosteum, which is firmly adherent to the calvarium, and the loose connective tissue, which is also known as the subgaleal layer. It receives its blood supply from the supratrochlear and supraorbital vessels.

Technique of Flap Harvest and Donor Site Closure. In the harvest of this flap, usually the oncologic nature of the resection requires that a bicoronal incision be outlined. Once the bicoronal skin incision is made, dissection is taken down to, but not through, the subgaleal layer. The scalp posterior to the incision is elevated in the subgaleal plane. This is done for a distance of 2 to 3 cm. This allows lengthening of the overall pericranial flap. An incision is then made in the pericranium at this level of posterior scalp elevation and then the anterior scalp flap is elevated in the subperiosteal plane. This is brought as far forward as the brow as is necessary to obtain the anterior craniotomy exposure. Once the ablation is completed and reconstruction begins, the outline of the pericranial flap is then made in the downwardly turned an-

terior scalp flap. This is widely based to capture the supratrochlear and supraorbital vessels. The flap is elevated by dissecting from distal to proximal in the subgaleal plane, mobilizing the pericranial flap off of the anterior scalp flap. It may then be draped into the ablative defect essentially along the separation of the nose from the intracranial cavity. This flap is usually placed inferior or on the nasal surface of any dural reconstruction. The pericranial flap is sewn into place posteriorly, usually by tacking it to the dura in the area of the planum sphenoidale. Although the pericranial flap will accept the skin graft and is highly vascularized, in most cases it is left to mucosalize on the nasal surface and no skin graft is necessary. Although the primary use of the pericranial flap is reconstruction of the anterior cranial base after craniofacial resection without orbital exenteration, it is also useful for repair of cerebrospinal fluid rhinorrhea after major skull base trauma that does not resolve spontaneously. In cases where a craniofacial resection is performed with orbital exenteration, the defect is usually reconstructed with free tissue transfer such as a rectus abdominis free flap.

FREE FLAPS IN HEAD AND NECK RECONSTRUCTION

Fascial and Fasciocutaneous Flaps

Radial Forearm Free Flap

The radial forearm free flap (Fig. 2–41) was first introduced as a fasciocutaneous flap in 1981 and subsequently used for

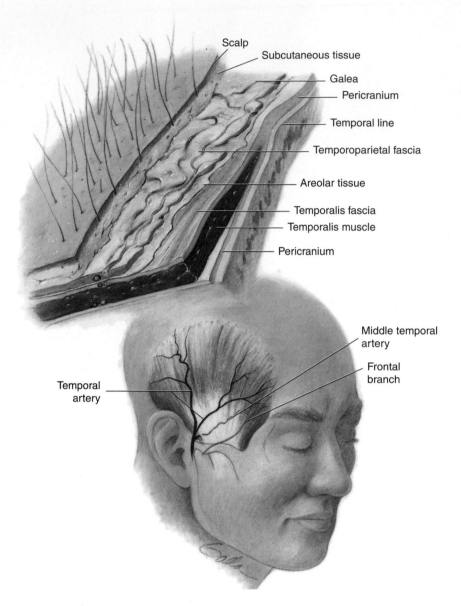

FIGURE 2-39. Anatomy of the temporoparietal region.

reconstruction of the oral cavity in 1983. This flap allows great flexibility in its use for head and neck reconstruction. It has a rich vascular supply from the radial artery. It is thin and pliable and has become the most commonly used soft tissue flap for head and neck reconstruction.

Anatomy. The radial artery arises from the brachial artery, just distal to the antecubital fossa. The vessel travels between the brachioradialis and the flexor carpi radialis muscles as it travels distally in the forearm. After emerging from deep to these two muscles, it travels in the lateral intermuscular septum of the forearm. It is through the lateral inner muscular septum that branches from the radial artery travel to reach the overlying skin and fascia. The artery is accompanied by a paired vein, its venae comitantes. These veins drain toward the antecubital fossa. In addition, the large cutaneous veins of the forearm, the cephalic vein and the basilic vein, also provide excellent outflow to this flap.

One may use either the superficial system or deep system of veins. Many surgeons prefer to take them as a single system by dissecting the venous outflow into the antecubital fossa to the communicating branch, which unites both systems. Typically then a single venous anastomosis will provide outflow to both superficial and deep systems.

The skin of the radial forearm free flap receives its sensory innervation by the lateral and medial antebrachial cutaneous nerves. The lateral antebrachial cutaneous nerve is the primary sensory nerve to the forearm. It closely follows the path of the cephalic vein. A sensate neurofasciocutaneous flap can be transferred by performing a neurorrhaphy from the lateral antebrachial nerve to a sensory nerve in the head and neck.

Flap Design and Harvest. Before using the radial forearm free flap, one must be certain that the ulnar artery adequately perfuses the palm and thumb. This can be assessed

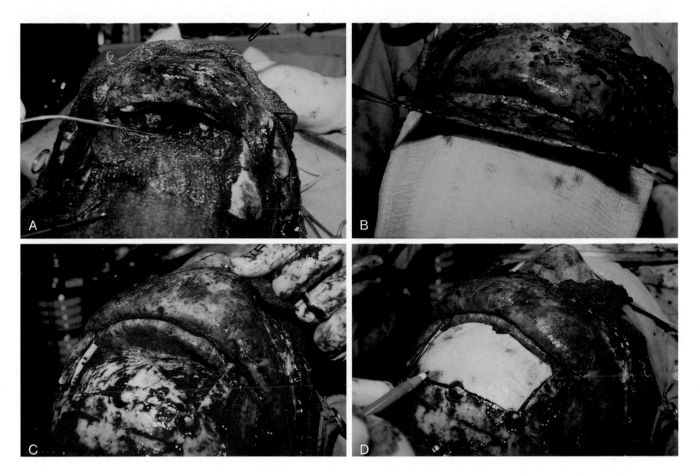

FIGURE 2-40. Clinical example of the pericranial flap for anterior cranial base reconstruction after craniofacial resection for esthesioneuroblastoma. *A,* Surgical defect; *B,* Pericranial flap elevated; *C,* Pericranial flap rotated into anterior cranial base defect; *D,* Craniotomy bone flap replaced.

using the Allen's test. In performing the Allen's test, both the radial and ulnar arteries are palpated at the wrist and occluded. The hand is then raised over the patient's head and is vigorously opened and closed allowing exsanguination of the palm. The palm is then brought to a neutral position, and the ulnar pulse is released. Within a few seconds, there should be a blush of blood into the thenar area. If not, the ulnar artery does not adequately supply the thumb and an alternative flap must be used.

Flap harvest begins by outlining its dimensions based on the template created from the surgical defect. This is designed so that the cutaneous portion of the flap overlies the distal radial artery. If the flap is to be designed as a buried flap for pharyngeal reconstruction, a modification can be made to allow exteriorization of a monitored segment. The radial artery as well as its draining cutaneous veins and the location of the medial and lateral antebrachial cutaneous nerves are outlined to be captured by the flap skin paddle. Before prepping the forearm, a tourniquet is placed around the arm just above the antecubital fossa. Just before flap harvest, the arm is then exsanguinated, and the tourniquet is inflated to 70 to 90 mm Hg greater than the patient's systolic pressure. Once the arm is exsanguinated, the flap is incised first along its radial aspect. Dissection continues medially until the lateral intermuscular septum is encountered. The plane of dissection in this flap elevation is immediately above the muscular fascia and peritenon of the muscle ten-

dons. The superficial branches of the radial nerve are identified and preserved. The ulnar aspect is incised and elevated in a subfascial plane until the lateral intermuscular septum is encountered. Between the tendons of the brachioradialis and flexor carpi radialis, the radial artery is identified in the distal forearm. The artery and its accompanying veins are ligated. The artery, intermuscular septum, and flap are then elevated from distal to proximal until the proximal end of the skin paddle is encountered. If the flap is being harvested with an ellipse to be used as an external cutaneous monitor, then an incision is made from the proximal end of the skin paddle to the monitored segment. The ellipse that is used as a monitor is incised down through the skin and dermis only. An incision is then made from the proximal aspect of the monitor toward the antecubital fossa. The skin in the intervening areas between the skin paddle and monitor is then elevated in a subdermal plane. This preserves a bridge of fascia between the skin paddle and the external monitor to ensure adequate vascularity to the skin monitor. The radial artery, venae comitantes, cutaneous draining veins, and antebrachial cutaneous nerves are then followed proximally as far as needed based on the distance of the defect to the recipient vessels in the neck. The tourniquet is then released, and the flap is allowed to perfuse. Bleeders along the flap and in the forearm are then ligated or cauterized. The flap is allowed to perfuse until it is ready to be transferred to the head and neck for reconstruction.

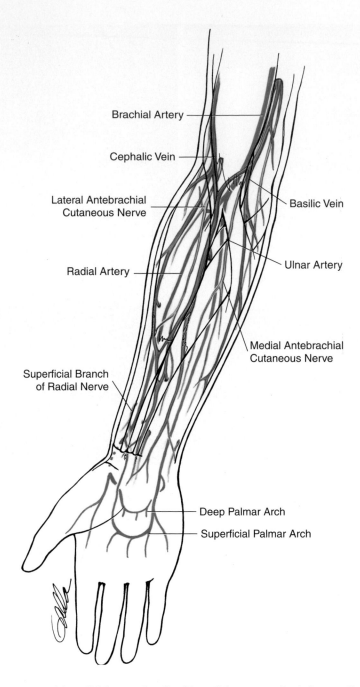

Brachial Artery

Cephalic Vein

Lateral Antebrachial
Cutaneous Nerve

Basilic Vein

Radial Artery

Ulnar Artery

Medial Antebrachial
Cutaneous Nerve

Superficial Branch
of Radial Nerve

Deep Palmar Arch

Superficial Palmar Arch

FIGURE 2–41. The neurovascular anatomy of the radial forearm free flap. The radial artery supplies inflow; outflow is either through the cutaneous veins of the forearm (usually the cephalic) or the venae comitantes of the radial artery. The lateral antebrachial cutaneous nerve is used most frequently as the neural supply to the flap.

The donor site closure is accomplished by undermining the edges of the wound in attempting to partially decrease the overall defect size by tacking the edges of the skin flaps to the soft tissue deficit. Attempts are made to cover the radial sensory nerve with the skin flaps in the dorsum of the forearm. A thick (0.018 inch) split-thickness skin graft is placed over the tendons and muscles of the forearm. A volar plaster splint is then used with an elastic bandage to immobilize the forearm in slight extension for approximately 5 days. The forearm is usually elevated to facilitate venous outflow.

Myocutaneous and Muscular Flaps

Rectus Abdominis Free Flap

The rectus abdominis free flap (Fig. 2–42), based on the deep inferior epigastric artery and vein, has assumed a major role in the reconstruction of major head and neck defects including defects of the base of skull. Because of its distant location from the ablative site, this flap facilitates simultaneous two-team surgery. Its vascular pedicle is reliable and large caliber and allows considerable flexibility in reconstruction of head and neck defects. It may be used either as

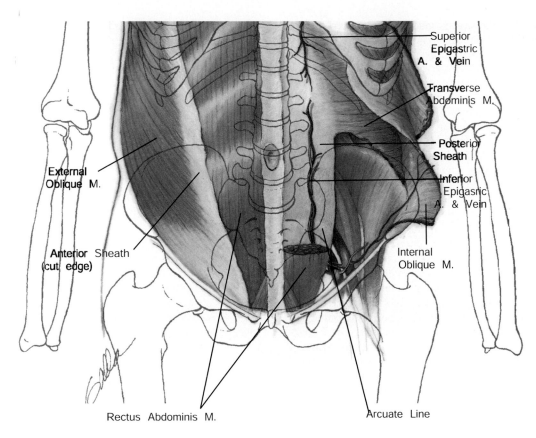

FIGURE 2–42. The rectus abdominis muscle has been removed from the rectus sheath. Note that the deep epigastric vessels are deep to the muscle. The arcuate line is noted midway between the umbilicus and the pubis.

a myocutaneous flap or as a muscle-only flap. Donor site morbidity is minimal.

Flap Anatomy. The rectus abdominis muscle originates from the pubis and inserts into the costal cartilage of ribs 5 to 7. Its primary function is that of a flexor of the trunk. The rectus abdominis muscle has two dominant vascular pedicles, the deep superior epigastric artery and vein and the deep inferior epigastric artery and vein. The deep superior epigastric artery is a terminal branch of the internal mammary artery and supplies the superior aspect of the muscle. The deep inferior epigastric artery is a branch off the external iliac artery. These two vessels run in a longitudinal direction to form an area of anastomosis above the umbilicus. The diameter of the deep inferior epigastric artery is approximately 2.5 to 3 mm and the diameter of the vein is 3 to 4 mm. It is the deep inferior epigastric artery and veins that are the primary vessels that supply the rectus abdominis free flap.

The rectus abdominis muscle is found within the rectus sheath in the anterior abdominal wall. The rectus sheath anatomy is critical to understanding harvest of this flap. The rectus sheath is divided into an anterior and a posterior layer. The anterior layer of the rectus sheath above the arcuate line is composed of a condensation of fascia from the external oblique aponeurosis and the anterior lamina of the internal oblique aponeurosis. The posterior layer of the rectus sheath above the arcuate line is composed of the posterior lamina of the internal oblique aponeurosis, the aponeurosis of the transversus abdominis muscle, and the transversalis fascia. Below the arcuate line, the anterior layer of rectus sheath is composed of the aponeurosis of the external oblique, internal oblique, and transversus abdominis muscles. The posterior layer of the rectus sheath below the arcuate line is composed of only transversalis fascia. The clinical implication of this anatomy is that if one removes the anterior layer of rectus sheath below the arcuate line, the rectus sheath is considerably weakened and requires prosthetic reconstruction. The arcuate line can be located halfway between the pubic symphysis and the umbilicus. The rectus abdominis muscle has three or four tendonous inscriptions that segmentalize the muscle. These areas represent fusion of the anterior layer of rectus sheath to the muscle and must be sharply dissected during the flap harvest. Musculocutaneous perforators that pass vertically through the muscle to supply the overlying skin are found in greatest abundance in the peri-umbilical area. The axial orientation of these perforators follows a line from the umbilicus to the tip of the scapula.

Flap Design and Harvest. The rectus abdominis muscle may be designed as either a muscle-only flap or a myocutaneous flap. When transferred as a myocutaneous flap, the skin paddle can be oriented vertically, directly over the muscle, or oriented obliquely with a portion of the flap overlying the external oblique aponeurosis lateral to the lateral border of the rectus sheath. When harvested as a muscle-only flap, a paramedian incision is made directly overlying the rectus abdominis muscle. The skin and subcutaneous tissue are incised, and the anterior layer of the rectus sheath is opened. The anterior layer of the rectus sheath is then opened in its entirety along the length of the rectus abdominis muscle. The muscle is then transected superiorly from its superior attachments at the costal margin and elevated from superior to inferior. The vascular pedicle may be identified on the lateral and deep surface of the muscle as the muscle is elevated out of the rectus sheath. The vascular pedicle is then followed proximally toward the external iliac vessels.

Typically when designing a rectus abdominis myocutaneous flap with a vertically oriented skin paddle, the paddle is outlined in the periumbilical area overlying the muscle above the arcuate line. The skin surrounding the paddle is incised down to and through the anterior layer of the rectus sheath. From the paddle, an inferior incision is made through the skin, subcutaneous tissue, and anterior layer of rectus sheath. The muscle is then exposed by opening the anterior layer of rectus sheath and its overlying subcutaneous tissue and skin. The same procedure is then performed along the superior aspect of the skin paddle. The muscle with its overlying skin may then be elevated out of the rectus sheath after transection of the superior most aspect of the muscle. The vascular pedicle is dissected inferiorly down to the external iliac vessels. The final portion of flap elevation requires separation of the inferior aspect of the muscle from its insertion onto the pubic symphysis and final pedicled dissection. Transection of the inferior most muscle facilitates final pedicle dissection.

When designing an obliquely oriented skin paddle of the rectus abdominis myocutaneous flap, the base of the skin paddle is in the periumbilical area. The oblique portion of the flap is oriented towards the tip of the scapula. The skin paddle is incised down to and through the level of the anterior layer of the rectus sheath except laterally. Laterally over the external oblique aponeurosis, a full fasciocutaneous flap is elevated and mobilized medially until the lateral border of the rectus sheath is encountered. Once the lateral border of the sheath is encountered, the lateral sheath incision is made just medial to the lateral border of the rectus sheath, thereby completing the fascial incision around the skin paddle. A vertical incision is then made inferior to the skin paddle through the skin and rectus sheath exposing the entire muscle. The flap dissection then proceeds as previously described.

Donor site closure of the rectus abdominis muscle-only flap where there has been no fascial sheath resection is very straightforward. Simply the anterior layer of the rectus sheath is approximated using heavy, nonabsorbable suture. The subcutaneous and cutaneous layers are then closed after placement of closed suction drains.

Closure of the donor site after myocutaneous flap harvest does require either a direct approximation of the medial and lateral borders of the rectus sheath in the area of fascial harvest or a reconstruction of the anterior sheath using mesh. An alternative treatment is to approximate the edges of the defect in the anterior layer of rectus sheath all above the arcuate line to the posterior layer of rectus sheath. This relies on the posterior layer rectus sheath above the arcuate line to be hardy enough to prevent hernia formation.

A potential disadvantage of the rectus abdominis donor site is incisional hernia. For this reason, meticulous closure of the rectus sheath is imperative. This flap is contraindicated in patients who have had extensive intra-abdominal surgery in whom the inferior epigastric vessels have potentially been damaged. The authors have used this flap successfully in patients who have undergone cesarean section delivery.

Latissimus Dorsi Flap

The latissimus dorsi flap (Fig. 2–43) may be used as either a pedicled or free flap to reconstruct a variety of soft tissue head and neck defects. This section will outline the latissimus dorsi flap dissection as if it were to be a free tissue transfer.

Anatomy. Latissimus dorsi muscle is a large muscle that takes origin from the spinous processes of the lower six thoracic vertebrae, thoracolumbar fascia, lumbar sacral spinous processes, the posterior iliac crest, and a lateral portion of the lower four ribs. It forms a single tendon to attach to the intertubercular groove of the humerus. Superiorly this is partially covered by the trapezius muscle, and on its deep surface it is superficial to the serratus anterior and external oblique muscles. The muscle is innervated by the thoracodorsal nerve. Its action is to adduct, medially rotate, and extend the upper extremity.

The thoracodorsal artery, which is a branch of the subscapular artery, is a primary vascular supply to the latissimus dorsi muscle. The subscapular artery divides in the axilla into the circumflex scapular and thoracodorsal arteries. The circumflex scapular artery courses over the scapular bone. The thoracodorsal artery continues inferiorly through the axilla along the undersurface of the latissimus dorsi muscle. On entering the muscle, the vessel divides into lateral and medial branches. The lateral branch is found 2.5 cm medial to the anterior margin of the muscle. The medial branch is found 3.5 cm inferior to the superior border of the muscle. The thoracodorsal artery does supply a branch to the serratus anterior muscle before it enters the latissimus dorsi muscle.

Flap Elevation and Donor Site Closure. The harvest of the latissimus dorsi muscle requires that the patient be placed in a lateral decubitus position. It is important to place axillary roll in the contralateral or dependent axilla to prevent stretch injury to the brachial plexus. The ipsilateral upper extremity is prepped and well into the cervical area as well as past midline and down past the area of the iliac crest. A sterile stocking is placed on the ipsilateral arm. The vascular pedicle to the latissimus dorsi muscle is located by drawing a line along the anterior border of the muscle 10 cm inferior to the axillary artery. The location of this pedicle as it enters the latissimus dorsi muscle can be confirmed with a Doppler ultrasound. The position of the skin paddle is influenced by the location and dimensions of the site to be reconstructed. The skin paddle should not extend beyond the muscle. Flap harvest begins by incising a line that parallels the lateral border of the latissimus dorsi muscle from the axilla. The anterior border of the muscle is identified and carefully reflected off the serratus anterior muscle. At this point, the vascular pedicle is identified on the undersurface of the

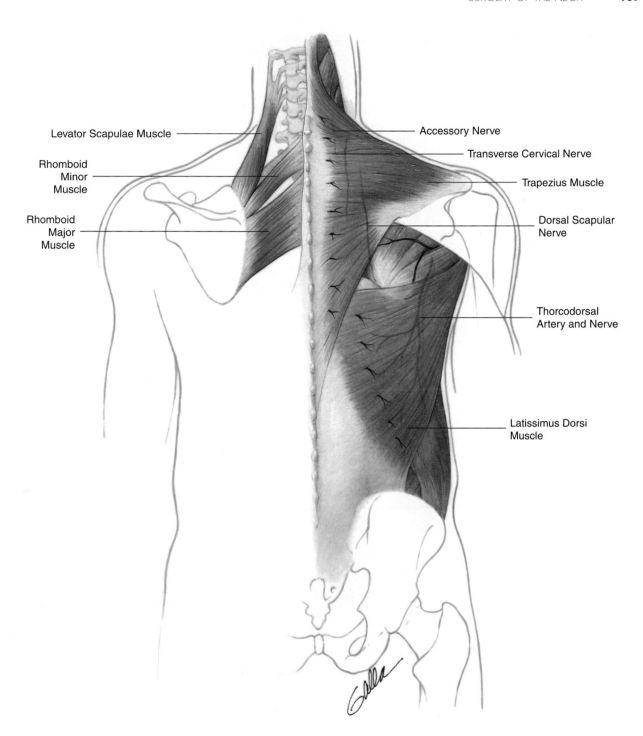

Levator Scapulae Muscle

Rhomboid
Minor
Muscle

Rhomboid
Major
Muscle

Accessory Nerve

Transverse Cervical Nerve

Trapezius Muscle

Dorsal Scapular
Nerve

Thorcodorsal
Artery and Nerve

Latissimus Dorsi
Muscle

FIGURE 2–43. Latissimus dorsi flap. The vascular supply to the latissimus dorsi muscle is through the thoracodorsal artery, a branch of the subscapular artery.

muscle and dissected superiorly into the axilla. Once the vascular pedicle can be identified, the remaining skin incisions around the skin paddle are completed. The skin is then elevated from around the skin paddle exposing the muscle in its entirety. The distal attachments of the latissimus dorsi muscle are then transected and the flap is mobilized to the axilla completely pedicled on its vascular supply. The donor site typically can be closed primarily. Suction drains are kept in the donor site for 5 to 7 days.

This flap is used primarily for large lateral skull base defects and in cases of total glossectomy reconstruction where the rectus abdominis muscle is not available. In the total tongue reconstruction, the potential exists to maintain muscle bulk by performing a neurorrhaphy to the stump of the hypoglossal nerve. This helps to prevent atrophy of the flap and maintains good bulk, which is critical to total tongue reconstruction. A disadvantage of this flap is that it does require the patient to be placed in a lateral decubitus position, which can make simultaneous two-team surgery difficult and increase overall operating time.

Composite Free Flaps

Scapular Osteocutaneous Flap

The scapular osteocutaneous flap (Fig. 2–44) was first recognized as a potential flap for composite soft tissue and bone reconstruction by Saijo in 1978. This flap was later popularized for oromandibular reconstruction by Schwartz. The authors found it useful for both oromandibular reconstruction as well as midface reconstruction.

Anatomy. The scapular flap is based on the circumflex scapular artery and vein, a branch off of the subscapular artery. The subscapular artery bifurcates into the thoracodorsal artery and the circumflex scapular artery. The circumflex scapular artery passes laterally through the triangular space that is formed by the long head of the triceps, the teres major muscle and the teres minor muscle. As the vessel passes through the triangular space, it supplies the

bone of the lateral border of the scapula. The vessel then terminates as horizontal and descending branches in the skin and fascia overlying the scapula. The horizontal branch is found 2 cm below the spine of the scapula and parallel to its horizontal course. The descending branch parallels the lateral border of the scapula and runs 2 cm medial to that border. The horizontal branch is referred to as the scapular pedicle, and the descending branch is referred to as the parascapular pedicle. The venous outflow to the flap is through its venae comitantes. These drain into the axillary vein.

Flap Design and Harvest. The harvest of the scapular free flap requires the patient to be placed in a lateral decubitus position. Important anatomic landmarks include the scapular spine, the lateral border of the scapula, and the triangular space. The authors usually mark the circumflex scapular artery as it passes through the triangular space by locating it with a Doppler flow meter. The entire upper extremity is prepared as is the shoulder up to the cervical area, the back to midline, and inferiorly down to the iliac crest. A sterile stocking is placed over the ipsilateral arm.

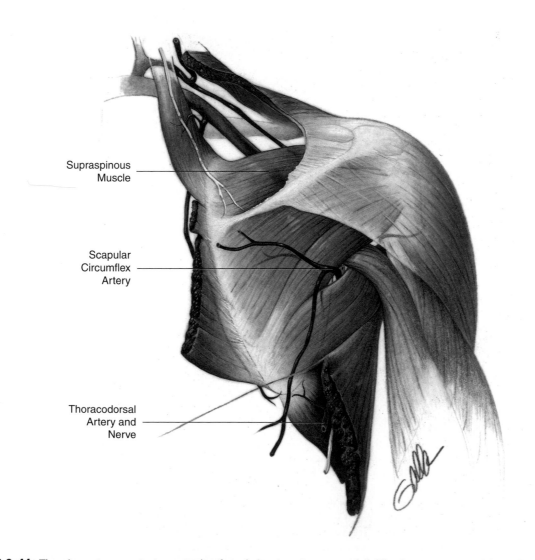

Supraspinous
Muscle

Scapular
Circumflex
Artery

Thoracodorsal
Artery and
Nerve

FIGURE 2–44. The subscapular artery is shown passing through the triangular space and dividing into transverse and descending branches. Note the angular branch from the thoracodorsal artery that supplies the bone of the angle of the scapula.

The cutaneous paddle is outlined depending on the needs of the defect. This may be oriented as a transverse or vertical paddle or may be demarcated as a single large bilobed flap. After the flap is incised, the elevation of the skin paddle proceeds from medial to lateral. Elevation occurs in a plane just above the fascia of the infraspinatus muscle. As the triangular space is approached, the branches of the circumflex scapular artery that supply the fasciocutaneous portion of the flap can be identified. At this point, the lateral most portion of the skin flap is incised. The teres major muscle may then be divided to allow dissection to follow the circumflex scapular vessels proximally to the subscapular artery. At this point, the infraspinatus muscle must be divided vertically from just below the scapular spine to its tip. The lateral border of the scapula is then harvested with a sagittal saw vertically in a direction that parallels the lateral border. The thickness of the bone harvest is dependent on the bony defect. A horizontal incision is then made, allowing full mobilization of the bony segment. This is made superiorly, and care must be used not to involve the glenoid fossa in this cut. Once the bone cuts have been made, the subscapularis muscle is divided sharply and the flap is now fully mobilized on its vascular pedicle. Flap dissection may be completed at the junction of the subscapular artery with the circumflex scapular artery, or, if further vessel length is needed, the thoracodorsal artery may be ligated distal to the circumflex scapular artery and the flap pedicle can be based on the subscapular artery. The subscapular artery may be dissected to the axillary artery. In cases in which a large soft tissue reconstruction is required, the thoracodorsal artery supplying the latissimus dorsi muscle can be preserved with the flap. This allows transfer of both the latissimus dorsi muscle flap and scapular osteocutaneous flap based in the single vascular pedicle.

Donor site closure of the scapular free flap requires a meticulous hemostasis. The authors usually do not reapproximate the teres major muscle. The subcutaneous and skin layers are closed, and two large suction drains are placed in the wound and left there for at least 7 days.

A major disadvantage of the use of the scapular osteocutaneous flap is related to potential donor site morbidity. When harvested as a bone flap, there is a potential for decreased range of motion morbidity of the upper extremity. It has been recommended that the scapular flap not be used in patients who have had a radical neck dissection with sacrifice of cranial nerve XI on the donor side.

Iliac Crest Osteomyocutaneous Flap

The iliac crest donor site (first described by Taylor) is based on the deep circumflex iliac artery and vein. This flap became popular for oromandibular reconstruction (Fig. 2–45) but was believed to be limited by the lack of flexibility allowed by the soft tissue component of the flap. Urken has subsequently modified this flap to include a vascularized internal oblique muscle paddle to improve the soft tissue component to this flap.

Flap Anatomy. The deep circumflex iliac artery and vein take origin from the external iliac vessels just before these vessels pass beneath the inguinal ligament. The deep circumflex iliac vein is found medial to the external iliac artery and must cross this artery to join the deep circumflex iliac artery as it travels toward the iliac crest. These vessels pass obliquely toward the anterior superior spine of the ilium, encased in a fibrinous canal formed between the transversalis fascia and the iliacus fascia. The vascular pedicle then pierces the fascia and the transversus abdominis muscle to lie between the transversus abdominis muscle and the iliacus muscle on the medial aspect of the iliac crest. These vessels supply the iliac crest bone and the skin that borders the lateral aspect of the iliac crest. The largest cutaneous perforator to the lateral iliac skin is the terminal branch of the deep circumflex iliac artery and is found 6 to 8 cm posterior to the anterior superior iliac spine. The ascending branch of the deep inferior epigastric artery and vein originate from the deep circumflex iliac vessels just medial to the anterior superior iliac spine. These vessels form a vascular pedicle on the deep surface of the internal oblique muscle and provide for an axial blood supply to the muscle.

Flap Design and Harvest. In almost all cases, a cutaneous component to this flap is incorporated so that an external skin monitor may be used. The cutaneous portion of this flap may be also used to reconstruct a cervical skin defect or alternatively may be used for intraoral soft tissue coverage.

In positioning the patient for an iliac crest free flap, it is important that the patient have a roll placed under the hip. The flap is outlined, with the lateral border of the iliac crest being identified first. The pulse of the femoral artery and approximate takeoff of the deep inferior epigastric artery and vein are noted and marked. The anterior superior iliac spine and the lateral border of the iliac crest are also marked. The cutaneous paddle is designed so it is centered 6 to 8 cm posterior to the anterior superior iliac spine and slightly cephalad to capture the dominant perforator that represents the termination of the deep circumflex iliac artery. A total of 15 to 18 cm of iliac bone may be harvested.

Flap harvest begins by incising the superior aspect of the elliptical skin paddle that overlies the iliac crest and lateral abdominal wall. Dissection is carried down to the level of the external oblique muscle. The external oblique muscle is then transected, leaving a 3-cm cuff of muscle attached to the medial border of the iliac crest. This preserves the cutaneous perforating vessels. The entire external oblique muscle is then elevated off the internal oblique muscle, exposing the latter. The superior, medial, and inferior attachments of the internal oblique muscle from the costal margin and rectus sheath are identified and taken down sharply. The internal oblique muscle is elevated away from the transversus abdominis muscle. The ascending branch of the deep circumflex iliac artery and vein are identified on the deep surface of the internal oblique muscle. The ascending branch is then traced proximally to the deep circumflex iliac artery and vein. These vessels are dissected to the external iliac vessels. The transversus abdominis muscle is transected, leaving a 3-cm cuff of muscle attached to the medial surface of the iliac crest, again to protect the cutaneous perforators. With the transection of the transversus abdominis muscle, the preperitoneal fat is exposed and mobilized medially away from the iliac crest. This now allows direct identification of the deep circumflex iliac artery and vein as it runs along the medial border of the iliac crest in a groove between the transversus abdominis muscle and iliac muscle.

Once the vessels are identified on the medial border of

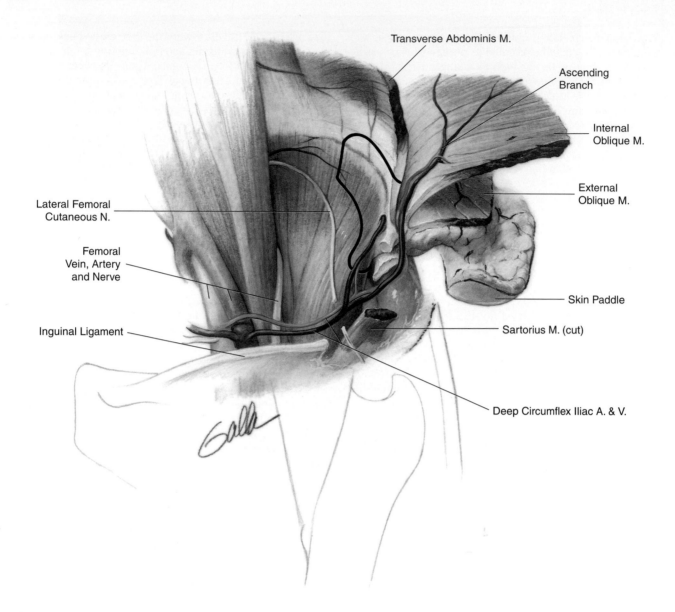

FIGURE 2-45. The blood supply to the iliac crest, internal oblique osseomyocutaneous flap. The DCIA gives off the ascending branch that it is an axial blood supply to the internal oblique muscle. The DCIA continues on the medial aspect of the iliac crest to supply the iliac bone and sends cutaneous perforators to supply the skin laterally.

the ilium, the inferior or lateral skin paddle incisions are made. Dissection is taken down to the lateral border of the iliac crest. The gluteal muscles and the muscles along the lateral aspect of the ilium are dissected in the subperiosteal plane exposing the entire iliac crest. The superior aspect of the iliac crest is then harvested. The length of bone harvested corresponds to the length of the defect being reconstructed. The vertical height of the harvested iliac crest is based on the height of the defect. Transection of the upper aspect of the iliac crest must be done with care so that the deep circumflex iliac artery and vein in the medial aspect of the iliac crest are not injured. Once saw cuts are made, final pedicle dissection is performed and the flap is essentially attached only by its vascular pedicle.

Donor site closure requires meticulous technique. After obtaining hemostasis, two drains are placed deep in the wound. The first layer of closure requires approximation of the transversus abdominis muscle to the iliacus muscle. This is closed using 0 Prolene. If the closure does not appear to be solid, holes may be drilled in the remnant of the iliac crest and a mattress suture may be placed through the transversus abdominis muscle and through the holes placed in the iliac crest bone. The second layer of closure approximates the external oblique muscle to tensor fascia lata and gluteus meatus muscle. The skin and subcutaneous layers are closed.

The greatest disadvantage of the iliac crest donor site is the morbidity. Patients require vigorous physical therapy to rehabilitate their gait. The vast majority of patients are able to resume normal gait after flap harvest. Another disadvantage of this flap is the potential for abdominal wall weakness and hernia formation.

Fibular Osteocutaneous Flap

The fibular free flap (Fig. 2–46) was first described as a potential donor site for vascularized bone transfer in 1975. It has subsequently gained popularity as a complete free flap for oromandibular reconstruction because of its ease of harvest and abundant length of bone available, up to 25 cm. This allows nearly total mandibular reconstruction.

Flap Anatomy. The fibular free osteocutaneous flap has its vascular supply based on the peroneal artery and vein. These vessels supply the fibula both through periosteal blood supply and through a nutrient artery. There are also septocutaneous perforators that supply the skin overlying the lateral aspect of the fibula to allow transfer of a reliable skin paddle with the bone. The origin of the peroneal artery is from the posterior tibial artery approximately 7 cm below the head of the fibula. The vessel is found in a fibrous canal between the tibialis posterior and flexor hallucis longus or alternatively may run in the flexor hallucis longus to descend along the medial aspect of the fibula. A nutrient vessel to the fibula is found 13.8 cm below the fibular head. Preservation of this vessel is not imperative for successful bony flap transfer. The peroneal vessel gives rise to septal, musculocutaneous, and septomuscular vessels that pass posterior to the fibula, either in the lateral intermuscular septum, behind the intermuscular septum, or within the muscles of the posterior compartment to reach the skin of the lateral leg. The greatest number of perforating vessels can be found at the junction of the middle and lower one third of the fibula. It has been reported that approximately 6.25% of specimens probably do not have reliable perforators to the overlying skin.

Flap Design and Harvest. In nearly all cases, a cutaneous paddle is outlined overlying the lateral aspect of the fibula usually at the junction of the middle and lower thirds. The head of the fibula is used as an important landmark for the common peroneal nerve, which lies in a subfascial position just inferior to the fibular head. The superior aspect of the skin incision is terminated inferior to this point. The long axis of the skin paddle is centered over the posterior aspect of the fibula, which corresponds to the location of the lateral intermuscular septum. When planning the incisions for this flap, approximately 8 cm of proximal and distal fibula should be left in place to avoid destabilizing the knee and ankle joints, respectively. A tourniquet is placed above the knee. The entire leg from the knee down is circumferentially prepped. The tourniquet is usually set at 340 mmHg. Dissection begins anteriorly with incision of the anterior component of the skin paddle and the vertical superior and inferior extensions. Dissection continues deeply until the peroneus muscle is encountered. The fascia of the peroneus muscle is incised and followed medially as the peroneus muscles are elevated anteriorly off the fibula. At this point, the septum between the lateral and anterior compartments is encountered and divided, exposing the anterior compartment muscles. The anterior compartment muscles are mobilized sharply off the innerosseus membrane. At this point, it is usually possible to identify the anterior tibial vessel and deep peroneal nerve, which are preserved. The interosseous membrane is then divided just medial to the fibula. At this point, proximal and distal osteotomies are made in the fibula which allows lateral retraction of the fibula. At the point of the distal osteotomy, the peroneal vessels are identified deep to the tibialis posterior muscle and are ligated. The peroneal artery is then followed from distal to proximal by dividing the tibialis posterior muscle covering it. Dissection continues to the junction of the peroneal artery and the posterior tibial artery. Perforators into the muscles medial to the vascular pedicle are identified and ligated. At this point, the tourniquet is released and the posterior limb of the skin incision is made down to the fascia overlying the soleus mus-

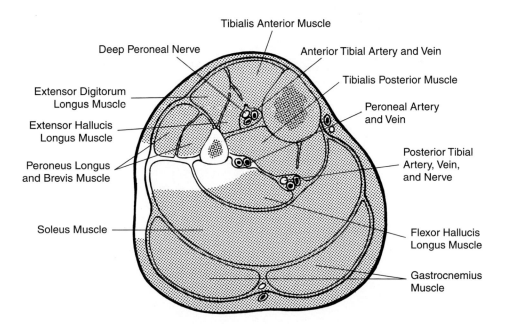

FIGURE 2–46. The peroneal artery supplies the fibula through both a medullary and periosteal blood supply. Septocutaneous and musculocutaneous perforators supply the skin overlying the lateral thigh.

cle. With lateral retraction of the fibula and its overlying skin paddle, an incision is made through the soleus muscle and through the flexor hallucis longus muscle. As this transection of muscle proceeds, care is used to check both on the medial and lateral aspect of the flap to see that a cuff of muscle is taken with the flap, therby ensuring protection of the cutaneous blood supply to the lateral skin paddle. The flap is then elevated on its peroneal vessels.

Donor site closure is straightforward. No attempts are made to recreate or to reapproximate the fascia of the compartments of the leg. The skin can usually be approximated primarily, however, at times a split-thickness skin graft is required to reconstruct the area from where the cutaneous paddle was harvested. A posterior splint is placed at the time of donor site closure and is left in place for 5 days after which the patient may begin partial weight bearing and then may increase ambulation as tolerated.

There are few disadvantages to the fibular osteocutaneous free flap. Initially it was believed that the skin paddle was not very reliable, but as its utilization is increased, it is clear that this is not the case. One disadvantage is limited flexibility of the skin paddle relative to the bone, but this is usually not a problem in most cases of oromandibular reconstruction.

All of the authors' patients undergo a preoperative magnetic resonance angiography of the lower extremities to assess the circulation to the distal lower extremity.

Chapter 3
Surgery of the Salivary Glands

WILLIAM W. MONTGOMERY   MACK L. CHENEY   MARK A. VARVARES

PAROTID GLAND

Surgical Anatomy

The parotid gland is the largest of the three salivary glands, weighing from 14 to 28 g. Microscopically it is classified as a compound tubuloalveolar gland of the serous type.

The parotid gland is flat and usually triangular in shape. It is bounded posteriorly by the mastoid process, anteriorly by the ramus of the mandible, superiorly by the zygomatic arch, and inferiorly by a line joining the tip of the mastoid process with the angle of the mandible. The wedge-shaped deep lobe extends inward toward the pharyngeal wall and lies in close approximation to the great vessels of the parapharyngeal space.

The gland is enclosed within a fibrous capsule that sends septa into the glandular substance, dividing it into lobules. The superficial layer (parotido-masseteric fascia) extends from the masseter muscle over the convex surface of the parotid gland and attaches to the lower border of the zygomatic arch superiorly and the cervical fascia over the sternocleidomastoid muscle posteriorly. The deep layer passes posterior to the gland, behind the ramus of the mandible, and fuses with the fascia of the posterior belly of the digastric muscle. The portion of the fascial sheet that extends from the styloid process to the posterior border of the mandible is called the stylomandibular membrane.

Of surgical importance is the parotid compartment, which consists of the space in which the nerves, vessels, and lymphatics associated with the gland lie (see Figs. 3–7 to 3–15). The compartment is formed by the bony and muscle boundaries. It may be divided into the following planes.

1. *The floor: The* styloid process, the transverse process of the atlas, the posterior belly of the digastric muscle, and the styloglossus, stylohyoid, and stylopharyngeus muscles form the floor of the parotid gland.

2. *Anterior plane:* Anteriorly, the compartment is bounded by the ramus of the mandible, covered inferiorly by the masseter muscle. Inferomedially, the internal pterygoid muscle inserts into the angle of the mandible, and the external pterygoid muscle inserts into the anterior surface of the temporomandibular joint and head of the mandible.

3. *Superior plane:* Superiorly, the boundaries are the external auditory meatus and the head of the mandible.

4. *Posterior plane:* Posteriorly, the compartment extends to the anterior surface of the mastoid process and the anterior border of the sternocleidomastoid muscle.

5. *Superficial plane:* Superficially, the compartment is bounded by the skin, superficial fascia, facial branch of the great auricular nerve, and lymph nodes.

In a comprehensive study of parotid anatomy, Gaughran pointed out that the parotid gland is really unilobar. However, superficial and deep portions of the gland are recognizable as subdivisions. In addition to the five surfaces of the parotid compartment mentioned above, other portions of glandular extensions have been described by Gaughran, as follows.

A. Superficial extensions
   1. Condylar process; medial to the temporofacial nerve rami and covers the base of the transverse facial vessels.
   2. Meatal process; rests on the meatal incisions of the cartilage of the external acoustic meatus.
   3. Posterior process; lies between the mastoid process and the sternocleidomastoid muscle, just lateral to the internal jugular vein.
B. Deep extensions
   1. Glenoid process; rests on the vaginal process of the tympanic part of the temporal bone.
   2. Stylomandibular process (carotid process); rests on the anterior surface of the styloid process. The external carotid hooks around the posterior border of this process, and the internal carotid lies medial to it, as does the lateral pharynx.

Arteries Located Within the Parotid Compartment
The *external carotid artery* ascends from under the cover of the digastric and stylohyoid muscles and lies in a groove on the deep surface of the glands. It enters the compartment at a point intersecting a line extending from the mastoid tip to the angle of the mandible. The *postauricular artery* is the first branch of the external carotid in the compartment. This artery usually lies deep and posterior to the facial nerve, but it may be found lateral to the nerve. It sends off an auricu-

lar branch at the anterior border of the mastoid process. The stylomastoid branch enters the canal deep to the seventh nerve. The external carotid artery ascends posterior to the stylomandibular process of the parotid and bifurcates into two terminal branches opposite the neck of the mandible. The first branch, the *internal maxillary artery,* courses forward between the sphenomandibular ligament and the mandibular neck. It passes forward between the sphenomandibular ligament and the mandibular neck. It passes through the stylomandibular fascia, then between the temporal muscle and lateral pterygoid muscle to enter the pterygoid space. The *superficial temporal artery* is the second terminal branch of the external carotid artery, originating opposite the neck of the mandible. It ascends under the cover of the parotid, giving off rami to the parotid. In its ascent, it is accompanied by the auriculotemporal nerve and lies intimately associated with the superficial temporal veins. The *transverse facial artery* is a branch of the superficial temporal artery. It originates in the region of the mandibular notch and may or may not traverse the parotid gland. In its forward course, it passes below the lower border of the zygomatic arch, lying 1 cm above the parotid duct. It is accompanied by zygomatic rami of the facial nerve and sends branches to the parotid, its duct, and the masseter muscle.

Veins Located Within the Parotid Compartment

The trunk of the *superficial temporal vein* is formed above the arch of the zygoma. It passes down into the parotid, uniting with the maxillary vein to form the posterior facial, or *retromandibular, vein.* Tributaries from the pterygoid plexus form the *internal maxillary vein.* It passes between the sphenomandibular ligament and neck of the mandible to form, with the superficial temporal vein, the *posterior facial vein.* The posterior facial vein then descends to the posterior parotid compartment, superficial to the external carotid artery, and runs along the dorsal margin of the ramus of the mandible. It divides into anterior and posterior branches. The anterior branch passes forward and unites with the *anterior facial vein* to form the *common facial vein.* The posterior branch joins the *postauricular vein* to become the *external jugular vein.* Of surgical importance is the fact that, as the postauricular vein emerges from the tail of the parotid gland, the lower branches of the cervicofacial division may be found anterior and superficial to the vein. Although variations do occur, most peripheral branches of the facial nerve are superficial to the venous system.

Nerves Located Within the Parotid Compartment

The auriculotemporal and facial nerves are included in the parotid compartment. The auriculotemporal nerve is a sensory branch of the posterior division of the mandibular nerve (fifth cranial nerve). It enters the parotid compartment on the medial side of the mandible and accompanies the superficial temporal artery between the auricle and condyle of the mandible. Gaughran notes the presence of communicating rami between the auriculotemporal nerve and the temporofacial division of the facial nerve. These rami lie close to the transverse facial and maxillary arteries, a potential source of trouble in parotid surgery.

Facial nerve rami of the auriculotemporal nerve communicate sensory fibers to the skin of the face, accompanying peripheral facial divisions. Postganglionic fibers provide se-

cretomotor fibers to the parotid gland. Preganglionic fibers arise in the ninth cranial nerve. Sensory fibers extend to the helix, tragus, external auditory meatus, tympanic membrane, and temporomandibular joint.

The facial nerve emerges from the skull by way of the stylomastoid foramen, which is strategically located between the mastoid process and the base of the styloid process. At this point, the nerve is about 3 to 4 mm in diameter and is easily identifiable. It lies 3 to 6 mm deep and medial to the tympanomastoid fissure. It takes an anteroinferior lateral course for 1 cm, at which point it enters the posterior border of the parotid gland between the superficial and deep portions.

Before its division, the facial nerve crosses the external carotid artery. The triangular process of the cartilaginous external auditory meatus points to the nerve branch trunk (see Fig. 3–9B). Three branches are given off: the postauricular nerve, a branch that goes to the posterior digastric muscle, and the stylohyoid muscle branch. As the facial nerve enters the parotid substance, it usually divides into the temporofacial and cervicofacial branches. The temporofacial division is anchored by rami from the auriculotemporal nerve. Terminal branching is variable. The most consistent pattern is one of temporal and zygomatic branches from the temporofacial division, and buccal, mandibular, and cervical branches from the cervicofacial division. Many patterns of anastomosis exist between these branches. The peripheral lower branches of the cervicofacial division usually lie superficial to the posterior and anterior facial vein.

Stensen's duct extends from the anterior border of the parotid gland and crosses over the external surface of the masseter muscle approximately 1 cm below the zygoma. Buccal and zygomatic branches of the facial nerve may lie in closer proximity to the duct. The transverse artery lies 1 cm above it. At the anterior border of the masseter muscle, the duct turns medially and pierces the buccal fat and buccinator muscle at the point called the buccinator dehiscence. It opens into the mouth through the parotid papilla, opposite the upper second molar.

Nodes Located Within the Parotid Compartment

Three groups of nodes are found within the parotid compartment. The first group is called the suprafascial group. Its nodes are found in the preauricular area. Members of the second group, the subfascial extraglandular nodes, are located preauricularly and infra-auricularly beneath the parotid sheath. Collectively, the first and second groups receive drainage from the temporal frontal region of the scalp, outer portions of the eyelid, and outer aspects of the ear. The lymph nodes of the deep group drain the upper and posterior parts of the nasopharynx, soft palate, and middle ear. Efferent vessels empty directly or indirectly into the jugular vein.

Inflammatory Diseases of the Parotid Gland

Acute Suppurative Parotitis

Diseases of the parotid gland can be divided into three types: inflammatory, obstructive, and neoplastic. Acute bacterial parotitis (parotid abscess) is an inflammation of the parotid gland that begins as a cellulitis and may progress to form an abscess. Early changes consist of localized inflammation of ductules with aggregations of white cells. Duct walls are destroyed, and parenchymal necrosis occurs. The small abscesses thus formed coalesce into larger areas of purulence, and infection may penetrate the fascial planes of the neck and face. Unopposed infection can result in facial paralysis, hemorrhage, septicemia, meningitis, brain abscess, or purulent temporomandibular arthritis.

Etiology. Bacterial parotitis can occur in the postoperative period after major surgery. Predisposing factors include old age, debilitating disease, dehydration, poor oral hygiene, carious teeth, stomatitis, and atropine-induced "dry mouth." Cellulitis or abscess formation may occur as a consequence of mechanical obstruction of Stensen's duct (calculi) or as a complication of systemic infection.

The usual offending organisms are coagulase-positive *Staphylococcus aureus and Streptococcus viridans.* The route of infection is generally accepted as being by retrograde flow up Stensen's duct. Blood and lymphatic spread from the tonsillar, peritonsillar, and precervical space may involve the deep lobe of the parotid.

Symptoms and Clinical Course. Signs and symptoms appear 24 to 36 hours after the onset of infection. Elevated pulse rate, temperature, and white blood cell count usually herald the onset of the infection. Severe pain is typical, and the patient may report trismus, particularly if the deep lobe of the parotid gland is affected. Tenderness on palpation and swelling of the parotid gland are present, with rubor and induration of the overlying skin. By the fourth to sixth day, unopposed infection will progress to abscess formation. Localized areas of fluctuant or abscess formation may be difficult to recognize because of the investing parotid fascia. It should be noted that fluctuation is a late sign. Stensen's duct orifice is edematous, and purulent material can be expressed from it. Unopposed abscess formation may result in a breakthrough into the temporomandibular joint, external auditory canal, face, or cervical planes. Computerized tomography (CT) will help determine whether an abscess has developed or if only diffuse inflammation is present.

Treatment. With the increasing incidence of penicillin-resistant strains of staphylococcus, early culture and sensitivity studies are mandatory. Duct secretions will contain the offending organism. Early recognition of this disease and appropriate antibiotic therapy are the key to successful treatment. Other measures include adequate hydration, discontinuance of anticholinergic drugs, and good oral hygiene.

The usual indications for surgical drainage are (1) increasing pain with early evidence of septicemia or central nervous system spread; (2) failure of medical treatment to be effective after 2 to 3 days; (3) fluctuation; (4) abscess breakthrough into adjacent areas; and (5) abscess seen on CT scan.

Surgical intervention before the 36-hour period after onset of symptoms has elapsed is usually unwarranted, unless an obvious abscess is detected. Two to 3 days are necessary for the multiple small abscesses of the parotid gland to coalesce. The incision and surgical technique are shown in Figure 3–1.

Non-Neoplastic Parotid Gland Disorders

Epidermic parotitis (mumps), an acute contagious disease of viral origin, is a frequently seen inflammatory disease of the parotid gland. Its highest incidence is in persons between 5 and 15 years of age. The incubation period is from 2 to 4 weeks. After a period of malaise and fever, tender swelling occurs in 70% of patients. The submandibular gland, pancreas, ovaries, testes, and prostate may also be involved. The central nervous system, breasts, and heart occasionally are affected.

Sjögren's syndrome is a progressive inflammatory disease of the parotid and lacrimal glands. The characteristic pathologic changes are atrophy of parenchymal tissue and replacement by lymphocytes and connective tissue. Women in the fourth decade of life are frequently affected. The cause is unknown.

In about 30% of cases, enlargement of the parotid gland is the first symptom. The submandibular gland may also be enlarged. Keratoconjunctivitis is a common first symptom. Patients also present with a beefy tongue, caries, and dry mucous membrane of the mouth, nose, or pharynx. Some patients (possibly as many as 70%) show joint changes, especially joint pain. There may be neuropathy, lymphadenopathy, and leukopenia. In addition, Raynaud's phenomenon may be present, and the liver and spleen may be enlarged. The pathology is basically an infiltration with T lymphocytes. There is also ductal hyperplasia; inspissated saliva can be seen in the ducts of the gland.

It is interesting that 10% of patients with rheumatoid arthritis have dry mouths. In the diagnosis of Sjögren's syndrome, rheumatoid factors, immunoglobulin M (IgM), and IgG levels are valuable. There can be a 15% false-positive rate with the Shirmer's test. Flow rate of the parotid and sialography are not diagnostic of Sjögren's syndrome, nor is the technetium radionuclide scan. Probably the best way to make the diagnosis is to perform a biopsy of the salivary glands by taking a portion of the lip or buccal mucous membrane. Others surgeons have performed biopsies of the lacrimal gland or the parotid gland; however, it seems to the authors that the buccal biopsy is the easiest method.

Kussmaul's disease is characterized by a benign unilateral recurrent swelling of the parotid gland. It is caused by mucinous or fibrous ductile plugs. Massage usually results in the extrusion of a plug from Stensen's duct, which is diagnostic of the disease.

Mikulicz's disease is a benign, self-limiting disease of varying duration and unknown cause. It is characterized by chronic enlargement of the salivary or lacrimal glands. Pathologic changes consist of parenchymal atrophy, lymphocytic infiltration, and ductile proliferation with islands of epithelial tissue.

Granulomatous diseases, such as tuberculosis, sarcoidosis, or mycotic disease, may appear clinically as primary parotid disease. Careful examination and history taking, as well as specific diagnostic tests, will identify the causative agent.

Toxic parotitis is caused by intoxication by mercury, copper, lead, iodine, or bromine. Uremia may produce a similar picture. The usual clinical presentation is chronic glandular swelling with hypersecretion and no constitutional symptoms.

Dysfunction of the parotid gland may be physiologic or

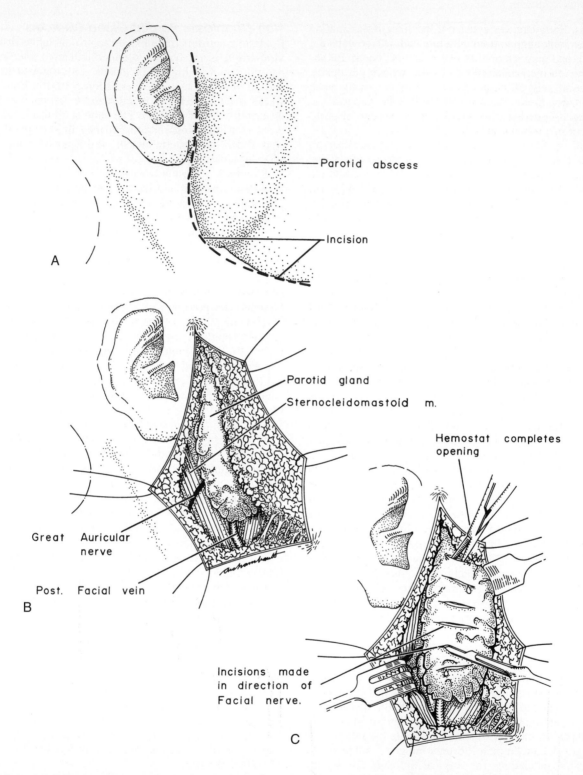

FIGURE 3-1. Parotid gland abscess. *A,* The skin incision begins in front of the tragus and follows the anterior border of the ear to a point 1 cm below the angle of the mandible. It is carried forward for 3 cm below the inferior margin of the mandible. *B,* The skin and subcutaneous tissues are reflected anteriorly until the entire lateral surface of the gland is exposed. Care must be taken to keep the dissection in a plane above the capsule, particularly in the anterior portion of the gland where branches of the facial nerve become superficial. *C,* Incisions are made on the surface of the parotid gland in the direction of the branches of the facial nerve. Deep dissection into the parenchymal tissue is accomplished with a "mosquito" hemostat. The hemostat is opened in the direction of the facial nerve to avoid injury and unnecessary bleeding. Numerous facial sheaths, in addition to the investing parotid capsule, compartmentalize parenchymal tissue. It is usually necessary to open more than one area of abscess formation. Penrose drains are inserted in appropriate locations, and the skin flap is packed with aureomycin-impregnated iodoform gauze. No attempt at primary skin closure is made.

pathologic. Ptyalism or hypersecretion may represent a physiologic response to a stimulation such as the cephalic phase of digestion or the infantile eruption of teeth. Pathologic secretion is associated with conditions such as metallic poisoning, stomatitis, gingivitis, glossitis, oral pharyngeal malignant disease, or Vincent's infection.

Decreased secretion is a common response to drugs such as atropine or propantheline bromide (Pro-Banthine). Hypofunction may also be secondary to febrile disease, myxedema, pernicious anemia, Plummer-Vinson syndrome, or emotional disorders. Prolonged loss of secretions results in xerostomia. The oral and pharyngeal mucosa is dry, red, and fissured. Glossodynia and loss of nutrition are frequent findings. Radiation therapy of the head and neck area frequently is responsible for this condition.

Metabolic conditions associated with nutritional deficiencies can result in asymptomatic enlargement of the parotid glands. Obesity, diabetes mellitus with liver disease, achalasia, anorexia nervosa, alcoholism, and inadequate nutrition are predisposing diseases. Microscopically, acinar cells are hypertrophied, and areas of parenchyma are replaced by fatty tissue. Sialography reveals a diminution of the terminal duct mass.

Benign hypertrophy is associated with thyroid dysfunction, diabetes, and menopause.

Duct Surgery of the Parotid Gland

Calculi of the Parotid Duct

Calculi are the second most common disease of the salivary glands that the surgeon is called on to evaluate. The order of frequency of salivary gland calculi is submandibular gland, 75%; parotid gland, 20%; and sublingual gland, 5%. Parotid calculi are most frequently found in Stensen's duct. Other, less frequently found locations are the secondary ductules, hilum, and parenchymal tissue.

Parotid calculi consist of inorganic salts of calcium, sodium, or phosphate. A nidus of bacteria, tissue debris, or foreign material is sometimes found. One theory of calculus formation is that inflammatory changes within the parotid ducts or gland give rise to a change in the nature of secretion. Increased viscosity and pH changes result in the precipitation of salts.

Pathologic changes that result from intermittent obstruction from calculous disease are hyperplasia or metaplasia of the duct epithelium, proximal dilation of the duct, fibrosis and stricture of the duct, acinar atrophy and fibrosis, recurrent acinar inflammation with cellulitis, abscess formation, and sinus or fistulous tracts from the duct or gland.

Symptoms, Diagnosis, and Clinical Course.

Calculous disease may or may not cause symptoms, depending on the size and number of calculi, their location, the presence of inflammation and infection, and stricture formation.

Characteristically, a stone blocking Stensen's duct distal to the buccinator muscle results in intermittent pain, swelling, and tenderness of the gland, particularly at meals. Saliva leaks around the stone and, as the stimulus for glandular secretion is removed, the swelling subsides. Occasionally, small stones or gravel are extruded.

Swelling of the duct around the stone, or the coexistence of an ascending infection, will result in an extended period of swelling with attending symptoms. Fever, with signs of local infection, ensues. The patient may report a foul oral discharge. Physical examination shows swelling and bluish erythema of the papillae. Bimanual palpation of Stensen's duct often reveals the presence of a calculus. Lacrimal probes are useful in locating a stone along the main course of the duct. The surgeon should try to use the largest possible lacrimal probe to avoid perforating the duct and creating a false passageway.

A calculus obstructing the intraglandular portion of Stensen's duct is not readily palpated either with a finger or a probe. When the main body of the gland is swollen without involvement of the accessory lobe, the obstruction is intraglandular. A patient with persistent swelling of a definitive portion of the gland sometimes presents a more difficult diagnostic problem. Swelling of the upper pole is rare; its usual cause is preauricular adenopathy. Swelling of the lower pole can be caused by calculus disease, adenopathy, or a parotid tumor. Distant metastasis may also be manifested as parotid swelling. Failure of the physical or radiologic examination to disclose the pathologic condition makes a biopsy mandatory. A fine needle biopsy is often of help here.

Treatment.

The surgical technique for removal of calculi of the parotid gland is shown in Figures 3–2 and 3–3.

Failure of duct resection to provide adequate outflow for parotid secretions presents a much more difficult situation. Some surgeons advocate reoperation and reanastomosis. Other procedures mentioned in the literature include reimplantation of the duct or plastic reconstruction using a buccal mucosal tube (Anderson and Byars, 1965). This operation is difficult and not always successful (Fig. 3–4). The authors recommend ligation of the proximal end of the duct once the surgeon is sure that the gland is free of infection (Fig. 3–5). This procedure has been shown to result in atrophy of parenchymal elements proximal to the point of ligation. Antibiotics are continued for 2 weeks after duct ligation. A localized narrowing occurring within the gland substance may occasionally be treated successfully by superficial parotidectomy. If all operative measures fail, a total parotidectomy should be considered.

Laceration of the Parotid Duct

Lacerations of the parotid duct are repaired by a technique similar to that used for reconstruction after resection of a stricture (Fig. 3–6).

Except when used as a separate procedure to resect a tumor of the parapharyngeal space not associated with the parotid gland, the intraoral approach is avoided whenever possible because of the increased chance for infection. Tumors from the scalp, face, ears, nasal cavity, and oropharynx may metastasize to the parotid gland or to the paraglandular lymph nodes. These tumors are usually squamous cell carcinomas, malignant melanomas, or, occasionally, sarcomas or cylindromas. Treatment should be aggressive, consisting of an adequate resection of the primary neoplasm,

Text continued on page 124

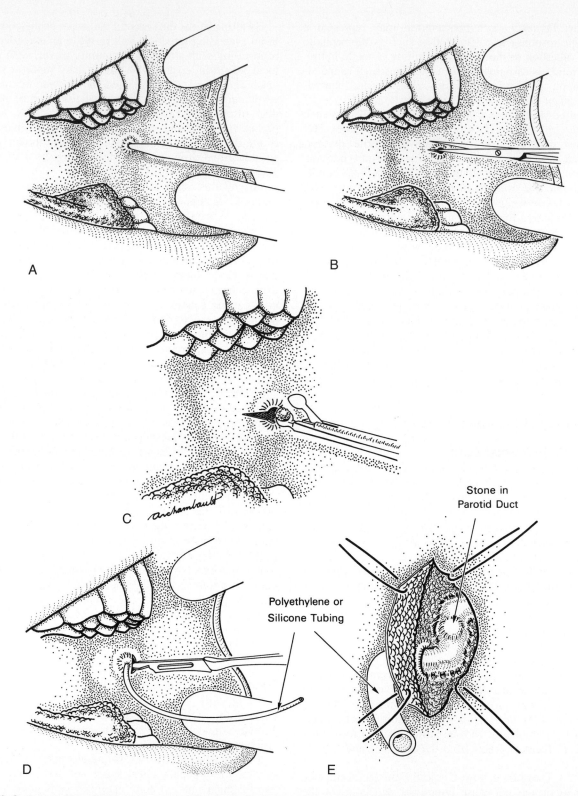

FIGURE 3–2. Stones of parotid duct. *A,* Stones are often situated in the parotid duct immediately proximal to the papilla. After a topical anesthetic has been applied, the orifice is dilated with a punctum dilator. *B,* One blade of iris scissors is inserted into the parotid duct after the orifice has been dilated. The distal duct and overlying mucous membrane are incised as shown. *C,* Following exposure of the distal parotid duct, the stone is readily available for removal with small-cupped forceps. *D,* Submucosal stones, which are situated in a more proximal position, can also be approached by the intraoral route. Polyethylene tubing is inserted into the parotid duct for a few millimeters only. After infiltration with a local anesthetic agent, a curved vertical incision is made just anterior to the papilla. *E,* Traction sutures are applied to the mucosal margins. The distal duct is identified and traced proximally in the submucosal tissue. Care must be taken to avoid pushing the calculus in a proximal direction during this dissection.

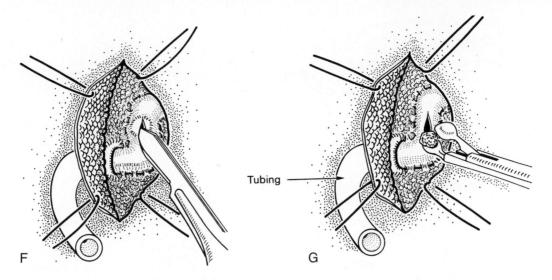

FIGURE 3-2. *(Continued) F,* A longitudinal incision is made in the parotid duct over the stone. Some surgeons advocate placing a ligature around the duct proximal to the stone so that it will not be displaced. *G,* The calculus is removed with small-cupped forceps, and the duct is irrigated with saline solution. It may or may not be necessary to approximate the margins of the mucous membrane incision.

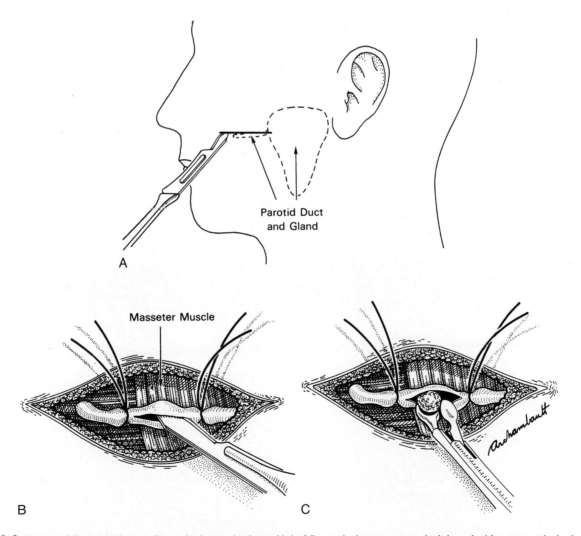

FIGURE 3-3. Stones of Stensen's duct. *A,* Stones in the proximal one third of Stensen's duct are approached through either a preauricular incision, as has been described for parotidectomy, or a horizontal cheek incision over the proximal duct. When elevating the cheek flap anteriorly, care must be taken not to damage the facial nerve fibers as they emerge from the anterior surface of the parotid gland. When making the horizontal incision over the parotid duct, it is well to remember that this structure lies immediately below a line extending from the tragus to a point that bisects the nasolabial region. An electrical nerve stimulator is essential for this dissection to avoid inadvertent damage to a branch of the facial nerve. Blunt dissection is used wherever possible. Once the duct is dissected and the stone is identified, temporary traction ligatures are placed around the duct proximal and distal to the site of the stone. This will serve to prevent any migration of the stone. *B* and *C,* A horizontal ductotomy incision is made, the stone is extracted, and the duct is irrigated with normal saline solution. The traction sutures are removed and the wound is repaired.

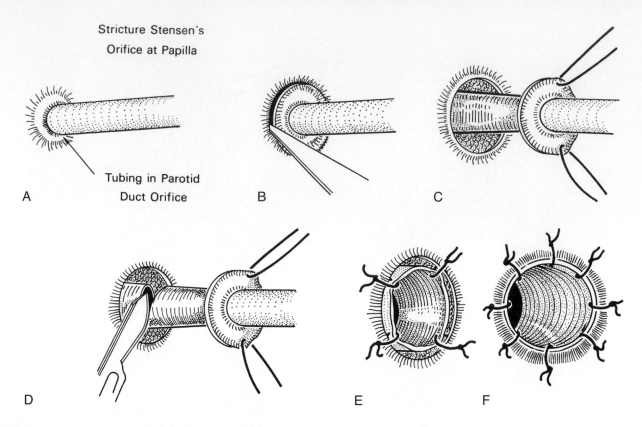

FIGURE 3-4. Strictures. *A*, Strictures at the papilla can often be repaired by inserting one blade of iris scissors into the duct after it has been dilated with a lacrimal dilator and making a longitudinal incision through the mucous membrane and duct as shown in Figure 3–2*A* and *B*. The mucous membrane of the duct is then sutured to the buccal mucous membrane with a very fine chromic or silk suture material. The stricture, however, may be proximal to the papilla. In such instances, polyethylene tubing is inserted into the parotid duct after the papilla is dilated in preparation for resection of the papilla. *B*, A circumferential incision is made around the papilla with a No. 11 blade. *C*, Traction sutures are placed as shown, and the duct is carefully dissected and pulled forward. *D*, The parotid duct is transected at right angles to its long axis at a point proximal to the stricture. *E* and *F*, A widely patent ductal orifice can be fashioned, as shown, by using No. 4-0 chromic catgut or No. 5-0 silk suture material.

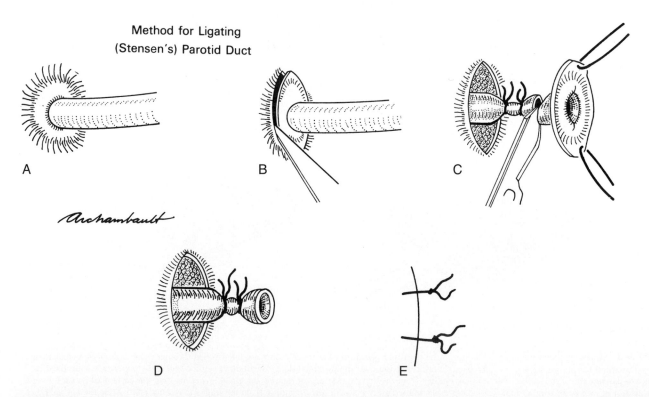

FIGURE 3-5. Method for ligating the parotid duct. *A*, Polyethylene tubing is inserted into the parotid duct after the papilla has been dilated with a lacrimal dilator. *B*, A circumferential incision is made around the papilla. *C*, Two No. 3-0 or 4-0 silk sutures are placed around the parotid duct, and the duct is transected distally. *D*, The distal portion of the parotid duct and papilla with its surrounding mucous membrane has been removed. *E*, The mucous membrane is repaired with No. 4-0 chromic catgut suture material.

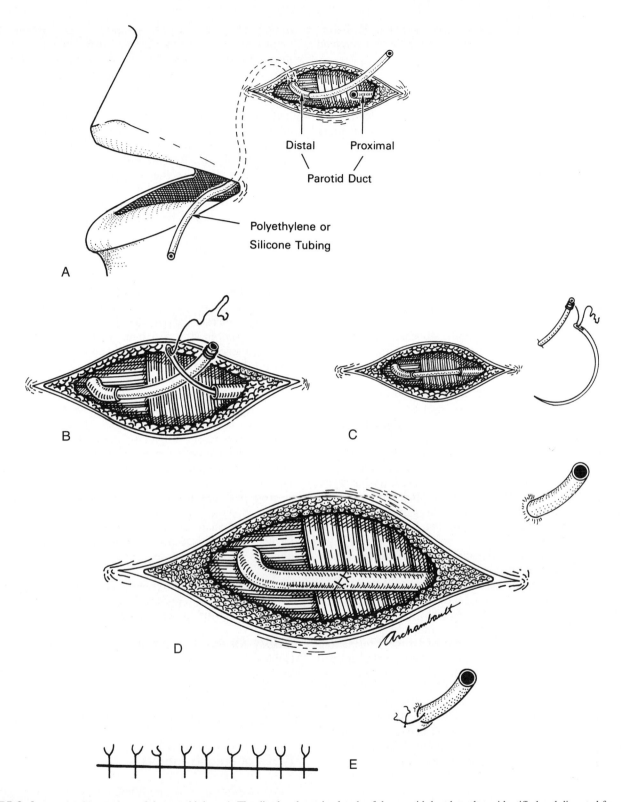

FIGURE 3–6. Repair of lacerations of the parotid duct. *A,* The distal and proximal ends of the parotid duct have been identified and dissected free. The papilla is dilated with a lacrimal dilator, and polyethylene tubing is inserted until it projects from the proximal end of the distal segment. *B,* Suture material is attached to the end of the polyethylene tube that projects from the proximal end of the distal parotid duct. This suture is applied to a large, curved, needle, which, in turn, is inserted into the distal end of the proximal duct. *C,* The needle and end of the polyethylene tube are brought through the adjacent skin. *D,* The polyethylene tubing is in place and the duct has been repaired with multiple No. 6-0 silk suture material. *E,* The wound has been repaired and the polyethylene tubing secured to the skin. The intraoral end of the polyethylene tube can be transected at the papilla so that it retracts into the duct and is not troublesome to the patient. This tubing should remain in place for approximately 2 weeks.

the parotid gland, and a block neck dissection. Radiation therapy is valuable when dealing with these malignant lesions.

Stricture, Laceration, and Ligation of the Parotid Duct

The causes for parotid duct stricture are (1) congenital narrowing; (2) poorly fitting dentures, with recurrent papillary inflammation; (3) recurrent duct inflammation with or without calculus disease; (4) poor oral hygiene; (5) trauma; (6) radiation fibrosis; and (7) surgery.

Calculi, chronic sialadenitis, sialectasia, and neoplasia should all be considered in the differential diagnosis of parotid duct stricture.

Treatment. Treatment depends on the location of the stricture and the degree of difficulty the patient is experiencing. A carefully obtained history may reveal the underlying cause for stricture formation. A CT scan will show the detail needed. Sialography may be necessary to locate the exact point of stricture.

If the obstruction is at the papilla, repeated dilatations at predetermined intervals may be all that is necessary. If these fail, the papilla can be incised in the manner described in the section on calculi (see Fig. 3–2).

If the above measures fail, some form of stomatoplasty is required. Small iris scissors are inserted into the papilla, and the distal portion of Stensen's duct is opened to a point at least 4 mm proximal to the stricture (see Fig. 3–2). Repair involves suturing the ductal mucosa to the oral mucosa after the duct and papillary edges have been beveled.

The authors prefer No. 5-0 chromic catgut for the repair and do not use a stent at this level. Another method for repair of a stricture at the papilla or distal parotid duct entails resection of the papilla and construction of a new orifice, as illustrated in Figure 3–4.

Strictures proximal to the buccopharyngeal dehiscence are approached through a standard preauricular incision or by way of a horizontal cheek incision made over the parotid duct (see Fig. 3–3). The extraglandular portion of the duct is identified, carefully avoiding branches of the facial nerve. A No. 50 Silastic tube is inserted into the parotid duct through the papilla up to the point of stricture formation. After the portion of the duct containing the stricture has been dissected from the surrounding soft tissue, it is resected. The proximal and distal ends of the duct are beveled. The Silastic tube is used to bridge the anastomosis, which is made with No. 6-0 chromic catgut or silk sutures. Care is taken not to pass the suture into the lumen because this predisposes the anastomosis to further stricture formation. The Silastic stent is left in place for 2 weeks.

Tumors of the Parotid Gland

Symptoms, Clinical Course, and Diagnosis

Tumors of the parotid gland usually are manifested as a preauricular or infra-auricular mass. Seventy-five percent of tumors arise in the tail or mid-portion of the gland. Both locations place the tumor grossly in the superficial lobe of the gland.

A bulging soft palate or lateral pharyngeal wall indicates involvement of the deep (median) parotid lobe. Deep-lobe tumors gave rise to earlier symptoms than superficial-lobe neoplasms owing to the limited space for expansion. The most frequent symptoms are pain referred to the ear or pharynx, a sensation of a lump in the throat, trismus, or difficulty in swallowing.

Parotid tumors appear in persons of all ages, from childhood to old age. However, in general, the greatest incidence of benign tumors is in the fifth decade of life, and that of malignant lesions in the sixth and seventh decades. Among all parotid masses, 70% are mixed tumors; 20%, carcinoma or sarcoma; 5%, miscellaneous tumors; and 5%, inflammatory masses.

Classically, a benign parotid tumor appears as a freely movable mass that is firm or cystic and occasionally nodular. The growth rate is slow, and benign tumors are painless. Benign tumors are solitary and do not invade locally. Those recurring after inadequate surgical excision are multiple and tend to spread throughout the glandular tissue.

A malignant parotid tumor is characterized by rapid growth. It is firm, sometimes fixed to the skin and surrounding structures, and tender. Facial nerve (branch) paralysis is present in 40% of patients with malignant parotid tumor. Evidence of cervical lymph node metastasis may be present. Malignant lesions involve the upper pole and retromandibular lobe more frequently than they involve other portions of the gland. Occasionally, the mandibular division of the trigeminal nerve may be involved. Local and distant metastasis is common with advanced lesions.

Local spread of malignant parotid tumors is variable. A rapidly growing or recurring malignant tumor may spread throughout the gland and surround musculature and trigeminal nerves. Adenocystic carcinoma is a frequent offender.

Any malignant parotid tumor is capable of invading cervical lymphatics. Squamous cell carcinoma is particularly prone to lymphatic spread. Hematogenous spread is often a later complication. Sites of distant metastasis include abdominal viscera, soft tissue, spine, scapula, long bones, and lungs.

Computerized axial tomography and magnetic resonance imaging (MRI) have become increasingly valuable in the diagnosis of parotid gland disease (Fig. 3–7).

Biopsy for Parotid Tumor

Controversy is still prevalent regarding the comparable merits of needle, incisional, excisional, frozen section, and permanent section biopsy for the diagnosis of parotid gland tumors. In general, the needle-biopsy technique is the first diagnostic step and most often conclusive.

Types of Parotid Tumors

Parotid tumors may be classified into the following groups:
 Tumors of epithelial origin
  Mixed tumors
   Benign
   Malignant
  Mucoepidermoid tumors (benign and malignant)
   Low-grade malignancy
   High-grade malignancy
  Squamous cell carcinoma
  Adenocarcinoma

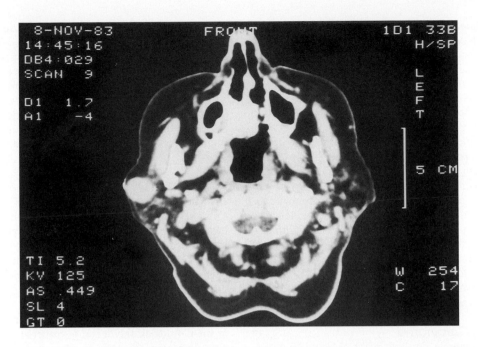

FIGURE 3–7. Axial computed tomography (CT) scan through the mid-portion of the parotid glands shows a homogeneous, oval-shaped sharply delimited tumor in the superficial portion of the right parotid gland anteriorly adjacent to the posterior margin of the masseter muscle. In an incisional biopsy, the incision should be made parallel to the direction of the facial nerve branches. The facial nerve stimulator is useful during this procedure. It is best to make the incision as anterosuperior to the ear as possible. Usually, a frozen-section diagnosis at the time of parotidectomy is satisfactory. At this time, the surgeon can make decisions concerning the facial nerve and neck dissection.

Adenocystic
    Variant forms
    Acinic cell type
Papillary cystadenoma lymphomatosum
Benign lymphoepithelioma
Oxyphil adenoma (onocytoma)
Sebaceous cell adenoma
Tumor of mesenchymal origin
    Angioma
        Benign hemangioma
        Malignant hemangioendothelioma
    Fibrosarcoma
        Metastatic tumor
        Melanoma
        Squamous cell carcinoma
        Lymphoma

Mixed Tumors

Mixed tumors of the parotid gland are the most common epithelial tumors. They consist of epithelial and connective tissue components in varying degrees, although most investigators believe them to be of epithelial origin.

Benign mixed tumors of the parotid gland are round, smooth, and freely movable. They grow slowly, although they may achieve a large size. They have a thin, delicate capsule with occasional projections extending into the surrounding parotid gland. This fact is clinically important in considering a safe surgical margin during excision.

Benign mixed tumors are more common in women than in men, with the peak incidence in the third and fourth decades of life.

Microscopically, benign mixed tumors are characterized by variable, diverse, structural histologic patterns. The growth

patterns frequently include strands, sheets, or islands of spindle and stellate cells, with a myoid configuration occasionally predominating. Tubular epithelial patterns with glandular areas, or a cylindromatous pattern, are frequently noted. Other variations include pseudocartilaginous structures, squamous metaplasia, calcification, oxyphilic cells, and palisading of the stroma. These tumors are usually amenable to surgical therapy, with 5-year cure rates of 78% to 84%.

The origin of malignant mixed tumors is debatable, but the common view is that these lesions arise from preexisting mixed tumors that have undergone malignant change. As with benign mixed tumors, the malignant type is found more frequently in women than in men, with the highest incidence in the fifth and sixth decades of life. The symptoms suggestive of malignancy are a preexisting mass that suddenly starts to grow rapidly, pain, and facial nerve paralysis. Cervical lymph node metastases occur in 15% to 20% of patients; however, if malignant disease develops after treatment for benign mixed tumor, 40% to 50% of these patients will have nodule metastasis. Sites of distant metastases include the lungs, bone, abdomen, brain, and reticuloendothelial system. Five-year survival rates vary from 55% to 65%.

Malignant mixed tumors tend to be larger than benign tumors. Necrosis, hemorrhage, and cyst formation occur frequently with these tumors. Histologically they may suggest adenocarcinoma, undifferentiated carcinoma, squamous cell carcinoma, spindle cell carcinoma, or sarcoma.

Mucoepidermoid Tumors

This group consists of mucus-secreting cells and epidermoid cells of ductal origin. The low-grade variety tends to be slow growing, less than 3 to 4 cm in size, well circumscribed, and partially encapsulated. Many pathologists believe that these are benign lesions and should be treated accordingly. The primary symptom is usually painless enlargement. The highest incidence is in persons in the fourth and fifth decades of life. Over 50% of the low-grade mucoepidermoid tumors contain mucinous cysts. Microcysts may coalesce into larger cysts, which may rupture into the surrounding soft tissue and give rise to an inflammatory reaction.

High-grade mucoepidermoid malignant tumors are poorly circumscribed, infiltrated, and larger than the low-grade variety. Cyst formation is uncommon. Metastasis to local lymph nodes occurs frequently.

Sixty to seventy percent of the low-grade malignant mucoepidermoid tumors are found in women; the incidence of high-grade tumors is equal in men and women. The primary symptom in high-grade malignant mucoepidermoid tumors is pain; 25% of patients will have facial nerve paralysis. Tumor growth is rapid, with regional node metastasis in 60% of patients and distant metastasis in about 30%. The 5-year surgical cure rate varies from 25% to 30%.

Squamous Cell Carcinoma

This is a rapidly growing, locally infiltrative tumor occurring in persons in the sixth and seventh decades of life. Its incidence is greater in men than in women. Typically, it has the usual characteristics of squamous cell carcinoma. The 5-year surgical survival rate varies from 30% to 40%.

Adenocarcinoma

The adenoid cystic variety is better known as a cylindroma. Grossly it resembles the benign mixed variety. It is well circumscribed and locally infiltrative. Histologically, it is characterized by anastomosing cords of epithelial cells to a cystic glandular pattern. Solid cords or epithelial cells may be abscessed, and the acellular cystic areas may contain mucoid or hyalinized deposits. The lesion is characterized by a slow growth rate. Metastasis to cervical nodes occurs in 30% of patients, with distant metastases as a much later development. The peak incidence is in the fifth and sixth decades of life. The 5-year survival rates vary from 20% to 25%.

Variant forms of adenocarcinoma include the anaplastic adenocarcinoma, which is characterized by small epithelial cells in clumps with a high degree of nuclear anaplasia and abundant connective tissue stroma.

Another variant form is the mucous adenocarcinoma, characterized by mucus-secreting cells resembling signet rings intermingled with small clumps of epithelial cells and mucinous products.

The acinic cell adenocarcinoma is a low-grade tumor that appears similar to a benign mixed tumor. Grossly, it is small, firm, movable, and encapsulated. The histologic pattern consists of acinar arrangements of epithelial cells in a scant fibrous-tissue stroma containing several vascular channels. The cells exhibit a fine granularity in their cytoplasm, with bluish staining properties.

Papillary Cystadenoma Lymphomatosum (Warthin's Tumor)

This tumor was first recognized by Albrecht in 1910 and later was described by Warthin in 1929. Grossly, it is a smooth, ovoid, soft inferiorly located parotid mass. It is well encapsulated and contains multiple cysts. Histologically, acinophilic epithelial cells line the cystic areas with papillary projections in a heavy lymphoid stroma. Malignant transformation has not been observed. It is thought that papillary cystadenoma develops from salivary gland tissue inclusions within lymph nodes lying either in the body of the parotid gland or adjacent to it. This tumor is more common in men than in women, with a peak incidence in the fifth and sixth decades of life. All patients survive with this tumor, but about 5% undergo tumor recurrences. Bilateral Warthin's tumors are not uncommon.

Lymphoepithelial Hyperplasia (Mikulicz's Disease)

This disorder may produce a diffuse enlargement of all or part of the parotid gland or it may be present as a discrete mass. Histologically, the lesion is composed of lymphocytic interstitial infiltrate with obliteration of the acinar pattern; occasional lymph follicles are noted. The lymphoid tissue is diffuse but well organized. Islands of proliferating epithelial cells simulating myoepithelial cells are occasionally found. The disorder occurs more frequently in women than in men. Its peak incidence is in persons 40 to 50 years of age. Occasionally both parotid glands are involved. The growth is slowly progressive and gives rise to pain around the ear or retromandibular area. Treatment by operation or radiation is effective.

Oxyphil Adenoma

This benign tumor is grossly well encapsulated and circumscribed, with occasional cystic areas noted on cut section. The eosinophilic oncocyte, characterized by a pink finely granular cytoplasm with small nuclei, is the predominant cell type. These cells are arranged in columns or cords. The lymphatic tissue does not present a characteristic pattern. The age of peak incidence is 60 to 70 years. Although the tumor is benign, it will recur if incompletely excised.

Tumors of Mesenchymal Origin

Tumors of mesenchymal origin arise from the supporting stroma and are extremely rare. They include angioma, benign hemangioma, malignant hemangioendothelioma, and fibrosarcoma. Because of the small number of cases, statistics on these tumors are not available.

Metastatic Disease

Conley and Arena in 1963 reported that malignant melanoma accounted for 46% of metastatic tumors to the parotid gland, and squamous cell carcinoma for 37%. The remaining 17% were from a variety of tumors. Five-year survival rates varied from 11.5% in patients with melanoma to 14.3% in patients with squamous cell carcinoma.

Parotidectomy

Preoperative Considerations

Successful management of parotid gland tumors depends on the surgeon's knowledge of parotid gland and facial nerve anatomy, surgical skills, and knowledge concerning the pathology, management, and prognosis, of parotid gland tumors.

Ninety percent of lesions found in the superficial lobe of the parotid gland are benign and can be resected by a superficial lobectomy, with minimal damage to the facial nerve. Most surgeons agree that enucleation of these tumors is never indicated and that the lesions should be resected with normal parotid gland tissue surrounding them. Sixty percent of these benign tumors are of the mixed variety.

Many surgeons resect benign cystic (Warthin's) tumors by performing a partial superficial lobectomy. Warthin's tumor can be diagnosed preoperatively by radioactive isotope technique, and MRI. Injury to the facial nerve branches is rare when the dissection is monitored with the facial nerve stimulator. However, the authors prefer superficial lobectomy for all benign tumors.

Benign swelling of the parotid gland may be the result of infection. These patients usually have a history of recurrent swelling and discomfort. Some surgeons perform a parotidectomy as therapy for this disease. The difficulty in dissecting the gland from the facial nerve must be taken into account when making the decision to treat the patient by this method.

It is noteworthy that in approximately 20% of a large series of patients with parotid tumors treated in several large medical centers the lesions were recurrent ones—either benign or malignant. The majority of the tumors were of the benign mixed type. Many recurrent tumors are multicentric. It is important to resect the old scar with recurrent benign mixed tumors. The skin over portions of recurrent mixed or malignant tumors that involves the subcutaneous layers must also be resected. A course of therapeutic radiation therapy is indicated after a second recurrence has been resected.

In patients with a rapid growth attended with discomfort, especially older patients, the presence of sarcoma or lymphoma must be suspected. Fine needle and incisional biopsies are indicated in these patients because, when the diagnosis is that of sarcoma or lymphoma, radiation therapy is the treatment of choice.

There is still some controversy as to whether to sacrifice the facial nerve when a malignant parotid tumor is treated surgically. Certainly, the rule is not hard and fast, for the tumor may be of low-grade malignancy and confined to the lateral lobe. In these patients, a diagnosis of malignant disease is usually made postoperatively. If a clear plane of cleavage can be established between the parotid tissue surrounding the tumor and the facial nerve and deep lobe of the gland, the facial nerve is preserved. When dealing with an obviously malignant tumor, especially when the patient has preoperative facial paralysis, the facial nerve branches are resected along with the entire parotid gland and tumor. Both the proximal and distal ends of the facial nerve are tagged with silk suture material if not grafted immediately.

A block neck dissection is indicated if the tumor is a squamous cell carcinoma or an adenocarcinoma. Squamous cell carcinoma has a high incidence of local recurrence and cervical metastasis, but not generalized spread. Adenocarcinoma has a high incidence of cervical and general metastases. If cervical metastasis is not present at the time of the operation, one or two lymph nodes may be taken from the infraparotid region and examined by frozen section biopsy. In general, malignant mixed tumors and mucoepidermoid carcinomas do not have a high incidence of cervical metastasis. A block neck dissection should be reserved for patients with palpably enlarged cervical lymph nodes or those shown on CT of the neck.

In patients with tumors involving the deep portion of the parotid gland, all branches of the facial nerve must be dissected in clear view and mobilized. Unnecessary retraction, stretching, and dissection with a sponge can cause paralysis. All dissection should be performed in the direction of the facial nerve branches. Bleeders are sponged gently, identified, clamped, and ligated. If necessary, branches of the nerve are sectioned to remove a deep lobe tumor. The cut ends of these branches are tagged with very fine silk sutures so that they may be easily identified and anastomosed after completion of the resection. Nerve sectioning and reanastomosis can ultimately preserve function, whereas stretching and injury of the nerve during the dissection can result in permanent facial paralysis. If there is a choice, it is best to transect the branch to the lower face rather than a superior branch because paralysis resulting in exposure of the eye causes severe complications. Special emphasis will be placed on facial paralysis and its management and repair in another section of this chapter.

Parotid gland tumors may extend to the lateral pharyngeal space by way of the stylomandibular tunnel. Tumors in the lateral pharyngeal space may also be completely independent of the parotid gland. In general, these tumors are difficult to manage surgically. If the tumor originates in the parotid gland, two (and possibly three) approaches are necessary. The facial nerve should be identified, and the superficial lobe should be resected. The submaxillary gland is resected to approach the region of the stylomandibular ligament. An intraoral incision and dissection may be required if the lateral pharyngeal extension is large or if the tumor extends to the base of the skull. It is usually not necessary to section the mandible anteriorly for exposure.

Surgical Technique

Successful parotid surgery is based on the following principles: (1) careful preoperative evaluation, (2) complete familiarity with the anatomy of the parotid gland and facial nerve, (3) complete removal of the parotid tumor, and (4) preservation of the facial nerve whenever possible.

General endotracheal anesthesia is administered by the oral route. The patient is positioned on his back with his face turned as far as possible to the side opposite the lesion. The temporal and preauricular areas are shaved before the skin is prepared. Four towels are used for the initial draping, leaving the face on the side to be operated on exposed. A plastic drape is attached anteriorly so that the face can be more closely observed during parotic surgery.

After the patient has been prepared and draped for the operation, the following anatomic structures should be either palpated or visualized.

1. Temporomandibular joint;
2. Preauricular skin crease;
3. Tragus;
4. Anterior surface of the cavum portion of the conchal cartilage;
5. Lobule of the ear;
6. Tip of the mastoid process;
7. Anterior border of the sternocleidomastoid muscle;
8. Angle of the mandible; and
9. Tip of the hyoid bone

The incision begins in the preauricular crease, just above the level of the tragus (Fig. 3–8A). It is directed posteriorly, at the level of the anterior attachment of the lobule of the

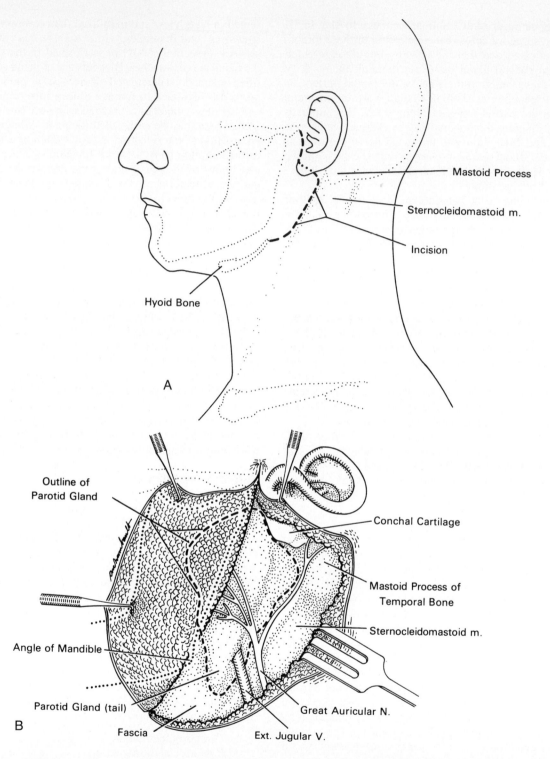

Mastoid Process

Sternocleidomastoid m.

Incision

Hyoid Bone

A

Outline of
Parotid Gland

Conchal Cartilage

Mastoid Process of
Temporal Bone

Sternocleidomastoid m.

Angle of Mandible

Parotid Gland (tail)

Great Auricular N.

B

Fascia

Ext. Jugular V.

FIGURE 3–8. Parotidectomy. *A,* The incision is begun in the preauricular crease, just below the temporomandibular joint and above the level of the tragus. At the level of the anterior attachment of the lobule of the ear it is directed posteriorly. At the tip of the mastoid process, it is again directed inferiorly along the anterior border of the sternocleidomastoid muscle to a level 2 cm below the angle of the mandible. From this point, it is carried forward to the tip of the hyoid. Hash marks are useful for orientation during closure. If a block neck dissection is to be included with the parotidectomy, the superior cervical incision must be extended anteriorly to the submental triangle. The vertical cervical incision begins over the sternocleidomastoid muscle and extends inferiorly to a point about 2 cm below the level of the clavicle in the midclavicular line. The posterosuperior portion of the anterior cervical flap must be handled with care because this area has poor circulation, and its viability could be jeopardized. *B,* The anterior flap has been reflected, exposing the entire parotid gland. It is not necessary at this point to identify the parotid duct or branches of the facial nerve as they emerge from beneath the anterior border of the gland.

ear. At the tip of the mastoid process, it is directed inferiorly along the anterior border of the sternocleidomastoid muscle to a level 2 cm below the angle of the mandible. From this point, it is carried forward to the tip of the hyoid bone. If a block neck dissection is to be included with the parotidectomy, the incision is continued anteriorly to the submental region. The remainder of the incision is similar to the Conley modification of the Schobinger incision (Chapter 2).

The anterior skin flap is elevated over the entire parotid gland with skin hooks (Fig. 3–8B). This plane is readily found in the layer of areolar tissue superficial to the periparotid fascia. As the flap is elevated in the region of the anterior aspect of the parotid gland, care should be taken not to injure the numerous branches of the facial nerve appearing from beneath the gland. It is not necessary at this time to identify Stensen's duct or to identify positively the branches of the facial nerve.

The lobule of the ear is elevated in a posterosuperior direction with a skin hook. The incision in the preauricular crease is developed to expose the perichondrium over the anterior surface of the cavum portion of the conchal cartilage and the cartilaginous external auditory canal. The dissection along the perichondrium is continued to the porus acusticus, or the beginning of the bony external auditory canal. A triangular portion of the conchal cartilage in this area is known as the "pointer." The pointer is directed posteroinferiorly toward the facial nerve. No attempt to identify the facial nerve is made at this time.

A skin flap is also elevated posteriorly, exposing the anterior border of the sternocleidomastoid muscle. The greater auricular nerve is identified as it courses in an anterosuperior direction. Near the anterior border of the sternocleidomastoid muscle, the nerve divides into an auricular branch and an anterior branch. The auricular branch is found coursing in a posterosuperior direction toward the mastoid tip and should be preserved. Auricular numbness will result if it is divided. The anterior branch is directed toward the angle of the mandible; it should be divided. In close proximity to the greater auricular nerve is the external jugular vein, which should be divided and ligated.

Evaluation of the Tail of the Parotid Gland. After the anterior branch of the greater auricular nerve and the external jugular vein have been divided, an incision is made in the fascia along the anterior border of the sternocleidomastoid muscle. The inferior limit of this incision is extended anteriorly 2 cm below the level of the mandible (Fig. 3–9).

The lobule of the ear is elevated posterosuperiorly. The dissection is continued over the perichondrium of the anterior surface of the cavum portion of the conchal cartilage. A projection of the conchal cartilage known as the pointer is located at the junction of the cartilaginous and bony external auditory canals. The posteroinferior point of this cartilaginous projection is pointed directly toward the facial nerve. No attempt to identify the facial nerve is made at this time.

A skin flap is elevated posteriorly, exposing the tip of the mastoid bone in the anterior border of the sternocleidomastoid muscle. The skin flap is elevated in a plane superficial to the fascia covering the parotid gland (see Fig. 3–8B). The

greater auricular nerve is easily identified on the lateral surface of the sternocleidomastoid muscle. It divides into the anterior and posterior branches. The anterior branch, which is directed toward the angle of the mandible, is divided. The posterior branch is preserved to avoid auricular numbness. The external jugular vein is found near the greater auricular nerve. This is divided and ligated at the anterior border of the sternocleidomastoid muscle.

The reflection of the parotideomasseteric fascia to the sternocleidomastoid muscle is elevated to expose the tail of the parotid gland (see Fig. 3–9A and B). The tail of the gland is elevated, and the common, anterior, and posterior facial veins are exposed. The tail of the gland is elevated from its bed in an anterosuperior direction, anterior to the sternocleidomastoid muscle. The dissection is continued superiorly until the posterior belly of the digastric muscle is identified. The anterior and posterior facial veins are ligated during this procedure. At this point, the external jugular vein and spinal accessory nerves are found deep and anterior to the anterior border of the sternocleidomastoid muscle. The hypoglossal nerve is situated inferior and deep to the posterior belly of the digastric muscle. The internal jugular vein, spinal accessory nerves, and the hypoglossal nerve should not be disturbed.

Identification of the Facial Nerve. Early positive identification of the facial nerve trunk or its divisions is the key to good parotid surgery. There are four techniques for approaching the facial nerve: anterior, superior, posterior, and inferior. Surgeons usually favor one of these and use it routinely. They should, however, be familiar with all of the techniques for facial nerve identification because the size and location of the tumor may render their usual approach impossible. Preservation of facial nerve function is of paramount importance during parotid gland surgery. A thorough knowledge of the anatomic relations of the facial nerve distal to the stylomastoid foramen is essential. If the proper techniques for identification are used and the dissection is aided by use of a facial nerve stimulator, injury can be avoided.

The *posterior technique* makes use of the conchal cartilage with its "pointer" extension at the junction of the cartilaginous and bony external auditory canals, the mastoid and styloid processes, the tympanomastoid fissure, the digastric and sternocleidomastoid muscles, and the transverse process of the atlas (Fig. 3–10).

The *inferior technique* makes use of the relationship of the posterior facial vein to the mandibular branch of the facial nerve. The inferior pole of the parotid gland is identified as shown in Figure 3–11. The pole is elevated in an anterosuperior direction, exposing the anterior and posterior facial veins. Positive identification of this branch is accomplished by blunt dissection directed superiorly between the tail of the gland and the posterior facial vein. The nerve is identified by using the facial nerve stimulator to produce a contraction of the depressor anguli oris muscle. The ramus mandibularis nerve is dissected posterosuperiorly to its junction with the lower division of the facial nerve.

Some surgeons prefer to identify the ramus mandibularis nerve at the posterior border of the submandibular gland. Here it lies superficial to the fascia over the mandibular gland and deep to the platysma muscle.

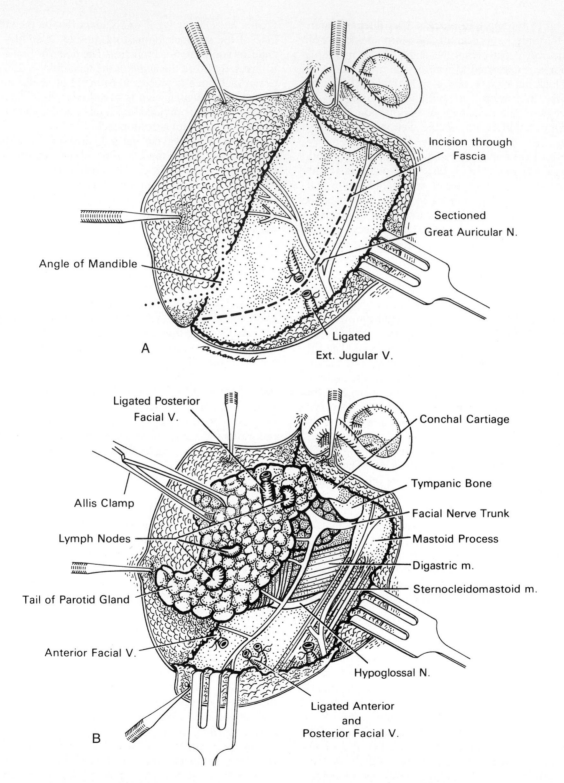

Incision through Fascia

Sectioned Great Auricular N.

Angle of Mandible

Ligated Ext. Jugular V.

A

Ligated Posterior Facial V.

Conchal Cartiage

Allis Clamp

Tympanic Bone

Lymph Nodes

Facial Nerve Trunk

Mastoid Process

Digastric m.

Tail of Parotid Gland

Sternocleidomastoid m.

Anterior Facial V.

Hypoglossal N.

Ligated Anterior and Posterior Facial V.

B

FIGURE 3-9. *A*, The external jugular vein and greater auricular nerves have been sectioned, and the anterior border of the sternocleidomastoid muscle is exposed. The parotideomasseteric fascia reflection is incised along the anterior border of the sternocleidomastoid muscle. The facial incision is continued anteriorly 2 cm below the level of the mandible.

B, The parotideomasseteric fascia has been elevated, exposing the tip of the parotid gland. As the tail of the parotid gland is elevated, the anterior and posterior facial veins become apparent. These are divided and ligated. The tail of the parotid gland is elevated in an anterosuperior direction, and the posterior belly of the digastric muscle is exposed as it extends in a posterosuperior direction beneath the sternocleidomastoid muscle.

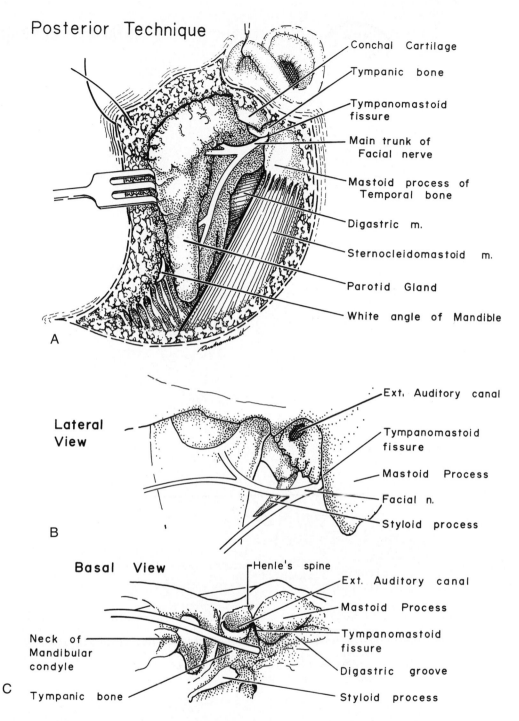

Posterior Technique

Labels (panel A):
Conchal Cartilage
Tympanic bone
Tympanomastoid fissure
Main trunk of Facial nerve
Mastoid process of Temporal bone
Digastric m.
Sternocleidomastoid m.
Parotid Gland
White angle of Mandible

A

Lateral View

Labels (panel B):
Ext. Auditory canal
Tympanomastoid fissure
Mastoid Process
Facial n.
Styloid process

B

Basal View

Labels (panel C):
Henle's spine
Ext. Auditory canal
Mastoid Process
Tympanomastoid fissure
Neck of Mandibular condyle
Digastric groove
Tympanic bone
Styloid process

C

FIGURE 3–10. Posterior approach to the facial nerve. The posterior technique for identification of the facial nerve is by far the safest and easiest unless the tumor lies between the mastoid process and the angle of the mandible. The structures in relation to this approach are described and illustrated in Figures 3–8 and 3–9. Having identified the triangular process of the conchal cartilage at its junction with the bony external auditory canal, the surgeon continues the dissection along the lateral surface of the tympanic bone until the tympanomastoid fissure is palpated (*A* and *B*). This fissure may also be identified by incising the fascia over the anterolateral portion of the mastoid bone and reflecting it anteriorly. It is in direct line with the stylomastoid foramen. Its inferior margin is considered to be approximately 4 mm from the trunk of the facial nerve as it emerges from the stylomastoid foramen (*C*). In addition to the "pointer" and the stylomastoid foramen, the transverse process of the atlas, styloid process, anterior border of the sternocleidomastoid muscle, and superior margin of the posterior belly of the digastric muscle are also useful landmarks. Noting these landmarks, dissections were conducted in the fatty-areolar tissue that lies lateral to the facial nerve. This dissection is conducted with a delicate hemostat and monitored with the facial-nerve stimulator. The hemostat is spread in an anteroposterior direction along the line of the facial-nerve trunk. There is usually no mistake when the facial-nerve trunk is identified because it stands out as a grayish white cord in contrast to the yellowish brown surrounding tissue. On rare occasions, a large tumor involving the entire parotid gland may displace the facial-nerve trunk laterally or posteriorly. In such instances, the facial nerve can be identified by first removing the lateral portion of the mastoid bone with a rotating cutting bur. The vertical portion of the facial nerve is identified and followed inferiorly to the stylomastoid foramen.

Inferior Technique

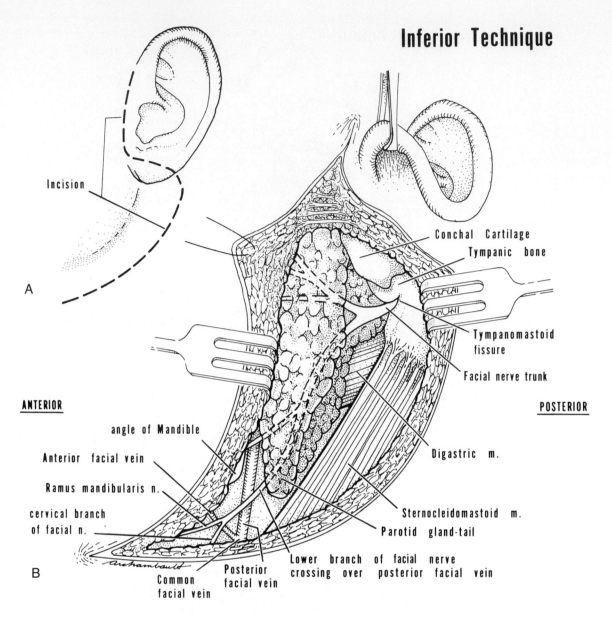

Incision

A

Conchal Cartilage

Tympanic bone

Tympanomastoid fissure

Facial nerve trunk

ANTERIOR

POSTERIOR

angle of Mandible

Anterior facial vein

Ramus mandibularis n.

cervical branch
of facial n.

Digastric m.

Sternocleidomastoid m.

Parotid gland-tail

Lower branch of facial nerve
crossing over posterior facial vein

Posterior
facial vein

Common
facial vein

B

FIGURE 3–11. *A* and *B,* Inferior approach to the facial nerve. The lower branch of the facial nerve invariably can be found immediately external to the posterior facial vein as it exits the lower pole of the parotid gland. This lower branch may divide into the ramus mandibularis and cervical branches before, or after, crossing the posterior facial vein. The lower branch of the facial nerve is then dissected proximally to the facial-nerve trunk. The posterior facial vein should not be confused with the external jugular vein, for the facial vein runs deep to the sternocleidomastoid muscle, whereas the external jugular vein lies superficial to this muscle. Elevation of the tail of the parotid gland greatly facilitates this dissection, which must be accomplished in a plane between the posterior facial vein and the parotid gland.

The *anterior approach* (Fig. 3–12) involves locating one or more branches of the facial nerve anterior to the parotid gland and tracing them back to the main trunk. The transverse or buccal branch of the facial nerve is almost invariably found just above Stensen's duct and approximately 1 cm below the zygomatic arch; it is not difficult to identify. The parotid duct is identified as it emerges from the anterior margin of the parotid gland. The buccal branch is found closely adjacent to the duct, either above or below it, and is positively identified by using the facial nerve stimulator. The buccal branch is then retracted posteriorly through the gland to the main temporofacial division.

The *superior technique* (Fig. 3–13) involves identifica-

tion of the superficial temporal artery and vein. These vessels are located by developing the incision in the preauricular crease in the region between the conchal cartilage and the head of the mandible. The superficial temporal artery and vein are dissected in an inferior direction to identify the temporofacial division of the facial nerve. Again, use of the facial nerve stimulator is essential for this dissection.

Another technique for identifying the facial nerve is to remove the tip of the mastoid bone, identify the vertical portion of the facial nerve, and then follow it out into the stylomastoid foramen. This route is especially valuable in patients who have a large tumor in the region of the stylomastoid foramen.

Anterior Technique

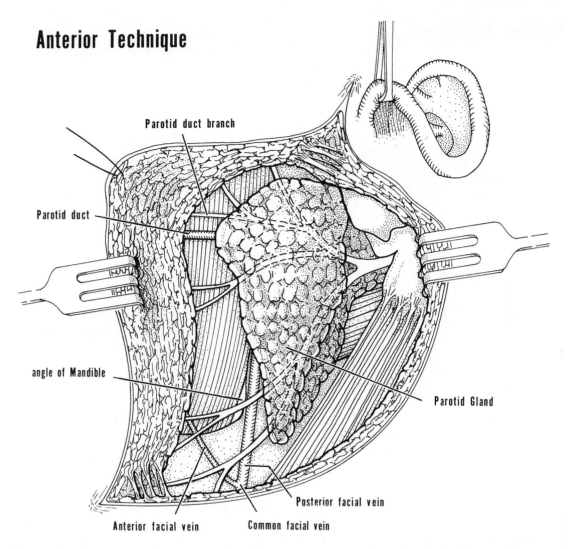

Parotid duct branch

Parotid duct

angle of Mandible

Parotid Gland

Anterior facial vein

Common facial vein

Posterior facial vein

FIGURE 3-12. Anterior approach to the facial nerve. The anatomy of the parotid duct is relatively consistent as it runs horizontally across the external surface of the masseter muscle, approximately 1 fingerbreadth below the zygoma. A portion of the buccal or zygomatic branch of the facial nerve invariably accompanies the parotid duct as it emerges from the anterior aspect of the parotid gland. The parotid duct is identified, and, using the facial-nerve stimulator, the zygomatic or buccal branch of the facial nerve is easily identified. This branch is followed proximally, the parotid gland being elevated as the dissection proceeds in a posterior direction. The zygomatic or buccal branch joins the superior division of the facial nerve, which in turn joins the main trunk posterior to the parotid gland. This dissection is somewhat difficult, but it is a technique well worth remembering when a tumor involves the posterior and inferior approaches to the facial nerve.

Superficial Lobectomy (Fig. 3–14A). The superficial lobe of the parotid gland is dissected in an anterior-to-posterior direction, superficial to the trunk, superoinferior division, and branches of the facial nerve (pes anserinus, or goosefoot). The tail of the gland is dissected anterosuperiorly before identifying the facial nerve. The entire posterior portion of the gland is dissected in a forward direction. The gland usually extends as high as the zygoma. At this point, the main trunk of the facial nerve has divided into the superior and inferior divisions. Directly in front of this division is the isthmus between the superficial and deep lobes. The isthmus is transected as early as possible.

Dissection immediately anterior to the isthmus should be conducted with care because of the anastomotic branches of the facial nerve in this region. The dissection is conducted mainly with a mosquito hemostat. The plane is dissected lateral to the facial nerve branches by blunt dissection. The fascia between the branches is carefully incised. Troublesome bleeders are carefully clamped and ligated as the dissection continues. A large number of clamps in the field of dissection are cumbersome and dangerous. McCabe and Work in 1967 described this technique as creating tunnels by incising the tissue between them. As the dissection proceeds toward the anterior margin of the gland, an area is approached in which the branches of the facial nerve have divided increasingly and become smaller caliber. Extreme care must be taken not to overmanipulate or stretch the facial nerve. As mentioned previously, a better return of function can be expected after dissection and reanastomosis than after injury or stretching of the nerve without section. Anteriorly, the parotid gland usually projects forward in the form of an accessory lobe adjacent to the parotid duct. This is followed forward to the anterior edge of the masseter muscle. The duct is divided and ligated at this point.

Superior Technique

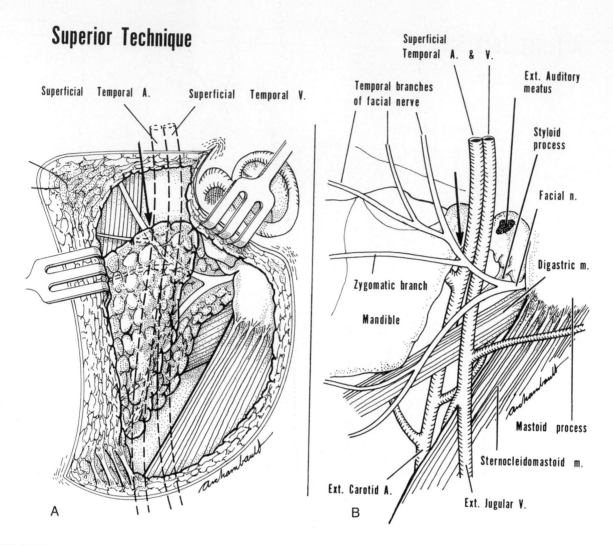

FIGURE 3-13. Superior approach to the facial nerve. The facial nerve can be identified by first extending the incision in the preauricular crease superiorly and elevating the flap anteriorly in a subcutaneous plane. The superficial temporal artery can be identified by its strong pulsations. The superficial temporal vein lies immediately posterior to this structure. The head and neck of the mandible can be identified by palpation. Just below this level, the superior division (temporofacial) of the facial nerve usually crosses over both the superficial temporal artery and vein. The nerve stimulator will facilitate this dissection.

Deep Lobectomy (Fig. 3–14B). The deep lobe of the parotid gland can be resected either along with the superficial lobe or separately. The latter procedure is simpler and safer unless the deep lobe is small and does not receive a number of penetrating blood vessels. Before resection of the deep lobe, the divisions and branches of the facial nerve in this region are carefully undetermined. The isthmus of the gland is grasped and retracted laterally (Fig. 3–15A). The deep lobe can easily be resected from the pterygoid fossa by blunt dissection unless it is penetrated by numerous branches of the internal maxillary artery. Arteries and veins entering the gland in this region should be carefully ligated. Inadvertent injury to the internal maxillary artery or vein can be troublesome. Many surgeons prefer to remove the deep lobe of the parotid gland piecemeal, between the divisions and branches of the facial nerve (Fig. 3–15B).

Closure. After completion of the parotidectomy it is wise to test all branches of the facial nerve and the main trunk with the facial nerve stimulator. The wound is carefully irrigated. All bleeders are carefully clamped and ligated.

Hemovac tubing is inserted, as shown in Figure 3–15C. This tubing should be kept away from direct contact with the facial nerve. The flaps are replaced. The wound is closed subcutaneously with No. 4-0 Dexon suture, and the skin is closed with either No. 5-0 or No. 6-0 polyethylene or nylon monofilament suture, or, better still, No. 6-0 fast-absorbing chromic catgut, using a continuous locking suture. If the fast-absorbing chromic suture is used, Mastisol is applied to the skin and Steri-strips are added to reinforce the suture line.

A dressing is not necessary when closed suction drainage is used. Leaving the wound uncovered allows for better observation and lessens the chance of pressure injury to the facial nerve. In addition, the discomfort of a tight surgical dressing is avoided.

Postoperative Care. The Hemovac closed suction drainage is discontinued after 48 hours. The skin sutures can be removed at the end of 1 week. The patient should be observed carefully during the first few postoperative days for the development of a hematoma. A salivary fistula may occur following a subtotal parotidectomy.

Parotidectomy

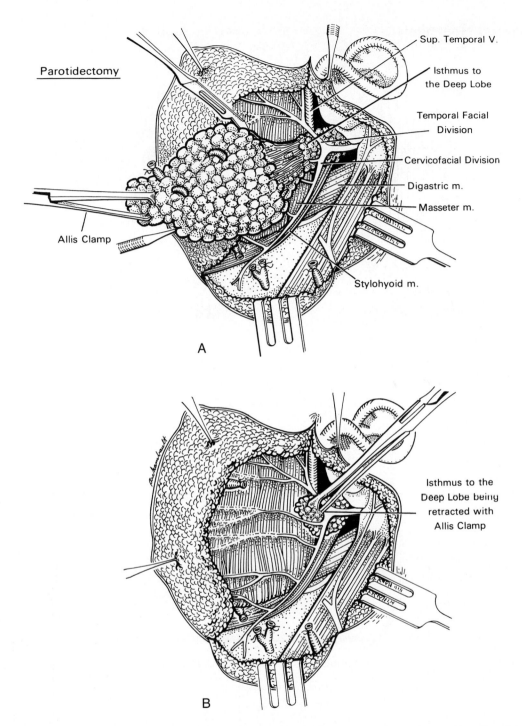

A

B

FIGURE 3-14. Parotidectomy (Continued). *A,* The parotid gland has been dissected from the trunk, divisions, and branches of the facial nerve. The anterior projection of the gland has been dissected free, and the parotid duct is being ligated. This dissection is conducted for the most part with a hemostat clamp. First, tunnels are created lateral to the branches. The fascia between the tunnels is incised as the gland is dissected forward. The facial-nerve stimulator is a useful adjunct to this dissection. *B,* The isthmus of the gland anterior to the temporofacial and cervicofacial divisions. It is important to clamp and ligate all troublesome bleeders, for a large number of hemostats in a bloody field render the dissection difficult and dangerous.

Reexploration for correction of a hematoma or salivary fistula is not advised during the immediate postoperative period because of the probability of facial nerve injury.

The management of facial nerve paralysis due to parotidectomy is discussed later in this chapter. The importance of protecting the eye by performing a lateral tarsorrhaphy and using methylcellulose eye drops is stressed.

Parotid Tumors of the Lateral Pharyngeal Space
(Fig. 3–16)

Tumors of salivary gland origin may occur in the lateral pharyngeal space. These may arise as separate tumors independent of the parotid gland; from the stylomandibular process of the parotid gland (deep to the stylomandibular membrane); or as a dumbbell tumor involving the deep lobe

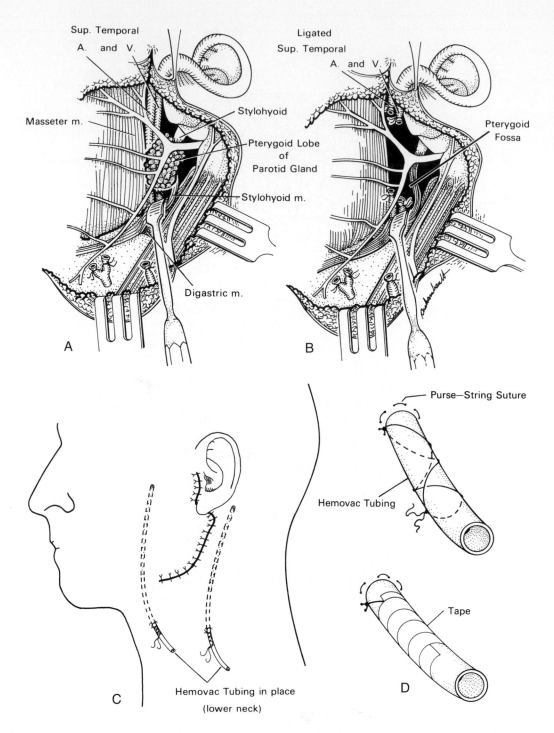

FIGURE 3–15. Parotidectomy (Continued). *A,* The temporofacial and cervicofacial divisions of the facial nerve and adjacent branches have been undermined. The isthmus is grasped with an Allis clamp and the deep (pterygoid) lobe of the parotid gland is being resected. This is accomplished by blunt dissection, care being taken to ligate all penetrating veins and arteries. Some surgeons prefer to remove the deep lobe piecemeal between the divisions and branches of the facial nerve. *B,* The trunk, divisions, and branches of the facial nerve are seen external to the fascia covering the masseter muscle. The posterior belly of the digastric muscle is being retracted posteroinferiorly, exposing the pterygoid fossa, which had been occupied by the deep lobe of the parotid gland. *C* and *D,* Hemovac tubing has been inserted and secured in place with silk suture material. The flaps have been replaced and repaired in two layers with No. 4-0 chromic catgut and No. 5-0 polyethylene sutures or 6-0 continuous mild chromic catgut suture. No dressing is necessary. This allows for better observation for complications, less chance for pressure injury to the facial nerve, and greater comfort for the patient.

of the parotid gland connected to a tumor in the parapharyngeal space by way of the stylomandibular membrane.

Generally, mixed tumors, occupying the lateral pharyngeal space and not connected to the parotid gland can be resected by way of a vertical incision in the lateral pharyngeal wall.

The exposure here is similar to that for a tonsillectomy. If, however, the tumor is large or extends to the base of the skull, the intraoral approach should be combined with an approach through the submandibular triangle after resection of the submandibular gland or by way of an anterior mandibulotomy.

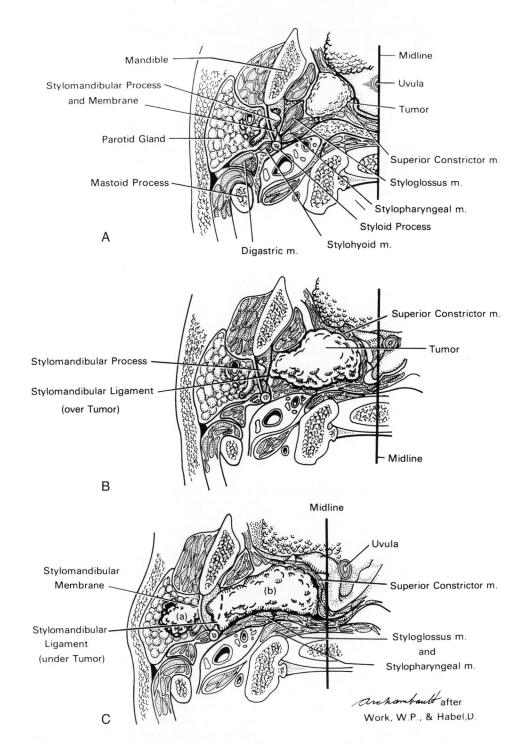

Mandible

Stylomandibular Process
and Membrane

Parotid Gland

Mastoid Process

Midline

Uvula

Tumor

Superior Constrictor m.

Styloglossus m.

Stylopharyngeal m.

Styloid Process

Stylohyoid m.

Digastric m.

A

Stylomandibular Process

Stylomandibular Ligament
(over Tumor)

Superior Constrictor m.

Tumor

Midline

B

Midline

Stylomandibular
Membrane

Stylomandibular
Ligament
(under Tumor)

Uvula

Superior Constrictor m.

Styloglossus m.
and
Stylopharyngeal m.

Archambault after
Work, W.P., & Habel, D.

C

FIGURE 3–16. *A,* Sketch of cross-section through the parotid gland at the level of the uvula (looking from above). The stylomandibular process is an extension of the parotid gland into the stylomandibular membrane. A mixed tumor of the lateral pharyngeal space is shown. Such lesions arise from a minor salivary gland and have no connection with the parotid gland. *B,* The tumor shown here arises from the retromandibular portion of the gland inferior to the stylomandibular ligament. It extends medially and superiorly to the lateral pharyngeal wall. *C,* This is the dumbbell tumor of the parotid gland. The lateral potion (a) of the dumbbell involves the deep lobe of the parotid gland, and the medial portion (b) extends to the lateral pharyngeal wall. The stylomandibular ligament is inferior to and at the level of the constricted portion of the dumbbell tumor.

Tumors arising from the inferior extension of the retromandibular portion of the parotid gland, and not involving the deep lobe of the parotid gland lateral to the stylomandibular membrane, are best resected with the combined parotid and submandibular approach. The facial nerve is identified. The cervicofacial division of the facial nerve is dissected free. (Removal of the tail of the parotid gland facilitates this dissection.) The skin incision is carried forward to expose the submandibular gland, which is resected (Figs. 3–17 to 3–20). Because the bulk of the tumor is in the parapharyngeal space, dissection is conducted mostly by way of the submandibular triangle. The facial nerve is carefully observed, as the posterior portion of the tumor, with surrounding normal parotid gland tissue, is resected.

Resection of the so-called dumbbell tumor is often rather difficult. Bimanual palpation and MRI scan is the best method for preoperative diagnosis of the tumor. The parotid extension can be palpated by applying pressure on the intraoral tumor. Also, the direction of the parapharyngeal tumor mass is deep, in the direction of the angle of the mandible. Resection of a dumbbell tumor is similar to that described for tumors arising from the inferior extension of the retromandibular portion of the parotid gland. However, if the portion of the dumbbell tumor involving the deep lobe of the parotid gland is large, then a superficial parotidectomy is essential to expose and prevent injury to the branches of the facial nerve. It may be necessary to use both the intraoral approach and the submandibular triangle approach to resect the parapharyngeal portion of the tumor, or to approach the tumor following a medial mandibulotomy.

SUBMANDIBULAR GLAND RESECTION

The diagnosis of submandibular gland disease is usually not difficult. The gland is easily examined by means of bimanual palpation. The presence of calculi can be established by routine radiographs of the floor of the mouth, CT scan, or submandibular duct sialography (see Chapter 1).

Indications

The most common indications for resection of the submandibular gland are proximally located calculi or a recurrent distal calculus of the submandibular (Wharton's) duct. Stricture of the submandibular duct, which may occur following a surgical procedure in the floor of the mouth or radiation therapy, is another indication for resection of the submandibular gland. Chronic submandibular sialadenitis can occur without the presence of calculi and may be an indication for resection. Primary tumors of the submandibular gland are not common; those found most often are cysts and adenomas. On occasion, a symptomatic benign hypertrophy of the submandibular gland occurs; it may be independent or associated with a similar hypertrophy of the parotid gland. Resection of the submandibular gland may also be indicated for exposure of underlying lesions involving the floor of the mouth or parapharyngeal tumors. A careful resection of the submandibular gland, with its surrounding lymph nodes, is an important part of a radical neck dissection.

Operative Procedure

General endotracheal anesthesia is preferred to local anesthesia. The patient's entire upper neck, horizontal portion of the mandible, and chin remain exposed with the patient draped for the operation. The inferior margin of the mandible is exposed for proper placement of the incision, and the chin remains in the operative field so that inadvertent stimulation of the ramus mandibularis nerve can be readily seen.

The horizontal skin incision is made along the lines of the chin, approximately 4 cm below the lower edge of the

horizontal portion of the mandible (Fig. 3–17A). It extends from the lateral aspect of the body of the hyoid bone to a point just anterior to the level of the mandibular angle. It is extended through the subcutaneous adipose layer, which varies greatly in thickness, the platysmal muscle, and the underlying superficial cervical fascia (Fig. 3–17B). The anterior border of the sternocleidomastoid muscle indicates the posterior extent of the incision. At this point, the superficial layer of deep cervical fascia external to the submandibular gland is apparent and not disturbed. A lower skin flap (Fig. 3–17C) is developed external to the fascia over the submandibular gland, exposing the intermediate tendon of the digastric muscle and the stylohyoid muscle. Following the tendon posteriorly, the common facial vein can be identified at the junction of the posterior belly of the digastric and sternocleidomastoid muscles (Fig. 3–18A). The common facial vein usually divides into the anterior and posterior veins at this point. The anterior facial vein is ligated and divided. The superior ligature should be left long, with a hemostat attached, so that it can be reflected superiorly. The fascia overlying the submandibular gland is incised in an anteroposterior direction at the inferior level of the gland (Fig. 3–18B). It is easily separated from the gland, unless repeated infections have occurred. As the fascia and anterior facial veins are reflected superiorly, the ramus mandibularis nerve is also retracted superiorly, external to the dissection that follows (Fig. 3–18C). Injury to this nerve should be avoided to prevent paralysis of the depressors of the lower lip and the resulting facial asymmetry, which is disturbing to the patient.

After the external surface of the gland has been exposed, the dissection is directed anteriorly (Fig. 3–19A). The anterior branches of the facial artery are encountered in this area and should be ligated and divided. The mylohyoid muscle is easily dissected from the anterior border of the submandibular gland. Its fibers run perpendicular to the fibers of the anterior belly of the digastric muscle.

The entire posterior border of the mylohyoid muscle is delineated and retracted anteriorly with a smooth blade retractor. The dissection is continued along the superior border of the submandibular gland (Fig. 3–19B). At this level, the anterior facial artery is encountered superficial to, through, or posterior to the submandibular gland and is ligated and divided. After the surgeon accomplishes this, the superior border can readily be freed by blunt dissection.

The next step is to identify positively the lingual nerve. This is accomplished by retracting the mylohyoid muscle anteriorly, grasping the anterosuperior aspect of the submandibular gland with a Babcock or Allison clamp, and retracting it in a posteroinferior direction. In so doing, the lingual nerve, which is tented down by the submandibular ganglion, is readily identified by its glistening white appearance (Fig. 3–19C). A mosquito-type hemostat is placed across the submandibular ganglion and its accompanying vein. These structures are transected below the clamp, and a ligature is applied above the clamp. This maneuver frees the lingual nerve, which retracts superiorly, out of the field.

The dissection is directed inferiorly. The intermediate tendon, anterior and posterior bellies of the digastric muscle, and the stylohyoid muscle are delineated (Fig. 3–20A). The submandibular gland is reflected superiorly, and, almost invariably, the hypoglossal nerve can be identified coursing

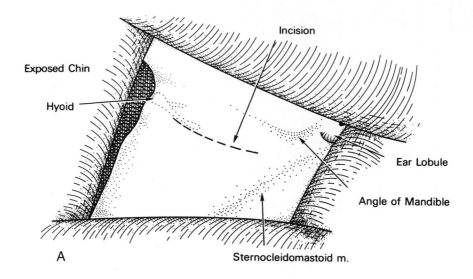

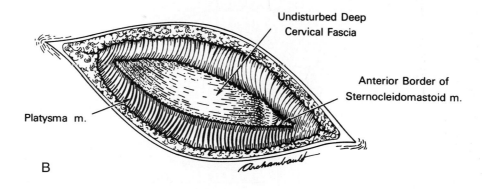

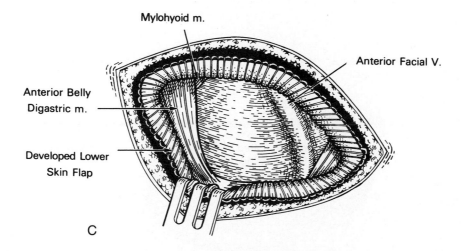

FIGURE 3-17. Submandibular gland resection. *A,* The upper half of the neck, the chin, and the lower border of the mandible should remain exposed as the patient is draped for the operation. The skin lesion is extended along a natural crease about 4 cm below the mandible from the lateral aspect of the hyoid bone nearly to the level of the mandibular angle. *B,* The incision is continued through the subcutaneous layer, which varies considerably in thickness, to the superficial layer of deep cervical fascia overlying the submandibular gland. *C,* Dissection is continued between the platysma and the superficial layer of deep cervical fascia, exposing the anterior belly and intermediate tendon of the digastric muscle and the anterior border of the sternocleidomastoid muscle.

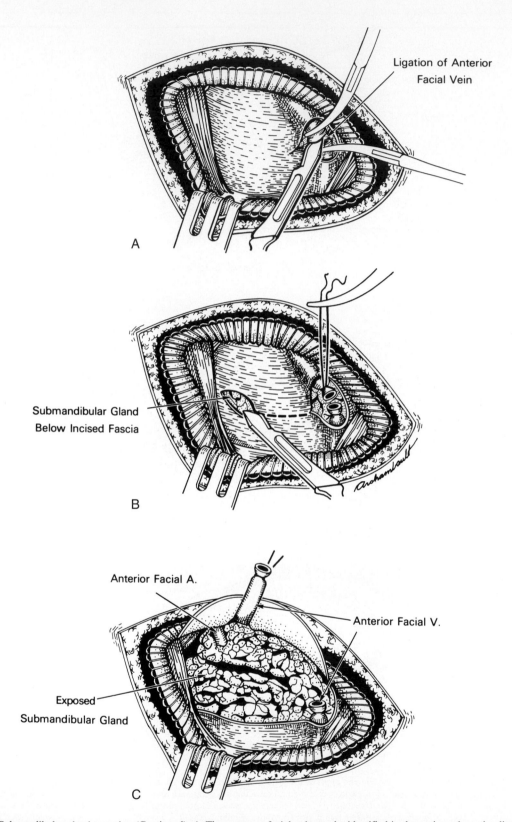

FIGURE 3–18. Submandibular gland resection (Continued). *A,* The common facial vein can be identified in the region where the digastric muscle meets the sternocleidomastoid muscle. At this point, the common facial vein is formed by the junction of the anterior and posterior facial veins. The anterior facial vein is divided and ligated. The ligature on the distal segment of this vein remains long and is clamped for superior retraction. *B,* The fascia overlying the submandibular gland is incised at about the same level as the skin incision. *C,* The anterior facial vein and overlying superficial layer of deep cervical fascia are carefully elevated over the submandibular gland. In so doing, the ramus mandibularis branch of the facial nerve is reflected superiorly away from the field of operation.

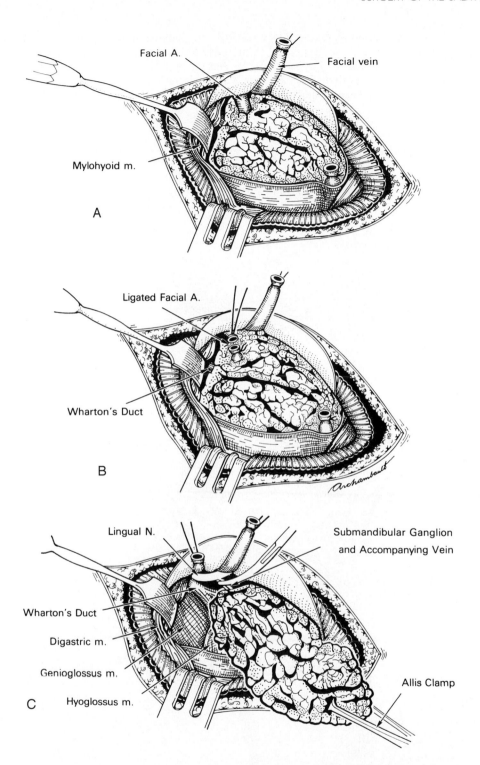

FIGURE 3-19. Submandibular gland resection (Continued). *A,* The posterior border of the mylohyoid muscle is dissected free from the submandibular gland and retracted anteriorly. Numerous small blood vessels may be encountered in this area. *B,* Dissection is continued along the superior and posterior borders of the submandibular gland. The facial artery is identified and ligated. This may be found coursing anterior to, through, or posterior to the gland. The remainder of the superior border is easily dissected. *C,* The lingual nerve is brought into view by retracting the mylohyoid muscle anteriorly and pulling the submandibular gland in a posteroinferior direction. The submandibular ganglion and its accompanying vein are clamped and divided. In so doing, the lingual nerve becomes reflected superiorly away from the surgical field.

in an anterosuperior direction just above and medial to the anterior belly of the digastric muscle (see Fig. 3–20A). The gland is carefully dissected from this structure. The submandibular duct is found immediately inferior to the lingual nerve (Fig. 3–20B). After this structure has been ligated and divided, the submandibular gland is elevated and retracted inferiorly to identify the genioglossus and hyoglossus muscles and the proximal end of the facial artery. The proximal end of the facial artery is ligated immediately above the digastric muscle (see Fig. 3–20A and B).

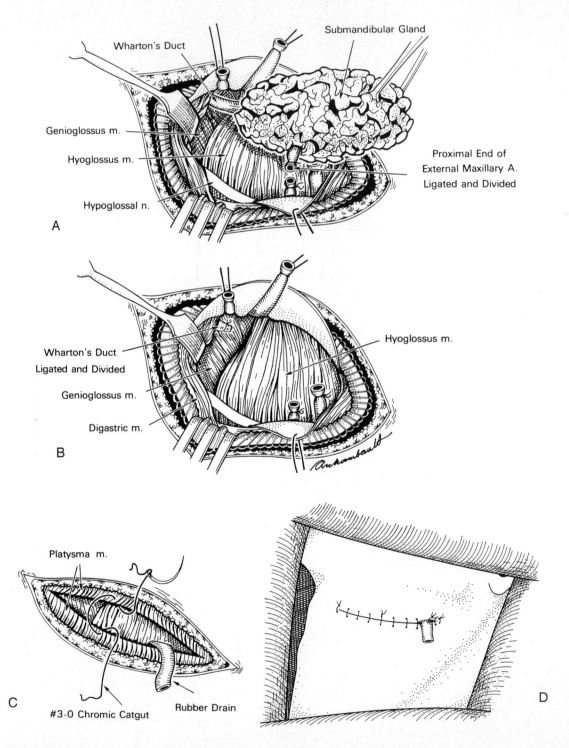

FIGURE 3–20. Submandibular gland resection (Continued). A, The intermediate tendon, anterior and posterior bellies of the digastric muscle, and the stylohyoid muscle are delineated. The inferior border of the submandibular gland is dissected free. The hypoglossal nerve is identified anteriorly as the anterior belly of the digastric muscle is retracted. The proximal portion of the facial (external maxillary) artery is ligated and divided. The submandibular gland remains attached only by the submandibular (Wharton's) duct. B, The submandibular duct is ligated and divided, and the gland is removed. The genioglossus and hyoglossus muscles are identified. C, The wound is closed in layers with No. 3-0 chromic catgut sutures. The platysma muscle should be carefully approximated. D, A Penrose drain is inserted posteriorly. The dermal layer is repaired by a subcuticular suture or interrupted sutures of No. 5-0 dermal suture material.

It is important to ligate the submandibular gland as far distally as possible to remove ductal stones. (Consider, for example, a 33-year-old man with a long history of submandibular gland infection and a stone in the submandibular duct. A submandibular gland resection was performed and he did well for 6 years, at which time pain and swelling again appeared in the submandibular triangle. A radiograph (Fig. 3–21) showed a stone in the distal duct that had not been resected in the procedure performed 6 years earlier.)

The entire field is palpated for enlarged lymph nodes. If any are present, they should be resected individually for examination.

The wound is carefully closed in layers with No. 3-0 or No. 4-0 chromic catgut sutures. It is important to carefully approximate the platysmal muscle (Fig. 3–20C). Drainage is accomplished by inserting either a Penrose drain or a single multiporous closed-suction drain, which should remain in place for at least 24 hours postoperatively. The skin is closed with No. 5-0 or No. 6-0 dermal suture to avoid excessive scarring (Fig. 3–20D). If minimal scarring is essential, a subcuticular stitch can be used.

FACIAL NERVE PARALYSIS

The facial nerve (Fig. 3–22 and Table 3–1) is the most frequently paralyzed nerve in the body. Paralysis of this nerve is a dreaded complication of intracranial, temporal bone, and parotid gland disease or surgery. It is a source of consider-

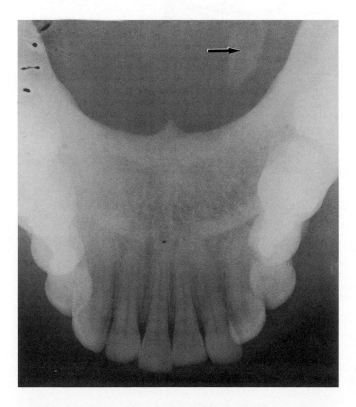

FIGURE 3-21. A stone *(arrow)* in the left submandibular duct that was not removed at the time of the submandibular resection. Eleven years later the site became infected, necessitating removal along with the remainder of the duct. This case points out the importance of removing the duct and stone at the time of gland resection.

able discomfort to patients because of the altered appearance of the face, the disturbed facial expression, the eye complications, the difficulty it causes with eating and drinking, and its effect on speech.

Etiology
Approximately 90% of cases of facial paralysis are caused by lesions in the temporal bone. The majority of these are diagnosed as idiopathic, or Bell's, facial palsy, which has been speculated as being caused by a virus, a microvascular disorder, or an autoimmune response. Other causes of intratemporal facial paralysis are herpes zoster oticus, fracture of the temporal bone, acute and chronic middle ear and mastoid infections, cholesteatoma, complication of a mastoid operation, diabetes, and tumors such as the glomus tumor, carcinoma, facial nerve tumor, and other less common lesions.

Involvement of the facial nerve in intracranial lesions is uncommon. Only 4% of cases of facial paralysis are caused by intracranial lesions. These lesions can be divided into three groups: supranuclear, nuclear, and posterior cranial fossa lesions. Supranuclear lesions, involving the cerebral cortex, can be the result of cerebrovascular accident, intracranial tumor, or trauma. Nuclear lesions are caused by tumors, inflammation, or aplasia. Facial nerve paralysis initiated in the posterior cranial fossa is most commonly caused by a cerebellopontine tumor, a meningeal lesion, a tumor of the petrous ridge, or fracture. Intracranial operations in which the posterior cranial fossa is involved can be complicated by facial nerve paralysis.

Paralysis of the extratemporal portion of the facial nerve (accounting for approximately 6% of facial paralysis) is undoubtedly the most dreaded complication of parotid gland surgery. Metastatic tumors and extension of disease from adjacent structures can involve the facial nerve. On occasion, acute or subacute infection of the parotid gland can result in facial nerve paralysis. Complete or incomplete facial paralysis associated with facial trauma is not uncommon.

Clinical Evaluation of the Paralysis

Evaluation of Degree
To evaluate the degree of paralysis, the patient is first observed for symmetry at rest (Fig. 3–23A and B). The frontal, ocular, and oral regions are then carefully evaluated for function and degree of paralysis. Is the paralysis complete or incomplete? If incomplete, is the distribution general? (It should be kept in mind that the function in the frontal region may be preserved in cases of cortical lesions and that isolated areas of function region may be preserved in cases of cortical lesions and that isolated areas of function are not uncommon in intracranial and extratemporal lesions.) The eye should be examined carefully to determine whether the cornea is protected by an adequate Bell's phenomenon and whether there is stasis of tears as a result of the lagophthalmos. Is the eye dry, and is the cornea ulcerated or painful? Swallowing liquids and chewing may present a problem and may result in ulceration of the buccal mucous membrane and drooling. The sagging face often causes considerable speech impediment, which should be evaluated and discussed with the patient. Unilateral nasal obstruction may accompany the facial paralysis.

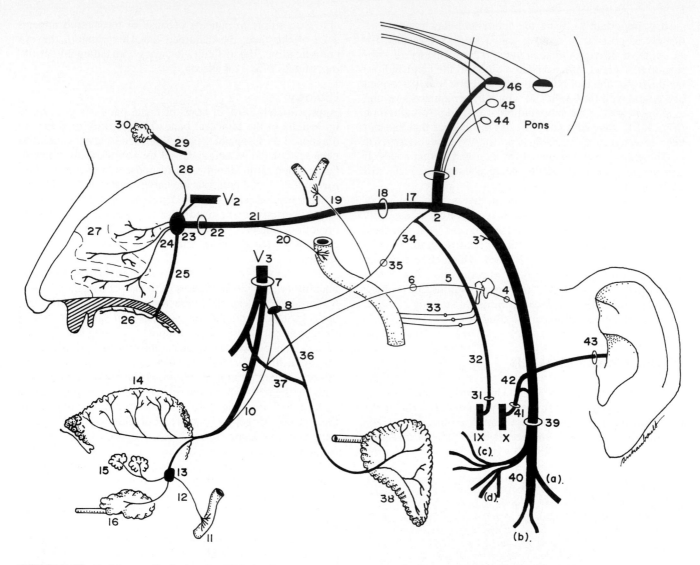

FIGURE 3–22. Facial nerve distribution. See Table 3–1 for numbers corresponding to the anatomic parts.

TABLE 3–1
Facial Nerve Distribution (see Figure 3-22 for numbers corresponding to the anatomical parts)

1. Internal auditory canal
2. Geniculate ganglion
3. Nerve to the stapedius muscle
4. Iter chordae posterius
5. Chorda tympani
6. Iter chordae anterius
7. Foramen ovale
8. Otic ganglion
9. Lingual nerve
10. Junction of chorda tympani and gland
11. Facial artery
12. Sympathetic fibers to ganglion
13. Submandibular ganglion
14. Distribution for taste, anterior
15. Sublingual glands
16. Submandibular gland
17. Greater superficial petrosal nerve
18. Hiatus canalis facialis superior
19. Sympathetic fibers from middle
20. Deep petrosal nerve (sympathetic infraorbital) fibers from carotid artery)
21. Nerve to vidian canal (middle fossa)
22. Vidian canal

23. Sphenopalatine ganglion
24. Postganglionic nerves to nasal
25. Greater palatine nerve
26. Postganglionic distribution to glands
   Palatal mycosa
   Sphenopalatine ganglion:
      Location: Pterygomaxillary fossa
      Distribution: 1. nasal mucosa
                      2. lacrimal gland
                      3. palitinal mucosa
   Otic ganglion:
      Location: just below foramen ovale
      Distribution: parotid gland
   Submandibular ganglion:
      Location: on hypoglossal muscle
      Distribution: submandibular and sublin-
      gual and taste and sensation to anterior
      two thirds of tongue
27. Nasal mucosa
28. Nerve to lacrimal gland mucosa
29. Lacrimal nerve
30. Lacrimal gland
31. Inferior tympanic canaliculus

32. Jacobson's nerve (branch of IX)
33. Caroticotympanicus nerves (sympathetic)
34. Lesser superficial petrosal nerve
35. Hiatus canalis facialis inferior
36. Postganglionic fibers to parotid lingual nerve
37. Auriculotemporal nerve
38. Parotid gland
39. Stylomastoid foramen
40. Facial nerve two thirds of tongue
   a. Postauricular branch
   b. Nerves to stylohyoid and posterior belly of digastric muscles
   c. Branches from the craniotemporal division (temporal-zygomatic)
   d. Branches from the craniocervical division (buccal-mandibular-cervical)
41. Mastoid canaliculus
42. Arnold's nerve (auricularis X)
43. Tympanomastoid fissure
44. Tractus solitarus (afferent from mucosa tongue)
45. Superior salivary nucleus salivary
46. VII nerve nucleus

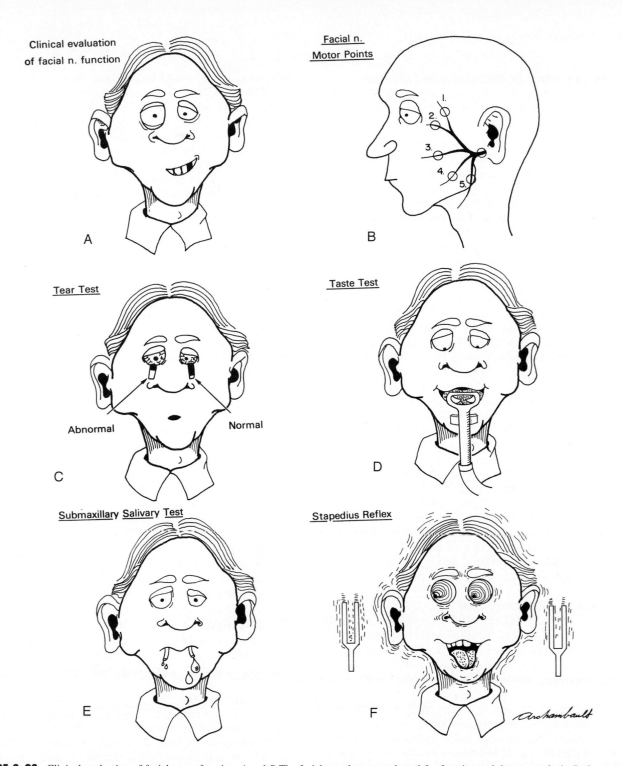

FIGURE 3-23. Clinical evaluation of facial nerve function. *A* and *B* The facial muscles are evaluated for function and degree paralysis. Is the eye adequately protected by Bell's phenomenon? Is there pooling of tears as a result of lagophthalmos? Is the eye dry? Does the patient drool? Does he have difficulty with chewing or speech articulation? If the frontal region is not involved a cortical lesion may be indicated. *C*, Lacrimation (Schirmer) test. This is used to determine the function of the greater superficial petrosal nerve (parasympathetic fibers). Two pieces of filter paper, 5 × 35 mm, are folded at right angles 5 mm from one end. After the examiner has made certain that there is no pooling of tears in the lower fornix, the patient is asked to gaze upward and the test strips are inserted over the lower eyelids at the junction of the middle and nasal one third. The strips are examined at the end of 5 minutes. A measurement of 15 mm is considered indicative of normal lacrimation. A measurement below 10 mm indicates abnormality if the measurement on the opposite side showed lacrimation to be normal. *D*, Taste test. Electrogustometry is a test of chorda tympani nerve function. The Urban Taste Tester, or a comparable battery-powered instrument, is used for quantitative evaluation of taste on the anterior two thirds of the tongue. Twenty to 40 μA are required to elicit taste in the young. This value increases to 150 μA with age. A difference of as little as 20 μA between the two sides is significant. A complete loss of taste is indicated by a current of 300 μA. *E*, Submaxillary Salivary Flow Test. The submandibular salivary flow tests the chorda tympani function and provides an accurate method to determine the ultimate course toward facial-nerve degeneration or to spontaneous recovery. A topical anesthetic is applied to the anterior floor of the mouth and a local anesthetic is infiltrated with a No. 25 to No. 30 needle beneath the frenulum. Both submandibular ducts are dilated with a punctum dilator, and No. 50 polyethylene tubing is inserted. This is accomplished by either beveling the end of the tube or inserting the tubing over a No. 5 suction tube obturator. Several drops of lemon juice are inserted in the anterior floor of the mouth to stimulate salivary flow. The number of drops of saliva obtained in approximately 2 minutes is counted. If the salivary flow on the affected side is 30% of normal compared with the opposite side, complete nerve degeneration is inevitable. *F*, Stapedius muscle reflex. Hyperacusis may indicate paralysis at or above the level of the nerve to the stapedius muscle. The test can be performed by striking two 500-cycle tuning forks with maximum intensity and simultaneously bringing one toward the right ear and the other toward the left ear. A more sophisticated method for demonstrating hyperacusis is with the use of the alternate binaural loudness test, an acoustic impedance meter, or a Zwislocki Bridge.

Electrical Testing of Facial Nerve Function

It is often difficult to stimulate the main trunk of the facial nerve as it exits from the stylomastoid foramen. It is more practical to use the five motor points (Fig. 3–23B).

1. The forehead and eyebrow are tested at a point 1 inch behind and slightly above the lateral aspect of the eyebrow.
2. The periorbital region can be tested at a point over the mid-zygomatic arch.
3. The cheek, upper lip, and nasal ala can be tested at a point midway between the base of the ear lobule and nasal ala.
4. The lower lip is tested by stimulating the ramus mandibularis nerve, at or slightly below the mandibular notch.
5. The cervical or platysmal area is tested by stimulating just posterior to the submandibular triangle.

When using *nerve excitability test* (NET), 3.5 to 5 milliamperes of current are usually necessary to stimulate the normal side, and also the involved (paralyzed) side if there is no reaction of degeneration. The degeneration is termed neurapraxia or a physiologic nerve block. A difference of 3 to 4 milliamperes between the normal and paralyzed side in the absence of any clinical improvement is significant, and indicates impending degeneration of the facial nerve.

The *maximum stimulation test* (MST) is probably more meaningful than the NET, as it is a more reliable method for evaluating facial nerve function and altered earlier during the process of facial nerve degeneration. A difference between the two sides can be detected by using the MST as early as 24 hours after the onset of paralysis, whereas an abnormal response to the NET may not be obtained until 48 to 72 hours after onset of nerve degeneration. The MST is carried out by increasing the current until the stimulus is uncomfortable. The facial muscle movements of the normal and involved side are compared during this testing. On occasion, the nerve trunk can be used in performing this test.

Lacrimation (Schirmer) Test

The tear test (Fig. 3–23C) is used to determine the function of the greater superficial petrosal nerve (parasympathetic fibers). Two pieces of filter paper, 5 mm wide and 35 mm long, are needed for this test. Each is folded 5 mm from one end, at approximately a right angle. Topical anesthesia is not required. The patient sits in a chair in front of the examiner and gazes upward. It is important to dry the lower fornix before testing because pooling of tears occurs with facial paralysis. The patient's lower eyelid is drawn downward, and the bent end of the strip is inserted over the lower eyelid at the junction of the middle and nasal thirds. The time at this point is noted. The strips are removed after 5 minutes, and the length of the moistened area is measured. A measurement of 15 mm is considered indicative of normal lacrimation. A measurement below 10 mm indicates an abnormality if a measurement of 15 mm was obtained on the opposite side.

Electrogustometry (Taste Test)

Chorda tympani nerve function can be evaluated by testing the taste sensation of the anterior two thirds of the tongue. Electrical methods provide the only quantitative measurement of taste function. The Taste Tester (Fig. 3–23D) is a practical battery-powered instrument for quantitative evalu-

ation of taste. As would be expected, there is considerable variation between the stimulus required for young and old patients. As a rule, 20 to 40 μA is required to elicit a response in the young, whereas up to 150 μA is required to elicit a response in elderly patients. The amount of current required for a response in the normal side is compared with that in the abnormal side. A difference of as little as 20 μA is significant. If no sensation of taste is initiated by a current of 300 μA, a total lack of chorda tympani function is indicated.

Submandibular Salivary Flow Test

Measurement of submandibular salivary flow (Fig. 3–23E) tests the chorda tympani function on the affected side compared with the normal side. The test should be performed as soon as possible following the onset of facial paralysis. May and Harvey suggest that repeated testing of submandibular salivary gland function is a more accurate method than the nerve excitability test for determining the ultimate course of facial nerve paralysis. In their series, if the salivary flow was 30% or less, of normal, compared with the opposite side, a complete nerve degeneration was inevitable.

A topical anesthetic is applied to the anterior floor of the mouth, and a local anesthetic is infiltrated using a No. 25 to No. 30 needle in the midline underneath the frenulum. This injection anesthetizes the area and elevates both papillae. The orifices of both submandibular ducts are dilated with a punctum dilator. The ducts are then probed to detect strictures or stones. A No. 50 polyethylene tube can be inserted into the submandibular duct by beveling the end or inserting the tubing over the obturator of a No. 5 suction tip. The tube is secured to the chin with tape. Several drops of lemon juice are inserted into the patient's mouth to stimulate salivary flow. The number of drops of saliva obtained in 2 minutes is counted, and comparison is made between the normal and the affected sides.

The Stapedius Muscle Reflex

Hyperacusis may indicate a paralysis at or above the level of the nerve to the stapedius muscle (Fig. 3–23F). Occasionally, a patient with facial paralysis will report hyperacusis. A simple office test for this condition is performed by striking two 500-cycle tuning forks with maximum intensity and simultaneously bringing one toward the right ear and the other toward the left ear. The effect of hyperacusis on the affected side will be obvious. A more sophisticated method for demonstrating hyperacusis is with an acoustic impedance rise at about 60 decibels. If not, the stapedius muscle is not functioning. The ABLB (alternate binaural loudness balance) test also can be used in cooperative patients to demonstrate hyperacusis.

Determining the Location of a Facial Nerve Lesion

Determining the location of a facial nerve lesion is often difficult. There are certain guidelines that will point to a specific area.

1. Supranuclear lesion. Supranuclear paralysis may be limited to the lower third of the face. Good muscle tone and a spontaneous smile may be present. Bell's phenomenon is

absent. Taste and lacrimation are normal. There may be other neurologic defects.

2. Nuclear lesion. Complete facial paralysis is often associated with sixth nerve paralysis. Lacrimation, salivation, and taste are not affected. A spontaneous smile is absent.

3. Posterior cranial fossa lesion. The vestibular and cochlear portions of the eighth cranial nerve may be involved. In these instances, facial paralysis is complete. Taste, lacrimation, and salivation may be altered. The fifth, ninth, tenth, and eleventh cranial nerves may be involved.

4. Geniculate ganglion lesion. Complete facial paralysis is present. Hyperacusis is present, and taste, lacrimation, and salivation are altered.

5. Tympanomastoid intratemporal lesion. The facial paralysis is complete, lacrimation is intact, and taste and salivation are altered.

6. Extratemporal lesion. Facial paralysis may be incomplete (there may be a branch or two spared). Taste, salivation, and lacrimation are normal.

Complications of Facial Nerve Paralysis

Paralysis of the orbicularis oculi muscle with resultant sagging of the lower lid (lagophthalmos) is, without doubt, the most troublesome feature of facial nerve paralysis. The patient is unable to approximate the lids, and there is pooling of tears in the fornix as a result of sagging of the lower lid. This results in intermittent blurring of vision and epiphora. The cornea is exposed, causing excessive evaporation of the tear film, drying of the eye, exposure keratitis, and corneal ulcer. Corneal ulcer is especially apt to occur when lacrimal function is decreased. It is extremely painful unless there is a simultaneous paralysis of the fifth nerve. Corneal ulcers can progress to perforation of the globe and blindness.

Immediate therapy is indicated when lagophthalmos is present. Patching of the eye is not too effective and, occasionally, can precipitate corneal ulceration when the eye remains open under the patch. Taping the lids together with Multipore Tape (3-M Company) is effective. The application of artificial teardrops and ointments is valuable as a short-term measure in keeping the cornea moist. A lateral tarsorrhaphy is indicated when the lagophthalmos is severe enough to prevent Bell's phenomenon from protecting the cornea. It is effective when properly executed (Figs. 3–24 to 3–39).

A lagophthalmos complicated by loss of corneal sensation (fifth nerve paralysis) requires the expertise of an ophthalmologist. A medial and lateral tarsorrhaphy will prevent corneal ulceration.

Tics, spasms, or contractures are the result of faulty regeneration. The contractures may result from replacement of atrophied muscle fibers with connective tissue. Synkinetic facial movements, such as the corner of the mouth being elevated when the patient closes his eye, is the result of fibers not following their original course during regeneration.

Unilateral lacrimation with mastication (crocodile tear syndrome) is the result of parasympathetic fibers originally supplying the parotid gland being misdirected to the lacrimal gland during regeneration.

The auriculotemporal syndrome (Frey's syndrome) consists of facial flushing and sweating over the parotid area

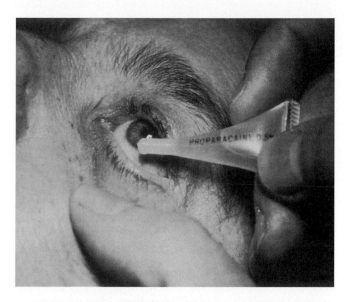

FIGURE 3-24. One drop of topical anesthesia (proparacaine, 0.5%) is placed in the eye and repeated in 5 minutes.

during mastication. It is the result of parasympathetic fibers, which were originally motor secretory to the parotid gland, being misdirected to the skin overlying the parotid gland during regeneration.

Not of least importance are the psychological and social difficulties that occur as a result of facial paralysis. The drooling with eating and drinking, the impaired speech, and the deprivation of effective facial expressions that patients with facial paralysis exhibit should be sufficient to initiate every effort for the restoration of function.

Lagophthalmos (inability to close the lids) results from paralysis of the orbicularis oculi muscle. The loss of the blink reflex and inability to close the lids results in a loss of movement of the tear film across the eye that moistens the very sensitive cornea. The flaccid lower lid resulting from loss of tone of the orbicularis oculi muscle produces an ectropion and poor drainage of tears. This, in addition to the increased evaporation of tears with the open eye, may result in damage to the corneal epithelium, which in turn leads to exposure keratitis, corneal ulceration and, on occasion, perforations. The patient's ability to look upward while attempting to close the eyelid (Bell's phenomenon) affects the incidence of exposure keratitis associated with paralysis of the orbicularis oculi muscle. Decreased tear production adds to this complication. It is thus wise to test tear production with the Schirmer test when decreased tear production is suspected.

A fifth nerve paralysis is a much more serious condition. The cornea is insensitive to pain, and thus there is no warning of exposure keratitis and corneal ulceration. The denervated epithelium is more easily injured, so ulcerations occur more readily. Once the ulceration has occurred, the denervated epithelium heals more slowly.

Management of Lagophthalmos
The use of drops and ointments is the simplest and most conservative management of the lagophthalmos and the dis-

comfort of the exposed cornea. Artificial tears, such as 1% methycellulose or polyvinyl alcohol, can be used every 1 or 2 hours. These usually do not produce blurred vision and can control the problem of dispersion of tears to cover the cornea. If the drops do not help, ointment is indicated. The ointment of choice is 0.5% erythromycin. This ointment is very effective but has the advantage of producing blurred vision. The ointment should be applied at bedtime, especially when the patient reports discomfort or when there is a poor Bell's phenomenon or decreased sensation of the cornea because of fifth nerve involvement.

The patient should wear protective glasses, such as wraparound goggles, especially when outdoors and exposed to wind and dust. The goggles actually form a humidity chamber. The humidity inside the chamber can be increased by adding a small piece of moist filter paper; however, this will fog the lens.

Taping of the lid is indicated in patients who do not have adequate ocular protection, patients who have pain, or patients with keratitis or corneal ulceration. Most patients with lagophthalmos should apply ointment at night and tape their lids closed. Clear plastic adhesive tape is best suited for this purpose. Tincture of benzoin is applied to the skin and allowed to dry before taping. When the tape is properly applied, there should be no sight with the eye.

A lateral tarsorrhaphy procedure or gold weight implanted in the upper lid is indicated in patients in whom recovery of the facial nerve is not expected for at least 3 months. It is also indicated in patients who have a poor Bell's phenomenon, severe lagophthalmos, dry eye, or a fifth nerve paralysis. A lateral and medial tarsorrhaphy is indicated in patients who have had repeated keratitis and corneal ulcers and patients who have both a dry eye and anesthesia of the cornea.

Other methods to protect the cornea of patients with a paralysis of the orbicularis oculi muscle include soft contact lens use, scleral shell, muscle transplant, palpebral spring implantation, and hypoglossal facial anastomosis. It is the authors' opinion that conservative management should be performed as long as the cornea is being properly protected and there is no anesthesia of the cornea and if there is a pos-

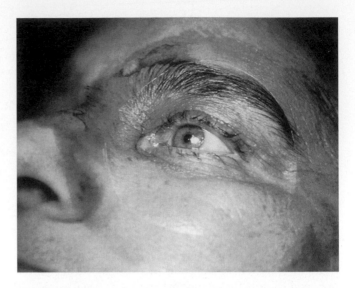

FIGURE 3–25. The eye is prepped with povidone-iodine (Betadine) solution and allowed to dry before a plastic drape is applied.

sibility that facial nerve function will return within a reasonable length of time. In other cases, the lateral tarsorrhaphy should be performed immediately, and a hypoglossal facial nerve anastomosis should be considered (1) in 9 months if the continuity of the facial nerve remains intact or (2) immediately if the nerve has been sectioned and anastomosis or grafting of the nerve is not possible.

Lateral Tarsorrhaphy

Technique. The technique of the lateral tarsorrhaphy operation will be given in considerable detail. When properly executed, this is the most effective method for protecting the eye. In addition, the result is not too cosmetically objectionable, and the procedure can be reversed easily when either facial nerve function has returned or the hypoglossal facial anastomosis becomes effective (approximately 6 months). The lateral tarsorrhaphy can be performed as an

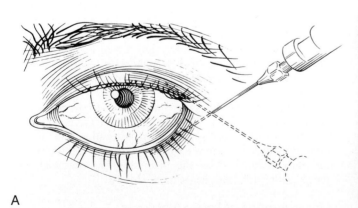

A

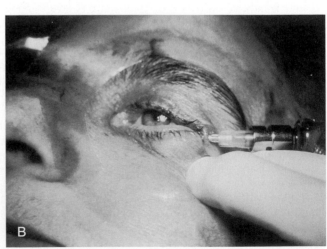

B

FIGURE 3–26. *A* and *B*, Local anesthesia (2% lidocaine with epinephrine 1:150,000) is injected from a point 5 mm lateral to the external canthus. The lateral half of both lid margins is infiltrated.

office procedure, in a minor procedure room, in the operating room, or even at the patient's bedside. The necessary equipment includes the following items:

povidone-iodine (Betadine) solution;
proparacaine 1%;
1% lidocaine (Xylocaine) with epinephrine;
normal saline solution;
0.5% erythromycin ophthalmic ointment;
No. 5-0 polyethylene suture (Dermalene);
No. 28 or No. 30 short hypodermoid needle;
2 mL syringe;
No. 15 Bard-Parker blade;
knife handle;
needle holder;
fixation forceps;
fine-toothed forceps;
scissors (straight iris, curved iris, suture)

Procedure. The lateral tarsorrhaphy procedure is performed with the patient in the supine position and the surgeon seated at the patient's side. Preoperative medication is not necessary. One drop of topical anesthesia, such as 1% proparacaine, is placed in the eye (see Fig. 3–24). This is repeated in 5 minutes. The eye is prepared with povidone-iodine (Betadine) solution, which is allowed to dry before applying a plastic drape (Fig. 3–25). The lid margins are anesthetized with 1% lidocaine with epinephrine. The injection of local anesthesia is begun at a point 5 mm lateral to the external canthus. The lateral half of each lid margin is infiltrated by gradually pushing the local anesthetic agent ahead of the needle point (Fig. 3–26A and B).

The upper lid margin is grasped with a fine-toothed forceps approximately 3 or 4 mm from the external canthus. The epithelium under the forceps is cut with straight or curved iris scissors, thus exposing the tarsal plate (Fig. 3–27). The external canthus must not be violated so that, if

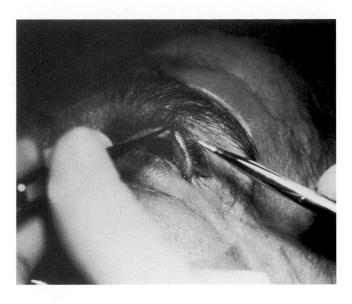

FIGURE 3–28. A strip about 6 mm long is cut from the upper lid margin and left intact medially.

function returns, the tarsorrhaphy can be reversed at a later date. A strip about 6 mm long is cut from the upper lid margin. This strip of epithelium is temporarily left intact medially (Fig. 3–28). A similar strip of epithelium is taken from the lower lid margin somewhat more medially placed than that of the upper lid (Fig. 3–29).

The two epithelium "handles" are grasped with forceps and pulled to bring the medial aspects of the two denuded areas together (Fig. 3–30A). This is a test to determine whether a sufficient length of lower lid margin has been resected to properly correct the lagophthalmos. Once the correct amount has been determined, the "handles" are removed (Fig. 3–30B). A monofilament No. 5-0 polyethylene suture supported by either plastic or rubber tubing (No. 90 polyethylene tubing or silicone rubber tubing) is best suited for

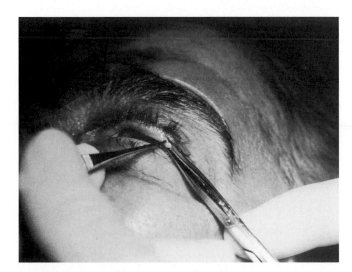

FIGURE 3–27. The upper lid margin is grasped with a fine-toothed forceps approximately 3 or 4 mm from the external canthus. The epithelium under the forceps is cut with a straight or curved iris scissors, thus exposing the tarsal plate.

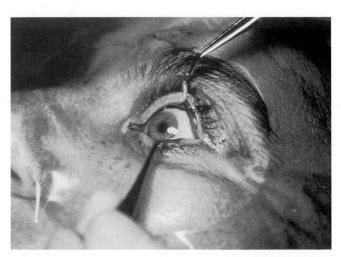

FIGURE 3–29. Epithelium over the margin of the lower lid is grasped 1 or 2 mm more medial as compared with the upper lid, and a strip of equal length is elevated.

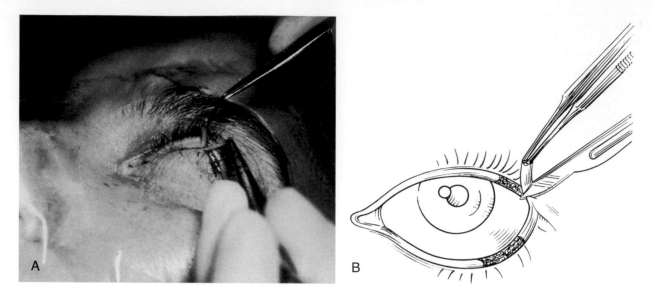

FIGURE 3–30. *A* and *B*, The two "handles" are grasped and pulled to bring the medial aspects of the two denuded areas together. This is a test to determine whether a sufficient length of lower lid margin has been removed to correct the lagophthalmos. Once the correct amount has been determined, the "handles" are removed.

this operation (Fig. 3–31). If the tubing is not used, the suture will be pulled free in a day or two by the levator palpebrae superioris, which is innervated by the third cranial nerve. The suture is placed as follows.

1. Down through the upper tarsal plate at the lateral margin of the denuded strip (Fig. 3–32);
2. Through the lateral aspect of the lower lid margin (Fig. 3–33);
3. Through a 6-mm-long piece of tubing (Fig. 3–34);
4. Up through the medial aspect of the lower denuded lid margin (Fig. 3–35);
5. Through the medial aspect of the upper denuded lid margin (Fig. 3–36);
6. Through a second 6-mm-long piece of tubing (Fig. 3–37); and, finally,
7. The suture is tied with multiple knots at the upper outer aspect of the repair (Fig. 3–38).

At the end of the repair (Fig. 3–39), blood is evacuated from the eye with normal saline solution. Once this has been accomplished, 0.5% erythromycin ointment is placed in the eye and the lids are closed. An eye patch is secured in place, with one strip of plastic tape.

The patient is instructed to apply erythromycin ointment

in the eye for 2 days, keeping the eye patched at all times. Thereafter, the patient should require no therapy unless there is an insufficient production of tears, in which case it would be necessary to continue the usage of artificial tears every 2 hours and the use of erythromycin ointment. It is very important to leave the tarsorrhaphy sutures in place for at least 2 weeks; otherwise, the scar between the lids becomes separated or stretched.

As soon as facial nerve function is restored, the lateral tarsorrhaphy is reversed by using local anesthesia as described above and separating the lids with a scalpel or scissors (see Fig. 3–39).

Facial Reanimation

The surgical management of facial nerve disorders requires an in-depth knowledge of the anatomy and physiology of this structure under normal and pathologic conditions. In addition, an understanding of how the dynamic parts of the face function in an integrated manner and of how disease and trauma result in a variety of complex clinical situations is critical to maximize the chances of optimal rehabilitation. Patients who are candidates for reparative surgery are pri-

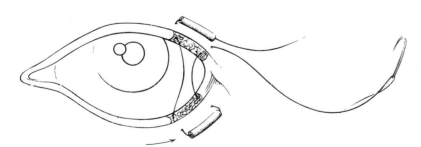

Direction of pull of lower lid

FIGURE 3–31. Sketch of lateral tarsorrhaphy procedure. No. 5-0 polyethylene suture is supported by plastic rubber tubing (No. 90 polyethylene or 0.03 × 0.065 inches silicone rubber tubing); otherwise, the sutures will be pulled free in a day or two by the levator palpebrae superioris.

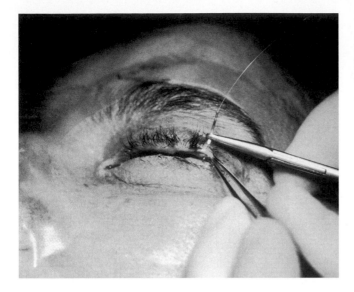

FIGURE 3–32. A suture (No. 5-0 Dermalene) is brought down through the lateral aspect of the denuded strip of the upper lid.

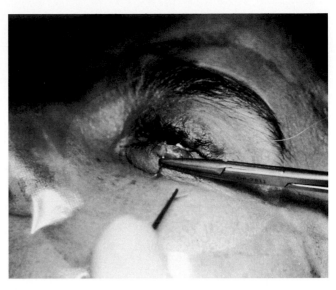

FIGURE 3–35. The suture is then brought up through the medial aspect of the denuded lower lid.

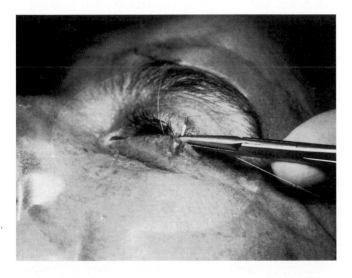

FIGURE 3–33. The suture is then brought through the denuded aspect of the lower lid margin.

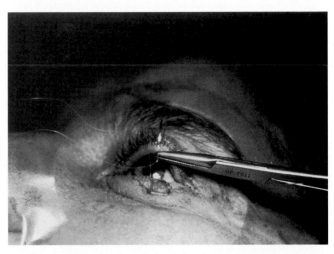

FIGURE 3–36. The suture is brought through the medial aspect of the denuded upper lid.

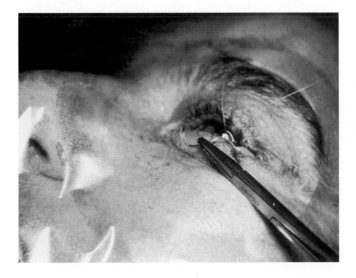

FIGURE 3–34. The suture is inserted through a piece of polyethylene tubing approximately the length of the denuded epithelium.

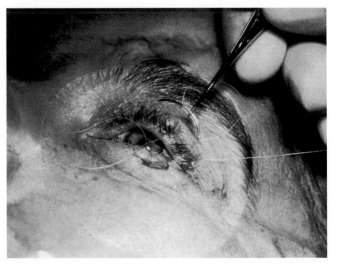

FIGURE 3–37. The suture is finally threaded through a second piece of polyethylene tubing.

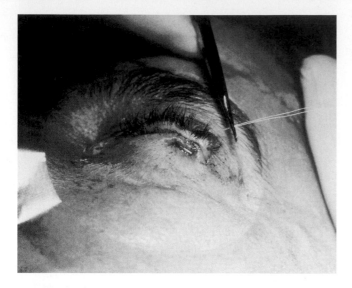

FIGURE 3–38. The suture has been tied with several knots and is being cut.

marily those with a nerve transection injury or long-standing facial paralysis (over 1-year duration) and no physical or electrical evidence of recovery. Conservative therapy with the expectation of spontaneous recovery usually is indicated in less severe injuries. A limited number of patients with congenital abnormalities of facial function and those suffering from hyperkinetic syndromes, including hemifacial spasm and blepharospasm, are candidates for surgical intervention. The surgical management of the paralyzed face varies and in many ways depends on the individual needs and desires of the patient. Other factors that must be considered before the formulation of a surgical plan are the causes and duration of the dysfunction, the patient's age, and the presumed condition of the facial nerve and muscles. The most important goals to be achieved are corneal protection, bilateral symmetry of the face at rest, and restoration of a symmetric smile. The surgeon must be certain that the patient is clear about the surgical objectives and be able to balance the importance of functional versus aesthetic objectives.

Facial Expression

Human communication depends largely on emotions conveyed through different facial expressions, resulting from the action of various muscle groups. Although there are 18 paired muscles involved with facial expression, clinical assessment of facial dysfunction primarily depends on the evaluation of the frontalis, orbicularis oculi, zygomaticus major, orbicularis oris, and lip depressor muscles (Fig. 3–40). Two functional elements are especially important in assessing facial dysfunction before treatment: the status of the nasolabial fold and the dynamics of smile formation.

The nasolabial fold consists of dense fibrous tissue, the levator muscles of the upper lip, and striated muscle bundles originating in the fold's fascia. The shape and depth of the nasolabial fold can vary greatly. Superiorly, the nasolabial fold begins where the alar nasi, cheek, and upper lip meet. From this point, the curve of the fold descends with a lateral orientation and terminates in the corner of the mouth. The fold can assume a straight, convex, or concave course. A smile is formed mainly by the levator muscles of the upper lip that pass through the orbicularis oris, inserting into the dermis and the vermilion line. A smile is divided into *two* stages. In the first stage, all the levator and fold muscles contract, elevating the upper lip to the nasolabial fold against the resistance given by the cheek fat, which limits the superior excursion of the upper lip. In the second stage, the levator superior, zygomaticus major, and caninus muscles raise the lip and the fold upward.

Smiles differ in their line of contracture, point of insertion, and the varying strengths of each muscle group. The interaction of these components results in one of three basic patterns: the zygomaticus major smile, the canine smile, and the full-denture smile. The zygomaticus major is the most common type, occurring 67% of the time; it is dominated by the zygomaticus major muscle (Fig. 3–41A).

The second most common is the canine smile, mainly caused by the action of the levator labii superioris; it occurs approximately 31% of the time (Fig. 3–41B). The least common is the full-denture smile, occurring in 2% of the population; it results from contraction of elevator and depressor muscles of the lips and the angles of the mouth (Fig. 3–41C). In this chapter, the House-Brackmann classification

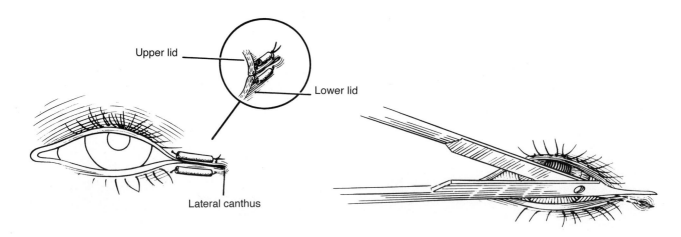

FIGURE 3–39. A sketch demonstrating the end result of the lateral tarsorrhaphy operation and reversal.

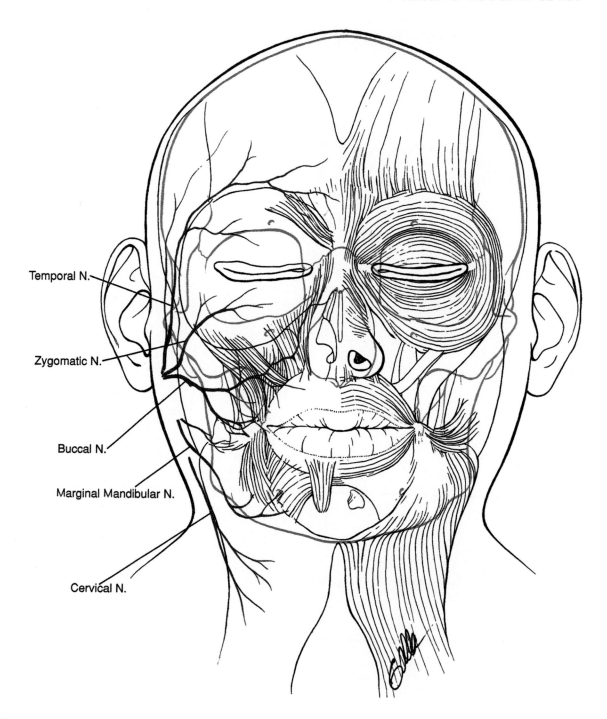

Temporal N.

Zygomatic N.

Buccal N.

Marginal Mandibular N.

Cervical N.

FIGURE 3–40. Peripheral distribution of the facial nerve. Distal to the stylomastoid foramen, the facial nerve branches into five major divisions at the pes anserinus. The nerve first bifurcates into upper and lower divisions. The upper division gives rise to the temporal and zygomatic branches and the lower to the buccal, mandibular, and cervical branches. The temporal branch serves the forehead musculature (frontalis, corrugator), and the zygomatic branch serves the orbicularis oculi. The buccal branch elevates the corner of the mouth, and the marginal mandibular serves the orbicularis oris and depressor labii oris. The cervical branch supplies the platysma.

is used throughout when referring to facial dysfunction and degrees of rehabilitation.

Techniques of Facial Nerve Repair

The most common situation in which facial nerve exploration is considered is following trauma, especially in the context of temporal bone fractures. Patients with immediate facial paralysis after temporal bone fracture proven by CT and electroneurography showing 90% or greater nerve fiber degeneration are candidates for surgical exploration. Occipital or frontal head injuries are the most common causes of transverse temporal bone fractures, which carry a 50% incidence of facial nerve paralysis. Patients with delayed-onset paralysis have an intact nerve; the dysfunction is likely

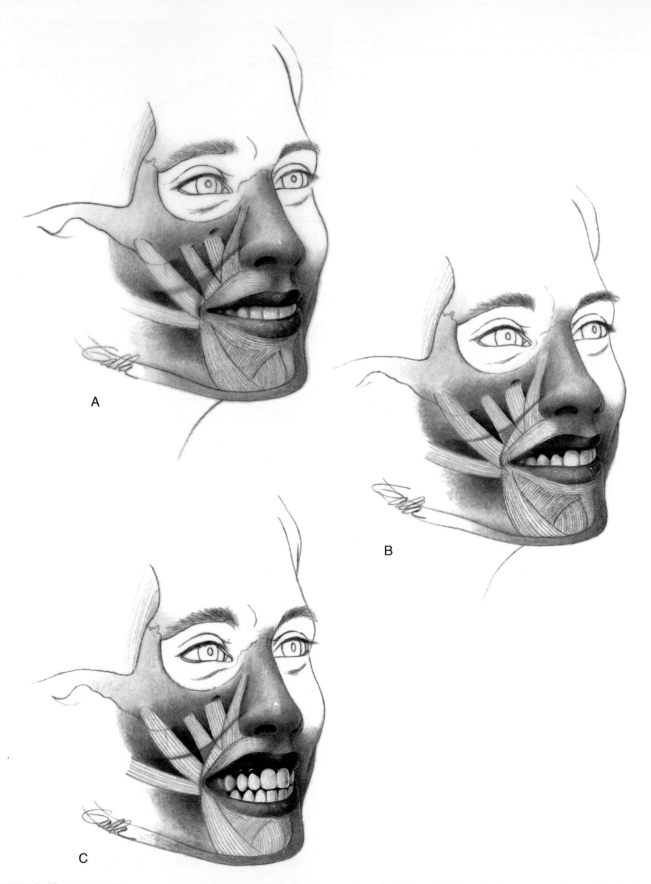

FIGURE 3–41. *A* and *B,* The most common type of smile is the zygomaticus major smile. It is produced by a dominant zygomaticus major muscle and the buccinator, which results in the corners of the mouth being elevated first. *B,* The canine smile results from a codominant levator labii superioris, which contracts first on initiation of a smile followed by activation of the zygomaticus major and buccinator for elevation of the corners of the mouth. *C,* The full-denture smile results from full activation of elevators and depressors of the lips and angles of the mouth, thus displaying both maxillary and mandibular teeth.

due to neurapraxia that tends to resolve spontaneously. Steroids (prednisone 60 mg per day initially, over a 10- to 12-day taper) often are used, but their benefit has yet to be proven conclusively in trauma. Routine supportive measures are included, especially eye protection with lubrication and taping, and in some cases tarsorrhaphy and gold weight implantation. Patients with immediate facial paralysis following temporal bone fracture are evaluated by fine-section (1.0 to 1.5 mm) CT scanning. Those in whom discontinuity of the facial canal is demonstrated are surgical candidates. There are no current controlled, prospective, randomized studies to support surgical decompression of all traumatic facial paralyses. The authors have found that it is best used in patients who have immediate paralysis with radiographic evidence of discontinuity of the fallopian canal and in patients with either delayed or immediate paralysis, with no evidence of nerve discontinuity, who fail to show signs of recovery.

Once a surgical decision is made and the patient is cleared of related injuries such as subdural hematoma, cervical spine fracture, and concussion, the appropriate route of access to the nerve is selected. When hearing is present in the involved ear, the middle fossa or transmastoid route is chosen depending on the site of injury. When audiometric and clinical examinations indicate anacusis, the translabyrinthine approach should be considered. Sites of facial nerve injury in both transverse and longitudinal temporal bone fractures most frequently involve the geniculate ganglion and labyrinthine segment. At exploration, the nerve often is found to be compressed or partially lacerated. In these cases, the nerve is to be decompressed and the epineurium is to be opened. If the nerve is completely transected or clearly devitalized, excision of the involved segment is performed, followed by primary repair or interposition (cable) nerve grafting. Suture reapproximation of nerve ends often is not necessary, or possible, for intratemporal defects. The graft should be interposed between two clean ends of the native nerve and stabilized with Surgicel and temporalis fascia. Signs of reinnervation begin to appear over the course of 6 months, continuing for 12 to 18 months thereafter. A House-Brackmann grade III level of recovery may be expected in the majority of cases.

Technique of Primary Nerve Repair

A neuron consists of a cell body with dendritic and axonal extensions. The axon is surrounded by a Schwann cell sheath. The communication between the axon of one nerve and the dendrite of another is termed a synapse. Individual axons are enclosed by a microscopic endoneurium and arranged in groups of fascicles, each of which is surrounded by a distinct perineurium. The fascicles and surrounding perineurium are enclosed by an inner loose areolar epineurium containing multiple vascular channels. The outer circumferential epineurium encloses bundles of fascicles and encases the entire peripheral nerve. Of these anatomic elements, two are crucial for the surgical correction of severed nerves: the outer epineurium, which is sutured in neural repair, (Fig. 3–42*A*) and the perineurium, which is sutured in fascicular repair (Fig. 3–42*B*). Peripheral nerve sheaths are well vascularized and include two

intracommunicative systems: (1) the perifascicular system, located in the epineurium and (2) the intrafascicular system, located in the endoneurium. Proximal to the stylomastoid foramen, the facial nerve usually is monofascicular.

A transected facial nerve is best repaired by primary end-to-end anastomosis. The nerve ends should be reapproximated without tension to prevent fibrous tissue growth into the anastomosis. In cases in which the pathology requires resection of 17 mm or less of the nerve's trunk, primary neurorrhaphy can still be accomplished by rerouting it. Given a stable patient, extratemporal facial nerve transection repair should be performed within the first 72 hours after injury to ensure distal segment excitability, thus facilitating its identification. After exposure of the severed ends, all devitalized tissue is removed with a fine scalpel. The epineural sheath then is approximated with 9-0 nonabsorbable sutures. Defects longer than 17 mm require placement of an interposition graft. Epineurial sutures should be used for repair of nerves divided within the temporal bone and proximal to the pes anserinus. Although fascicular sutures would appear to be ideal to maintain the precise anatomic direction of the fibers, they are difficult to place and most surgeons do not use them. Furthermore, the extratemporal nerve lacks sufficient identifiable topographic orientation to be useful in fascicular repair, and the nerve is monofascicular proximal to the stylomastoid foramen. During repair, the surgeon should take small bites of the epineurium so that the underlying nerve substance is not distorted or injured. This is best accomplished by careful preparation of the nerve before suturing by removing all fibrous tissue and debris from the epineurium. In intratemporal repair, the horizontal segment rarely is accessible to suture repair; therefore, the nerve ends should be carefully approximated and held in place with Surgicel.

Interposition Grafting

Cable grafts are used when the nerve cannot be reapproximated or the repair is under tension. The most common donor grafts are the ipsilateral greater auricular nerve and sensory nerves of the superficial cervical plexus. Other graft sources are the sural and the medial antebrachial cutaneous nerves. The greater auricular nerve is ideal for defects less than 6 cm in length. The only contraindication to its use is the presence of malignancy in the surgical field. The graft must be carefully harvested, cleaned with normal saline solution, and set at the repair site following removal of extraneous tissue and complete hemostasis. The results of cable grafting generally are favorable. The quality and quantity of axonal regrowth are best when repair is done as soon as possible *after* disruption of the nerve. Negative factors are poor technique, infection, anastomotic tension, and poor graft match. Radiotherapy delays reinnervation but does not impede it. In most cases, return of movement is first noted 6 months after surgery. Usually improved muscle tone precedes voluntary movement. Recovery often is heralded by a tingling sensation in the facial skin (Tinel's sign) and improved tone. Movement usually is first noted in the middle third of the face and over time extends superiorly toward the eye. Improvement may be expected over the course of 12 to 18 months. Movement tends to lack coordination, resulting in a variable degree of synkinesis. A House-Brack-

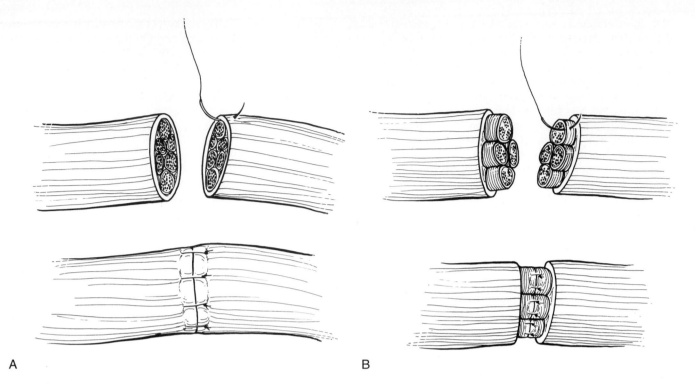

A

B

FIGURE 3–42. Extratemporal facial nerve transection repair.

mann grade III recovery level is expected in the majority of cases.

Nerve Graft Harvesting

Greater Auricular Nerve.   Several features make the greater auricular nerve (Fig. 3–43) particularly useful in facial nerve reconstruction. These include proximity to the facial nerve, cross-sectional diameter, and limited functional morbidity following its harvest. Its usefulness is limited in the reconstruction of long defects and of branching nerve gaps because it rarely yields more than two divisions, which are of small caliber and often short.

The greater auricular nerve runs over the sternocleidomastoid muscle at a point midway between the mastoid tip and the angle of the mandible. The nerve will bisect a line drawn between these two points at the anterior aspect of the sternocleidomastoid muscle, posterior to the external jugular vein. It may be harvested through an extension of a postauricular incision or a separate neck incision.

Sural Nerve. The sural nerve (Fig. 3–44) is commonly used in peripheral nerve repair. The factors that contribute to its utility are its length (40 cm), accessibility, and relatively low morbidity deriving from its sacrifice. Two teams may work simultaneously at the donor and recipient sites thereby reducing surgical time. On the negative side, the caliber of this nerve is variable (often too large), making graft approximation difficult, and the scar resulting from its harvest may be unsightly.

The sural nerve is formed by the union of the medial sural cutaneous nerve and a single communicating branch of the lateral sural cutaneous branch of the peroneal nerve. The

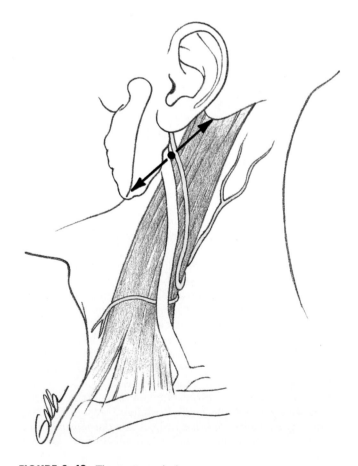

FIGURE 3–43. The greater auricular nerve.

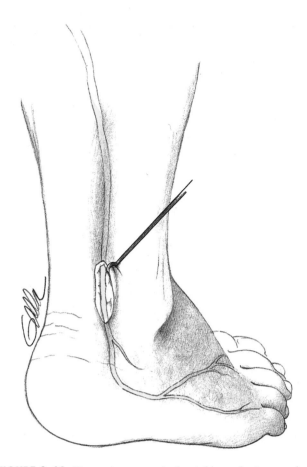

FIGURE 3-44. The sural nerve can be located in a subcutaneous plane posterior to the lateral fibular malleolus. It runs in parallel with the small saphenous vein.

dominant contributor, the medial sural cutaneous nerve, arises from the tibial nerve in the popliteal fossa between the superior heads of the gastrocnemius muscle. The nerve runs deep to the muscular fascia for a variable distance down the posterior calf and then pierces the fascia to lie in close association with, but deep to, the short saphenous vein at the lateral malleolus. The nerve and vein run in a lateral compartment between the lateral malleolus and the tendon of the calcaneus. At this point, the nerve divides into several branches that pass around the malleolus distally and supply the skin of the foot. The nerve is devoid of major branches until it divides into two dependable branches on the lateral aspect of the foot. As the nerve courses proximally over the lateral head of the gastrocnemius muscle, it can be traced in a superficial plane over the muscular fascia if additional nerve graft length is required.

The nerve may be harvested through multiple transverse incisions or a longitudinal incision. Nerve and tendon strippers may be used to isolate and harvest the nerve from the lower leg. The sural nerve is identified through a small incision posterior to the lateral malleolus and then dissected proximally with the stripping instrument. Proximal division can be accomplished by placing gentle longitudinal traction on the nerve and then using the cutting edge of the instrument to sever it. This technique is only appropriate when a simple nonbranching nerve graft is required. Peripheral

branches of the nerve cannot be preserved when using this instrument. A direct approach to the nerve is achieved through a longitudinal incision starting behind the lateral malleolus and then extending it up the leg until adequate nerve length is obtained. Neuroma formation at the distal end of the transected nerve is a potential complication. It may be prevented by suturing the distal end of the nerve within the body of the gastrocnemius muscle.

Medial Antebrachial Cutaneous Nerve. The medial antebrachial cutaneous nerve (MACN) (Fig. 3–45) is a sensory nerve of the arm that has been used extensively for the repair of peripheral nerve defects in the extremities and recently has been reported as a useful choice for facial nerve repair.

The MACN arises from the medial cord of the brachial plexus, adjacent to the ulnar nerve. It carries fibers from the eighth cervical and first thoracic nerves. It lies medial to the axillary artery and, more distally, anterior and medial to the brachial artery. At the junction of the middle and lower thirds of the arm, it pierces the brachial fascia medially and becomes closely associated with the basilic vein. At this point, it divides into anterior and posterior (ulnar) branches. The branches travel parallel to the basilic vein until the posterior branch turns toward the ulna. The anterior branch divides into three to five branches between 6 cm proximal and 5 cm distal to the elbow.

The anterior branch of the MACN may pass superficial or deep to the medial cubital vein and divide into several branches that are distributed to the anterior and medial surfaces of the forearm as far as the wrist. The posterior branch passes posteriorly, anterior to the medial condyle of the humerus, and divides into branches to supply the skin on the posteromedial aspect of the forearm.

Important topographic landmarks for harvesting this nerve are the medial epicondyle of the humerus, the biceps tendon, and the basilic and medial cubital veins. The fascial plane separating the biceps brachii muscle and the triceps brachii muscle should be palpated and outlined. The use of a proximal sterile tourniquet allows for easy identification of the basilic vein. The upper extremity is prepped and draped from the axilla to the wrist. The donor site can be continuous with the head and neck ablative field. The donor area can be accessed by a second surgical team at the time of surgical ablation, thus expending reconstruction.

A longitudinal lazy (S) incision is made from the mid-arm to the mid-forearm, just medial of the mid-sagittal plane of the extremity. Dissection is begun superiorly through the subcutaneous tissue. The basilic vein is always identified where it pierces the brachial fascia to become superficial. The vein is always the best landmark for identifying the MACN, as the nerve runs in close association with this vessel. In approximately 50% of specimens, the nerve will travel superficial to the medial cubital vein at the elbow.

Once the nerve is identified, its anterior branches are traced distally until an adequate length of nerve and branching pattern are obtained. The anterior branch of the nerve divides distally into three to five large branches. In patients with a thick adipose layer in the upper arm, the dissection of the nerve and vein may be more difficult. It is important not to dissect deep to the muscular fascia because this may

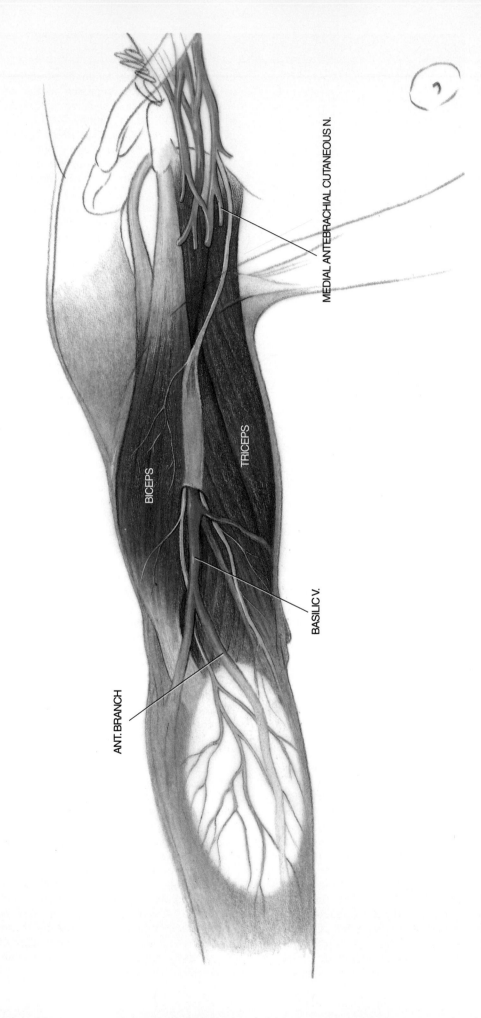

FIGURE 3–45. The medial antebrachial cutaneous nerve arises primarily from the medial cord of the brachial plexus with contributions from the ventral rami of eighth cervical and the first thoracic nerve. As it enters the arm, it lies superficial to the brachial artery and lies in close proximity to the basilic vein. At the elbow, it divides into posterior and anterior branches that supply sensation to the ulnar aspect of both the flexor and extensor surfaces of the forearm.

risk injury to the median nerve that lies directly deep to the MACN.

The wound is closed in two layers. No drain is necessary, and the upper extremity is dressed with a compressive wrap. Dissection of this nerve results in an average nerve graft of 18.7 cm (if the dissection is taken proximally to the origin from the medial cord), with a potential length of 24 to 26 cm. Proximally the nerve graft diameter averages 3 to 4 mm.

The donor site has the advantage that the incision is well concealed on the medial aspect of the arm. The cutaneous sensory innervation distribution includes that distal arm anteromedially, the antecubital fossa, the posterior olecranon, and the area from the midline of the forearm ventrally to the midline dorsally. Leaving the posterior branch intact ensures that sensation over the elbow and medial border of the forearm remains intact.

The sensory deficit over the forearm is normally limited to a 6 × 6 cm area of the forearm, which decreases over a 6- to 12-month period and usually recovers fully by 3 years.

The truncal and divisional diameters of this graft are similar to that of the facial nerve and its branches, thereby providing an excellent size match for both the proximal and distal neurorrhaphy. The distal branching pattern provides four to six branches for facial nerve repair, thereby eliminating the need for multiple grafts. In addition, MACN grafts may be used when the greater auricular nerve is the field of tumor. They have the advantage, over the sural nerve, of rapid postoperative rehabilitation because ambulation is unimpaired and the risk of cellulitis is avoided in patients with peripheral vascular disease.

Reinnervation Techniques
In cases of known facial discontinuity in which primary repair or cable grafting is impossible, reinnervation of the facial nerve should be considered. Because muscle atrophy and structural degeneration of the nerve proceed rapidly, early reinnervation produces more favorable results. In patients with intracranial injury or idiopathic or traumatic facial paralysis in which neural continuity is preserved but function has not returned spontaneously, it is best to wait at least 1 year before considering surgical reinnervation. In the paralyzed face with potential recovery of function, electromyography often demonstrates evidence of polyphasic reinnervation potentials. The lack of reinnervation potentials and normal action potentials and the presence of fibrillation potentials 1 year after injury provide evidence of permanent denervation and are prerequisites to reinnervation surgery. In patients who present long after the injury (more than 2 years) and in whom electromyography shows no reinnervation potentials, a muscle biopsy should be performed. This is important because evidence of atrophy and neurofibrosis in the muscle are predictive of a poor functional result following reinnervation surgery and are indications for rehabilitation with muscle transfer techniques.

Facial reinnervation has been performed with the hypoglossal, contralateral facial, trigeminal (motor), and spinal accessory nerves. The accessory and trigeminal nerves are seldom used. Sacrifice of the spinal accessory nerve results in trapezius muscle paralysis and significant shoulder morbidity. The motor branch of the trigeminal is very difficult to access except during infratemporal approaches, and experience with it as a reinnervation source is limited. Hypoglossal-facial reinnervation remains the most practical and frequently used method of facial nerve reinnervation.

Hypoglossal-Facial Anastomosis (Alternate Technique)
The technique is contraindicated when there is ipsilateral vagal paralysis because it may result in severe swallowing dysfunction. A modified Blair parotidectomy incision is made in the preauricular crease and extended inferiorly to the cervical crease approximately 2 to 3 cm.

Below the Mandible. The facial nerve is identified between the styloid process and the mastoid tip and then dissected distal to the pes anserinus. To identify the hypoglossal nerve, the sternocleidomastoid muscle is retracted posteriorly and followed superiorly to identify the posterior belly of the digastric muscle. Once this muscle is retracted superiorly, the hypoglossal nerve is found coursing inferiorly. The hypoglossal nerve is within 2 to 3 cm of the main trunk of the facial nerve (see Fig. 1–35) and can be identified as it gives rise to the ansa hypoglossis. It may be electrically stimulated to document tongue motion. The nerve is followed anteriorly and medially into the tongue musculature and freed of fascial attachments. The hypoglossal nerve is transected distal to the ansa hypoglossis and the facial at the stylomastoid foramen.

Anastomosis of the nerve is performed as described for primary anastomosis. The two stumps should be free of the tension and cut sharply to allow for precise coaptation. The ends should be approximated with 9-0 epineural sutures in each quadrant. A modification of this technique is the partial XII-VII transfer, which limits tongue atrophy and dysfunction. A donor nerve, usually the greater auricular, is harvested. One end of the graft is sutured to the proximal segment of a partially severed 12th nerve and the other to the trunk of the severed 7th nerve (Figs. 3–46 and 3–47).

In approximately 6 months, the patient can be expected to show improved facial tone and symmetry. Rehabilitation then focuses on teaching the patient to smile by moving the tongue. The goal is to achieve as close a symmetric smile pattern as possible. Mass movement can be decreased with exercise and biofeedback training. A blink reflex cannot be reproduced, and corneal exposure and xerophthalmia may require adjunctive lid procedures.

Cross-Facial Nerve Grafting
The goal of this procedure is to reinnervate the paralyzed side using a cross-over graft from the contralateral facial nerve. This is accomplished most commonly with a sural nerve graft, which connects the distal segments of the paralyzed side to a corresponding branch of the contralateral healthy facial nerve. Approximately 25 to 30 cm of sural nerve is necessary for this procedure. When successful, the technique results in restitution of the emotional smile and synchronous eye blinking. The disadvantages are that the sural nerve has to be secured from a second surgical site, and, most importantly, there is surgical violation of the normal facial nerve. Four techniques for cross-facial nerve grafting have been described. Scaramella transects the buccal division of the normal side and routes the sural nerve graft subcutaneously under the lip into the stump of the fa-

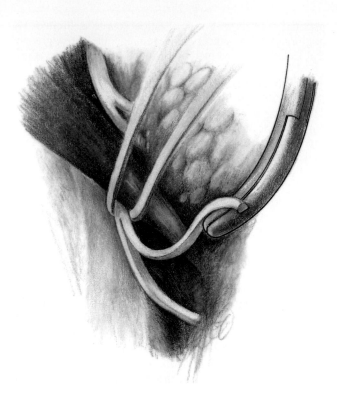

FIGURE 3–46. The hypoglossal nerve is split distal to the ansa hypoglossi. A 30% section is taken from the superior aspect of the nerve trunk.

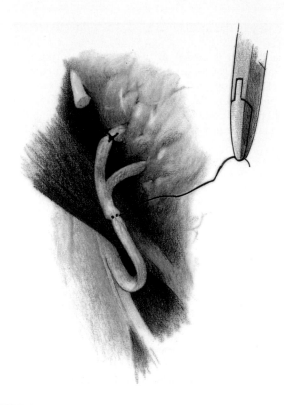

FIGURE 3–47. The main trunk of the facial nerve is divided, and the split segment of hypoglossal nerve is reflected superiorly and anastomosed to it.

cial nerve on the paralyzed side. Fisch uses dual grafts, in which a branch of the zygomaticus of the normal side is transected and attached to the zygomaticus portion of the paralyzed side while the buccal division of the normal side is cable grafted to the marginal mandibular division of the paralyzed side. Anderl advocates four separate grafts from the temporal, zygomatic, buccal, and marginal mandibular divisions of the normal nerve grafted to the corresponding individual divisions on the paralyzed side. Baker and Conley transect the entire lower division, including the marginal mandibular and cervical branches on the normal side, and graft them to the main trunk of the nerve on the paralyzed side. A separate jump graft is used to reinnervate the lower branches of the facial nerve on the normal side.

Reanimation Techniques

In cases in which mimetic muscles are atrophic, as demonstrated by biopsy and histologic study, or when early facial reanimation is desired, innervated regional muscle transfers should be considered. The temporalis and masseter are the most frequently used muscles because they are regional and can be transferred with their nerve supply. Most surgeons prefer to use them for oral reanimation and rehabilitate the eye separately with upper lid gold weight implantation and lower lid suspension.

The temporalis muscle transfer provides movement and improves symmetry to the paralyzed side of the mouth. It is short and thin and has contractile capabilities ranging from 1 to 1.5 cm. The middle 2 to 2.5 cm of the muscle is best suited for transfer as the length is adequate and resists the forces of soft tissue fibrosis. The internal maxillary ar-

tery provides vascular supply to the undersurface of the muscle and the trigeminal nerve (V2) innervation to the muscle in an Arcadian pattern. Exposure of the temporalis muscle is gained through an incision running from the mid-portion of the superior auricular helix to the superior tem-

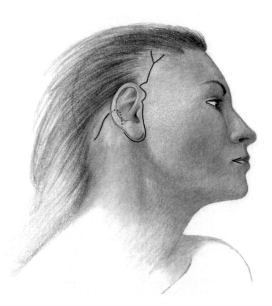

FIGURE 3–48. The incisions used for access to the temporalis muscle include preauricular incision, which can be extended into the postauricular sulcus and posterior hairline, if necessary. In addition, there is a tangential incision made over the mid-section of the temporalis muscle to allow access to the temporoparietal fascia and the temporalis muscle.

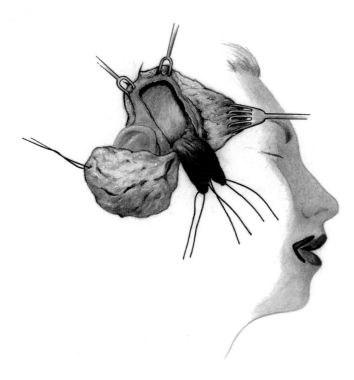

FIGURE 3–49. A temporoparietal fascial flap is harvested before elevation of the temporalis muscle. This is based on the superficial temporal artery and vein and is mobilized laterally before transfer of the midportion of the temporalis muscle.

poral line (Fig. 3–48). Superiorly the incision extends 5 to 6 cm above the hairline and inferiorly to the pretragal area to allow soft tissue dissection in the mid-face. A temporoparietal fascia flap should be harvested before exposing the temporalis fascia because this flap is used to recontour the donor site defect (Fig. 3–49). Thereafter, a 4.5-cm area is undermined, extending from the zygomatic

arch to the oral commissure. At the time of oral commissure, a vermilion incision is made extending 1.5 to 2 cm along the upper and lower lips to expose the lateral aspect of the orbicularis muscle. A subcutaneous tunnel is then developed between the upper incision and the oral commissure. It is considered complete when the surgeon is able to pass the index and medial fingers through it (Fig. 3–50). In cases in which the anatomy is restricted, a rhytidectomy flap may be used to facilitate the transfer. The central temporalis muscle flap is detached from its origin at the temporal line and elevated with at least 2 cm of underlying pericranium (Fig. 3–51). The vascular and neural supplies to the muscle flap are preserved. A centrally placed incision represents the point of attachment of the transferred flap at the commissure. The flap is sutured into the orbicularis muscle using 3-0 Prolene sutures (Fig. 3–52). Overcorrection of the commissure and nasolabial fold is critical. The second or third molar of the upper dental arch should be exposed at the completion of the procedure (Fig. 3–53). The wound is closed with 6-0 nylon sutures at the oral commissure. The previously developed temporoparietal fascial flap is used to fill the donor site defect (Fig. 3–54). A Penrose drain and a conforming dressing are placed for 24 to 36 hours. The procedure can provide oral support within 6 weeks. Movement is achieved by clenching the jaws; however, the resulting contraction is not physiologic, and rehabilitation requires physical therapy. Regardless of the degree of preserved innervation, some atrophy of the transfer will occur, particularly in elderly and debilitated patients. Additional procedures, such as partial wedge resection of the lower lip and redundant nasolabial fold excision, often are needed for cosmetic and functional reason.

Physical Therapy After Surgical Reanimation

Physical therapy often is necessary after surgical rehabilitation of the paralyzed face, especially after hypoglossal-facial nerve anastomosis, temporalis muscle transposition, and

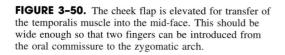

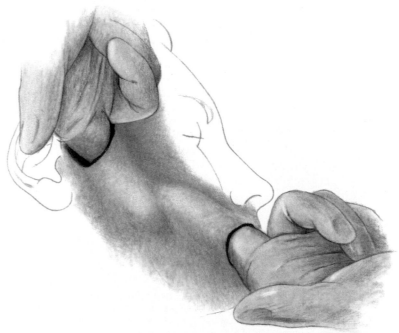

FIGURE 3–50. The cheek flap is elevated for transfer of the temporalis muscle into the mid-face. This should be wide enough so that two fingers can be introduced from the oral commissure to the zygomatic arch.

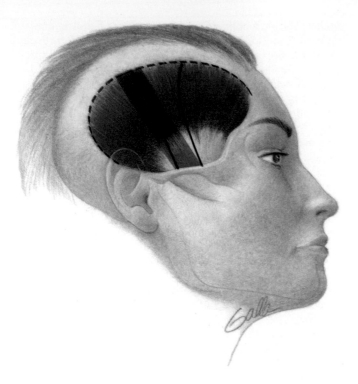

FIGURE 3-51. The temporalis muscle is elevated with muscular fascia and underlying pericranium. The orientation of the muscle can be varied to accommodate individual smile patterns. The dark segment indicates the most common segment used for transfer, which accentuates a horizontal smile pattern. The more vertically oriented pattern is well suited to provide additional midline elevation of the lip, mimicking a type II smile pattern.

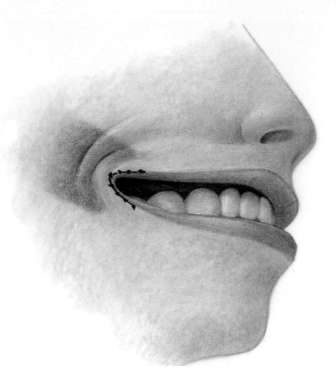

FIGURE 3-53. The resting tension at the completion of muscle transfer should be exaggerated. It is common for the second or third molar of the upper dental arch to be exposed at the completion of the procedure.

free muscle transfer and for patients with synkinesis after primary nerve repair.

The primary goals of physical therapy are the achievement of facial symmetry at rest, improved mouth control for a symmetric smile, and reduced synkinesis. Emphasis is on isolation of muscle contraction and in achieving specific facial movements with a reduced effort. Biofeedback helps motor

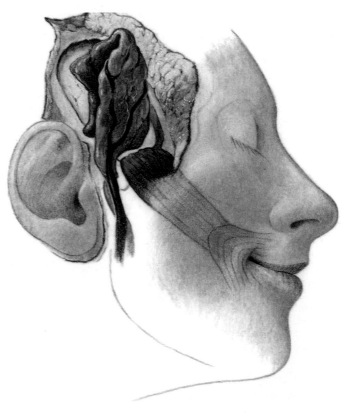

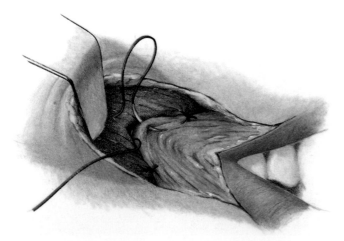

FIGURE 3-52. The distal end of the temporalis muscle flap should be sutured to the lateral aspect of the orbicularis oris muscle with Prolene suture. It is important that muscle-to-muscle contact be achieved, as this is believed to improve the dynamic nature of the procedure.

FIGURE 3-54. After completion of the transfer over the zygomatic arch and stabilization of the orbicularis oris muscle, the temporoparietal facial flap is used to recontour the donor site. This is draped into the temporal fossa and stabilized with a 4-0 clear polydioxanone suture. Special attention is given to creating a proper transitional zone between the muscle at the zygomatic arch and the donor defect.

learning and programming with diminished sensory input and aids in the development of cortical impulses involved in voluntary movement. Visual techniques are implemented using a mirror or with electromyographic feedback.

After hypoglossal-facial nerve anastomosis, patient education is centered on understanding the relationship between tongue action and the resulting facial movement. The ultimate goal is to achieve effective muscle strength and control to produce meaningful facial movement.

In Temporalis Muscle Transposition. Isometric exercises are initiated 2 to 3 weeks postoperatively. The patient is taught to develop a symmetric smile by biting down, thereby tightening the temporalis muscle segment on the affected side while trying to control movement on the unaffected side. The exercise regimen is gradually advanced to include speaking and smiling, which require contraction of jaw and cheek muscles on the operated side without biting down. This pattern of muscle contracture is challenging and requires time, a high degree of motivation, and regular sessions to master. Patients are advised to practice frequently at home in front of a mirror. Regular follow-up is indicated to ensure that correct movement patterns are being achieved.

Chapter 4
Surgery of the Cervical Esophagus

WILLIAM W. MONTGOMERY   MARK A. VARVARES

Cervicogastric tubal alimentation is an alternate method to the gastrostomy or nasogastric route for maintaining nutrition when normal deglutition is impaired. This method of feeding is indicated (1) for patients with prolonged dysphagia after head and neck operations; (2) for patients having mechanical obstruction secondary to unresectable or recurrent tumor above the cervical esophagus; (3) during and after radiation therapy in patients with lesions of the upper air and food passages; and (4) for patients with neurologic diseases with complicating dysphagia.

Nasogastric tube feedings are satisfactory for maintaining nutrition for short periods. However, prolonged use of a nasogastric feeding tube has many disadvantages. The unsightliness of a tube projecting from the nose often confines patients and prevents them from appearing in public. The tube commonly causes nasal irritation and rhinorrhea. Nasopharyngeal and pharyngeal discomfort are common. Irritation of the posterior cricoid and cricoarytenoid joint region produces local pain and pain radiating to the ear.

The complications and inconveniences of a gastrostomy are well known. Leakage around the tube often results in dermatitis. Patients must partially disrobe and assume their recumbent position during feedings.

TEMPORARY ESOPHAGOTOMY TECHNIQUE

A simple and efficient technique to make a cervical esophagotomy of short duration is the use of the Yankhauer suction apparatus. A Yankhauer suction apparatus is inserted into the hypopharynx by way of the mouth under general anesthesia. The tip of the Yankhauer suction is directed to the inferior anterolateral aspect of the pyriform sinus. This maneuver outdents the cervical skin. The tip of the suction is palpated with a finger on the neck. There is surprisingly little tissue between the tip of the Yankhauer and the tip of the finger.

After ensuring that there are no pulsations in this area, an incision is made to expose the tip of the Yankhauer suction. The tip of the suction is pushed through the incision so that the tip of a nasogastric feeding tube can be connected to the tip of the suction with a strong suture.

The tip of the nasogastric feeding tube is pulled out of the mouth and disconnected from the Yankhauer suction tip.

Using the aid of a laryngoscope, the tip of the nasogastric feeding tube is inserted postcricoid into the esophagus. The authors find this to be a very brief and excellent technique for performing a cervical esophagotomy.

CERVICAL ESOPHAGOSTOMY

Although the indications for cervical esophagostomy are similar to those for a cervical esophagotomy, esophagostomy is more suitable than esophagotomy for patients with long-standing or permanent dysphagia. The cutaneous esophageal communication will not close if the feeding tube is inadvertently removed with cervical esophagostomy, as it will with a cervical esophagotomy. The tube is more easily changed. After the operation has healed, the tube can be changed either by the patient or by a person caring for the patient.

Surgical Technique

After a nasogastric feeding rube has been inserted, a skin incision is made anterior to the sternocleidomastoid muscle, at the level of the lower half of the thyroid cartilage (Fig. 4–1A) using the skin lines in this region as a guide.

The anterior border of the sternocleidomastoid muscle is delineated so that it may be retracted laterally. The carotid sheath is identified by blunt dissection and retracted laterally. The larynx is retracted to the opposite side, and the dissection is continued until the prevertebral fascia and vertebral bodies have been identified. A vertical incision is made through the inferior pharyngeal constrictor muscle posterior to the posterior border of the thyroid lamina (Fig. 4–1B).

The posterior border of the thyroid lamina is retracted anteriorly and to the opposite side, exposing the upper portion of the cervical esophagus and the pyriform sinus. At this point, the nasogastric feeding tube can be palpated through the esophageal wall. The wall of the lower portion of the pyriform sinus is grasped with a Babcock clamp, and a vertical incision is made into the lumen (Fig. 4–1C). Stay sutures are placed around the incision so that the mucous membrane can be retracted laterally (Fig. 4–2A).

The mucous membrane is sutured to the skin incision

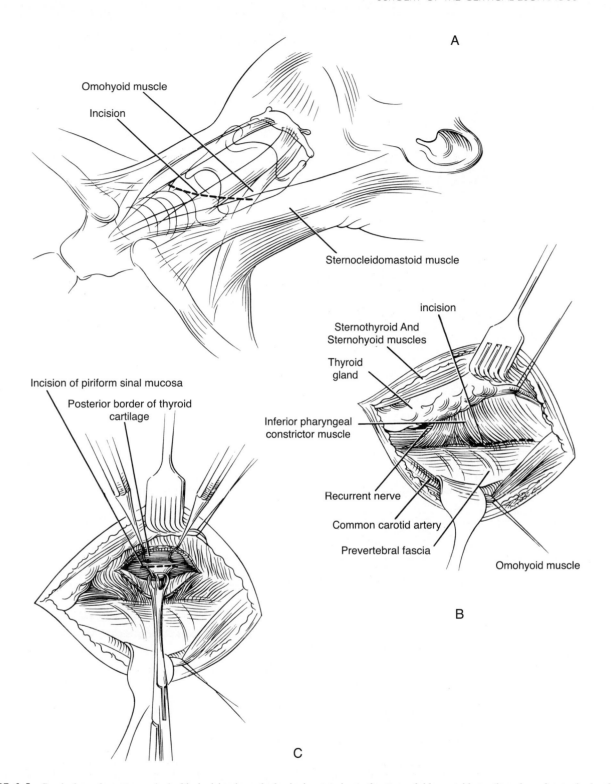

FIGURE 4–1. Cervical esophagostomy. *A,* A skin incision is made, beginning anterior to the sternocleidomastoid muscle and running to the level of the lower half on the thyroid cartilage. *B,* A vertical incision is made through the inferior pharyngeal constrictor muscle, posterior to the posterior border of the thyroid lamina, while retracting the larynx to the right. *C,* The wall of the lower portion of the pyriform sinus is grasped with a Babcock clamp, and a vertical incision is made in the inferior aspect of the mucosa of this sinus.

with No. 5-0 nylon or silk sutures, thus forming the esophagostomy. The esophagostomy should be fashioned in the superior aspect of the skin incision so that the tract will be directed inferiorly (Fig. 4–2B).

The remainder of the incision is repaired in layers. A drain is not necessary unless the surgeon believes that the operative field has been contaminated or anticipates postoperative bleeding. The esophagostomy sutures should remain in place for 10 days. The patient is shown the technique for changing the feeding tube 2 weeks after the operation.

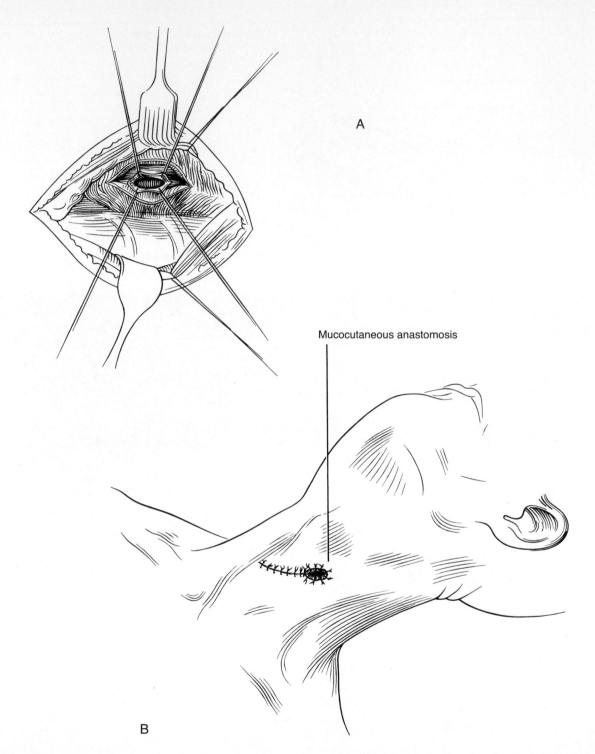

FIGURE 4-2. Cervical esophagostomy. *A,* Stay sutures of No. 00 chromic catgut are placed around the incision so that the mucous membrane can be retracted laterally. *B,* The margins of the mucosa of the pyriform sinus have been sutured to the superior aspect of the skin incision. This provides a tract lined with mucous membrane that descends to the postcricoid region. The remainder of the skin incision is repaired in layers. A drain is not usually necessary unless it has been difficult to control bleeding.

CRICOPHARYNGEAL OR INFERIOR CONSTRICTOR MYOTOMY AS TREATMENT FOR DYSPHAGIA

Dysphagia, a symptom the otolaryngologist is often called on to evaluate and treat, may result from a variety of causes, including trauma, infection, tumor, and neurologic disor-

ders. It is often characterized by the inability of the pharyngeal musculature to propel the bolus into the upper esophagus. This is caused partly by dysfunction of the pharyngeal musculature and partly by the absence of a coordinated reflex relaxation of the cricopharyngeal muscle.

Mills reported the successful use of the cricopharyngeal myotomy in patients with dysphagia accompanying bulbar palsy, whereas Peterman reported some temporary relief in patients with oculopharyngeal muscular dystrophy. Blakeley, Garety, and Smith noted good results in several patients with various types of dysphagia, including oculopharyngeal muscular dystrophy.

When treating the patient with dysphagia due to muscular dystrophy, it is necessary to section the lower portion of the inferior constrictor muscle as well as the cricopharyngeal muscle. The results after inferior constrictor myotomy with oculopharyngeal muscular dystrophy have been very gratifying.

A cricopharyngeal myotomy should be performed routinely in conjunction with any partial or supraglottic laryngectomy after resection of a pharyngeal diverticulum. It is often impossible for patients undergoing these procedures to resume adequate deglutition if myotomy is omitted. A cricopharyngeal myotomy can be performed either when a partial laryngectomy is carried out or as a separate procedure. Because a radical neck dissection is often necessary when a subtotal laryngectomy is performed, the cricopharyngeal and inferior constrictor muscles are readily accessible for section at that time. A myotomy as a separate operation is performed as described in the legends of Figures 4–3 to 4–5.

The patient can resume a soft diet on the second postoperative day if the mucous membrane has not been perforated during the operation. If the membrane has been perforated, the patient's nutrition should be maintained by a nasogastric feeding tube for at least 1 week after the operation.

An inferior constrictor myotomy is indicated post-laryngectomy for spasm of this muscle, which prevents good esophageal speech or speech after a tracheoesophageal shunt operation (see Chapter 12). Botulism toxin can also be used to control these spasms.

HYPOPHARYNGEAL—ESOPHAGEAL DIVERTICULUM (ZENKER'S DIVERTICULUM)

Etiology

There are several theories about the etiology of hypopharyngeal-esophageal diverticula, including (1) spasm of the cricopharyngeal muscle, (2) congenital defects in the supporting muscles of the cervical esophagus, and (3) congenital defects between the components of the inferior constrictor muscle. Anatomically, these diverticula can be divided into three groups, as shown in Figure 4–6.

A herniation may occur between the upper fibers of the cricopharyngeal muscle and the inferior fibers of the inferior constrictor muscle. It is believed to be the result of either an incoordination between the cricopharyngeal and inferior constrictor muscles or a spasm of the cricopharyngeal muscle. This is the most common site for a hypopharyngeal diverticulum.

A diverticulum can occur just below the cricopharyngeal muscle where the circular esophageal musculature is somewhat deficient.

The cricopharyngeal muscle is made up of two parts: an upper oblique portion and a lower transverse, or sphincteric, portion. The upper portion is innervated by the vagus nerve through the pharyngeal plexus. The lower portion is innervated by a branch of the recurrent laryngeal nerve. An asynergy between these two muscles results in a herniation or pulsion posteriorly between them.

The hypopharyngeal diverticulum (Fig. 4–6), regardless of the exact site of its development, first projects posteriorly and then to the left, in the space between the prevertebral and the pretracheal fascia. The exact reason for the protrusion to the left is not known. One possible explanation is that the cervical esophagus has a slight convexity to the left and the carotid sheath lies more laterally in the left side of the neck than in the right.

Signs and Symptoms

A hypopharyngeal diverticulum occurs in middle-aged and elderly patients. It may remain asymptomatic for many years.

The first symptom of a hypopharyngeal diverticulum is often a gurgling sensation when the patient drinks. As the disease progresses, the patient may have dysphagia caused by partial obstruction of the cervical esophagus and eructation or regurgitation after swallowing food. Aspiration may occur while the patient is eating or between meals. Nocturnal aspiration is not uncommon and is accomplished by severe coughing spasms. Aspiration can lead to acute or chronic pulmonary infection. The patient may also have a history of weight loss.

Diagnosis

Diagnosis of a hypopharyngeal diverticulum is confirmed by barium swallow studies (Fig. 4–7). The size, shape, and location of the sac, as well as the patency of the cervical esophagus, can be determined. Spasm of the cricopharyngeal muscle may be noted during fluoroscopy.

Preoperative Management

The patient is carefully evaluated for the presence of acute or chronic pulmonary infection. In addition to the cuffed endotracheal tube in the trachea, a No. 8 or No. 9 endotracheal tube is inserted into the esophagus as shown in Figure 4–3A.

Surgical Treatment

Incisions
The hypopharyngeal diverticulum may be approached by an incision made along the anterior border of the sternocleidomastoid muscle (Fig. 4–3B and C). The incision is carried through the platysmal muscle. Flaps are elevated in a subplatysmal plane anteriorly and posteriorly. The anterior cutaneous nerve is identified in the superior aspect of the exposure and is preserved.

An incision is made through the superficial layer of deep cervical fascia anterior to the sternocleidomastoid muscle (see Fig. 4–4). The latter is retracted laterally, exposing the omohyoid and sternohyoid muscles. The omohyoid muscle is transected, and the upper and lower segments are retracted

Text continued on page 172

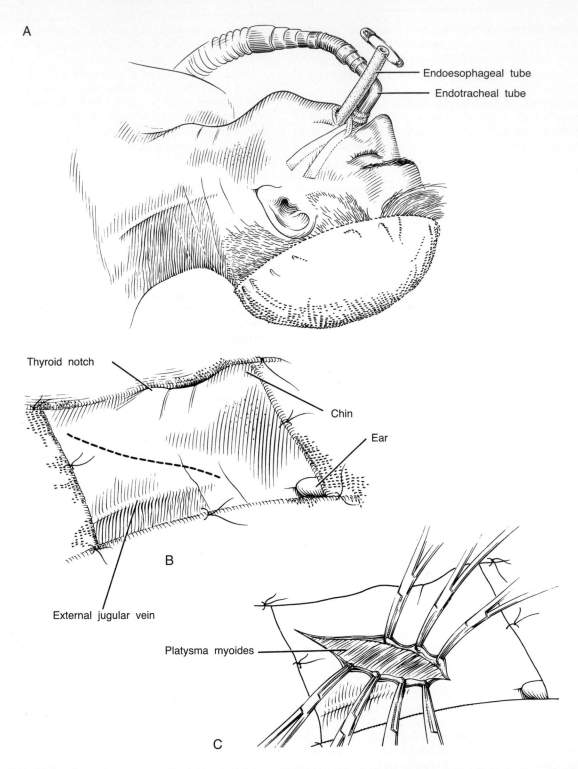

A

Endoesophageal tube
Endotracheal tube

Thyroid notch

Chin

Ear

B

External jugular vein

Platysma myoides

C

FIGURE 4-3. Inferior constrictor myotomy. *A,* The operation is performed with the patient in a supine position and with his head turned to the right and slightly extended. The anesthetic is administered by way of an endotracheal tube. A No. 8 or No. 9 long endotracheal tube is inserted into the cervical esophagus. *B,* An incision is made along the anterior border of the left sternocleidomastoid muscle as shown. This extends nearly to the sternoclavicular joint. *C,* The incision is carried through the platysma myoides, and the anterior border of the sternocleidomastoid muscle is exposed. The fascia anterior to this muscle is carefully incised so that the muscle can be retracted laterally.

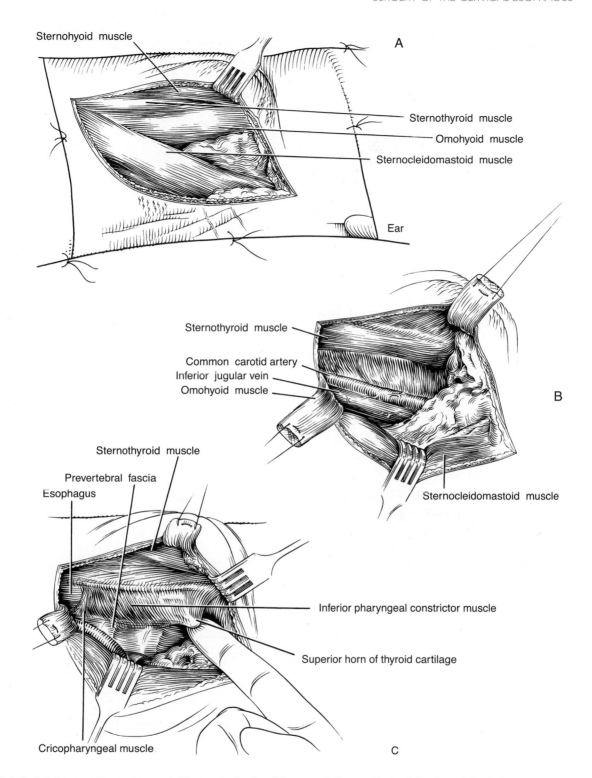

FIGURE 4–4. Inferior constrictor myotomy. *A,* The anterior border of the sternocleidomastoid muscle has been delineated, and the anterior belly of the omohyoid muscle is seen crossing the field obliquely. The sternothyroid and the sternohyoid muscles are also identified. *B,* The sternothyroid muscle and thyroid gland are retracted medially. It is usually necessary to divide the anterior belly of the omohyoid muscle and the middle thyroid vein to obtain adequate exposure. The contents of the carotid sheath are identified so that they may be retracted laterally. *C,* The inferior constrictor muscle is identified. The plane of cleavage is established between this and the prevertebral fascia. As the larynx is rotated to the right, the superior horn of the thyroid cartilage becomes apparent. The full length of the inferior constrictor muscle, including the cricopharyngeal muscle, is thus exposed.

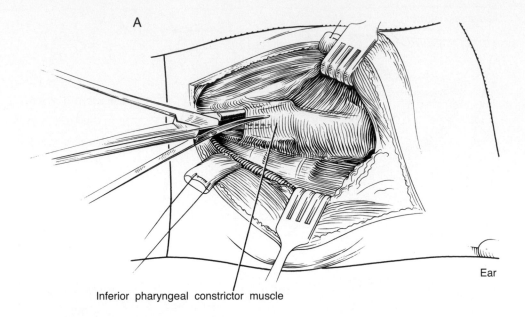

A

Inferior pharyngeal constrictor muscle

Ear

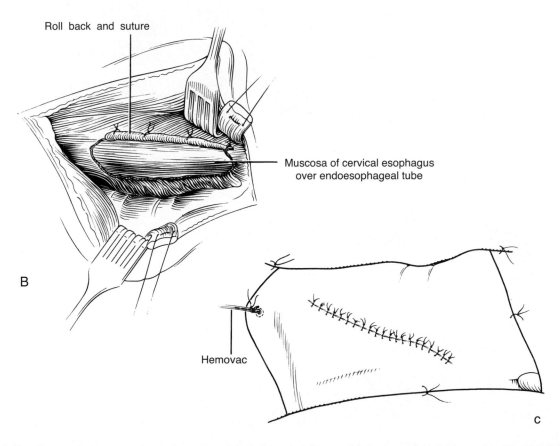

Roll back and suture

B

Muscosa of cervical esophagus
over endoesophageal tube

Hemovac

C

FIGURE 4–5. Inferior constrictor myotomy. *A*, Sectioning of the inferior constrictor muscle begins at the inferior margin of its cricopharyngeal portion. The muscle can be sectioned with scissors, as shown, if the plane of the cleavage can be established between the muscle and the mucous membrane. When dealing with neuromuscular disorders such as oculopharyngeal muscular dystrophy, this plane is difficult to establish and thus there is a real danger of inadvertently perforating the mucous membrane. In such instances, the entire inferior constrictor muscle must be painstakingly sectioned with a No. 15 Bard-Parker blade. The presence of an endotracheal tube in the cervical esophagus greatly facilitates this procedure. *B*, The anterior margin of the sectioned inferior constrictor muscle must be reflected and sutured anteriorly. This ensures against reunion of the sectioned muscle. *C*, The exposure is closed in layers with chromic catgut and dermal sutures. The sectioned ends of the anterior belly of the omohyoid muscle should be sutured together. Hemovac tubing is inserted into the depths of the dissection with its dermal exit just below the clavicle. This reduces the possibility of hematoma formation and eliminates the necessity of a pressure dressing.

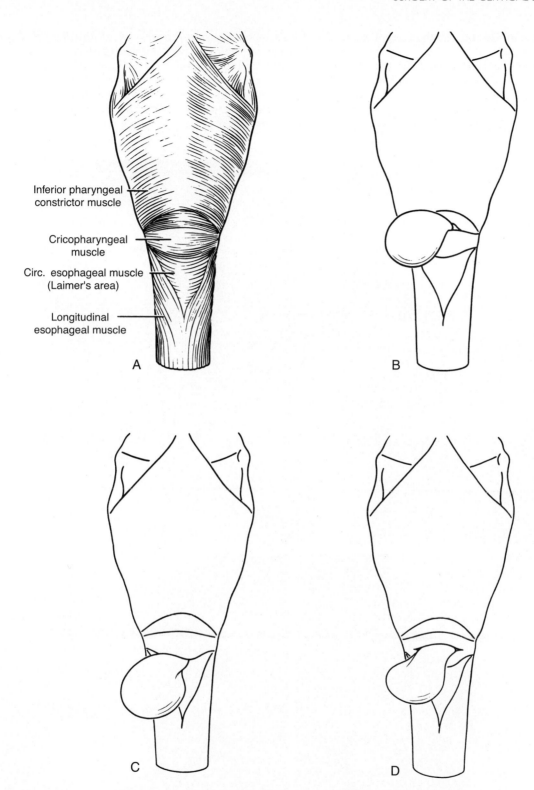

Inferior pharyngeal
constrictor muscle

Cricopharyngeal
muscle

Circ. esophageal muscle
(Laimer's area)

Longitudinal
esophageal muscle

A

B

C

D

FIGURE 4–6. Hypopharyngeal diverticulum. *A,* The muscles posterior to the larynx and cervical esophagus are shown. These are the inferior pharyngeal constrictor, the cricopharyngeal, and the circular longitudinal esophageal muscles. *B,* A diverticulum occurring between the fibers of the inferior constrictor muscle and the cricopharyngeal muscle is depicted. This is the most common site for a hypopharyngeal diverticulum. *C,* A diverticulum occurring below the cricopharyngeal muscle, where the circular esophageal musculature is somewhat deficient, is shown. *D,* A diverticulum is shown projecting between the upper oblique and lower transverse portions of the cricopharyngeal muscle. An asynergy between these two muscles may be the result of a herniation at this level.

away from the field with No. 00 chromic catgut sutures (Fig. 4–4B).

The superior aspect of the thyroid gland becomes visible after retracting the omohyoid muscle. The superior thyroid artery is identified. It may be divided, and ligated, if necessary. The carotid sheath, along with the ansa hypoglossi, is retracted laterally. The ansa hypoglossi may be transected

for adequate exposure if necessary. With finger dissection, a plane is established between the inferior constrictor muscle and the prevertebral fascia (Fig. 4–4C). The posterior border of the left thyroid cartilage is palpated. Rotation of the larynx to the opposite side will increase the exposure and allow visualization of the cervical trachea and esophagus. It may be necessary to divide the middle thyroid vein,

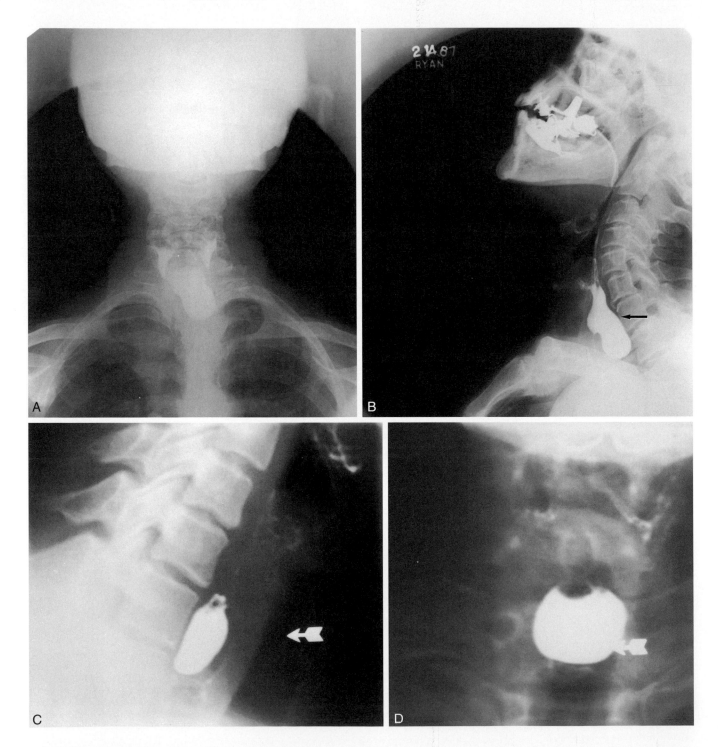

FIGURE 4–7. Hypopharyngeal diverticulum. *A,* Anteroposterior barium-swallow radiograph showing a moderately large hypopharyngeal diverticulum in a 74-year-old woman. The pyriform sinuses are normal. As in most cases, the diverticulum extends to the left of the midline. *B,* A lateral barium-swallow radiograph showing the diverticulum and its site of origin. The sac is found at a higher level during the operation because the radiographic image is taken with the patient in the upright position and the sac is filled with barium. *C* and *D,* Barium-swallow radiograph showing a smaller sac in a 59-year-old woman. This had been symptomatic for 6 months. Although the sac appears to be in the midline, it was approached surgically from the left side.

which empties into the jugular vein, and the inferior thyroid artery to obtain adequate exposure, especially when a large or inferiorly positioned sac is being dissected.

Occasionally, it may be difficult to locate the sac as it is invested by fascia. In general, the sac is found somewhat higher than it is shown on the radiographs because they are taken when the patient is erect and the operation is performed with the patient supine. If the sac extends inferiorly to the thoracic inlet and into the upper mediastinum, it is important to identify the recurrent laryngeal nerve before dissecting the fascia from the sac. This nerve is found in the lateral tracheoesophageal groove. A nerve stimulator can be used to locate it if necessary. The technique for resecting and repairing the hypopharyngeal diverticulum is described and illustrated in Figures 4–8, 4–9, 4–10 and 4–11.

The authors have found in the past that resecting the sac can become complicated, especially if the mucous membrane of the pharynx or cervical esophagus is inadvertently entered. Thus, for the past 15 years after dissecting the sac free, the authors, using three No. 2-0 silk sutures, have plicated it superiorly with excellent results.

Wound Closure
The omohyoid muscle is reapproximated. The platysma is closed with No. 3-0 chromic catgut, and the skin is repaired with either No. 5-0 nylon interrupted sutures or No. 6-0 mild chromic continuous suture. If 6-0 myochromic is used, it should be covered with Mastisol and Steri strips. A closed suction drainage system is used (Fig. 4–5C).

Postoperative Care

The patient should receive only liquids for the first 12 hours, follow a soft diet for a few days, and then resume a regular diet.

If the mucous membrane has been violated, then a nasogastric feeding tube is used for 5 to 7 days. At this point, radiographic studies made with contrast material are used to test the cervical esophagus potency and detect any possible leaks.

Possible Complications

Hemorrhage
Hemorrhage is not common when closed-suction drainage is used. If it does occur, the wound should be opened and packed. Blind clamping at a bleeding site is inadvisable because of the possibility of injury to structures such as the recurrent laryngeal nerve.

Leakage
Leakage is manifest by pain and swelling in the operative region. The wound should be opened and packed with antibiotic impregnated iodoform gauze. It is not advisable to attempt secondary repair at this time. The authors have not seen leakage with the plication technique.

Injury to the Recurrent Laryngeal Nerve
Injury to the recurrent laryngeal nerve may be temporary or permanent. Immediate repair is not advised.

Recurrence of Diverticulum
Recurrence of the diverticulum is rare. The authors have not seen it with a plication technique.

Stricture of the Cervical Esophagus
This complication is uncommon even if a fistula forms during the postoperative period. Bougienage is the treatment of choice if the stricture persists for more than 3 months.

RECONSTRUCTION OF THE CERVICAL ESOPHAGUS

Twenty percent of all carcinomas of the esophagus occur in the cervical region. Statistics for resection of carcinoma of the cervical esophagus show consistently low cure rates. The unfavorable results are probably owing to the fact that the disease is often undiagnosed until it is well advanced; therefore, resections are not sufficient to encompass the area of involvement.

The first report of an attempted reconstruction of the cervical esophagus was made by Czerny in 1877. The operation was unsuccessful. There have been many techniques reported since then. The two techniques presented in this chapter are reconstruction of the cervical esophagus using the forearm free-flap technique and also a two-stage procedure using the cervical skin. The gastric pull-up procedure for reconstructing the cervical esophagus is not described in this book. The results following the gastric pull-up operation are good even when radiation therapy has been administered to the cervical region. The operation requires both a head and neck surgeon and a thoracic surgeon and is difficult to perform if the patient has a feeding gastrostomy.

Technique for Two-Stage Reconstruction After Laryngoesophagectomy With or Without a Radical Neck Dissection

First Stage
A U-shaped superiorly based cervical flap is used for a laryngoesophagectomy without radical neck dissection. The incision is modified (Fig. 4–12A) when a radical neck dissection is added to the procedure. A horizontal cervical skin flap may also be used (Fig. 4–15). After removal of the surgical block, incisions are made in the flap for construction of the pharyngostoma and esophagostoma (Fig. 4–12B). The pharyngostoma is constructed before replacement of the skin flap. If the pharyngeal orifice is too large, it may be sutured laterally on each side with No. 2-0 Vicryl on a curved cutting needle to narrow it to the proper diameter. The incision for the esophagostoma can be placed in a more superior position than that shown in Figure 4–12A. The sutures used to construct the inferior aspect of the pharyngostoma pass through skin, prevertebral fascia, and pharyngeal mucosa. This secures the pharyngostoma to the prevertebral fascia and prevents any leakage of saliva behind the skin bridging the pharyngostoma and esophagostoma. An adequate bridge of skin between the esophagostoma and tracheostoma facilitates dissection at the time of the second-stage procedure. However, this bridge of tissue is not essential. A specially

Text continued on page 179

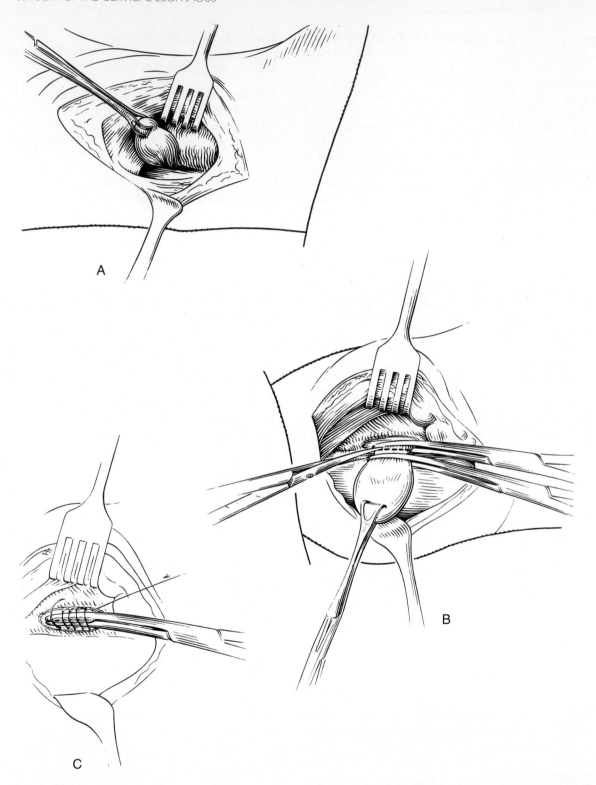

FIGURE 4-8. Hypopharyngeal diverticulum—resection of sac with a narrow neck. The surgical approach to a hypopharyngeal diverticulum is identical to that described and illustrated for inferior constrictor myotomy (Figs. 4–3 and 4–4). *A,* This sac is identified by establishing a plane between the inferior constrictor muscle and the prevertebral fascia. A rotation of the larynx to the opposite side increases this exposure. A nasogastric feeding tube can be palpated in the cervical esophagus. The sac is usually invested by fascia, which makes its location difficult to determine. The fascia is carefully dissected from the diverticulum to the level of its junction with the esophageal mucosa. If the sac extends inferiorly to the thoracic inlet, the recurrent laryngeal nerve must be identified before the dissection of this fascia. *B,* Clamps are placed across the neck of the sac. The neck is sectioned between the two clamps. *C,* A continuous No. 3-0 chromic catgut suture is placed through the base of the diverticulum and over the clamp.

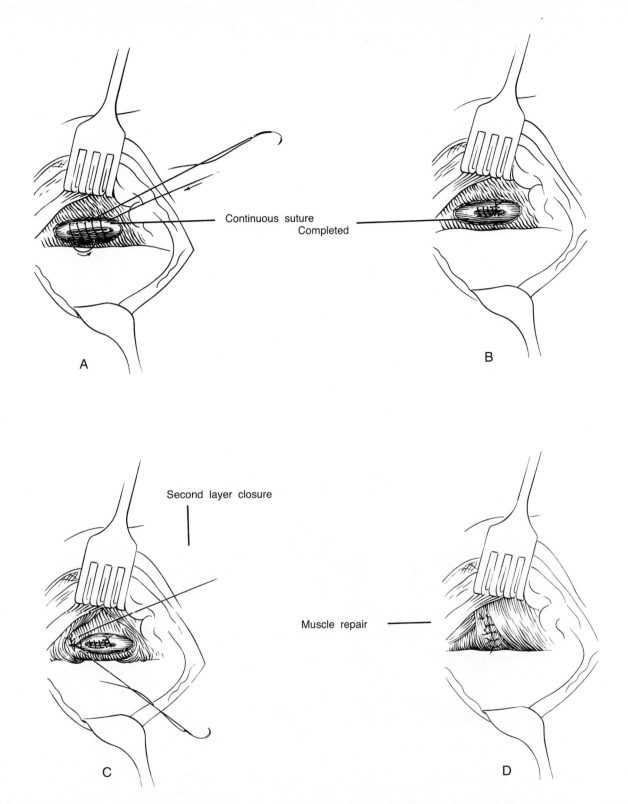

FIGURE 4–9. Hypopharyngeal diverticulum—resection of a sac with a narrow neck. *A,* The last suture is returned in the opposite direction halfway along the repair, as shown, to facilitate tying and bunching of the suture line. *B,* The continuous-suture closing is tied, thus completing first-layer repair of the mucous membrane. *C,* A second layer of interrupted No. 3-0 chromic catgut sutures is used to reinforce the first continuous layer. *D,* The final layer of the closure repairs the muscle defect. A posterior cricopharyngeal myotomy is accomplished at this time.

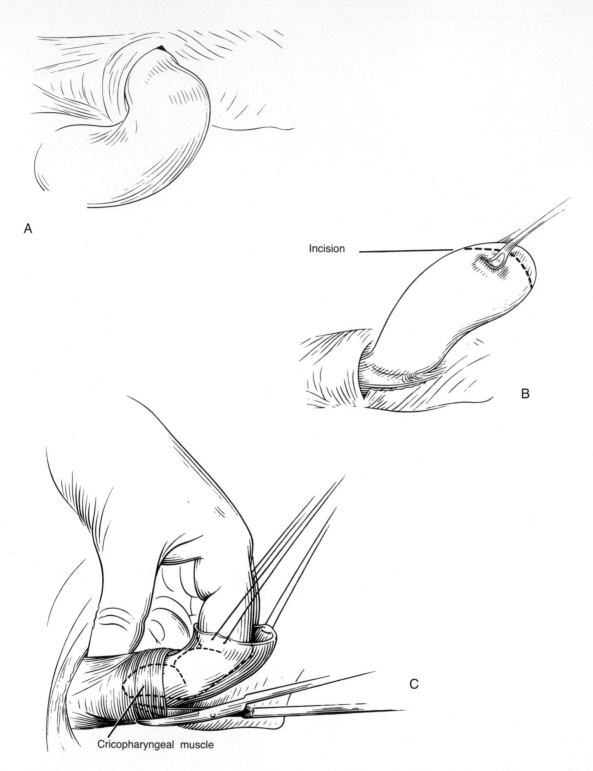

Incision

A

B

Cricopharyngeal muscle

C

FIGURE 4-10. Resection of a sac with a large neck. *A,* As much of the investing fascia around the diverticulum is dissected as possible without caus-ing injury to the cervical esophagus. *B,* The diverticulum is retracted superiorly with a Babcock clamp. The sac is opened at its apex. *C,* Traction su-tures of No. 2-0 chromic catgut are placed in the periphery of the opening at the apex of the diverticulum. The surgeon's index finger is placed in the diverticulum, and the junction of the diverticulum and the cervical esophagus can be palpated. This allows for a more complete dissection of the invest-ing fascia from the sac and prevents inadvertent removal of the esophageal wall, which will result in postoperative stricture. The fibers of the cricopha-ryngeal muscle are sectioned with this finger in place.

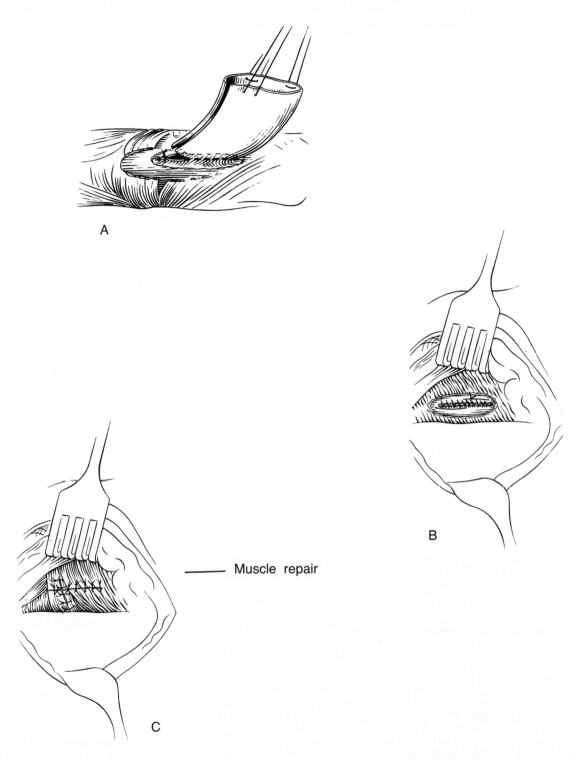

Muscle repair

FIGURE 4-11. Hypopharyngeal diverticulum. *A,* An incision is made along the length of the sac to its junction with the cervical esophageal mucosa. The sac is amputated at this junction. The resulting defect in the cervical esophagus is repaired with No. 3-0 chromic catgut sutures as the dissection progresses. *B,* A second layer of reinforcing sutures has been applied. *C,* The muscle defect is repaired with interrupted No. 3-0 chromic catgut sutures as the third layer of closure. The sectioned omohyoid muscle is reapproximated. The remainder of the surgical exposure is repaired in layers with No. 3-0 catgut and dermal sutures. Closed-suction drainage is inserted as shown in Figure 4–5C.

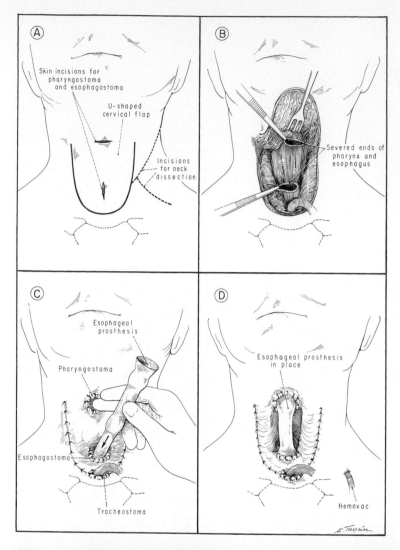

FIGURE 4–12. Laryngoesophagectomy—first stage. *A,* A U-shaped cervical flap based superiorly is used for a laryngoesophagectomy without radical neck dissection. This incision is modified when a radical neck dissection is added to the procedure. *B,* After removal of the surgical block, incisions are made in the flap for construction of the pharyngostoma and esophagostoma. *C,* The pharyngostoma is constructed before replacement of the skin flap. If the pharyngeal orifice is too large, it may be sutured laterally on each side with No. 2-0 Dexon to narrow it to the proper diameter. The sutures used to construct the inferior aspect of the pharyngostoma pass through the skin, prevertebral fascia, and pharyngeal mucosa. This secures the pharyngostoma to the prevertebral fascia and prevents any leakage of saliva behind the skin bridging between the pharyngostoma and esophagostoma. *D,* The plastic esophageal tube, used to bridge the gap between the pharyngostoma and esophagostoma, is first inserted into the esophagostoma and then up into the pharynx.

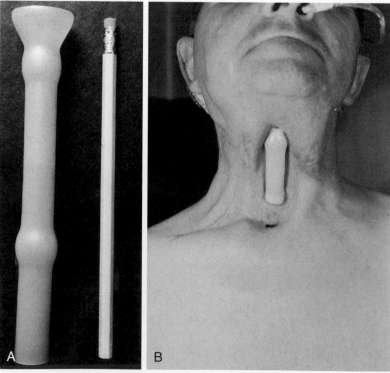

FIGURE 4–13. *A* and *B,* The Montgomery silicone esophageal tube (Boston Medical Products, Inc., Westborough, MA) is used to bridge the gap between the pharyngostoma and esophagostoma after laryngoesophagectomy. The upper funnel-shaped end fits into the pharynx and prevents downward displacement of the tube. The bulbous dilation just below the upper flared end is situated inferior to the pharyngostoma and prevents upward displacement of the tube. The lower dilated portion of the tube is situated below the esophagostoma and assists in preventing reflux of gastric contents into the cervical region.

designed esophageal tube (Boston Medical Products, Westborough, MA) (Fig. 4–13) is inserted through the esophagostoma inferiorly and into the pharynx superiorly (Fig. 4–12C and D). This tube is constructed of medical-grade silicone and has three functions: (1) It eliminates the problem of profuse salivary leakage by way of the pharyngostoma (a few patients have been able to eat and drink with this tube in place); (2) it maintains a widely patent pharyngostoma and esophagostoma (the authors and colleagues have had no instance of postoperative stenosis after use of the esophageal stent); (3) it creates a trough between the pharyngostoma and the esophagostoma, thus facilitating the second-stage procedure (see also Chapter 5).

The horizontal cervical skin flap is described in detail in Figure 4–15.

Second Stage

The second stage is performed 4 to 6 weeks after the first, depending on the rapidity of healing. The plastic esophageal tube is removed as the patient is being prepared for the operation. A circumferential, oval-shaped incision is made that includes the pharyngostoma and esophagostoma (Fig. 4–14A). The distance between the vertical limbs of this incision is obtained by measuring the circumference of the pharyngostoma and esophagostoma and adding approxi-

mately 1.5 cm. The missing link of cervical esophagus is constructed with a linear vertical suture line of No. 2-0 Vicryl. Closely placed, interrupted sutures are inserted (Fig. 4–14B and C). A nasogastric feeding tube is inserted either immediately before or after this suturing. Some surgeons prefer to insert a salivary bypass tube along with the feeding tube when performing the second-stage reconstruction.

A cervicothoracic skin flap (Fig. 4–14C) is outlined using an opening 4 × 4-inch gauze sponge for measuring. A margin of $1\frac{1}{2}$ inches is added to the measured length of this flap and 1 inch to the measured width. A delayed or nondelayed flap may be used. There is no advantage to the delayed flap if the dissection is performed with care. The pedicled flap can be elevated rapidly to the supraclavicular area. At this point, it is imperative to preserve every possible vessel entering and leaving the flap. Vicryl sutures (No. 2-0) are placed subcutaneously to advance the flap into its cervical position. Tension should not be placed on these sutures. A split-thickness skin graft is then taken from the thigh to cover the defect in the upper chest and lower cervical regions (Fig. 4–14D). The Hemovac is inserted, and the skin edges are sutured with nylon suture. Figure 4–16 is a postoperative photograph of the results of reconstruction of the cervical esophagus after laryngoesophagectomy and a left radical neck disssection.

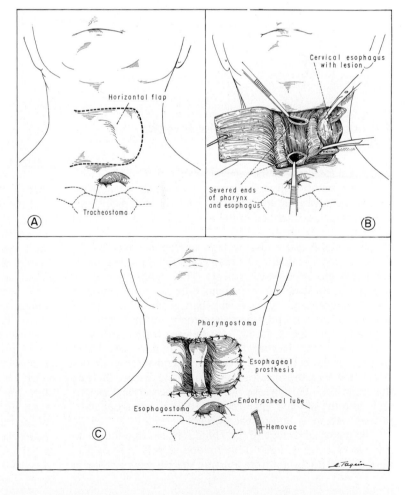

FIGURE 4-14. Cervical esophagectomy for recurrent carcinoma after laryngectomy. Horizontal cervical skin flap. First stage. *A,* A horizontal cervical pedicled flap is elevated. The extent of the lesion is outlined by palpation. *B,* The cervical esophagus is transected at least 2 cm below the lesion. A plane of cleavage is established behind the esophagus and anterior to the prevertebral fascia. From below, the tissue block is dissected superiorly in this plane. The carotid sheaths are the lateral limits of this block dissection. The specimen is removed by amputation at the hypopharyngeal level. *C,* The nonbased end of the horizontal pedicled skin flap is sutured in place. Before reattachment of the superior and inferior aspect of the skin flap, the pharyngostoma and esophagostoma are constructed with No. 3-0 Vicryl sutures. Hemovac tubing is inserted. After plastic esophageal tubing has been cut to an estimated length, it is inserted.

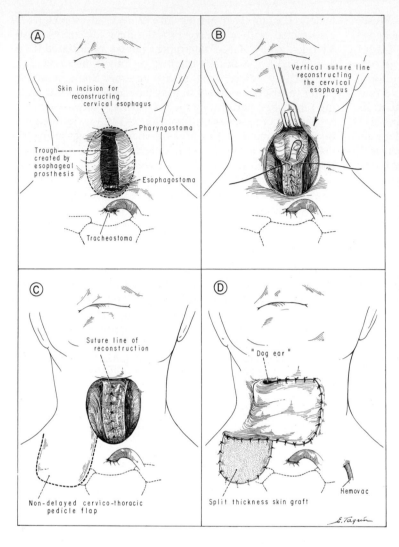

FIGURE 4–15. Reconstruction of cervical esophagus-second stage. The second stage is performed 4 to 6 weeks after the first, depending on the speed of healing. The plastic esophageal tube is removed as the patient is being prepared for the operation. *A,* A circumferential, oval-shaped incision is made to include the pharyngostoma and esophagostoma. The distance between the vertical limbs of this incision is obtained by measuring the circumference of the pharyngostoma and esophagostoma and adding approximately 1.5 cm. *B,* The missing link of cervical esophagus is constructed by placing a linear vertical suture line of No. 3-0 chromic catgut. Closely placed interrupted sutures prevent leakage. A nasogastric tube is inserted either immediately before or after this suturing.

C, A cervicothoracic pedicled skin flap is outlined by using an opened 4 × 4–inch gauze sponge for measuring. One and one-half inches are added to the measured length and 1 inch to the measured width. The pedicled flap can be elevated to the supraclavicular area with rapidity. At this point, it is imperative to preserve every possible vessel entering and leaving the pedicled flap. Chromic catgut sutures (No. 3-0) are placed subcutaneously to advance the flap into its cervical position. No tension should be placed on the sutures. *D,* A split-thickness skin graft is then taken from the thigh to cover the defect in the upper chest and lower cervical regions. The Hemovac is inserted, and the skin edges are sutured with No. 4-0 or No. 5-0 nylon suture. Reconstruction of the cervical esophagus after laryngectomy using a horizontal cervical skin flap is shown in Figure 4–14.

Reconstruction Using a Radial Forearm Fasciocutaneous Flap

The radial forearm fasciocutaneous flap in combination with the Montgomery salivary bypass tube (see Chapter 5) for reconstruction of the hypopharynx and cervical esophagus is performed as described in Figures 4–17, 4–18, 4–19, and to 4–20.

The radial forearm fasciocutaneous flap is a useful technique for reconstruction of the hypopharynx and the cervical esophagus in selected patients. This technique may be used for reconstruction in patients who have undergone a total laryngectomy and cervical esophagectomy or in those who have had a subtotal pharyngectomy and in whom the larynx remains intact. It may also be used for patients who have had a total laryngectomy but who have developed stenosis of the neopharynx. As in all reconstructive procedures, however, the oncologic control of the disease dictates the reconstruction. Disease far distal in the cervical esophagus into the thoracic inlet requires a total laryngopharyngoesophagectomy and gastric pull-up.

The major advantage of the radial forearm free flap is its reliable vascularity, large caliber blood vessels, ease of harvest, donor site distant from ablative site allowing two-team surgery, minimal donor site morbidity, easy tubulation of the pliable soft tissue, and the potential for excellent neopharyngeal or tracheoesophageal speech.

The vascular anatomy and harvest techniques for the radial forearm free flap are discussed in Chapter 2.

Flap design, when used with pharyngoesophageal reconstruction, varies with the size of the defect. The authors have successfully reconstructed defects from the level of the nasopharynx to the thoracic inlet. Estimating the length of the flap is necessary for successful reconstruction of the defect. This can usually be estimated at the time of laryngoscopy and esophagoscopy. Once the length of the defect is determined, the donor arm is prepared by placing a tourniquet above the elbow and prepping sterily. In most cases, the flap harvest is done simultaneously with ablation. The flap is outlined, and the dimensions are driven by the length of the defect as determined and a width of 6 to 8 cm. The flap is centered over the radial artery and cephalic vein in the distal forearm. In most cases, a proximal skin monitor is incorporated into the flap harvest to allow physiologic monitoring of the flap in the perioperative period. Once the flap design is outlined on the donor site, the arm is exsanguinated with an elastic bandage and the tourniquet is inflated to a pressure of 90 mm of mercury above the patient's baseline sys-

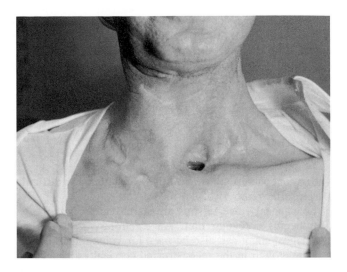

FIGURE 4-16. A postoperative photograph shows the results of reconstruction of the cervical esophagus after laryngoesophagectomy and a left radical neck dissection.

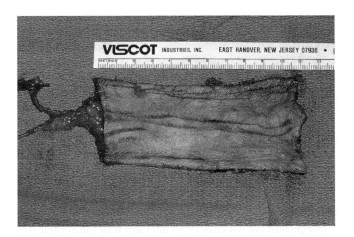

FIGURE 4-17. Harvested radial forearm free flap, 8 cm wide and a length equal to the length of the pharyngoesophageal defect.

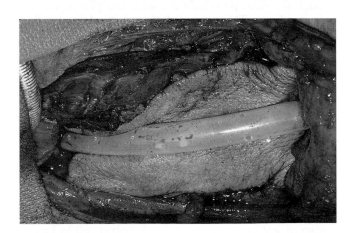

FIGURE 4-18. Flap insertion begins with suturing of the superior and inferior margins and placement of the Montgomery Salivary Bypass Tube.

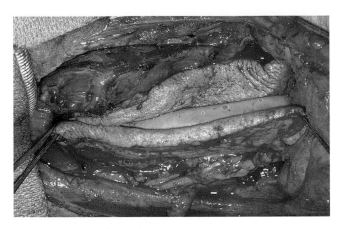

FIGURE 4-19. Tubulation of the flap around the salivary bypass tube (see Chapter 5).

tolic pressure. The flap is then harvested as described in Chapter 2.

If the flap is harvested in its entirety and the ablation is still proceeding, then it is possible to tubulate the forearm in situ in the donor site. This is done using a 3-0 Vicryl suture on a tapered needle with the edges inverted into the lumen. In place, the salivary bypass tube may facilitate this donor site tubulation.

Once ablation has been completed, the forearm flap is taken from its donor site by ligating the feeding artery and draining vein. The flap is taken to the neck where it is inset. A salivary bypass tube is placed through the defect transorally. This is secured to the nasal septum by way of a red rubber catheter attached to the upper aspect of the bypass tube that is passed through the nasal cavity and sutured to the nasal septum in the vestibule. The flap is completely tabulated in the case of the total laryngopharyngectomy defect.

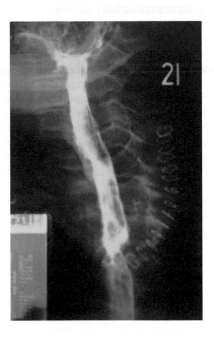

FIGURE 4-20. Postoperative barium swallow radiograph demonstrating a patent repair.

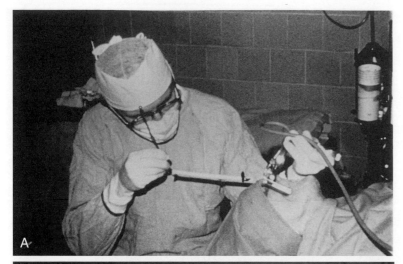

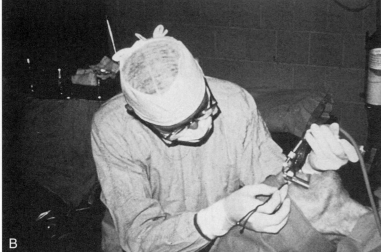

FIGURE 5-10. *A,* A standard Jackson laryngoscope is used to expose the hypopharynx. An endotracheal-tube stylet has been inserted into the bypass tube and crimped at its proximal end. *B,* The salivary bypass tube has been inserted into the cervical esophagus. At this point the stylet and laryngoscope are removed. The upper end of the bypass tube is pushed into place with the index finger.

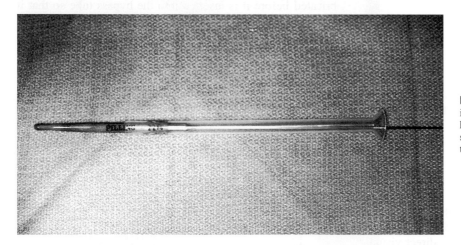

FIGURE 5-11. A salivary bypass tube has been inserted over a No. 22 French filiform bougie that has been thoroughly lubricated. This is often the simplest way to insert a salivary bypass tube when treating a stricture of the cervical esophagus.

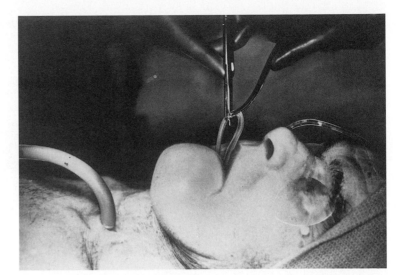

FIGURE 5–12. To remove the salivary bypass tube, the feeding tube is grasped in the oropharynx and the loop pulled out of the mouth. This loop of feeding tube is cut.

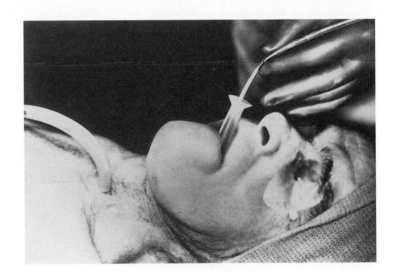

FIGURE 5–13. The upper portion of the feeding tube has been removed from the nose, and the bypass tube and distal portion of the feeding tube are being pulled from the mouth.

Chapter 6
Surgery of the Trachea

WILLIAM W. MONTGOMERY

HISTORY OF TRACHEOTOMY

The first detailed reports of tracheotomy are provided by Galen and Aretaeus in the second and third centuries A.D. At the beginning of the Christian era, the trachea was known as the "rough artery" (*tracheia arteria*), to distinguish it from blood vessels, which were believed to contain air as well as blood. Not until the 19th century was "trachea" accepted as a term designating the air tube extending from the larynx to the bronchi. It is not known whether surgeons of the early Christian era actually attempted the operation. It is strongly suspected that the operation was more often proposed than performed.

Goodall (1934), in a thorough search of the literature, could find records of only 28 successful tracheotomies performed before 1825. The infrequent use of the operation was apparently because of (1) limited knowledge of the anatomy; (2) lack of surgical experience; and (3) the threat of "loss of face" if the patient should die during or after the operation. Early reports of tracheotomy imply that it was often performed on patients who were near death from suffocation. It is not surprising that the success rate was poor under such circumstances. Even as late as the 18th century, phlebotomy was the accepted first choice in treatment.

The first reported successful tracheotomy was performed in 1546 by Antonio Muso Brasovolo, an Italian physician, who performed the procedure to relieve a pharyngeal or laryngeal abscess when the barber-surgeon attending the patient refused to undertake the operation. The next reference to a successful tracheotomy appears in 1620, nearly 100 years later.

In 1620, Nicolas Habicot removed a blood clot from the larynx by means of a tracheotomy and is thus credited with the first successful removal of a foreign body from this organ. In a more interesting operation, he effected the release of a foreign body through the intestinal tract. A 14-year-old boy had swallowed nine gold pieces wrapped in cloth to prevent them from being stolen. A tracheotomy released the restriction in the airway caused by compression of the trachea by the cloth containing the gold pieces, which was lodged in the esophagus. The bundle with the gold pieces was then pushed into the stomach with a lead sound and was later recovered as it departed from the lower intestine.

In 1766, Caron, at St. Germain en Lay, performed a tracheotomy on a 7-year-old boy to remove a bean. This was the first successful tracheotomy in a child to be recorded.

Detharding, in 1714, recommended a tracheotomy for persons who apparently had drowned (Fig. 6–1). This treatment was again recommended for drowned persons by de-Bouteau in 1783 "in order that all the water may be got out of the lungs and that warm air may be blown in and out of them by means of a tube."

In 1732, Chovell used the operation in an attempt to cheat the hangman. He performed a tracheotomy on a prisoner the night before the prisoner was condemned to hang. Needless to say, the prisoner did not survive.

During the early 19th century, Bretonnear and Troussear demonstrated that tracheotomy could be successfully used to relieve distress due to obstruction of the trachea caused by diphtheria.

Moreau, in the 17th century, was the first to perform a tracheotomy with the patient in the recumbent position. Until this time, the operation had been performed with patients in the sitting position with their neck in hyperextension.

A transverse skin incision was used until the time of Fabricius (16th century), who condemned this approach because of the danger of cutting blood vessels and because it provided inadequate exposure of the trachea. The vertical incision was usually of moderate length. The vertical incision became the rule after this and retained its popularity until the present time. DeGarengeot recommended that the incision extend from the symphysis of the chin to the sternum. He must have been a courageous surgeon, because he is credited with being the first to divide the thyroid isthmus to expose the trachea (1720). Early surgeons were afraid of hemorrhage from the thyroid isthmus; hence, the operation was either a "high" or "low" tracheotomy (above or below the isthmus).

There is some confusion regarding the nomenclature with reference to tracheotomy and tracheostomy, just as there is between gastrotomy and gastrostomy. A *tracheotomy* is an operation during which an incision is made in the skin of the anterior neck and the anterior tracheal wall. The resulting tract between the skin and trachea is bridged with a tracheotomy tube. A *tracheostomy* is an operation during which the distal end of the transected trachea, or an opening in the anterior tracheal wall, is sutured to the skin of the anterior neck. The resultant opening is referred to as a tracheostoma

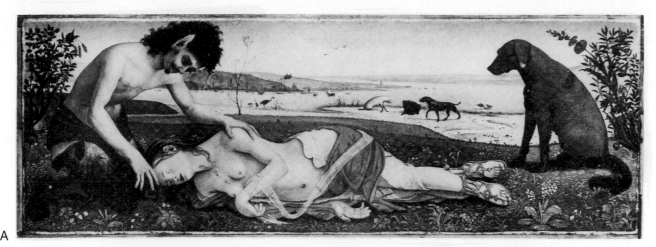

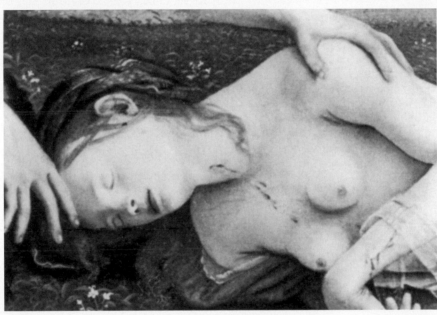

FIGURE 6-1. *A,* Among the paintings of the earlier Italian schools in the National Gallery, London, is one by Piero di Cosima, showing the body of a woman lying on the banks of an estuary or river. Kneeling at her head is a satyr and seated at her feet is a dog of the Labrador retriever type. *B,* In her neck is a wound, which closely resembles a tracheostomy incision. If it can be accepted that this is a painting of a tracheostomy orifice, it is one of the earliest to be found. (From Holborow, 1959)

and usually does not require a tracheal tube. If it does, it is referred to as a tracheal or laryngectomy tube. I suspect that this effort will not change otolaryngologists and others from referring to a tracheotomy as tracheostomy.

EARLY TRACHEOTOMY TUBES

There is no mention of the tracheotomy tube before the writings of Fabricius in the 16th century. Fabricius, who never performed a tracheotomy, describes the tube as small, straight, and short, with two wings at the outer end to prevent the tube from sliding into the trachea. "It should not be too wide lest too much air gets into the lungs." The surgeons of this era stressed that the tube must not touch the posterior wall of the trachea.

Guilio Casserio, a pupil of Fabricius, described a curved tube with several holes for air in its lower portion. The

curved (quarter circle) tube has been in use since that time. Casserio's tube was made of silver; also recommended at that time were gold and lead tubes. A less likely tracheotomy tube was the one fashioned from a goose's quill by Ferriere in 1784.

In 1730, Martin credits a layman with the idea of an inner tube to keep the tracheotomy tube clear of mucus without removing the outer tube from the trachea.

When the tracheotomy became the treatment of choice for laryngeal diphtheria in the middle of the 19th century, many improvements were made to the tracheotomy tube. In 1855, Chassaignac invented a sharp-pointed hook with a groove on the inferior surface of the shaft. The hook was inserted below the cricoid cartilage to draw the trachea upward. A bistoury was then passed along the groove and into the trachea. Many modifications of this idea have been introduced subsequently, including, more recently, the Rockey tracheotome and the Sierra tracheotome. Luer invented the movable shield. The valved tube was first introduced by Bourdilat and was modified in 1869 by Fuller. A valved tracheotomy tube in use today was introduced by Tucker. Most tracheotomy tubes used today are fashioned from plastic (Tracoe and Shiley). If a speaking valve is indicated, it is applied to the external end of the tracheotomy tube. I have been unable to find the source of our friend and foe, the inflatable cuffed tracheotomy tube.

INDICATIONS FOR TRACHEOTOMY

In general, the indications for tracheotomy may be classified as (1) respiratory obstruction, (2) secretory retention, and (3) respiratory insufficiency.

Respiratory Obstruction

Trauma
Facial fractures (especially mandibular) can be complicated by edema, hematoma, or hemorrhage of the airway above the larynx and can necessitate a tracheotomy. External or internal injury to the larynx or cervical trachea may result in respiratory obstruction. Symptoms of respiratory obstruction following trauma may occur immediately after the injury or develop slowly over a period of days or weeks.

Foreign Bodies
Respiratory obstruction from foreign bodies usually occurs in children, in whom beans, buttons, beads, and other objects may be aspirated and become lodged in the larynx. A bolus of meat is probably the most common foreign body to become lodged in the adult larynx.

Irritants and Corrosives
Respiratory obstruction can result from damage to the pharyngeal, laryngeal, and cervical tracheal mucous membrane by steam, irritant gases, corrosive liquids, burning gases, or hot air from fire.

Infections
Infections in the upper respiratory tract may progress to obstruction. The most common cause for inflammatory obstruction is acute laryngotracheobronchitis. This condition occurs predominantly in young children in association with an apparent upper respiratory infection. The obstruction is caused by inflammatory edema of the mucosal lining of the larynx, trachea, and bronchi and also by thick tenacious secretions. Hoarseness, croupy cough, stridor, dyspnea, restlessness, fever, and prostration occur as the disease progresses. An increase in the respiratory rate and retraction of the suprasternal notch during inspiration are signs that should alert the physician to the need for immediate action. A tracheotomy can be avoided by providing antibiotic and steroid therapy before the situation progresses to the point of an emergency.

Congenital Anomalies
Congenital anomalies of the upper respiratory tract may necessitate a tracheotomy. Obstruction may result from malformations above the larynx, such as choanal atresia (the newborn is usually unable to mouth breathe). Malformations of the larynx include supraglottic fusion, laryngeal webs, cysts, atresia, deformities of the cricoid cartilage, and limited or absent laryngeal function. Congenital lesions below the larynx include esophageal atresia, tracheoesophageal fistula, vascular rings, and abnormalities of the great vessels.

Vasomotor Incidents
Vasomotor incidents occurring in association with angioneurotic edema or drug sensitivity may promote obstruction in the upper airway, necessitating a tracheotomy.

Laryngeal Dysfunction
Impaired abduction of the larynx may limit the airway sufficiently to necessitate a tracheotomy. Impaired abduction occurs with bilateral paralysis of the recurrent laryngeal nerve, cricoarytenoid arthritis, and conditions that produce laryngeal tetany or spasm. The onset of airway obstruction from these causes may be either acute or slow and insidious.

Cysts and Neoplasms
Cysts and neoplasms of the upper respiratory tract can result in airway obstruction. Benign (subglottic hemangioma) and malignant lesions of the larynx are included in this group.

Secretory Retention

Inadequate clearance of secretions from the tracheobronchial tree can result in obstruction of the lower airway and alveolar hypoventilation. This type of hypoxia develops more slowly than that associated with other types of respiratory obstruction. The causes for secretory retention are numerous and, in general, are associated with the patient's inability to cough, improper deglutition with aspiration, and the inability to expectorate. The situation is usually quite obvious when aspiration, neuromuscular disorders, and a depressed cough are observed. Restlessness is often an early symptom. Respirations are shallow and jerky because of the patient's apprehension of impending aspiration. As the hypoxia progresses, the patient becomes confused, depressed, and lethargic. On examination, rales and rhonchi are heard throughout the chest. Tachycardia and hypotension develop as the situation progresses. Cyanosis either appears late or is not present. Because there is inadequate alveolar oxygen saturation and excessive carbon dioxide accumulation, determinations of the blood pH, P_{CO_2}, oxygen saturation, P_{O_2}, and chloride are indicated. Oxygen therapy alone is not sufficient treatment because carbon dioxide accumulation may continue and result in respiratory standstill. A cuffed tracheotomy tube, frequent aspiration of secretions, and respiratory assistance may be indicated until the cause of the disorder can be determined and, if possible, treated. Endotracheal intubation is an effective technique for suctioning the trachea and providing assisted ventilation. However, endotracheal intubation produces much more discomfort than the cuffed tracheotomy tube, and there is a significant incidence of injury to the larynx and trachea with its prolonged use.

Respiratory Insufficiency

A tracheotomy may be indicated to assist and maintain respiration even when there is no obstruction or secretory retention in the airway. This situation is usually associated with central or neuromuscular disorders. The purpose of the tracheotomy is to allow positive-pressure respiration and to reduce airflow resistance and the dead space. Intratracheal intubation may be used for short periods with relative safety. However, prolonged intubation may initiate laryngeal or tracheal stenosis.

MANAGEMENT OF AIRWAY OBSTRUCTION

Acute Complete Obstruction

Endotracheal Intubation
Whenever possible, either a bronchoscope or an endotracheal tube should be inserted by the intralaryngeal route. Unfortunately, such equipment is usually not available when the emergency arises. When properly executed, endotracheal intubation is the fastest method for establishing an airway, thus avoiding a traumatic, hurried tracheotomy. No anesthesia is required for such an intubation. After intubation, a general anesthetic may be administered while an orderly tracheotomy is performed. The incidence of complications during the tracheotomy is reduced when a bronchoscope or endotracheal tube is present in the trachea.

Cricothyrotomy (Laryngotomy)
When endotracheal intubation is not possible, making an incision through the cricothyroid membrane best relieves an obstructed airway.

Technique. The patient's neck is placed in extension by inserting a roll of fabric under the shoulders, or the neck is brought over the knee of the "squatting" surgeon. The surgeon quickly identifies the position of the thyroid notch with his or her index finger. This finger should then descend in the midline to the prominence of the cricoid cartilage. The depression of the cricothyroid membrane is identified, and a mark is made in the midline with the fingernail (Fig. 6–2A). A vertical incision is made in the middle over the thyroid and cricoid cartilages as the subcutaneous vessels are retracted from the midline with the thumb and index finger (Fig. 6–2B). As the wound is spread by finger dissection, the cricothyroid membrane can be readily identified. The cricothyroid membrane is incised horizontally as close as possible to the cricoid cartilage to prevent bleeding from the cricothyroid arteries (Fig. 6–2C). The cricothyroid space is widened by inserting either the handle or the blade of the knife into the horizontal incision and rotating it 90 degrees (Fig. 6–2D). A tracheotomy tube or a silicone tracheal cannula is inserted.

In the past we have been taught that it is essential to perform an orderly tracheotomy as soon as possible after the laryngotomy, for a prolonged cricothyrotomy can result in perichondritis, subglottic edema, and cicatricial stenosis. This may not be true. I have kept silicone tracheal cannulas in patients with cricothyrotomy for more than 25 years without complications in cases where a conventional tracheotomy is not possible because of an inferiorly displaced larynx.

Imminent Airway Obstruction

Emergency Tracheotomy
An emergency tracheotomy is indicated when respiratory obstruction is too severe to allow time for an orderly tracheotomy, when facilities are not available for insertion of a bronchoscope or endotracheal tube, or when the surgeon believes that the patient cannot survive a few minutes of increasing hypoxia without brain damage. The operation is difficult to perform on patients with a short, thick neck or with disease in the tracheotomy site or on an infant whose trachea is soft and difficult to identify by palpation.

Technique. The patient's neck is placed in hyperextension so that the larynx and trachea are prominent. This also allows the trachea to be elevated in relation to the suprasternal notch (Fig. 6–3A). The trachea is placed in prominence and fixed in the midline as the surgeon's thumb and index finger push the adjacent musculature and great vessels laterally beneath the sternocleidomastoid muscle. The position of the thyroid notch, cricoid cartilage, and cricothyroid membrane is quickly identified.

Any patient needing an emergency tracheotomy does not require local anesthesia. A vertical incision is made in the midline from the level of the cricothyroid membrane almost to the suprasternal notch. It should be made through the subcutaneous tissues to facilitate subsequent finger dissection (Fig. 6–3B). The incision is widened with the surgeon's index finger or with the knife handle. The index finger of the opposite hand identifies the prominence of the cricoid cartilage and the beginning of the trachea. A small horizontal incision is made immediately beneath the cricoid cartilage through the pretracheal fascia (Fig. 6–3C), which allows this finger to dissect onto the anterior surface of the trachea. With firm pressure, it is usually possible in this manner to dissect the thyroid isthmus downward to expose the three upper tracheal rings. The surgeon's finger is moved slightly to his or her side so that the vertical midline incision can be made through the second and third tracheal cartilages (Fig. 6–3D). A hemostat or tracheotomy dilator is introduced into the trachea, and a tracheotomy or endotracheal tube is inserted. If respiratory assistance is not necessary, the next step is to ligate all vessels. If respiratory assistance is necessary, temporary hemostasis can be obtained by packing gauze firmly into the wound and around the cannula. The skin closure should not be tight around the tracheotomy tube, thus avoiding subcutaneous emphysema.

Impending Respiratory Obstruction

Orderly Tracheotomy
An orderly tracheotomy is the operation of choice for impending asphyxia and the other nonemergency indications mentioned.

Technique. Whenever possible, an orderly tracheotomy should be performed with an endotracheal tube in place and the patient under general anesthesia.

The patient is placed on the operating table as shown in Figure 6–3A. A pillow, sandbag, or rolled sheet is placed under the patient's shoulders to effect the greatest promi-

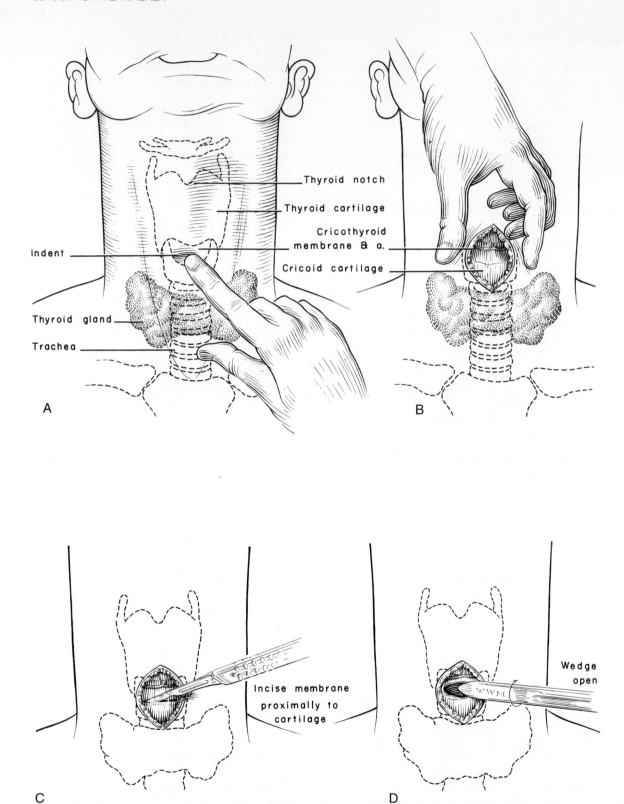

FIGURE 6-2. Cricothyrotomy (laryngotomy). *A*, The patient's neck is placed in hyperextension by inserting a roll of fabric under the shoulders or by placing the dorsum of the neck over the knee of the "squatting" surgeon. In so doing, the thyroid notch becomes prominent anteriorly. The surgeon identifies the position of the thyroid notch with his index finger. This finger descends in the midline to the prominence of the cricoid cartilage. The depression of the cricothyroid membrane is identified above the superior margin of the cricoid cartilage. A mark is made in the midline at this level with the fingernail. *B*, A vertical incision is made in the midline over the thyroid and cricoid cartilages. Vessels are retracted from the midline with the thumb and index finger of the opposite hand, as shown. *C*, As the wound is spread apart by finger dissection, the cricothyroid membrane becomes readily apparent. The cricothyroid membrane is incised horizontally as close as possible to the cricoid cartilage to prevent bleeding from the cricothyroid arteries. *D*, The cricothyroid space is widened by inserting either the handle or the blade of the knife into the horizontal incision and rotating it 90 degrees. This establishes an airway. A tracheotomy tube is temporarily inserted if one is available. A cricothyrotomy can be accomplished in 15 to 30 seconds.

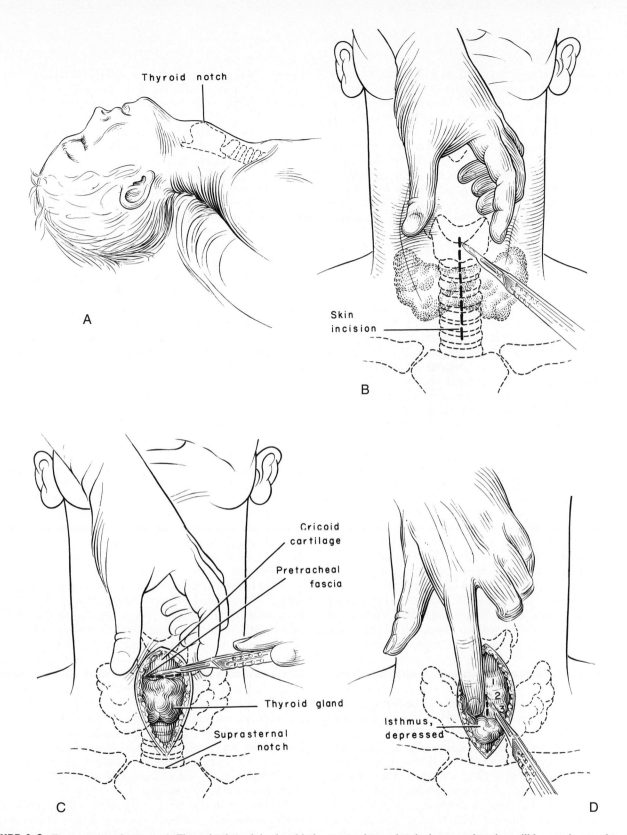

FIGURE 6-3. Emergency tracheotomy. *A,* The patient's neck is placed in hyperextension so that the larynx and trachea will be prominent and to allow the trachea to be elevated in relation to the suprasternal notch. *B,* The trachea is placed into prominence and fixed in the midline as the thumb and index finger of the surgeon's left hand push the adjacent musculature and vessels laterally beneath the sternocleidomastoid muscle. The anterior midline positions of the thyroid notch, cricoid cartilage, and cricothyroid membrane are quickly identified. A vertical incision is made in the midline from the level of the cricothyroid membrane nearly to the suprasternal notch. This incision is carried directly through the subcutaneous tissue. *C,* The incision is widened with the surgeon's index finger of his right hand or with a knife handle. The index finger of the left hand identifies the prominence of the cricoid cartilage. A small horizontal incision is made immediately beneath the cricoid cartilage through the pretracheal fascia. The left index finger is inserted into this incision to the space between the thyroid isthmus and the trachea. With firm pressure, the thyroid isthmus is dissected inferiorly by finger dissection to expose the upper three tracheal rings. *D,* The index finger of the left hand is moved slightly to the operator's left so that a midline vertical incision can be made through the second and third tracheal rings. A hemostat or tracheotomy dilator is introduced into this incision while a tracheotomy or endotracheal tube is inserted into the tracheal lumen. Once an airway has been established, all bleeding can be controlled in an orderly fashion. This operation can be accomplished in 1 or 2 minutes.

nence of the trachea and larynx. If an endotracheal tube or bronchoscope has not been inserted and the patient has any degree of severe dyspnea, he or she should not be placed in this position until the local anesthetic has been injected and the preparations have been completed.

A local anesthetic is injected subcutaneously in the region of the proposed vertical incision. The deeper tissues over the cricoid and trachea are injected in the midline.

I no longer advocate the horizontal (Fig. 6–4A to C) incision for a tracheotomy. The cosmetic result is no better (and often worse) than a vertical incision, it is much more difficult to adjust the level of the tracheotomy tube, and it is much more difficult to close the incision after the tracheotomy tube is removed.

A vertical incision is made from above the level of the cricoid arch to the suprasternal notch. The vertical incision is carried through the platysma muscle, exposing the sternohyoid muscles. Superior and inferior undermining is accomplished by blunt dissection superficial to the fascia covering the sternohyoid muscles. At this point, the sternohyoid muscles, median raphe, and the anterior jugular veins can be seen. A vertical incision is made in the median raphe between the sternohyoid muscles from the level of the cricoid cartilage into the inferior aspect of the dissection (Fig. 6–4B). The sternohyoid and underlying sternothyroid muscles are retracted laterally, exposing the cricoid cartilage and thyroid isthmus.

To perform a tracheotomy at the proper level, it is often necessary to transect and ligate the thyroid isthmus. Occasionally, the isthmus is small or so placed that ligation is not necessary. A small horizontal or vertical incision is made through the pretracheal fascia over the inferior aspect of the cricoid cartilage. The position of the vessels in this area will usually indicate to the surgeon the proper location for this incision (Fig. 6–4C). A small hemostat is inserted in this incision and directed inferiorly behind the thyroid isthmus and anterior to the trachea (Fig. 6–5A). After the proper plane of cleavage between the thyroid isthmus and trachea has been determined with the small hemostat, a larger hemostat is inserted to completely separate the thyroid isthmus from the anterior tracheal wall by blunt dissection (Fig. 6–5B). A large hemostat is placed on each side of the thyroid isthmus, which is then divided with a knife or scissors (Figs. 6–5C and D). The thyroid isthmus is suture ligated on each side with 2-0 chromic catgut or 3-0 Vicryl suture material (Fig. 6–6A).

A short No. 20 hypodermic needle is used to inject 2 mL of 4% lidocaine (Xylocaine) or 4% cocaine solution into the lumen of the trachea (Fig. 6–6B). A tracheal hook or large skin hook is inserted into the tracheal lumen between the first and second tracheal rings. Retraction in an anterosuperior direction will stabilize the trachea and greatly facilitate the incisions for the tracheal fenestration (Fig. 6–6C).

In my opinion, a tracheal fenestration is preferable to a simple horizontal or vertical incision of the trachea or to one of the flap techniques. A fenestration minimizes the danger of posterior displacement of portions of the tracheal cartilage with subsequent tracheal stenosis.

There are a number of ways to fashion a tracheal fenestration. If the tracheal rings are not ossified, the fenestration can be accomplished by making a circular incision with a No. 15 knife blade and removing the incised tissue in one

piece. Usually it is necessary to make cruciate incisions as shown in Figure 6–6D. The four triangular flaps of tissue are then removed by means of a Ring punch (Fig. 6–7A), forceps, or a knife (Fig. 6–7B). I now routinely use the tracheal trephine fenestrator to fashion an opening in the anterior tracheal wall. A No. 6 tracheotomy tube fits nicely into this fenestration. If a larger tube is indicated, the opening can be enlarged by making a small lateral incision on each side, while using a larger tracheal fenestrator. A sterile tracheotomy tube with obturator in place is inserted into the trachea (Fig. 6–7C). The obturator is removed, and the lateral aspects of the horizontal incision are loosely approximated with one or two sutures. Iodoform gauze may be loosely packed around the tube for hemostasis (Fig. 6–7D). Sufficient space should be left around the tube to minimize the danger of subcutaneous emphysema. A tracheotomy tube can be secured in place with two silk sutures on each side or with tracheotomy tape (Fig. 6–7E). The ends are tied on either side of the neck with a square knot. The inner cannula is inserted. A tracheotomy dressing is applied, and a moist 4 × 4-inch sponge is suspended, covering the tracheotomy tube, over a second tape around the patient's neck.

CARE AFTER TRACHEOTOMY

The inner cannula should be removed and cleaned every 2 to 3 hours for the first 3 days and as needed thereafter. It should be washed with hot soap and water; a pipe cleaner or a piece of 1-inch gauze bandage attached to a sink faucet is used to clean the inner surface. The cannula is rinsed with alcohol and then sterile water before being reinserted. A small humidifier attached to the tracheotomy tube provides extra humidification.

In addition to the tracheotomy dressing, a moist 4 × 4 sponge is suspended anteriorly to the tracheotomy tube (see Figs. 6–10D and E). The sponge should be changed frequently and should not be allowed to become dry.

If possible, the patient should be placed in a private room with the windows and doors closed so that the temperature (75°F) and humidity (90%) can be more easily controlled. A humidifier should run continuously. Cool humidification is preferable to steam. If crusting occurs, 1 or 2 mL of normal or hypotonic saline solution can be instilled into the trachea every 2 hours. A mucolytic agent, such as acetylcysteine (Mucomyst) solution can be inserted into the trachea every 3 to 4 hours as therapy for severe crusting. Again, a small tracheotomy tube humidifier attached to the tracheotomy tube is very helpful.

Suctioning should be accomplished with a sterile soft-rubber catheter. A Y-tube or opening in the catheter is necessary to allow insertion of the catheter into the trachea without suction. Suction is applied only during withdrawal of the catheter. Prolonged or frequent suctioning should be avoided. It may be necessary to suction every hour or so for the first few days because of the increased bronchial secretions initiated by the presence of the tracheotomy tube.

The tracheotomy tube should be changed on the sixth or seventh postoperative day (Fig. 6–8). A change before this time is usually not necessary and may be complicated by bleeding or difficult reinsertion of the tube.

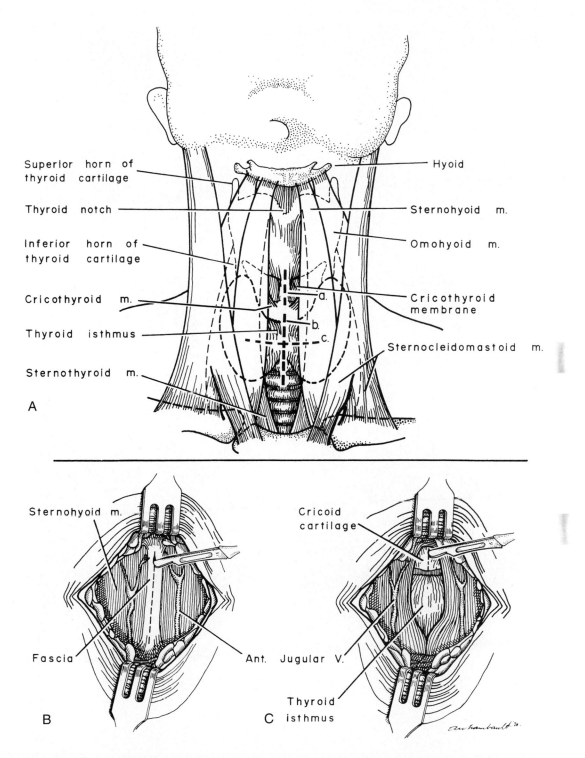

FIGURE 6-4. Orderly tracheotomy. *A,* This sketch illustrates the relationships of the various incisions used to approach the upper airway to the thyroid cartilage, cricoid cartilage, thyroid isthmus, and trachea. A vertical incision is used to approach the cricothyroid membrane and to carry out an emergency cricothyrotomy (*a*). A vertical incision is used for an emergency tracheotomy; this incision extends from the cricothyroid membrane to a point well below the thyroid isthmus in the anterior midline (*b*). A horizontal incision over the thyroid isthmus can be used for an orderly tracheotomy. However, I prefer the vertical incision. This incision is made approximately 2 cm below the cricoid cartilage and should be at least 5 cm long (*c*). *B,* The vertical incision has been carried through the platysma muscle, exposing the sternohyoid muscles. Additional exposure is obtained by undermining superiorly and inferiorly, with blunt dissection, above the fascia covering the sternohyoid muscles. The sternohyoid muscles, median raphe, and anterior jugular veins should be in view. A vertical incision is made in the median raphe between the sternohyoid muscles from the level of the cricoid cartilage to the inferior aspect of the dissection. The sternothyroid muscles are separated in a similar fashion, exposing the inferior aspect of the cricoid cartilage and the thyroid isthmus. *C,* The thyroid isthmus has been exposed. Occasionally the isthmus is small and so placed that entrance into the trachea can be gained without division of the isthmus. The thyroid isthmus should be approached from above by making a small vertical or horizontal incision through the pretracheal fascia over the cricoid cartilage.

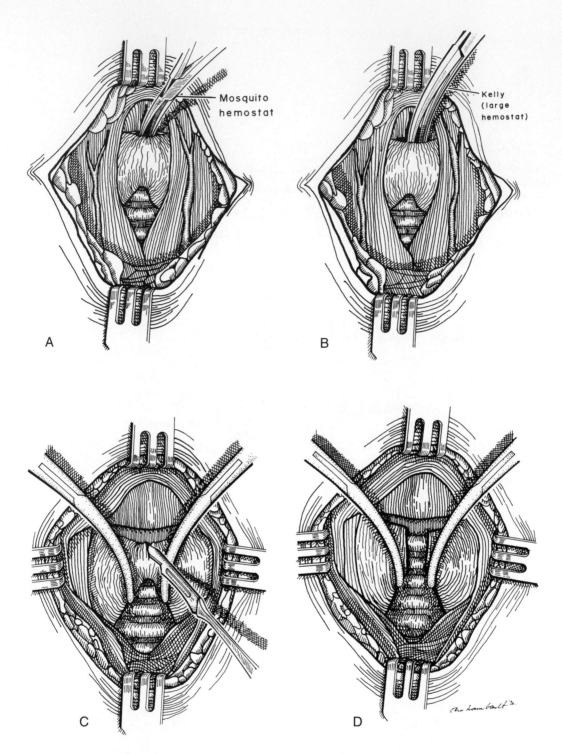

FIGURE 6–5. Orderly tracheotomy, *continued. A,* A small hemostat is inserted into the incision over the cricoid cartilage. By dissecting firmly against the inferior border of the cricoid cartilage and anterior wall of the trachea, a plane can be established between the thyroid isthmus and trachea, without producing troublesome bleeding from the thyroid isthmus. *B,* A larger hemostat is inserted to complete the separation between the thyroid isthmus and anterior tracheal wall. *C,* A large hemostat has been placed on each side of the thyroid isthmus, which is then incised with a knife or scissors. *D,* The thyroid isthmus has been divided in the midline.

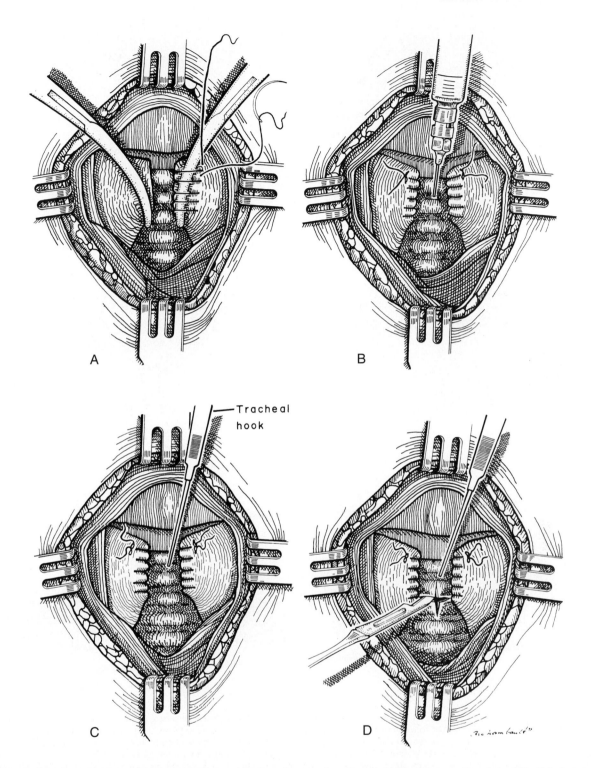

FIGURE 6-6. Orderly tracheotomy, *continued*. *A,* The thyroid isthmus is suture-ligated on each side with a running stitch of No. 2-0 chromic catgut or 3-0 vicryl sutures. Note that the last suture is returned in an opposite direction through the thyroid isthmus to facilitate tying it after the hemostat has been removed. *B,* A short No. 20 hypodermic needle is used to inject 2 mL of 4% lidocaine (Xylocaine) or cocaine solution into the tracheal lumen. The aspiration of air indicates that the needle has been properly placed into the tracheal lumen. *C,* A tracheal hook has been inserted into the tracheal lumen between the first and second tracheal rings. The trachea is retracted in an anterosuperior direction. *D,* A cruciate incision through the intercartilaginous membrane and two tracheal rings can be made with a knife, unless the tracheal rings are ossified.

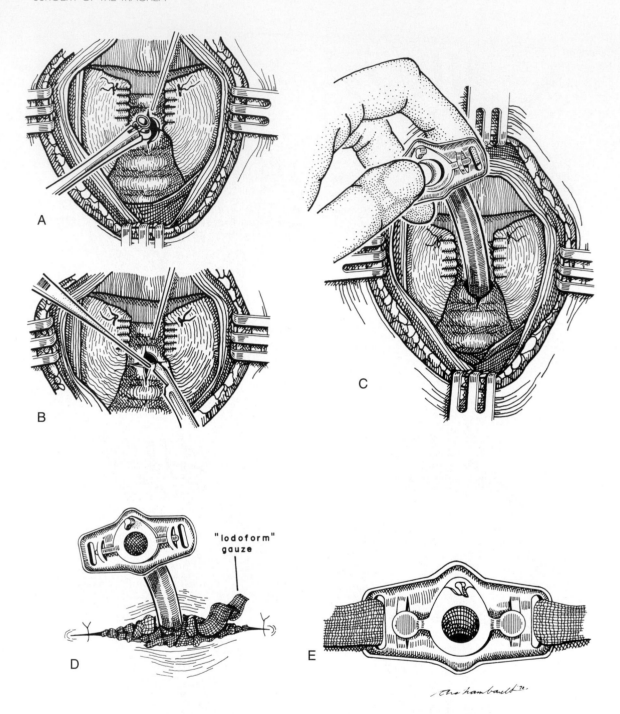

FIGURE 6–7. Orderly tracheotomy, *continued. A,* The four triangular flaps of tissue are removed with a ring punch, making certain that this tissue does not fall into the triangular lumen. *B,* The triangular flaps of tissue can also be removed with forceps and a knife or with scissors. *C,* A sterile tracheotomy tube with an obturator in place is inserted through the fenestration in the anterior tracheal wall and into the tracheal lumen. *D,* The obturator has been removed, and the lateral aspects of the horizontal incision have been loosely approximated with one or two dermal sutures. Iodoform gauze is packed in the incision around the tracheotomy tube for hemostasis. *E,* A tracheotomy tape has been passed through each side of the faceplate of the tracheotomy tube and secured on either side of the neck with a square knot. The inner cannula has been inserted and locked in place. A tracheotomy dressing is then applied, and a moist 4- × 4-in sponge is suspended in front of the tracheotomy tube over a second tracheotomy tape around the patient's neck.

The tracheotomy tube is observed for signs of infection. If infection is present, a culture is taken and the patient is given the appropriate antibiotics.

If the tracheotomy tube will be in place for a prolonged period, the patient (or the parents, if the patient is an infant) is carefully instructed in tracheotomy care. This allows the patient to leave the hospital at an earlier date.

The tracheotomy tube should be removed as soon as possible, especially in children, to prevent complications and dependence. In adults, the tracheotomy tube is plugged for at least 24 hours before its removal. In children, and especially in infants, it may be necessary to insert smaller and smaller tracheotomy tubes before a full plug is inserted before decannulation.

When the tube is removed, a pressure dressing is placed over the wound to occlude the fenestration. The tracheotomy tract usually closes spontaneously in 2 to 3 days. If the tracheotomy tube has been in place for a prolonged period, the tract may be lined with skin. In such instances, the dermal tract is removed after making an elliptical incision around the tracheotomy opening. The skin surrounding the elliptical incision is undermined, and the tract is closed in two or three layers.

Method for Changing the Tracheotomy Tube

Special instructions from a doctor or nurse and supervised practice are required before the patient changes his or her own tracheotomy tube. The opening in the neck (see Fig. 6–8A) is directly connected to the trachea, which makes insertion of a tracheotomy tube a simple maneuver.

To remove the tracheotomy tube, the tracheotomy tape is untied and the shield or faceplate of the tracheotomy tube is grasped with the thumb and index finger and pulled forward and downward. The spare clean tube, with the tracheotomy tape applied, should be ready to be inserted before the tracheotomy tube is removed. A very light film of mupirocin ointment (Bactroban) is applied to the surface of the tracheotomy tube to facilitate ease of insertion. The tracheotomy tape can be applied to the tube as a single or double strand, as shown in Figures 6–8B and C.

When inserting the tracheotomy tube, the patient faces a mirror and grasps each side of the tube's faceplate with a gentle inward pressure. Again, it is important that the spare tube be inserted with a gentle inward pressure and that the spare tube be inserted immediately after the dirty tube is removed.

After the tracheotomy tube has been secured in place and the tracheotomy tape tied, a gauze sponge should be applied over the tube as shown in Figures 6–8D and E.

Method for Suctioning (FIGURE 6-9)

The amount of mucus secretion varies. It increases when the patient has a cold, when the air in the home is dry, or when the tube is irritating. Suctioning may be necessary to control the mucus.

A portable suction machine may be rented from a medical or surgical supply house. The patient will receive instructions on its use when the machine is rented. As a rule, the rubber catheter should not be inserted beyond the inner end of the tracheotomy tube unless specific instructions to do so have been given by the physician.

If a suction machine is not available, a bulb syringe and a catheter can be purchased at a drugstore and used for suctioning (see Fig. 6–9).

Instructions

1. Assemble the equipment as shown in Figure 6–9.
2. Hold the catheter in one hand and the bulb attached to the syringe in the other hand.
3. Squeeze the bulb before inserting the catheter into the tracheotomy tube to expel the air in it.

4. Release the rubber bulb; the mucus will be drawn into the catheter and syringe.
5. Clean the equipment by washing it in soap and water. This equipment should be boiled frequently to maintain cleanliness.

The patient may need to wear a gauze tracheotomy bib under the tracheotomy tube, especially if there is drainage around the tube. Often, sterile gauze tracheotomy bibs are available from the hospital's central sterile supply department.

MANAGEMENT OF COMPLICATIONS OF TRACHEOTOMY OPERATION

Avoidance of Emergency Tracheotomy

The surgeon should use good clinical judgment in deciding whether a tracheotomy should be performed. The operation should not be delayed until the situation becomes an emergency. The time to transport the patient to the operating room and perform an orderly tracheotomy is when the surgeon is wondering whether a tracheotomy should be performed. Whenever possible, a bronchoscope or endotracheal tube should be inserted and the tracheotomy performed in an orderly manner with the patient under general anesthesia.

Apnea After Tracheotomy

A markedly decreased respiratory rate, or apnea, may occur after the tracheotomy in a patient with chronic laryngeal obstruction. In cases of chronic laryngeal insufficiency, a build-up of carbon dioxide and a lowering of oxygen tension in the alveoli and blood have occurred. Thus, the stimulus for respiration is changed from lack of oxygen to increased carbon dioxide. After the tracheotomy is performed, the patient has free exchange, inspiring atmospheric air, and the blood level of carbon dioxide abruptly decreases. This abrupt decrease in the carbon dioxide content of the blood results in a loss of stimulus for breathing and, thus, apnea. The respiratory center in the medulla is sufficiently anoxic not to change immediately from carbon-dioxide stimulation to oxygen-lack stimulation. When performing a tracheotomy on a patient with a chronic laryngeal obstruction, apnea may be prevented by one of two methods. The first is by partially obstructing the tracheotomy tube so that the change of oxygen saturation and carbon dioxide loss is more gradual. The second relies on having a cuffed tracheotomy or endotracheal tube available so that when hypoventilation or apnea does occur, artificial ventilation can be provided until the crisis has passed.

Severe Hypotension

In addition to the hypotension associated with aerophagia and other pulmonary complications of the tracheotomy, hypotension may result from a sudden decrease in the carbon dioxide level of the blood after the operation. In these patients, the high carbon dioxide content in arterial blood be-

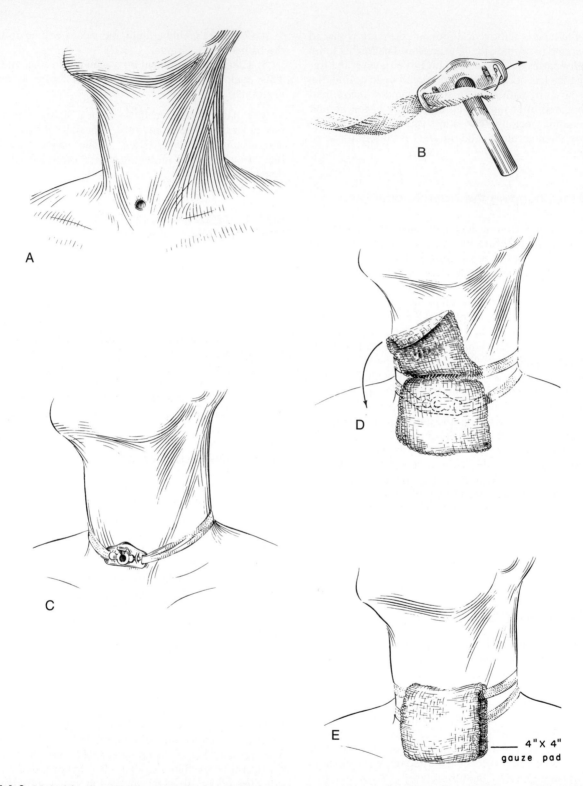

FIGURE 6-8. Method for changing the tracheotomy tube. *A,* This sketch shows the opening in the front of the neck. There is a direct tract from this opening into the trachea, which makes the insertion of the tracheotomy tube a simple maneuver. *B,* There are two methods for application of the tracheotomy tape to the tube. The figure demonstrates the one-strand technique. The end of the tracheotomy tape is inserted through the slot on one side from the front to back and then out the opposite slot in a reverse direction. *C,* The double-strand technique for application of the tracheotomy tape is illustrated. The knot can be tied either on the side or back of the neck according to the patient's preference. *D,* After the tracheotomy tube has been secured in place, it is best to apply some form of protective shield to prevent foreign material from entering the tracheotomy orifice. A single strand of tracheotomy tape is tied around the neck above the tracheotomy tube. A 4- × 4-in gauze square is suspended from this tape to cover the tracheotomy tube. *E,* The 4- × 4-in gauze square is now covering the tracheotomy tube. The gauze may be moistened to increase the humidity to prevent crusting within the tracheotomy tube. Plain 4- × 4-in gauze pads* are preferred to those containing a layer of cotton batting.

*Gauze sponges, 4- × 4-in (16 ply), are manufactured by Carolina Absorbent Cotton Co., Charlotte, N.C. 28200, and also by Johnson & Johnson (No. 7624).

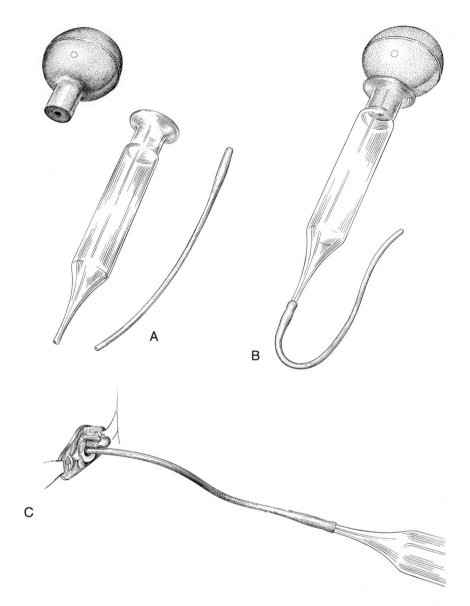

FIGURE 6–9. Method for suctioning when a machine is not available. *A,* A bulb syringe, rubber bulb, and suction catheter. *B,* The rubber bulb and suction catheter have been attached to the bulb syringe. *C,* To suction, the catheter is held in one hand and the bulb attached to the bulb syringe in the other hand. The bulb is squeezed before the catheter is inserted into the tracheotomy tube. When the rubber bulb is released the mucus will be drawn into the catheter and bulb syringe.

fore the tracheotomy, by its action on the medullary centers, produces an elevation in blood pressure. Treatment consists of the administration of intravenous fluids and vasopressors.

Hemorrhage

Hemorrhage may occur during the tracheotomy procedure. Some individuals have an extensive anterior jugular system. The veins in these patients can be avoided by dissecting as near to the midline as possible.

Bleeding from the thyroid isthmus, which is another source for hemorrhage, can be avoided by carefully transecting and suture-ligating the thyroid isthmus before incising the trachea. At times, bleeding from the tracheal wall can be quite troublesome. It is best controlled with the use of suction and cauterization. If a suction apparatus is not available in the operating room, bleeding from the trachea can be controlled by inserting a tracheotomy tube that is large enough to fit tightly against the margin of the tracheal fenestration.

Hemorrhage may be caused by injury to abnormally positioned large veins or arteries in the region of the tracheotomy site. The aortic arch can be high in children and in the elderly. Cervical hyperextension during the tracheotomy elevates the aortic arch and its branches into the surgical field. The various branches of the aorta may be abnormally distributed to the region selected for the operation. To avoid this uncommon and often fatal complication, the surgeon should search frequently during the operation for any unusual pulsations. Blind dissection in the suprasternal region should be avoided. In general, the thyroid isthmus should be dissected very carefully, particularly at its lower border.

Profuse Bronchorrhea

Profuse bronchorrhea may follow irritation caused by insertion of the tracheotomy tube or by endotracheal aspiration. Vigorous endobronchial aspiration may lead to a reduction of the intra-alveolar pressure and an increase in pulmonary blood pressure. In a poorly compensated patient, overzealous endobronchial suctioning may produce pulmonary edema and its complications.

Subcutaneous Emphysema

Closing the subcutaneous wound too tightly around the tracheotomy tube invites subcutaneous emphysema. At times, the emphysema may become severe, extending from the eyebrows to the abdomen. It can be prevented or controlled by packing iodoform gauze, impregnated with an antibiotic ointment, around the tracheotomy tube or by inserting a cuffed tracheotomy tube.

Injury to the Recurrent Laryngeal Nerve

Injury to the recurrent laryngeal nerve can be prevented by use of proper surgical technique and by avoiding an emergency tracheotomy. Attempts to repair a sectioned recurrent laryngeal nerve are futile.

Pneumothorax or Pneumomediastinum

Pneumothorax can be avoided by placing the dissection high and in the midline. If the pleura is incised during the tracheotomy, the incision should be sutured if possible. Chest discomfort with pneumothorax may be mild or severe and retrosternal or precordial in position. Subcutaneous emphysema may be noted in the suprasternal notch. A crackling noise (Hamman's sign) is heard over the precordial area in association with systole, the respiratory rate increases, and breathing is labored. Radiograph examination provides the diagnosis; the air is best seen in the oblique lateral views. Most patients respond to conservative management: administration of oxygen, antibiotics, and sedatives. A chest tap or mediastinotomy is indicated in patients with pneumothorax who have a sudden change in their vital signs, manifested by shock, rapidly spreading subcutaneous emphysema, and deteriorating respiratory function. Tubes are inserted and connected to water-seal drainage.

Atelectasis

Atelectasis usually results from the aspiration of blood or other foreign material into the bronchi during the tracheotomy. Occasionally, the tip of the tracheotomy tube will be directed into the mainstem bronchus, resulting in collapse of the opposite lung. Use of an overlong tracheotomy tube should be avoided in children. Frequent aspiration of bloody tracheal secretions and instructing the patient to take deep breaths will frequently prevent atelectasis.

Tracheoesophageal Fistula

This is an unusual complication of the orderly tracheotomy, but it may frequently accompany the emergency stab-type tracheotomy. To avoid this complication, the emergency stab-type tracheotomy should be performed through the cricothyroid membrane, at which level the posterior wall is protected by the posterior cricoid lamina, and followed, as soon as possible, by an orderly tracheotomy. A tracheoesophageal fistula may also result from an ill-fitting tracheotomy tube that rubs against and erodes the posterior tracheal wall.

Aerophagia

Occasionally, and especially in infants, continual swallowing is noted after a tracheotomy. Older patients have attributed the attempts to swallow continually to the sensation of having a lump in the throat. Abdominal distention soon becomes apparent, and the patient repeatedly vomits small amounts of fluids. Dyspnea occurs as the diaphragm is elevated by abdominal distention. This complication has been reported to result in hypotension, shock, and even death.

The diagnosis is made by percussion of the abdomen, which elicits tympani, and radiographic examination of the abdomen, which demonstrates a large air bubble in the stomach and bowel. The treatment of choice is decannulation as soon as possible or replacement of the tracheotomy tube with a tube of a different shape to prevent the sensation in the throat. The electrolyte balance is evaluated, and a nasogastric tube is inserted to relieve the distention. Oral feedings are avoided until active peristalsis resumes.

Dislocation of the Tracheotomy Tube

The tracheotomy tube has a tendency to tilt forward when the tracheotomy skin incision is low in the neck, especially when a horizontal skin incision was used. The dislocation occurs as the patient's neck is changed from the operative position of hyperextension to the position of flexion, during which the trachea descends and the tracheotomy tube is pulled from the tracheal fenestration. Another more common cause for dislocation of the tube is tracheotomy tape that is improperly tied or placed loosely around the neck. Cervical emphysema or edema may also be responsible for dislocation. The tube can also become dislodged when it is changed, or it can be inserted into a false passage. To prevent dislocation, only experienced personnel should be allowed to change a tracheotomy tube in the immediate postoperative period.

Reinsertion is often difficult when a tracheotomy tube is dislocated during the early postoperative period. My technique is to insert the left index finger into the tracheotomy tract, find the opening in the anterior tracheal wall by palpation, and insert the tracheotomy tube with the right hand, along the left index finger and into the trachea.

Recurrent Respiratory Obstruction

The various causes of this complication are treated or avoided by the following measures.

1. Inspissated secretions in the tracheotomy tube are treated by frequent care of the tracheotomy tube.

2. Tracheal crusting is avoided by proper humidification.

3. Dislocation of the tracheotomy tube is avoided by selecting a tube of the proper size and length for each patient and by securing it in place properly.

4. Obstruction by secondary hemorrhage is avoided and treated as outlined above.

5. Ulceration of the anterior wall of the trachea by the end of the tracheotomy tube, erosion of the innominate artery, or ulceration of the carina with the formation of granulation tissue and obstruction of the airway are avoided by proper placement of the tracheotomy orifice. A tracheotomy that is too low may lead to any of these complications, especially in infants.

Subglottic Edema and Tracheal Stenosis

These complications can be prevented by incising the trachea below the second tracheal ring. Prophylactic antibiotic and steroid therapy, in addition to proper wound care, will prevent secondary edema and infection and most likely will prevent subglottic edema and tracheal stenosis.

Treatment of subglottic edema and tracheal stenosis consists of lowering the tracheotomy tube if it is too high. The use of tracheal dilators is said to be valuable, but it has been ineffectual in my experience. The management of subglottic stenosis is discussed in Chapter 16.

Tracheitis Siccus

Tracheitis siccus is prevented by proper cold humidification of the patient's room. Measures are taken to avoid secondary infection of the tracheotomy wound. A moist sponge is placed over the tracheotomy orifice. The tracheotomy tube should be removed as early as possible. Crusts are removed with suction or forceps. High negative pressure should be avoided when suctioning with a Y-tube or when a hole in the catheter is occluded with a finger. Frequent cleansing of the inner cannula of the tracheotomy tube is essential. Acetylcysteine (Mucomyst) can be instilled into the trachea to dislodge crusts. Ringer's solution or normal saline solution (1 mL) is inserted into the tracheotomy tube every half hour to soften crusts. Crusting can often be rapidly resolved by instilling hypotonic (0.4%) saline solution at the rate of 4 drops per minute. Expectorants such as saturated solution of potassium or syrup of hydriodic acid are useful.

Pneumonia

Pneumonia, which frequently follows a tracheotomy, is avoided by using an uncontaminated suction catheter. If it does occur, appropriate antibiotics are administered.

Dysphagia

It has been reported that the laryngeal mucosa can become desensitized by the diversion of air currents from the larynx to the tracheotomy orifice, which can result in aspiration during deglutition. Difficulty with swallowing may also be caused by compression of the esophagus by either an ill-fitting tracheotomy tube or a tracheotomy tube with an inflated cuff.

Keloid Formation

Keloids are more likely to form when the tracheotomy wound has been infected than when it has remained free of infection. When present, keloids should be excised or injected with triamcinolone diacetate. When a keloid follows a vertical incision, a Z-plasty repair offers the best result.

Difficult Decannulation

Some infants and small children who seemingly have regained an adequate airway after a tracheotomy develop cyanosis when the tracheotomy tube is removed. The mothers of such patients should be trained in tracheotomy care, and the children should not be discharged. The size of the tracheotomy tube can be gradually decreased until finally a blank or plugged tube is used. The child should be observed carefully in the hospital for 24 to 48 hours after removal of the blank tube.

Nonclosure of Fistula After Decannulation

If the tracheal fistula will not close when the usual methods for closure have been used, adhesives, pressure dressings, and suturing may be necessary. A vertical incision heals much more rapidly than a horizontal one. A long-standing tracheotomy orifice often requires operative closure. The operation is performed several weeks after decannulation. After horizontal elliptical excision of the dermal orifice and resection of the dermal tracheotomy tract, the wound is closed in two or three layers.

Chapter 7
Tracheotomy and Tracheostomy Tubes

WILLIAM W. MONTGOMERY   STUART K. MONTGOMERY

The surgeon should be familiar with a variety of tracheostomy and tracheal tubes. Most surgeons use plastic tracheostomy and tracheal tubes today, mainly because they are less expensive than the sterling silver and stainless steel tubes. Acquiring a working knowledge of several types of plastic and metal tracheostomy tubes, whether they are cuffless, cuffed, or fenestrated, involves little effort and pays big dividends. In our practice, we have been successful with the following tracheostomy tubes.

METAL TRACHEOSTOMY TUBES

The main advantages of metal tubes are durability and a wide variety of lengths and curvatures. Figure 7–1 shows variations in curvature and length among the more commonly used metal trach tubes.

The Jackson tracheostomy tube (Pilling, Fort Washington, PA) (Fig. 7–2) is probably the most widely used metal tube. It is available in sizes ranging from No. 00 to No. 12, in short, regular, and long lengths. If surgeons are limited to one type of metal tracheostomy tube, the Jackson type is undoubtedly the best choice because it serves well in most cases. The Jackson tube is made with either a rotating or a swivel lock.

The Luer tracheostomy tube (Pilling) (see Fig. 7–1) is a short tube that is more acutely curved than the Jackson tube. It is supplied with a swivel lock and is especially useful in patients who cannot tolerate longer tracheostomy tubes. The Luer tube is available in sizes ranging from No. 00 to No. 10.

The Tucker tracheostomy tube (Pilling) (Fig. 7–3) has a contour similar to that of the Jackson tube, except that the curve is a full 90-degree arc. The Tucker tube is supplied with a swivel lock in sizes ranging from No. 00 to No. 10. A Tucker valved inner tube is available for regular length tubes in No. 4 through No. 10.

The Hollinger tracheostomy tube (Pilling) (see Fig. 7–1) is attached to the neckplate at an acute downward angle of 65 degrees rather than the usual 90 degrees. Sizes 0 and 1 are for use in infants weighing as little as 4 lb. The Hollinger tube is available in sizes up to No. 8 and is acceptable for use in adults, except those with very deep tracheas. The funnel-shaped opening allows easy insertion of aspirating catheters.

PLASTIC AND SILICONE TRACHEOSTOMY TUBES

Cuffless Tracheostomy Tubes

Cuffless, nonfenestrated tubes are used for routine tracheotomies. They are supplied with a variety of inner cannulas and an obturator. The Shiley cuffless tube (Mallinckrodt, Inc., St. Louis, MO) (Fig. 7–4) is available in sizes 4 through 10 in even sizes only. Disposable inner cannulas are available and feature snap-lock connectors. These disposable inner can-

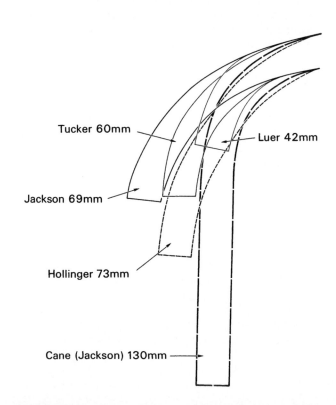

FIGURE 7–1. Lengths and curvatures of metal tracheostomy tubes, illustrating the variations in curvature and length of commonly used No. 6 metal tracheostomy tubes. With a knowledge of these variations, the surgeon can select an alternate tracheostomy tube when the one used is ill fitting.

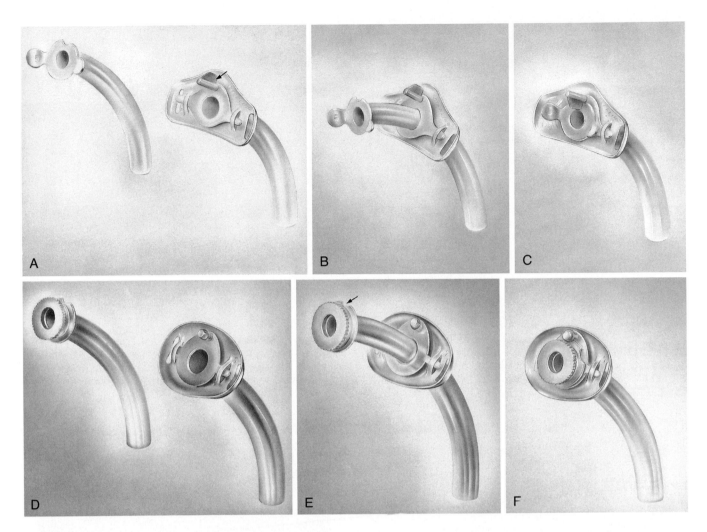

FIGURE 7–2. Jackson tracheostomy tube. *A,* A sterling-silver Jackson tracheostomy tube consists of an outer tube and an inner cannula. The outer tube is shown on the right. The slots on either side of the neckplate are situated so that the tracheostomy tape placed around the neck can secure the tracheostomy tube in place. The neckplate is loosely secured to the tracheostomy tube to minimize the movement of the tracheostomy tube within the trachea. A swivel lock (*arrow*), attached to the tracheostomy tube, serves to lock the inner cannula (shown on the left) in place after it has been inserted. *B,* The inner cannula is being inserted into the tracheostomy tube. *C,* The inner cannula is now in place. The swivel lock has been rotated either clockwise or counterclockwise 180 degrees to secure the inner cannula in place. *D,* A Jackson tracheostomy tube with a rotating lock device is shown with its inner cannula. The rotating lock provides quick and easy removal of the inner tube. There is less chance for snagging of gauze wipes and a lessened bulk with this type of lock than with a swivel lock. *E,* When the inner cannula is being inserted into the tracheostomy tube, the notch (*arrow*) in the rim of the plate on the inner tube should be rotated to the 12 o'clock position before the cannula is inserted. *F,* The inner cannula has been inserted and the notch rotated slightly in a clockwise direction.

nulas facilitate tracheotomy care but can be more expensive in the long run compared with the standard inner cannulas.

The TRACOE *twist* cuffless tracheostomy tube (TRACOE Medical GmbH, Frankfurt, Germany) (Fig. 7–5) is made from medical-grade plastic material, which is flexible at room temperature and becomes more pliable at body temperature. It has an anatomically shaped swivel neckplate, which moves around 2 axes, horizontal and vertical. It allows for a greater range of motion for the patient. TRACOE *twist* tubes are supplied with inner cannulas and are available in sizes 4 through 10.

Pediatric Tracheostomy Tubes

Pediatric tracheostomy tubes are generally more flexible. The Shiley pediatric tube (Mallinckrodt) (Fig. 7–6) is available in sizes 3.0 to 6.5. It is a single-lumen tube with no in-

ner cannula; thus, frequent changing and suctioning are necessary. It is supplied with an obturator.

The TRACOE *comfort* pediatric tracheostomy tube (see Fig. 7–5) is a flexible tube with a slightly tapered shaft, eliminating the need for an obturator. It is available with a variety of inner cannulas that can be removed for tube maintenance. Inner cannula styles include low-profile, 15-mm connectors and two types of speaking valves (Fig. 7–7). Extra-long lengths are also available. TRACOE *comfort* pediatric tubes start at size 3.

Cuffed Tracheostomy Tubes

Cuffed tracheostomy tubes, fenestrated and nonfenestrated, are indicated for patients who are aspirating or require positive pressure ventilation. Both Shiley (Fig. 7–8) and TRACOE *twist* (Fig 7–9) offer low-pressure cuffed tubes

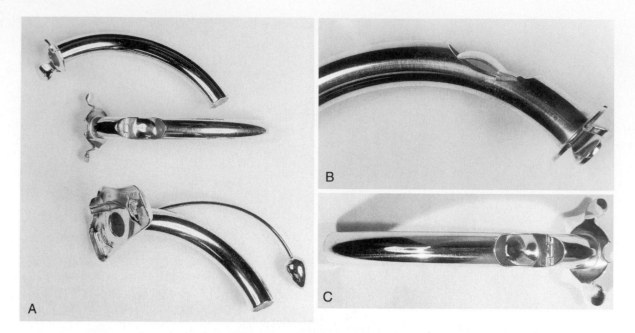

FIGURE 7-3. The Tucker valved tracheostomy tube. *A,* A No. 5 Tucker valved tracheostomy tube. There is an extra inner tube into which the Tucker valve has been constructed. The Tucker valve is worn during the daytime so that the patient may enjoy normal coughing and speech. The other inner tube is worn while the patient is sleeping. *B,* A close-up side view of the Tucker valve in the open position. *C,* The Tucker valve in the open position viewed from above.

with a variety of inner cannulas and obturators in either fenestrated or nonfenestrated models.

LARYNGECTOMY TUBES

Laryngectomy tubes are shorter in length than tracheostomy tubes. The Shiley laryngectomy tube (Fig. 7–10) is supplied with several inner cannulas and is available in sizes 6, 8, and 10. The TRACOE *twist* laryngectomy tube (Fig. 7–11) is available in sizes 5 through 10 and features a multi-directional swivel neckplate. The Singer laryngectomy tube (Boston Medical Products, Westborough, MA) (Fig. 7–12)

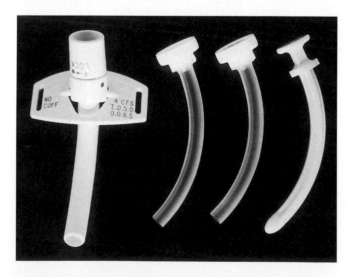

FIGURE 7-4. The Shiley cuffless tracheostomy tube. The set comes with three inner cannulas and an obturator. One inner cannula has an extension that can be attached to anesthesia or humidification tubing. The second inner cannula is flush against the neckplate, primarily for better cosmesis. The third has an obstructed lumen to be used as a plug, for example, during the process of decannulation. All three inner cannulas lock in place with a clockwise twist. The Shiley comes in sizes 4, 6, 8, and 10.

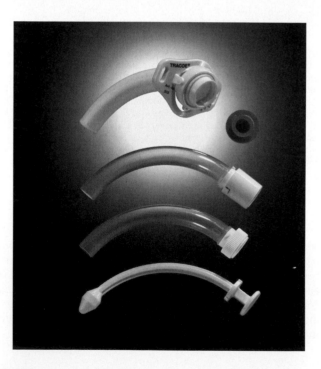

FIGURE 7-5. The TRACOE *twist* cuffless tracheostomy tube. The set comes with the outer tube, inner cannula with 15-mm connector (for attachment to anesthesia or humidification tubing), a low profile inner cannula with plug for decannulation, obturator, and neck strap. Inner cannulas lock in place with a clockwise twist. TRACOE twist tubes are available in sizes 4, 5, 6, 7, 8, 9, and 10.

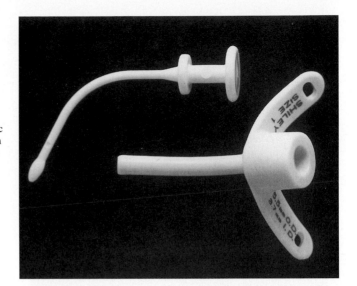

FIGURE 7–6. The Shiley pediatric tracheostomy tube. The Shiley pediatric tracheostomy tube comes in sizes 3.0 (4.5 mm o.d.; 3.0 i.d.) to 6.5 (9.0 mm o.d.; 6.5 mm i.d.). It does not have an inner cannula; thus, frequent changing and suctioning are necessary.

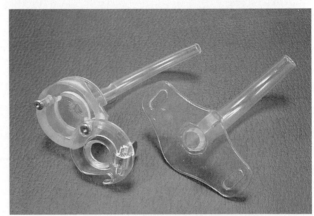

FIGURE 7-7. The TRACOE *comfort* pediatric tracheostomy tube. TRACOE *comfort* pediatric tubes are available in sizes 3 (6.4 mm o.d.; 2.5 mm i.d.) through 6 (10 mm o.d.; 8.5 mm i.d.). Inner cannulas and extra-long lengths are available.

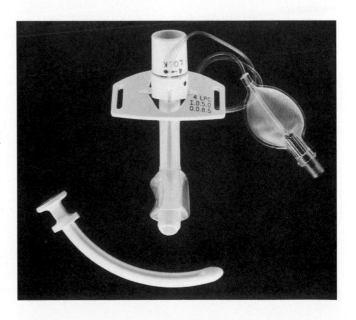

FIGURE 7-8. The Shiley low pressure cuffed tracheostomy tube. The Shiley low-pressure cuffed tube is recommended for aspiration, when assisted ventilation is required, or following laryngeal surgery to put the larynx at rest. It is available in sizes 4, 6, 8, and 10.

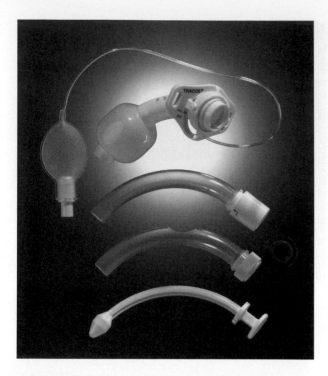

FIGURE 7-9. The TRACOE *twist* low pressure cuffed tracheostomy tube. The set comes with the outer tube, inner cannula with 15 mm connector (for attachment to anesthesia or humidification tubing), a low profile inner cannula with plug, obturator, and neck strap. Neckplate can swivel 360°. Inner cannulas lock in place with a clockwise twist. TRACOE *twist* cuffed tubes are available in sizes 4, 5, 6, 7, 8, 9 and 10.

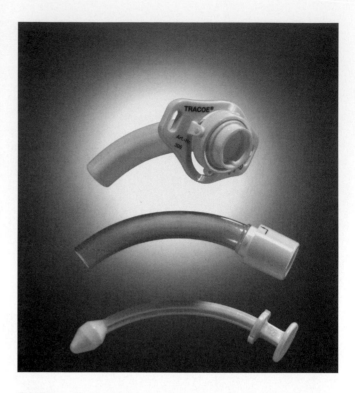

FIGURE 7-11. The TRACOE *twist* laryngectomy tube. The set comes with the outer tube, inner cannula with 15 mm connector (for attachment to anesthesia or humidification tubing), obturator, and neck strap. Inner cannulas lock in place with a clockwise twist. TRACOE twist laryngectomy tubes are available in sizes 5, 6, 7, 8, 9 and 10.

is a flexible silicone tube with no inner cannula and is available in 7 diameters and 4 lengths (28 different sizes).

SPECIAL PURPOSE TRACHEOSTOMY TUBES

Moore Tracheostomy Tube

When there is a narrowing or obstruction below the level of a regular tracheostomy tube, the Moore tracheostomy tube

(Fig. 7–13*A* and *B*) is quite useful. This tube is made from flexible silicone and is available in sizes 6 and 8. It has a standard long length of 115 mm and is nonfenestrated. The Moore tube, supplied with two different inner cannulas and an obturator, can often be a lifesaver.

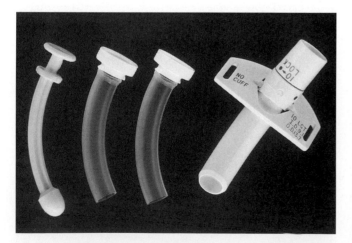

FIGURE 7-10. The Shiley laryngectomy tube. The Shiley tracheostomy (laryngectomy) tube (sizes 6, 8, and 10) is used when there is difficulty maintaining the patency of the tracheostoma.

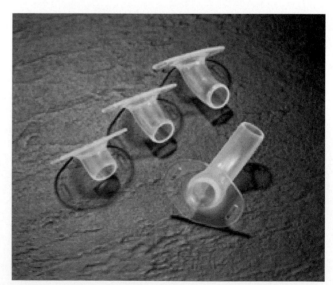

FIGURE 7-12. The Singer laryngectomy tube. The Singer laryngectomy tube is a flexible silicone tube with no inner cannula and is available in seven diameters and four lengths (28 different sizes).

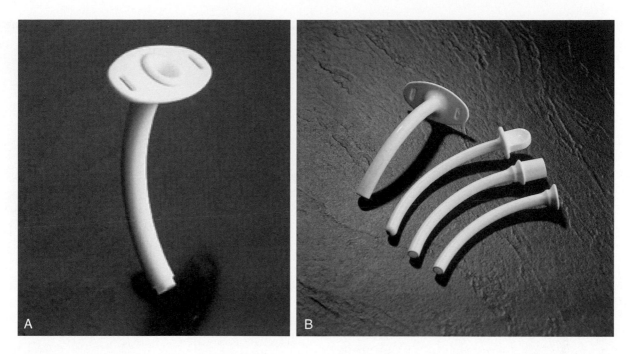

FIGURE 7-13. The Moore tracheostomy tube. *A,* The Moore tracheostomy tube is made from flexible silicone and is available in sizes 6 and 8. *B,* It has a standard long length of 115 mm, is nonfenestrated, and is supplied with two different inner cannulas and an obturator. It can be shortened if necessary.

TRACOE Comfort Tracheostomy Tubes

TRACOE *comfort* tracheostomy tubes are designed for long-term tracheostomy use and are constructed of a unique flexible transparent material. The tubes become pliable with body temperature, which aids in tube compliance with the tracheal anatomy. The tubes are available in a wide variety of sizes, lengths, and inner cannula styles. The standard length tubes (Fig. 7–14) are used for routine tracheostomy care, and the extra-long-length tubes (Fig. 7–15) provide an extended length to bypass tracheal stenosis.

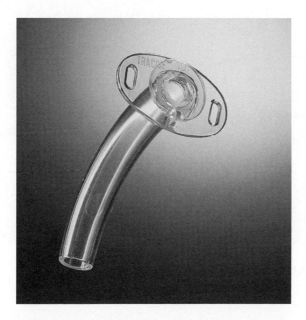

FIGURE 7-14. The TRACOE *comfort* standard length tracheostomy tube. The standard length tubes are used for routine tracheostomy care and are available in sizes 3 (6.4 mm o.d.; 2.5 mm i.d.) through 14 (18.2 mm o.d.; 12 mm i.d.). Available inner cannulas include low profile, 15 mm connector, and two types of speaking valves.

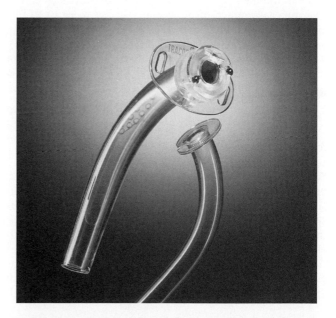

FIGURE 7-15. The TRACOE *comfort* extra-long-length tracheostomy tube. The extra-long-length tubes are used for bypassing tracheal stenosis and are available in sizes 5 (9.0 mm o.d.; 4.0 mm i.d.) through 14 (18.2 mm o.d.; 12 mm i.d.). Available inner cannulas include low profile, 15 mm connector, and two types of speaking valves.

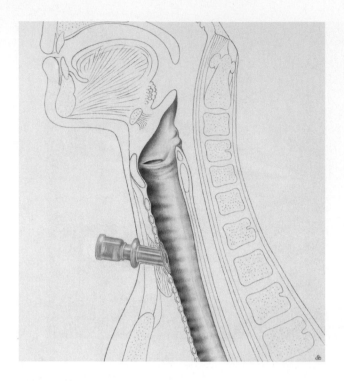

FIGURE 7-16. The Montgomery long-term cannula. The main advantage of the cannula is that there is no foreign body projecting into the trachea since the cannula flange extends only to the inner surface of the anterior tracheal wall. The Montgomery long-term cannula is shown with speaking valve.

Montgomery Tracheal Cannula

The Montgomery Long-Term Cannula (Boston Medical Products, Inc, Westborough, MA) is designed to be used in place of the tracheostomy tube in patients with sleep apnea. The main advantage of the cannula is that there is no foreign body projecting into the trachea because it extends only to the inner surface of the anterior tracheal wall (Fig. 7–16). The cannula can be used with all tracheostomies except those requiring assisted respiration and when aspiration is present. A complete description of the system can be found in Chapter 8.

Speaking Valves

Speaking valves have been designed to allow tracheostomy tube patients to vocalize without the need for finger occlusion. The valves provide one-way airflow, opening on inspiration and closing on expiration to redirect the airflow through the larynx for speech. The Montgomery Tracheostomy Speaking Valve (Boston Medical Products, Inc) (Fig. 7–17) fits the standard 15-mm connector end of tracheostomy tubes and inner cannulas. The valve uses a thin silicone diaphragm for low resistance and features a cough

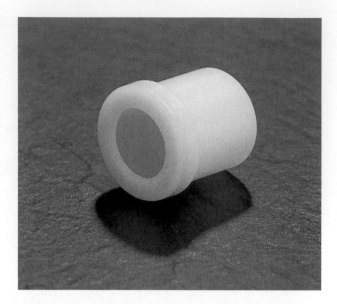

FIGURE 7-17. The Montgomery tracheostomy speaking valve. The tracheostomy speaking valve features a low-resistance diaphragm and cough release mechanism.

release mechanism, which is easily reset by the patient. There is also a valve available for ventilator-dependent patients, the VENTRACH Speaking Valve (Boston Medical Products, Inc) (Fig. 7–18). It connects to the 15-mm connector end and has a 22-mm body to accommodate standard ventilation equipment.

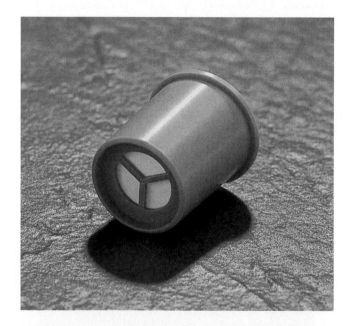

FIGURE 7-18. The Montgomery VENTRACH speaking valve. The VENTRACH speaking valve is designed to reside "inline" between the tracheostomy tube and ventilation equipment for ventilator-dependent patients.

Chapter 8
Montgomery Tracheal Cannula System

WILLIAM W. MONTGOMERY   STUART K. MONTGOMERY

The Montgomery Tracheal Cannula System (Boston Medical Products, Inc., Westborough, MA) (Fig. 8–1) provides long-term access to the tracheal airway in situations that require an artificial airway or when access is needed for pulmonary hygiene. The system can be used to create a new tracheotomy or to replace a long-term tracheostomy tube. The components of the system used to create a tracheostomy are a surgical instrument to incise a circular opening in the tracheal wall and a "short-term" tracheal cannula (surgical procedure described later). For long-term or permanent tracheostomies, there is a "long-term" tracheal cannula and an instrument (STOMEASURE, Boston Medical Products) (Fig. 8–2) to measure an existing tracheostomy for size selection.

The Montgomery Tracheal Fenestrator (Boston Medical Products, Inc.) (Fig. 8–3) is a two-piece surgical stainless steel instrument consisting of a trephine knife that fits over an inner sleeve. The cutting edge of the trephine knife is designed to both cut and saw. The cutting effect is for the soft tissue of the anterior tracheal wall, and the teeth are used to cut through ossified cartilage. The suction holds the inner sleeve against the tracheal wall while the cutting end of the fenestrator is slowly rotated. The core of removed trachea either adheres to the inner sleeve or passes up the suction tubing. The fenestrator cuts a circular opening slightly smaller than that of the cannula to ensure a snug fit. The tracheal fenestrator is supplied in sizes 4, 6, 8, and 10.

The Montgomery Short-Term Tracheal Cannula (Boston Medical Products, Inc.) (Fig. 8–4) was originally designed to be used in place of a tracheostomy tube in patients with sleep apnea. The cannula is constructed of medical grade silicone. It is now more widely used in all incidents in which a tracheotomy is indicated, with the exception of when aspiration is present or positive-pressure breathing is indicated. The uniquely designed thin inner flange of the cannula is shaped to fit snugly against the contour of the inner anterior tracheal wall. No tube projects into the tracheal lumen. The flange, the only portion of the cannula to remain intraluminal, is placed at a 27-degree angle to the long axis of the cannula. The vertical dimension of this flange is much longer than its width. This shape permits it to fit snugly against the concave contour of the anterior intraluminal tracheal wall and helps prevent rotation once it is in place.

The short-term cannula is supplied in an extra-long length designed to be trimmed once in place, depending on the patient's neck thickness. There are circumferential rings on the shaft of the short-term tracheal cannula that create a series of ridges and grooves. The three ridges adjacent to the flange are in the shape of circumferential barbs. These inner ridges allow the tracheal cannula to be inserted easily but prevent it from being displaced anteriorly once it is fixed in place. The grooves between the ridges serve to secure a faceplate or ring

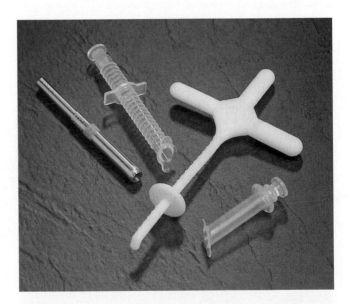

FIGURE 8-1. The Montgomery tracheal cannula system. The tracheal fenestrator (*left*) is a surgical steel instrument that incises a precise circular opening for proper placement of the tracheal cannula. The fenestrator has a serrated blade to penetrate both tissue and cartilage. The inner sleeve of the fenestrator attaches to standard suction tubing and removes the incised core of the trachea. The short-term cannula (to the right of the fenestrator) is placed in the new tracheotomy and left in place for several weeks. It is then replaced by the long-term cannula. The tracheostomy measuring device (STOMEASURE) (cross-shaped device) measures both the length and diameter of an existing tracheostomy. These dimensions are then used to select the corresponding long-term cannula. The long-term cannula (*lower right*) has a highly polished surface to permit and encourage growth of epithelium both from the trachea and the skin of the tracheotomy tract.

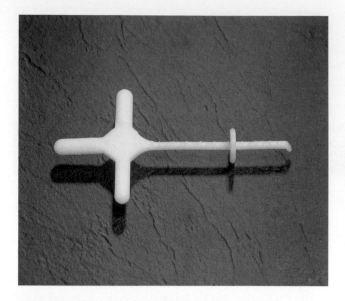

FIGURE 8-2. The Montgomery STOMEASURE. A stoma measuring device, the STOMEASURE has been developed to accurately measure the tracheal stoma diameter and length for fitting of a long-term cannula.

washer in the desired position according to the thickness of the wall between the trachea and the anterior cervical skin.

The cannula has a longitudinal groove along its shaft to allow drainage of serum and the products of inflammation that may occur during the immediate postoperative period. The groove also serves to identify the inferior aspect of the tube, thus being a reference point to indicate whether the cannula has been accidentally rotated out of its proper position. The longitudinal groove should always be at the 6 o'clock position. The wing-shaped faceplate secures the cannula in place at the time of surgery. It is sutured to the skin on each side with one 3-0 silk suture. The plug is used to obstruct the cannula once the cannula airway is not needed. It is fixed in place simply by twisting the plug in a

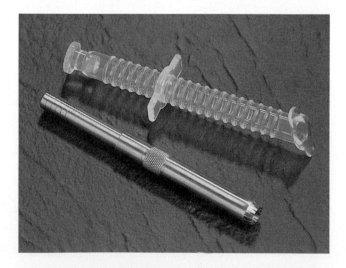

FIGURE 8-3. The Montgomery tracheal fenestrator is shown with the corresponding short-term cannula.

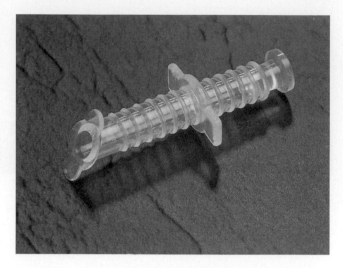

FIGURE 8-4. The Montgomery short-term cannula is shown with the wing-shaped faceplate and plug attached. The inner flange of the cannula is designed so that the vertical dimension is greater than the horizontal dimension. This design allows for ease of insertion into the opening of the anterior tracheal wall and also helps prevent rotation of the cannula once it is in place. The flange is fashioned at a 27-degree angle to the long axis of the cannula so that the cannula will project straight forward or in a slightly superior direction when inserted.

clockwise direction after insertion. The plug has a head so that it cannot be introduced too far into the tracheal cannula.

After the Montgomery short-term cannula has been in place for 1 week to 10 days, the faceplate can be replaced by the ring washer. The washer is less bulky and prevents

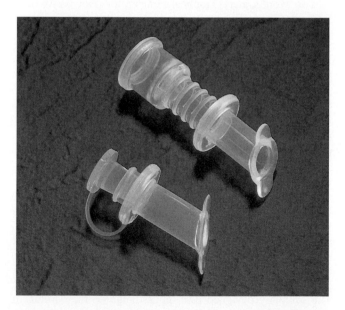

FIGURE 8-5. The Montgomery long-term cannula is shown with two configurations: *top* with speaking valve attached for hand-free speech; and *bottom* trimmed with the plug inserted for a low profile suitable for a sleep apnea patient. The long-term cannula differs from the short-term cannula in that the three circumferential barbed ridges adjacent to the inner flange are omitted. The smooth portion between the angled flange and the ring washer varies in length and resides in the tracheostoma. It helps establish a smooth epithelialized stoma and permits ease of insertion and removal by the patient. There are 24 sizes.

irritation of the skin surrounding the Montgomery tracheal cannula. The ring washer is supplied attached to the plug with a silicone lanyard, which can be easily removed using scissors if so desired. After 4 to 6 weeks, the short-term cannula should be removed and replaced with the appropriate-sized long-term cannula.

The Montgomery long-term cannula (Fig. 8–5) differs from the short-term cannula in that the circumferential barbs are omitted and replaced by a smooth shaft. This smooth portion resides in the tracheostoma and serves to encourage the growth of epithelium to create a smooth stoma.

The long-term cannula can be used after initial insertion of the short-term cannula or as a replacement for an exist-

ing tracheostomy tube. The long-term cannula is supplied in sizes 4, 6, 8, and 10, with six lengths for each diameter (a total of 24 sizes).

PLACEMENT OF THE SHORT-TERM CANNULA

A vertical tracheotomy incision (Fig. 8–6A) is used to insert the Montgomery tracheal cannula. This incision is essential for proper vertical alignment of the cannula when applying the skin sutures. The median raphe between the sternohyoid and sternothyroid muscles is identified and in-

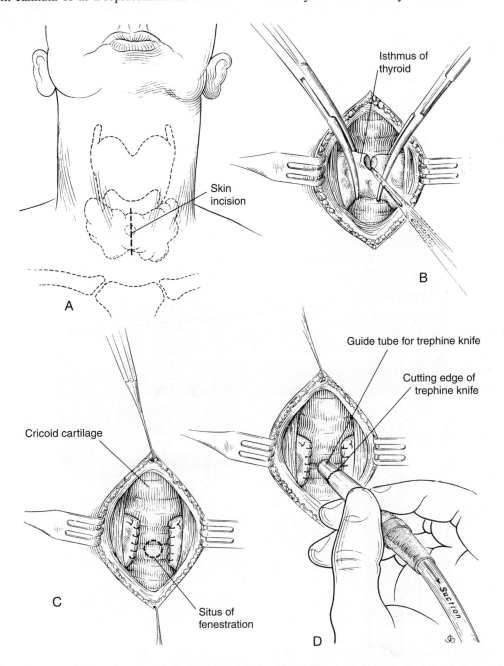

FIGURE 8–6. *A,* A vertical skin incision is made to expose the thyroid isthmus. *B,* It is divided and suture-ligated. *C,* The divided segments have been dissected away from the anterior tracheal wall. The site for the fenestration is indicated. *D,* The tracheal fenestrator has been placed over its inner sleeve, which is in turn connected to suction tubing and placed against the anterior tracheal wall.

cised. The thyroid isthmus is divided and ligated with sutures (Fig. 8–6B). The anterior wall of the trachea is exposed so that the fenestration can be made at the proper level (Fig. 8–6C). The fenestration of the anterior tracheal wall is made with the tracheal trephine fenestrator (Figs. 8–6D and 8–7).

To use the tracheal fenestrator, the inner sleeve is first attached to suction tubing. The fenestrator is placed over the inner sleeve so that the inner sleeve projects beyond the cutting edge of the fenestrator (Fig. 8–7D). The projecting edge of the inner sleeve is then placed against the anterior tracheal wall, to which it immediately adheres because of the negative pressure. The outer sleeve with cutting edge is advanced and rotated to incise the anterior tracheal wall (Fig. 8–8A). The core of trachea removed either adheres to the end of the inner sleeve or is aspirated into the suction tubing.

The advantages of this instrument over the previous methods for making a tracheotomy fenestration are that it is simpler, it is less traumatic to the trachea, and a perfectly round fenestration can be made in the anterior tracheal wall (Fig. 8–8B).

To insert the end of the Montgomery tracheal cannula into the trachea, its end is compressed with a curved hemostat. In so doing, the end forms a point (Fig. 8–8C) that can easily be inserted into the lumen of the trachea (Fig. 8–8D). The tracheal cannula is then pulled anteriorly until the inner flange fits snugly against the intraluminal anterior tracheal wall (Figs. 8–9, 8–10A and B).

The wound is closed in layers above and below the Montgomery short-term cannula (Fig. 8–10C). The faceplate is applied over the tracheal cannula and is advanced until it fits fairly closely, but not too tightly, against the skin (Fig. 8–10D). The faceplate is secured in place with one 3-0 silk suture on each side. Anesthesia or oxygen can be administered by the tracheal cannula as the patient recovers from general anesthesia. If there is a significant loss of air superiorly into the upper respiratory system or if anesthesia is to be continued, a Fogarty catheter is inserted and inflated superior to the level of the Montgomery tracheal cannula.

POSTOPERATIVE CARE OF THE SHORT-TERM CANNULA

The faceplate is left in place for 7 to 10 days or until the tracheotomy incision has healed. It is advisable to clean under the faceplate twice a day using cotton-tipped applicators saturated with 1:1 hydrogen peroxide/normal saline

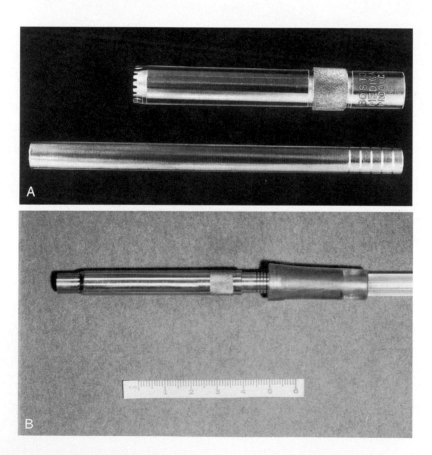

FIGURE 8–7. *A*, The tracheal fenestrator consists of an outer trephine knife that fits over an inner sleeve. The tracheal fenestrator incises a circular opening 2 mm less than the outside diameter of the corresponding Montgomery tracheal cannula; the trachea stretches so that it will easily allow the tracheal cannula. The cutting edge of the trephine knife is designed so that it can both cut and saw. The cutting effect is for the soft tissues of the anterior tracheal wall, and the teeth are used to saw through ossified cartilage. The fenestrator is available in sizes 4, 6, 8, and 10. *B*, The inner sleeve fits snugly inside the trephine fenestrator. The serrated end of the inner sleeve fits into standard suction tubing.

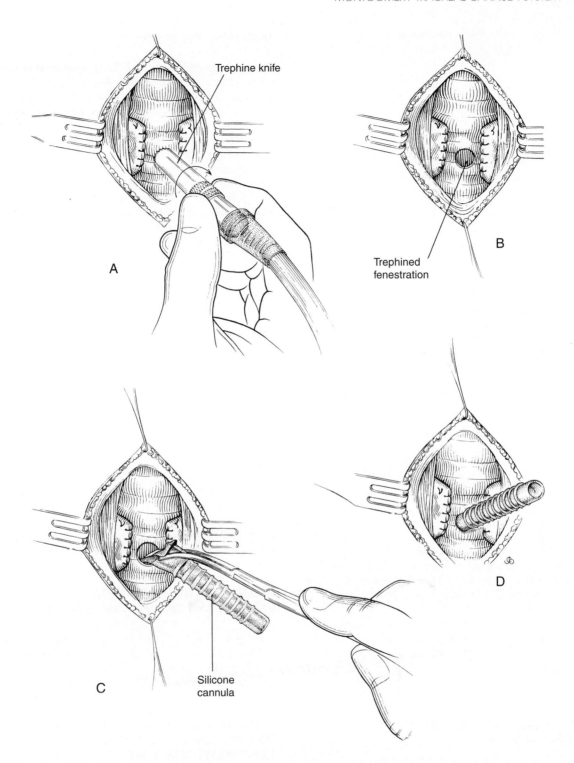

FIGURE 8–8. *A,* Once the inner sleeve has become adherent to the anterior tracheal wall by suction, the outer, or trephine, portion of the tracheal fenestrator is advanced to the tracheal wall. A core of tracheal wall is cut by rotating the fenestrator in a clockwise direction. The suction will prevent the core from falling into the tracheal lumen. *B,* The anterior tracheal wall has been fenestrated. *C,* The flanged end of the tracheal cannula is grasped with a curved hemostat and inserted through the fenestrated tracheal wall. *D,* The flange is now intraluminal.

solution. Pat dry the area and apply Betadine or an equivalent ointment. The faceplate is removed, and a ring washer is applied to the same groove (Fig. 8–10*E*). The cannula can be shortened to a convenient length at this time simply by cutting it with straight scissors or by using a No. 10 surgical blade. The ring washer prevents medial displacement of the tube and is less irritating to the skin around the tracheotomy than the faceplate. Again, note the position of the longitudinal groove, which should be at the 6 o'clock position.

Postoperatively, a lateral soft tissue radiograph or xeroradiograph of the larynx and trachea is obtained to make

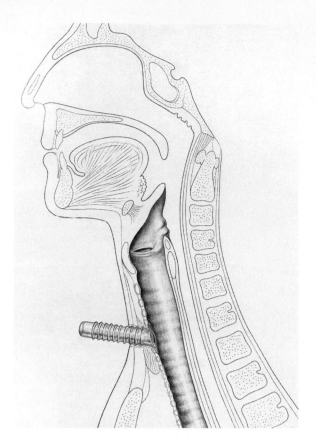

FIGURE 8–9. The main advantage of the silicone tracheal cannula is that there is no foreign body projecting into the trachea because the cannula flange extends only to the inner surface of the anterior tracheal wall.

certain that the inner flange is in position and firmly against the inner aspect of the anterior tracheal wall (Fig. 8–11).

It is important to inspect the cannula periodically to ensure that the longitudinal groove is in its proper inferior location (6 o'clock).

The inside of the cannula can be cleaned with a cotton-tipped applicator or suctioned if necessary. The cannula should be plugged when it is not needed to assist or replace the upper airway. The plug is inserted with a slight twist.

THE MONTGOMERY LONG-TERM TRACHEAL CANNULA

After 4 to 6 weeks, the short-term cannula should be removed and replaced with the appropriate-sized long-term cannula. The shaft of the long-term cannula between the inner flange and the first outer ring varies in length and has a highly polished surface (Fig. 8–12A). This surface permits and encourages growth of epithelium from both the trachea and the skin to line the tissue of the stoma and allows for ease of removal and insertion of the cannula by the patient or physician. The ring and groove system allows the placement of one or more ring washers to adjust the length (Fig. 8–12B).

Measuring the Stoma

To ensure proper fitting of the long-term cannula, the tracheal stoma should be measured. The STOMEASURE (Boston Medical Products, Inc.) (Fig. 8–13), a stoma-measuring device, has been developed to accurately measure the tracheal stoma diameter and length for fitting of a long-term cannula. The three short-tapered stems are used to determine the diameter of sizes 6, 8, or 10. The long graduated stem has an angled end, which simulates the 27-degree angle flange of the cannula. Once the stem is inserted into the stoma and slightly withdrawn to seat the angled end against the anterior tracheal wall, the ring washer is slid up against the skin. The STOMEASURE is removed, and the measurement under the ring washer is noted. These measurements can be obtained as an office procedure.

To measure stoma diameter, each short-tapered stem is gently inserted into the stoma until the correct diameter is determined (Fig. 8–14). Lubrication can be used if necessary. The stems correspond to sizes 6, 8, and 10. If the size 6 stem is too large, a size 4 long-term cannula series is now available.

To measure stoma length, the washer is installed and slid to the number "8" on the scale. The flanged end is inserted into the trachea, with care taken not to advance too far to the posterior wall of the trachea. Once the flanged end is inside the trachea, the STOMEASURE is gently retracted until the flange has engaged the anterior tracheal wall. While maintaining this position, the washer is advanced until it reaches the skin (Fig. 8–15). The STOMEASURE is removed, and the number on the shaft directly under the washer is noted and recorded on the patient's record for future reference. This length measurement is compared on the long-term cannula selection chart, and the corresponding long-term cannula is selected (Table 8–1).

INSERTING THE LONG-TERM CANNULA TO REPLACE THE SHORT-TERM CANNULA

After 4 to 6 weeks, the short-term cannula should be removed and replaced with the appropriate long-term cannula. The long-term cannula is inserted in the same manner as the short-term cannula.

INSERTING THE LONG-TERM CANNULA TO REPLACE AN EXISTING TRACHEOSTOMY TUBE

This procedure can be performed in the physician's office if the tracheal stoma is well established and the patient can tolerate the changing procedure. Otherwise, it is best performed with the patient under general anesthesia. The existing tracheostomy tube is first removed. The stoma is then measured as described earlier. Usually the existing tracheotomy tract is directed posteroinferiorly. If general anesthesia is used, this tract can be straightened by a single vertical midline incision in the skin inferiorly and in the trachea superiorly. The flange end of the cannula is compressed with

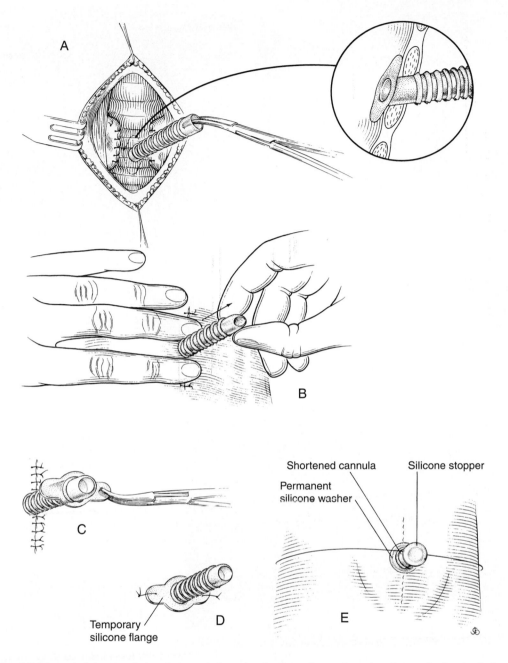

FIGURE 8–10. *A* and *B*, The end of the cannula is pulled anteriorly so that the flange fits snugly against the anterior intraluminal tracheal wall. *C*, Following repair of the incision, the faceplate is advanced to the groove adjacent to the skin surface. *D*, The faceplate is secured to the skin with one No. 3-0 silk suture through each wing. An endotracheal tube can be inserted into the Montgomery tracheal cannula as the patient recovers from anesthesia. *E*, The faceplate has been removed and replaced by the ring washer. The cannula can be shortened by cutting it in a groove with straight scissors.

a curved hemostat to form a point that can be easily inserted into the lumen of the trachea. The cannula is then inserted into the tracheal lumen. Once inserted, the cannula is pulled anteriorly until the inner flange fits snugly against the intraluminal anterior tracheal wall. The tube is rotated so that the longitudinal groove is at the 6 o'clock position. The plug/ring set is installed on the cannula and advanced until it rests against the skin. One or two ring washers may be used to "fine tune" the length (see Fig. 8–12B). The external portion of the cannula can be shortened by cutting it with straight scissors or a scalpel blade. It is best to leave a length

of at least two rings anterior to the ring washer. This will enable the tube to be grasped when the ring washer, plug, or speaking valve is applied.

PATIENT MAINTENANCE OF THE LONG-TERM CANNULA

Many patients are able to remove, clean, and reinsert their cannulas with ease, which greatly simplifies cannula care (Figs. 8–16 through 8–21).

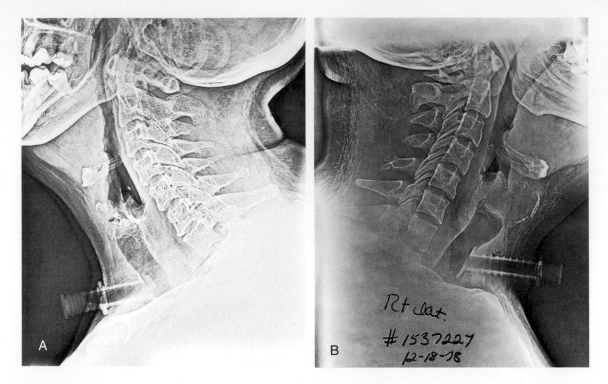

A

B

FIGURE 8-11. If there is uncertainty as to the position of the inner flange, a lateral neck x-ray or xeroradiograph is taken. Xeroradiographs showing inner flange of the Montgomery long-term cannula (*A*), and the Montgomery short-term cannula fitting snugly against the anterior intraluminal trachea (*B*).

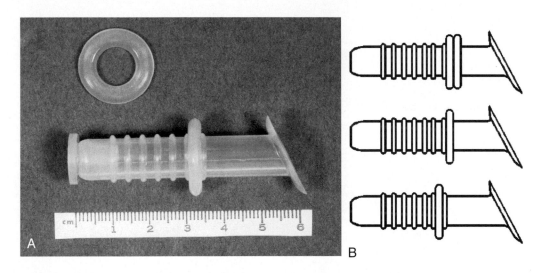

A

B

FIGURE 8-12. *A*, The Montgomery tracheal cannula for long-term use is shown. It differs from the short-term cannula in that the shaft of the long-term cannula between the inner flange and the first outer ring varies in length and has a highly polished surface. *B*, The stoma length of the long-term cannula can be fine-tuned by ring washer placement. The ring washer is shown in various positions depending on the distance between the anterior tracheal wall and the skin.

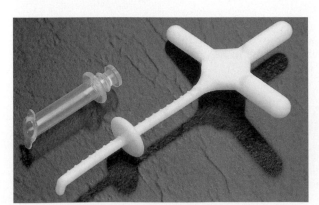

FIGURE 8-13. The Montgomery STOMEASURE. The STOMEASURE is shown with the corresponding long-term cannula. The three short tapered stems are used to determine the diameter of the stoma. The long graduated stem has an angled end, which simulates the 27-degree angle flange of the cannula and is used to determine the stoma length.

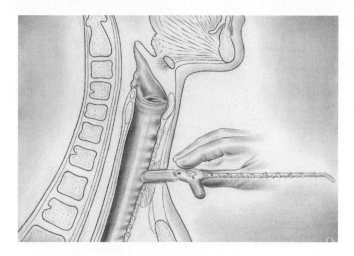

FIGURE 8-14. Measuring stoma diameter using the Montgomery STOMEASURE.

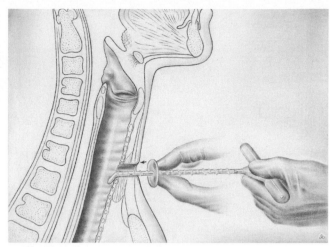

FIGURE 8-15. Measuring stoma length using the Montgomery STOMEASURE.

TABLE 8-1
Long-Term Cannula Selection Chart

STOMEASURE (Scale No.)	Stoma (Length, mm)	Size 4 (9 mm od)	Size 6 (11 mm od)	Size 8 (12 mm od)	Size 10 (13 mm od)
2.0	17–25	330425	330625	330825	331025
2.5	17–25	330425	330625	330825	331025
3.0	25–33	330433	330633	330833	331033
3.5	33–41	330441	330641	440841	331041
4.0	33–41	330441	330641	440841	331041
4.5	41–49	330449	330649	330849	331049
5.0	49–57	330457	330657	330857	331057
5.5	49–57	330457	330657	330857	331057
6.0	57–65	330465	330665	330865	331065
6.5	57–65	330465	330665	330865	331065

od—outside diameter.

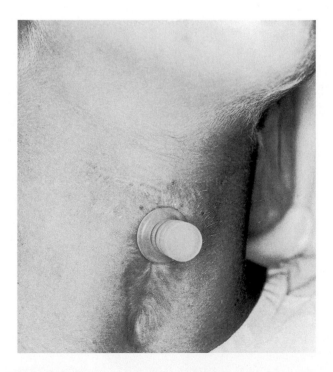

FIGURE 8-16. This patient is using a plugged Montgomery long-term cannula after repair of glottic and subglottic stenosis and removal of the Safe-T-Tube. During this period of cannula use (two weeks), she learned to remove, clean, and reinsert it.

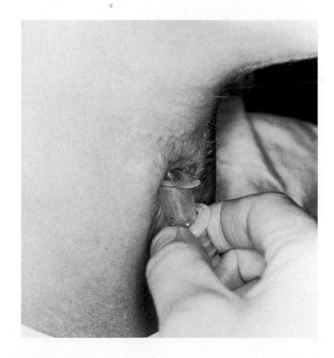

FIGURE 8-17. The cannula is removed by simply pulling it forward.

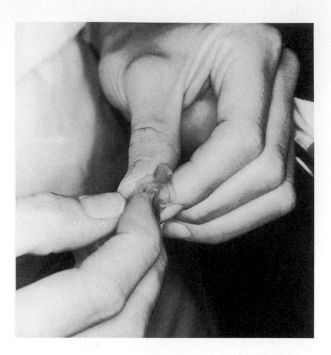

FIGURE 8–18. The lower, or inferior, inner flange is pressed into the lumen with the index finger.

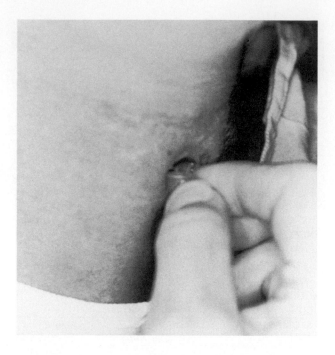

FIGURE 8–20. The end of the cannula has been pushed into the lumen and pulled gently forward, engaging it into proper position. It awaits application of the ring and insertion of the plug.

SPEAKING VALVES FOR THE MONTGOMERY TRACHEAL CANNULA

Speaking valves (Fig. 8–22) are available that can be attached to the Montgomery tracheal cannula in patients with insufficient inspiratory airways and adequate expiratory airways. An example of this is a patient with bilat-

eral vocal cord paralysis in the position of the adduction. The housing of the valve mechanism is constructed from silicone or plastic that is denser than that used in the Montgomery tracheal cannula. The valves are designed to allow cannula patients to vocalize without the need for finger occlusion. The valves provide one-way airflow using a thin silicone hinged diaphragm that opens on inspiration

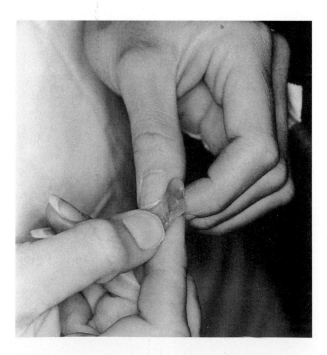

FIGURE 8–19. The inner end of the cannula is squeezed together, greatly reducing its size. This narrow pointed end of the cannula is easily slipped into the tracheotomy tract.

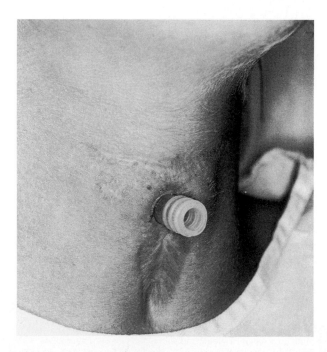

FIGURE 8–21. The cannula in place.

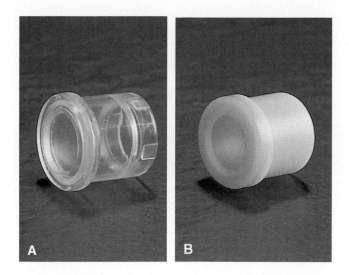

FIGURE 8–22. The Montgomery cannula speaking valves. *A*, Silicone. *B*, Medical grade plastic.

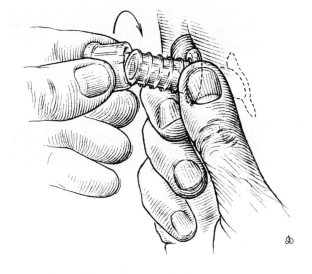

FIGURE 8–23. Attaching the speaking valve to the cannula.

and closes on expiration. A unique cough release feature allows excessive air pressure to escape through the valve by displacing the diaphragm anteriorly. The displaced diaphragm is then easily reset by the patient's fingertip. The valves are available in two models: silicone and medical grade plastic. The valve is applied to the Montgomery tracheal cannula by inserting it over the cannula, which has been shortened to the desired length (Fig. 8–23). It is held in place by four prongs that fit into the groove of the cannula.

Chapter 9
Tracheal Stenosis

WILLIAM W. MONTGOMERY

The incidence of segmental loss of cervical trachea has increased markedly in recent years. This is partly the result of both an increased incidence of treatment, by tracheal intubation and tracheotomy, of patients with severe injuries who require assisted ventilation and an increase in the number of patients undergoing complex cardiovascular and pulmonary operations. The incidence and recognition of acute and chronic cervical tracheal stenosis resulting from external trauma, as well as improved methods for resuscitation immediately after injury, has also added to the number of patients requiring surgical repair of tracheal stenosis.

ETIOLOGY OF CERVICAL TRACHEAL STENOSIS

Figure 9–1A and Table 9–1 describe the etiology and classification of tracheal stenosis.

Stenosis Above the Tracheotomy Orifice

Intubation
A hurried and misdirected intubation can result in severe injury to either the larynx or cervical trachea. Most often this injury occurs laterally in the subglottis or the cervical trachea. The site of trauma is denuded epithelium and is subsequently secondarily infected, which leads to loss of cartilaginous support in this area. Occasionally, the tracheal wall may be perforated during intubation. Stenosis usually results from a granuloma formed at the site of the injury (see Fig. 9–1B).

The specimen shows loss of tracheal mucosa and exposed tracheal cartilage at the level of the inflated tracheotomy cuff (*lower arrow*). This would have resulted in tracheal stenosis if the patient had survived.

Incorrect Placement of Tracheotomy Site
A superiorly placed tracheotomy, one just under, through, or above the cricoid cartilage often results in stenosis caused by subglottic edema, granulation tissue formation, or loss of anterior tracheal support.

Trauma During the Operation
The anterior wall of the trachea above the tracheotomy site may be injured during emergency tracheotomy. The result is a buckling-in of the anterior tracheal wall and an anteroposterior narrowing of the trachea, or a loss of support of the anterior cartilaginous wall, medial displacement of the lateral tracheal walls, and, finally, anteroposterior slitlike stenosis.

External Trauma of the Cervical Trachea
Stenoses of varying widths, configurations, and lengths can result from external trauma. These differ according to the size, shape, site of impact, and weight of the instrument producing the trauma. A slight blow to the anterior wall of the trachea inflicted with a blunt object might result in a minimal buckling-in of the anterior wall or bowing of the lateral walls. Such defects produce insignificant airway impairment. In contrast is the unique injury caused by the trachea striking a linear object, such as a rope, while the subject is traveling at high speed. This type of injury can result in complete transection of the trachea and separation of the superior and inferior segments, with or without an external wound. These stenoses are classified as being above the tracheotomy site because an emergency tracheotomy is invariably performed below the level of stenosis.

Stenosis at the Tracheotomy Site

Excessive trauma to the anterior cartilaginous support of the trachea inflicted during a hurried tracheotomy can result in stenosis of this area. Many surgeons believe that placing an H incision in the anterior tracheal wall during tracheotomy is inadvisable because this can result in buckling-in of superior and inferior tracheal wall flaps and stenosis at the tracheotomy site. It is best to make a carefully placed circular incision, slightly larger than the tracheotomy opening.

For the most part, stenosis at the tracheotomy site results from local chondritis and loss of cartilaginous support, along with the formation of polyps and granulation tissue. Stenosis at the site of the tracheotomy is most often not recognized until an attempt is made to perform decannulation. The compromised airway may become apparent immedi-

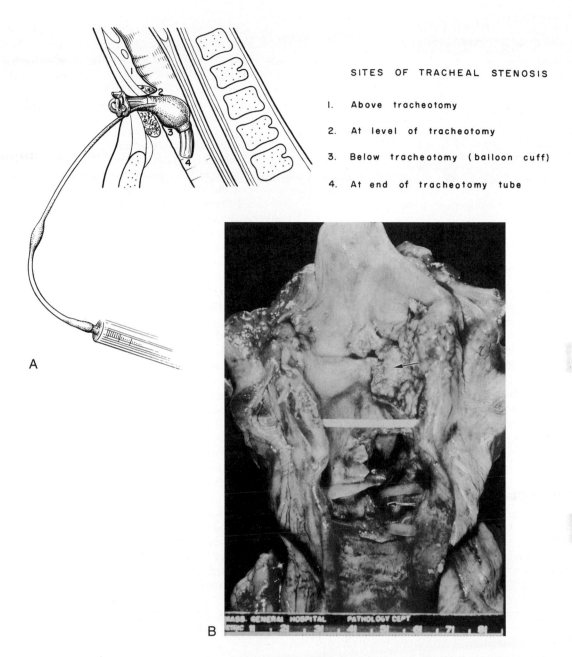

SITES OF TRACHEAL STENOSIS

1. Above tracheotomy

2. At level of tracheotomy

3. Below tracheotomy (balloon cuff)

4. At end of tracheotomy tube

A

B

FIGURE 9-1. *A,* Classification of cervical tracheal stenoses. *1.* Above the tracheotomy orifice. This type of stenosis results from buckling-in of the anterior tracheal wall, loss of anterior tracheal support, or a granuloma. *2.* At the level of the tracheotomy orifice. This occurs as a result of polyp and granulation formation at the tracheotomy site. A loss of cartilaginous support may also occur at this level. *3.* Below the tracheotomy orifice. This almost invariably is caused by incorrect use of a cuffed tracheotomy tube. *4.* At the end of tracheotomy tube. This usually occurs in the anterior tracheal wall and is caused by pressure from the end of the tracheotomy tube. Ulceration is followed by secondary infection and formation of a granuloma or chondritis, with resulting loss of cartilaginous support. *B,* A 61-year-old man was admitted to the medical service of a hospital with airway obstruction due to an undiagnosed carcinoma of the larynx (*upper arrow*). The laryngeal carcinoma was detected when a life-saving emergency tracheotomy was performed. However, central hypoxia had produced sufficient damage to require assisted respiration. The patient died 6 days after hospital admission.

ately after removal of the tracheotomy tube or may not be evident until days or weeks after decannulation.

Stenosis Below the Tracheotomy Site

Prolonged use and improper management of the cuffed endotracheal tube or cuffed tracheotomy tube accounts for stenosis that usually occurs just below the tracheotomy site. Initially there is damage to the tracheal mucous membrane by exces-

sive and prolonged pressure exerted from the inflated cuff and the superior and inferior motion of the inflated cuff against the tracheal wall during assisted ventilation (see Fig. 9–1B). The degree of underlying damage is proportional to the type and amount of secondary infection. Ultimately, exposure of the cartilaginous tracheal rings and loss of support at this level occurs. In such cases, the impaired airway will become apparent soon after decannulation. Usually gradual fibrosis occurs, with symptoms beginning 2 to 3 weeks after decannulation. Stenosis may also result in this area from development of a granu-

TABLE 9–1
Etiology of Cervical Tracheal Stenosis

Above the tracheotomy orifice:
  Trauma during intubation
  Incorrect placement of the tracheotomy site
  Traumatic tracheotomy above the tracheotomy orifice
  External trauma to the cervical trachea
At the level of the tracheotomy orifice:
  Trauma during the operation
  Infection, with formation of polyps and granulation tissue
  Loss of cartilaginous support anteriorly or laterally
Just below the tracheotomy orifice:
  Ulceration due to pressure at the site of the inflated tracheotomy cuff
  Formation of a granuloma
  Loss of cartilaginous support with resultant tracheal malacia or fibrous
    stenosis
At the end of the tracheotomy tube (usually anteriorly):
  Formation of a granuloma
  Loss of cartilaginous support

loma, loss of anterior tracheal support, and collapse of the lateral walls, which produces an anteroposterior slitlike stenosis.

Stenosis at End of Tracheotomy Tube

Injury to the trachea may occur from pressure exerted by the end of a tracheotomy tube. The ulceration of the mucosa becomes secondarily infected. A granuloma may develop that narrows the airway. Chondritis is followed by loss of support and a more serious type of tracheal stenosis.

PREVENTION OF TRACHEAL STENOSIS

Prolonged intubation, especially in patients with injury to the larynx or trachea, can be a significant causative factor in stenosis of the larynx or trachea. Patients who are receiving intermittent mandatory ventilation and continuous positive airway ventilation should undergo extubation as soon as possible. Unless patients are unable to protect their airways from aspiration or have an airway obstruction, they can undergo extubation at an earlier date, based on their gas exchange values. Consideration of extubation based on conventional respiratory-mechanics criteria for extubation can result in unnecessarily prolonged intubation.

A high tracheotomy should be avoided. A tracheotomy tube placed immediately below the cricoid cartilage can result in airway obstruction due to subglottic and upper tracheal edema. If a high tracheotomy has been performed, the fenestration should be lowered and the patient should be given prednisone and antibiotics systematically (Fig. 9–2).

Occasionally, because of its anatomic structure, a patient's trachea will not accommodate the curvature of a specific tracheotomy tube. In such instances, the tip or lower end of the tube will strike against the anterior tracheal wall and cause ulceration followed by granuloma formation. If detected early, the selection of a tracheotomy tube with a more suitable curve may resolve this problem. If the patient complains of excessive coughing, mucous secretions, or discomfort just below the suprasternal notch when the tracheotomy is inserted, there is a strong possibility that the shape or length should be considered as the cause.

The nonemergency operation should not be hurried or misdirected. The fenestration in the anterior tracheal wall must be placed below the level of the second tracheal ring. A circular fenestration of the anterior tracheal wall, of a diameter slightly larger than the tracheotomy tube to be used, is ideal and will prevent the buckling-in defect of the anterior trachea.

Any signs of infection at the tracheotomy site should be thoroughly investigated by means of culture and sensitivity tests, and specific antibiotic therapy should be instituted. The incidence of infection associated with acute and subacute stenosis of the trachea is high. The organisms usually involved are coagulase-positive *Staphylococcus aureus, Escherichia coli*, and *Proteus bacilli*. Usually ciprofloxacin (Cipro), 500 mg, twice daily, and amoxicillin (Augmentin), 875 mg, twice daily, will resolve these infections. The treatment should be continued for at least 2 weeks.

Proper management of the cuffed tube is essential in preventing tracheal stenosis. Some reports indicate that the cuff should be deflated for 5 to 10 minutes every hour. Proper tracheotomy care is essential with a cuffed tube, especially when assisted ventilation is used. The entire tracheotomy tube should be changed frequently. A sterile suction catheter and sterile gloves are used each time the tracheal secretions are aspirated.

An obstruction of the trachea at the end of the tracheotomy tube can be most distressing. This should be suspected when the patient complains of intermittent respiratory difficulty and the need to frequently adjust the tracheotomy tube. An immediate bypass of this area by inserting an endotracheal tube or a Moore Tracheostomy Tube (Boston Medical Products, Inc) through the tracheotomy tube may be lifesaving.

If there are symptoms of an impaired airway after a tracheotomy tube has been removed, the trachea should be immediately evaluated by obtaining anteroposterior and lateral radiographs of the trachea. An axial computed tomography scan of the trachea may be necessary to more accurately evaluate the stenosis.

DIAGNOSIS OF A CERVICAL TRACHEAL STENOSIS

The anteroposterior (with copper filtration) and the lateral neck radiography studies of the cervical trachea with the patient's head in full extension are essential to outline the air column of the cervical trachea. Fluoroscopy is used for identifying tracheal malacia. The segment without support will collapse during inspiration. Computed tomography and magnetic resonance imaging scans may be required for additional detail. Laryngoscopy and bronchoscopy help to determine the exact level of the stenosis as its location is measured by comparing it with the level of the vocal cords and the existing tracheotomy orifice.

TREATMENT OF ACUTE TRACHEAL STENOSIS

Much of the early management of acute tracheal stenosis has been mentioned under the sections on etiology and prevention.

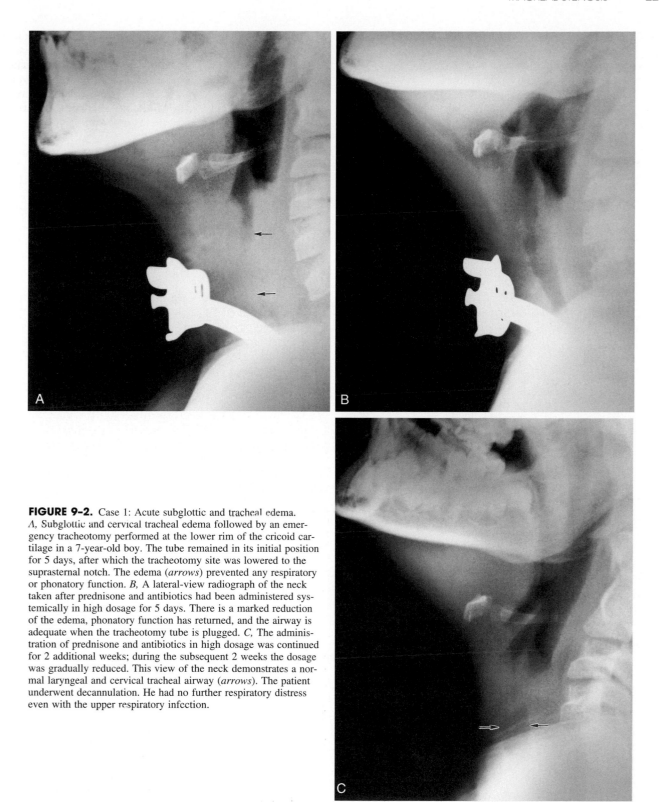

FIGURE 9–2. Case 1: Acute subglottic and tracheal edema. *A,* Subglottic and cervical tracheal edema followed by an emergency tracheotomy performed at the lower rim of the cricoid cartilage in a 7-year-old boy. The tube remained in its initial position for 5 days, after which the tracheotomy site was lowered to the suprasternal notch. The edema (*arrows*) prevented any respiratory or phonatory function. *B,* A lateral-view radiograph of the neck taken after prednisone and antibiotics had been administered systemically in high dosage for 5 days. There is a marked reduction of the edema, phonatory function has returned, and the airway is adequate when the tracheotomy tube is plugged. *C,* The administration of prednisone and antibiotics in high dosage was continued for 2 additional weeks; during the subsequent 2 weeks the dosage was gradually reduced. This view of the neck demonstrates a normal laryngeal and cervical tracheal airway (*arrows*). The patient underwent decannulation. He had no further respiratory distress even with the upper respiratory infection.

Granulomas in the cervical trachea that interfere with the airway are resected endoscopically by way of an anterior commissure laryngoscope or a bronchoscope. Microlaryngoscopy with use of the laser is often helpful. Granulomas should be approached by way of an existing tracheotomy orifice when possible. A steroid injection into the site of the origin of the granuloma is useful as a prophylactic measure to prevent recurrence of granulation-tissue formation. Topical use of mitomycin-c (3%) has demonstrated success in preventing recurrent stenosis when applied for 3 minutes on a saturated pledget.

If an acute airway problem is the result of a crushing injury to the tracheal cartilaginous rings, the treatment of choice is open reduction and stenting with a silicone Montgomery Safe-T-Tube (Boston Medical Products) (Fig. 9–3). This allows maintenance of the tracheal lumen while the cartilages heal in their correct anatomic position. The duration of stenting is directly proportional to the degree of trauma and varies from a few weeks to 2 months.

As mentioned previously, stenosis at the lower cervical or upper thoracic trachea occurring at the end of the tra-

cheotomy or endotracheal tube can be an acute emergency. As a first step in its treatment, an endotracheal tube is inserted beyond the area of stenosis to a more distal position in the trachea. Subsequently, a tube is inserted to bypass the area of obstruction. A Moore Tracheostomy Tube, which is made of soft silicone, or a Montgomery Thoracic Safe-T-Tube can be used to bypass the area of stenosis.

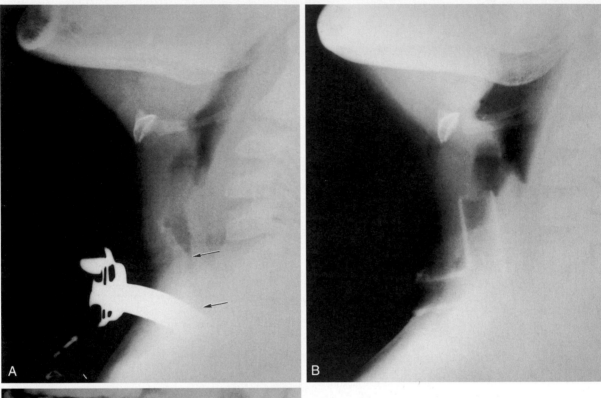

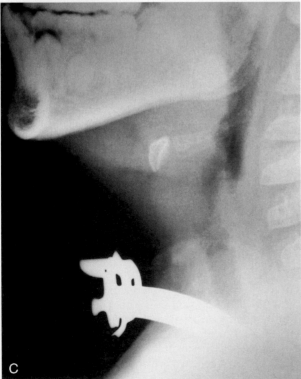

FIGURE 9-3. Case 2: Acute tracheal stenosis with unilateral laryngeal paralysis. *A*, The tracheal stenosis (*arrows*) involves nearly the entire cervical trachea. This radiograph was taken 2 weeks after a severe penetrating injury that split the patient's cervical trachea, cricoid cartilage, and larynx. The stenosis results from a buckling-in, or collapse, of tracheal cartilaginous support. A tracheotomy tube is located just above the suprasternal notch. *B*, A silicone tracheal Safe-T-Tube is in place after repair of the cervical tracheal stenosis. The posteriorly displaced cartilaginous rings were returned to their anatomic positions. A silicone tracheal Safe-T-Tube, with a diameter slightly in excess of the normal tracheal lumen, was chosen for stenting. With this in place, there was a slight vertical gap in the trachea anteriorly; this was repaired with sternohyoid muscle and fascia (see Figs. 9–13 and 9–14). *C,* A lateral radiograph of the neck taken immediately after removal of the silicone Safe-T-Tube, which had remained in place for 2 months, showed the tracheal lumen to be adequate. A tracheotomy tube was left in place for 2 weeks because of the possibility of a recurrent stenosis.

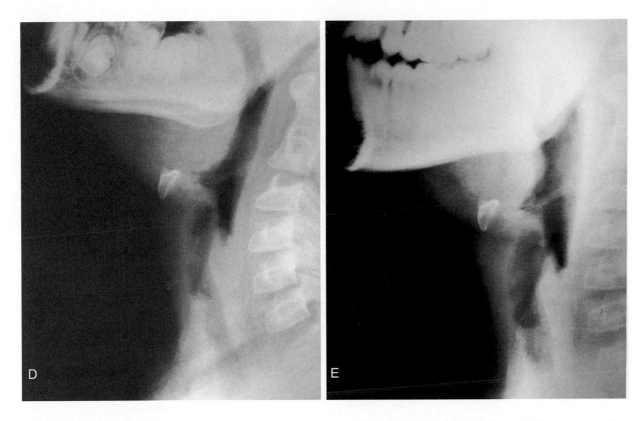

FIGURE 9–3. *Continued D,* A lateral radiograph of the patient's neck taken 1 year after repair of the acute tracheal stenosis. The scar tissue makes the tracheal air column appear irregular. The airway is adequate, even when the patient exercises strenuously. *E,* A lateral radiograph of the neck taken 5 years after the injury demonstrates a normal tracheal airway. The patient's voice remains hoarse because of irregularity and paralysis of the left larynx.

Once the emergency situation is resolved, the patient is transferred to the operating room, where the granuloma is carefully resected through a bronchoscope. Again, the injection of a steroid into the site of origin and 3-minute application of pledget saturated in mitomycin-c may prevent recurrent formation of granulation tissue. All possible conservative measures should be used to correct this low tracheal obstruction; segmental resection in this area is a major undertaking and still carries a significant mortality rate.

Dilatation and bougienage are frequently mentioned in the literature as being helpful when treating a patient with tracheal stenosis. Surgeons at the Massachusetts Eye and Ear Infirmary have found tracheal dilatation to be unsatisfactory and occasionally harmful.

SURGICAL REPAIR OF STENOSIS ABOVE THE TRACHEOTOMY TUBE

When the stenosis is caused by a tracheotomy having been placed immediately below the cricoid cartilage, the tracheotomy orifice is moved to as low a level as possible. If the impaired airway is the result of subglottic edema, and there is no buckling-in or loss of tracheal rings, then no further therapy other than lowering the tracheotomy site may be necessary. Acute or subacute subglottic and tracheal stenoses that result from edema will resolve more rapidly when the patient is given large doses of prednisone and antibiotics systemically after the tracheotomy orifice has been lowered.

A buckling-in deformity of the tracheal rings above the tracheotomy site is not uncommon in patients with stenosis at this level. Again, a new tracheotomy orifice is placed in as inferior a position as possible (Fig. 9–4). This facilitates the administration of an anesthetic during the operation and places the tracheotomy fenestration as far as possible from the site of repair.

A midline vertical skin incision should be used for this procedure (see Fig. 9–4*A* and *B*). The margin of the tracheal incision is retracted with small hooks. With this exposure, it is usually possible to replace the tracheal rings in their anatomic position. However, if there is extensive fibrosis, it is necessary to make additional vertical incisions in, or through, the involved cartilaginous rings at several points (see Fig. 9–4*C*). After this repair, a silicone Safe-T-Tube, of sufficient diameter to completely fill the tracheal lumen, is inserted (see Fig. 9–4*C*). The tube will serve to stent the repaired trachea in its anatomic position. Sutures are not necessary to close the tracheal incision. The muscular, subcutaneous, and dermal layers are carefully approximated.

The lower horizontal section of the trachea demonstrates the tracheal cartilages replaced in their anatomic position and stented by the extratracheal portion of the silicone tracheal Safe-T-Tube.

The repair of stenosis in the anterior wall of the trachea above the tracheotomy site, which results from loss of the anterior aspect of the tracheal rings, causes an anteroposterior slitlike stenosis (Fig. 9–5). The lateral tracheal rings are intact (see Fig. 9–5*A*). A vertical midline incision is made in the anterior wall of the trachea so that the entire area can

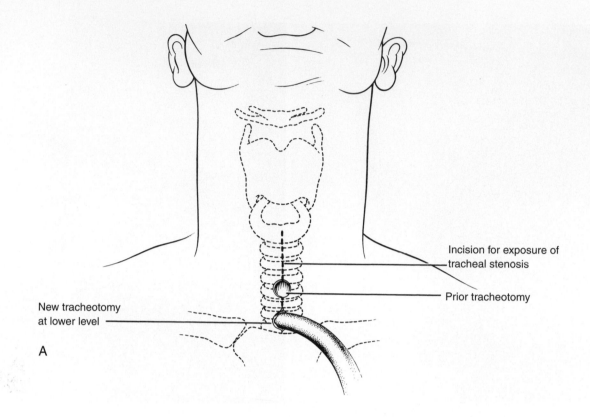

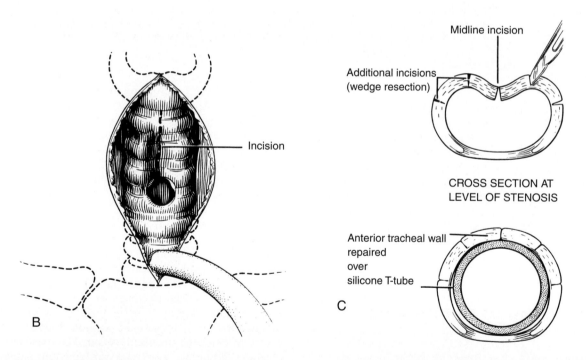

FIGURE 9–4. Tracheal stenosis occurring above the tracheotomy orifice. *A,* In most patients with tracheal stenosis a vertical midline incision is used. The incision begins in the superior midline of the existing tracheotomy orifice. The new tracheotomy fenestration is made immediately above the suprasternal notch, both for the administration of an anesthetic during the operation and to serve as an exit for the extratracheal portion of the silicone tracheal Safe-T-Tube. *B,* A vertical midline incision is also used to open the trachea at the level of stenosis. *C,* The upper horizontal section through the trachea demonstrates the midline incision and also the additional incisions that may be necessary to replace the cartilaginous tracheal rings in their anatomic position.

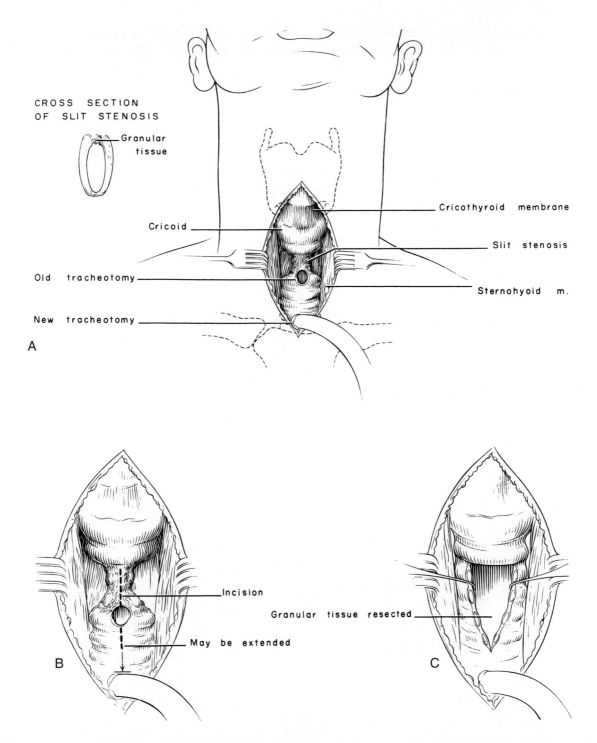

FIGURE 9-5. Tracheal stenosis occurring above the tracheotomy orifice. *A,* Loss of the anterior portion of one or more rings of the tracheal cartilage above the tracheotomy site results in collapse of the lateral walls towards the midline. This results in a slitlike stenosis. Scar tissue, or granulation tissue formed anteriorly, adds to the narrowing of the airway. A cross-section of this stenosis is shown to the left. A new tracheotomy orifice made at a lower level, just above the suprasternal notch, is shown. The entire length of the stylohyoid muscles is carefully dissected in this area. These muscles are to be used for reconstruction of the anterior wall of the trachea. An endotracheal anesthesia tube is introduced by way of the lower tracheotomy fenestration. *B,* An anterior vertical midline incision is made in the area of stenosis, beginning at the upper rim of the old tracheotomy orifice. This is best made with a No. 15 knife blade. The tissue to be cut may be relatively thin scar tissue, or there may be rather extensive granulation tissue present. A vertical midline incision is also made below the old tracheotomy site. This latter incision is made for exposure. It may be extended to the lower tracheotomy orifice, if necessary. *C,* The fibrous and granulation tissues have been resected. The lateral walls of the trachea are retracted with small skin hooks.

be exposed (see Figs. 9–5*B* and *C*). As the lateral walls of the trachea are retracted laterally, the defect becomes apparent.

A Montgomery Safe-T-Tube is inserted that completely fills the normal trachea, leaving an area of dehiscence anteriorly (Fig. 9–6*A*). There are several ways to repair the de-

hiscent area above the new tracheotomy. The simplest is to dissect the sternohyoid muscles and suture them over this defect (Figs. 9–6*B* and *C*). The sternohyoid muscles can be overlapped before they are sutured together to make a thicker wall.

Occasionally, the area void of mucous membrane in the

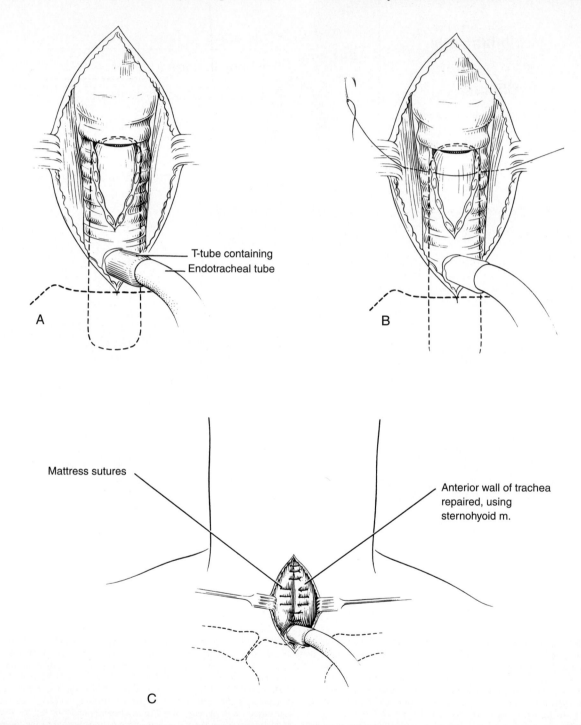

T-tube containing
Endotracheal tube

A

B

Mattress sutures

Anterior wall of trachea repaired, using sternohyoid m.

C

FIGURE 9–6. Tracheal stenosis occurring above the tracheotomy orifice. *A*, A Safe-T-Tube of a size that will fit the tracheal lumen completely and allow maximum lateral displacement of the trachea in the stenotic area has been inserted. The trachea between the area of stenosis of the new tracheotomy site may be opened (*broken line*) to facilitate insertion of the Safe-T-Tube. The external limb of the Safe-T-Tube exits by way of the lower tracheal opening, and the administration of an anesthetic is continued by way of an endotracheal tube inserted into this portion of the Safe-T-Tube. *B*, Mattress sutures are placed through the sternohyoid muscles and margins of the tracheal defect. The sternohyoid muscles are thus used to cover the defect in the anterior tracheal wall. It is best to place all the sutures before any are tied. *C*, The sternohyoid muscles have been approximated in the midline. It is not necessary to place mattress sutures above and below the area of stenosis. The remainder of the wound is closed in layers, and closed-suction drainage is applied.

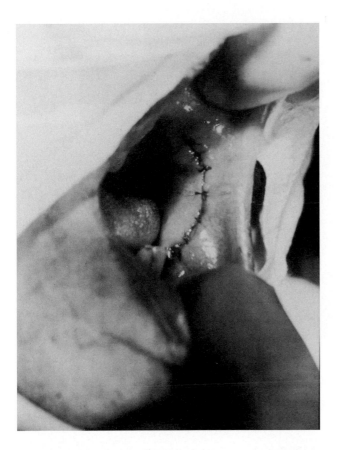

FIGURE 9–7. A photograph of the repair after resection of a large buccal mucosal graft. The incisions should avoid the parotid duct papillae and orifice.

in the recovery area after the patient awakes from general anesthesia. Plugging the Safe-T-Tube prevents dehydration of tracheal secretions and eliminates frequent suctioning, which is irritating to the trachea. Plugging the external limb of the Safe-T-Tube allows the patient to breathe and speak in a normal fashion.

CASE STUDY 9-1

Tracheal Stenosis With Anterior Wall Collapse

A 4-month-old infant was admitted to the hospital with acute respiratory distress complicating an upper respiratory tract infection. A tracheotomy was necessary. The infection rapidly subsided, but attempts at decannulation were unsuccessful.

A second tracheotomy was performed at a lower level 6 months later. Again, attempts to decannulate the trachea were unsuccessful.

Two years after the original tracheotomy, a lateral neck radiograph (Fig. 9–8A) showed tracheal narrowing above the tracheotomy orifice. A third operation was performed at the Massachusetts Eye and Ear Infirmary. During this procedure, after the trachea had been split anteriorly, the stenosis was found to be caused by a collapse of the anterior tracheal wall. The tracheal rings were incised so that they could be replaced to their anatomic position (Fig. 9–8B). A Montgomery Safe-T-Tube was inserted. The trachea has remained patent to the present date (Fig. 9–8C).

area of stenosis is too extensive for spontaneous re-epithelialization. In such cases, a mucous graft or split-thickness skin graft can be used for epithelial cover under the muscle repair. Large mucous membrane grafts can be obtained from the buccal region after the papilla and orifice of Stensen's duct have been identified (Fig. 9–7). After the buccal mucous membrane graft has been obtained, the margins are undermined slightly, and repair is accomplished by primary closure in a vertical suture line. No cosmetic defect will result in the donor site, and postoperative discomfort is minimal. A mucosal graft may also be obtained from one side of the nasal septum. The mucosal layer of the nasal septum is dense, and subsequent shrinkage of the graft is minimal. A *split-thickness* skin graft is best obtained from the supraclavicular region because it is near the field of operation and lacks hair. Large split-thickness skin grafts should be avoided because of subsequent tracheal crusting. The graft is sutured to the margins of the defect after the Safe-T-Tube has been inserted. The graft is then covered with muscle layer. This repair usually heals well in 3 or 4 weeks, and the Safe-T-Tube can be removed.

The Montgomery Safe-T-Tube serves as both a stent and a tracheotomy tube. When treating an infant or small child, it is advisable to use the pediatric-type Safe-T-Tube. The external limb slants superiorly. This makes it easier to keep the tubal airway patent.

It is essential to plug the external portion of the Safe-T-Tube as soon as possible after the operation. It can be done

COMPLETE STENOSIS OF THE CERVICAL TRACHEA

The ideal treatment for patients with circumferential stenosis of the cervical trachea and loss of mucosal continuity is sleeve resection of the stenotic portion and end-to-end anastomosis. In young patients, who have relative elasticity of the annular rings of the trachea, a gap in the tracheal continuity of up to 3 cm can be closed without release techniques. Up to an extra centimeter can be gained with the patient's head in extreme flexion. The tension (over 1,000 g) on the suture line of an anastomosis after a sleeve resection of more than 3 cm is sufficient to result in recurrence of the stenosis in a significant percentage of patients. An accurate approximation of the cut ends of the trachea is essential to prevent recurrent stenosis. A mucosa-to-mucosa approximation with supporting intracartilaginous sutures is an ideal repair technique. The end-to-end anastomosis may be complicated by disruption or an air leak at the suture line or a stricture of the lumen at the site of the anastomosis. Dissection of the trachea from its surrounding fascia adds little to the degree of mobilization and probably interferes with the blood supply. If the mucosa of the posterior tracheal wall is not involved and is intact, it need not be disturbed. In such instances, a wedge, rather than a sleeve, resection is performed. It is very important that the patient's neck remain in the position of flexion for at least 10 days post-

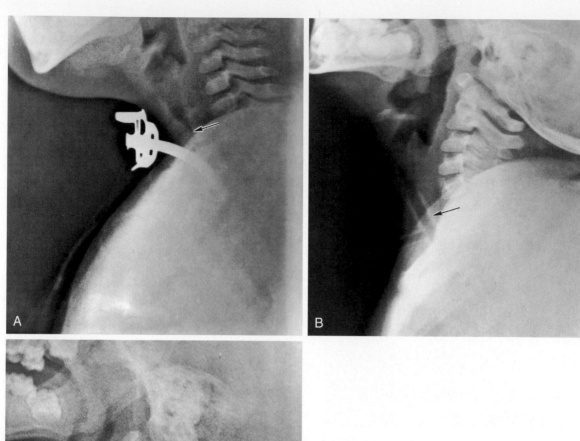

FIGURE 9–8. Tracheal stenosis with anterior wall collapse. *A*, A tracheal stenosis above the tracheotomy orifice caused by posterior displacement or buckling of the cartilaginous rings in an infant 2 years and 10 months of age. The stenosis (*arrow*) had been present for 2 years. *B*, The stenosis has been corrected by returning the cartilaginous rings to their anatomic position and providing support for them with a silicone Safe-T-Tube (*arrow*). *C*, A lateral-neck radiograph taken 4 years after repair of the tracheal stenosis. The child has had no further difficulty with respiration or phonation.

operatively. Return to normal cervical motility should be gradual.

Techniques for Gaining Extra Length for a Primary Anastomosis of the Trachea

There are three methods for gaining extra length for a primary anastomosis to avoid excessive tension on the suture line. The first method is a superior mobilization of the distal trachea from the thorax (Fig. 9–9). The intrathoracic operation carries the danger of a mediastinal dissection. During the lengthening procedure, the right hilus is mobilized and the pulmonary ligament is divided. The pulmonary vessels are freed from the pericardium. Finally, the left mainstem bronchus is sectioned distal to the carina and reattached to the tracheal bronchial system by an end-to-end anastomosis with the right main-stem bronchus. Up to 6 cm of superior mobilization can be accomplished with this procedure.

Another method for obtaining additional length for an end-to-end anastomosis of the trachea without excessive suture line tension involves releasing the larynx from its attachment to the hyoid bone Fig. 9–10) or sectioning the muscles attached to the superior aspect of the hyoid bone (Fig. 9–11 and Fig. 9–12). Either technique provides inferior mobilization of the superior tracheal segment. Up to 5 cm of tracheal mobilization can be achieved. The author prefers the suprahyoid release technique because its use in his patients has resulted in no interference with swallowing. The infrahyoid release is followed by a high incidence of interference with deglutition (probably caused by stretch injury of the superior laryngeal nerves).

Text continued on page 239

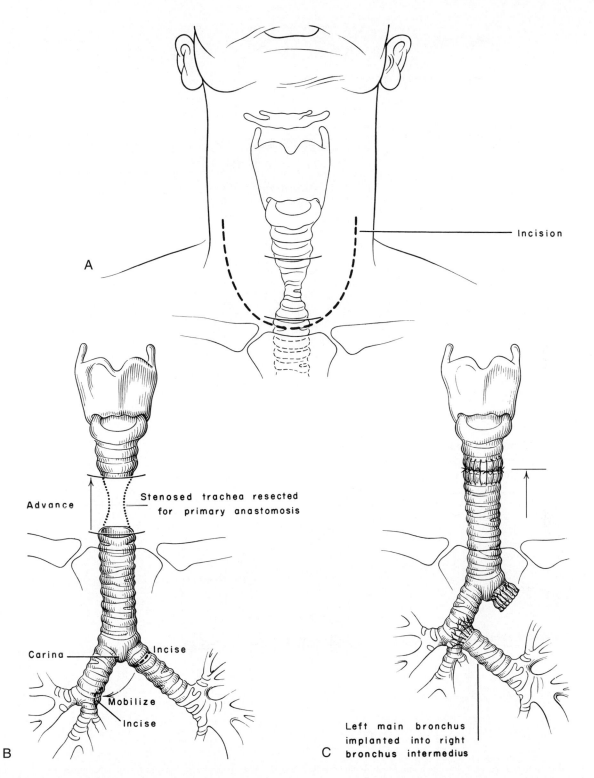

A

Incision

Advance

Stenosed trachea resected
for primary anastomosis

Carina

Incise

Mobilize

Incise

B

C

Left main bronchus
implanted into right
bronchus intermedius

FIGURE 9–9. Intrathoracic (inferior) tracheal release. *A,* A U-shaped flap is elevated to expose the area of stenosis in the cervical trachea. After resection of the portion of trachea involved in the stenosis, the distance between the remaining ends is measured. The ends then are retracted towards each other to measure the amount of tension produced inferiorly and superiorly when they are approximated with the neck in hyperflexion. *B,* The intrathoracic technique for superior mobilization of the trachea (Grillo). During this lengthening procedure, the right hilus is mobilized and the pulmonary ligament is divided. The pulmonary vessels are freed from the pericardium. *C,* A left mainstem bronchus has been anastomosed to the right middle-lobe bronchus by an end-to-side anastomosis. This will allow up to 6 cm of superior mobilization.

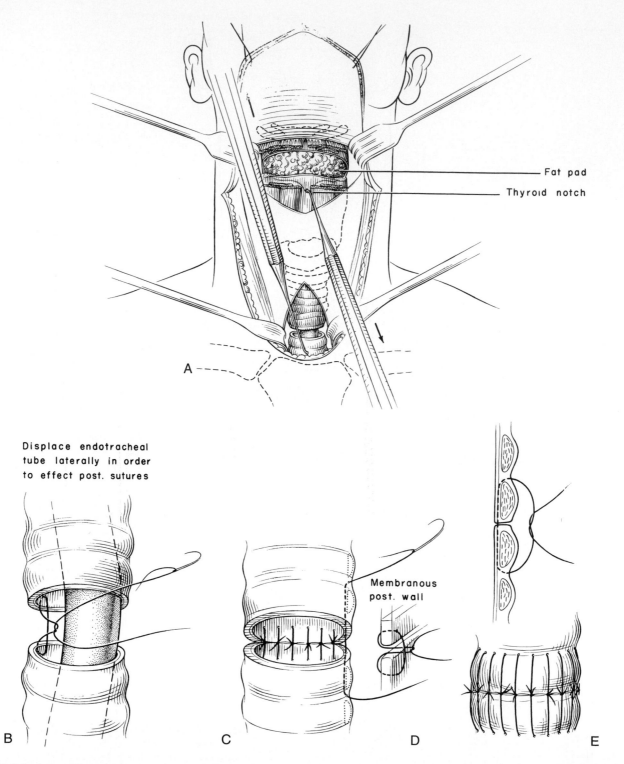

Fat pad

Thyroid notch

Displace endotracheal
tube laterally in order
to effect post. sutures

Membranous
post. wall

B   C   D   E

FIGURE 9-10. Laryngeal release below the hyoid level. *A,* The release below the level of the hyoid bone has been accomplished, thereby causing the larynx and proximal trachea to drop. Anastomosis of the trachea can be most readily performed by retracting the larynx inferiorly and the distal segment of trachea superiorly. *B,* Anastomosis of the membranous portion of the trachea is performed first. The sutures can be tied from an anterior position, as shown. *C,* The membranous portion of the trachea has been repaired. The knots of the sutures are seen in this illustration. These retract through the site of anastomosis and ultimately take their position on the posterior surface of the membranous trachea. The lateral and anterior walls of the anastomosis are repaired in two layers. The larger suture is placed above the tracheal rings through the annular ligament in a downward direction, posterior to the cartilage in a submucosal plane, and then in a similar route through the distal tracheal segment. The illustration to the right is a close-up of the technique used when suturing the membranous posterior tracheal anastomosis so that the knot of the suture will migrate to the posterior wall of the membranous trachea. *D,* A cross-section of the suture, which encompasses a tracheal ring of both the distal and proximal tracheal segments. It is important to place this suture between the cartilage and mucosal layer so that it will not project into the tracheal lumen. *E,* The completed anastomosis.

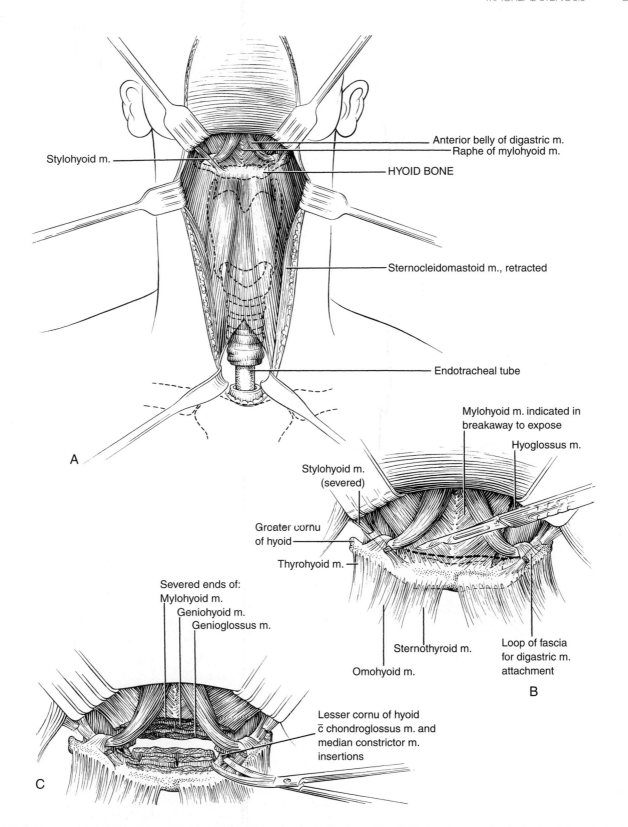

Stylohyoid m.

Anterior belly of digastric m.
Raphe of mylohyoid m.

HYOID BONE

Sternocleidomastoid m., retracted

Endotracheal tube

A

Stylohyoid m.
(severed)

Greater cornu
of hyoid

Thyrohyoid m.

Mylohyoid m. indicated in
breakaway to expose

Hyoglossus m.

Sternothyroid m.

Omohyoid m.

Loop of fascia
for digastric m.
attachment

B

Severed ends of:
Mylohyoid m.
Geniohyoid m.
Genioglossus m.

Lesser cornu of hyoid
c̄ chondroglossus m. and
median constrictor m.
insertions

C

FIGURE 9–11. Laryngeal release above the hyoid bone. *A,* An endotracheal tube shown bridging the gap between the proximal and distal tracheal ends after the tracheal stenosis has been resected. An anterior cervical skin flap has been elevated to the suprahyoid region. The anterior belly of the digastric muscle, the mylohyoid muscle, and the stylohyoid muscle are identified. *B,* The muscle attachments to the superior surface of the hyoid bone are transected, exposing the preepiglottic space. The tendinous portion of the digastric muscle between its anterior and posterior bellies is identified. The stylohyoid muscles are transected at this point. *C,* The lesser cornua of the hyoid bone are palpated and transected with heavy scissors. Note that the mylohyoid, geniohyoid, and genioglossus muscles are separated from the hyoid bone, exposing the preepiglottic space.

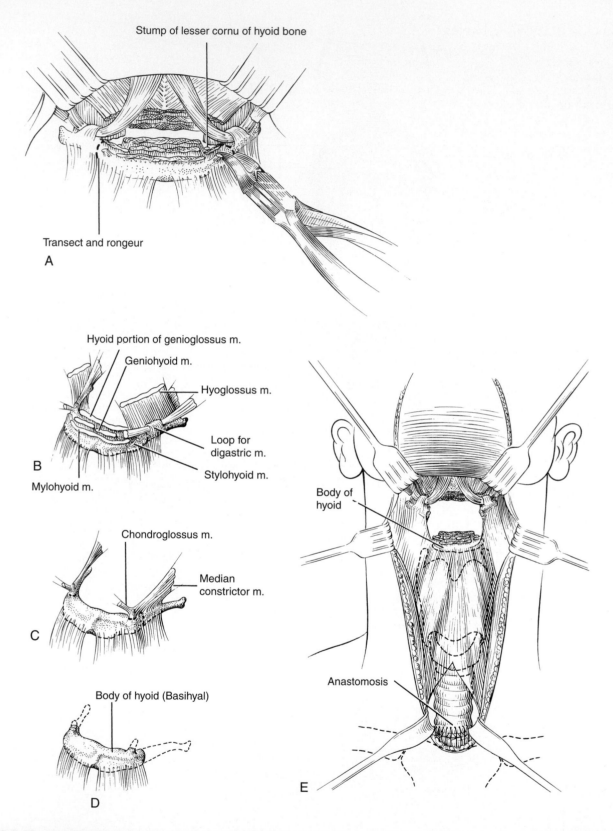

FIGURE 9–12. Laryngeal release above the hyoid bone. *A,* The dotted lines indicate the point where the hyoid bone is sectioned, separating its body from the greater horn on each side. *B,* An oblique view showing the site for the hyoid bone incision immediately anterior to the tendinous attachment of the digastric muscle to the hyoid bone. *C,* An oblique view illustrating the relationship of the chondroglossus and median constrictor muscles to the bone incisions that separate the greater and lesser cornua of the hyoid bone from its body. *D,* The greater and lesser cornua of the hyoid bone have now been separated from the body of the hyoid bone and its inferior muscle attachments. *E,* At the termination of the operation, the body of the hyoid bone has dropped inferiorly along with the thyroid cartilage, cricoid cartilage, and proximal segment of trachea. An anastomosis of the distal to the proximal trachea has been accomplished.

Technique of Laryngeal Release Above the Hyoid Bone

After the body of the hyoid bone is exposed using the U-shaped skin flap (see Fig. 9–11A), the muscle attachments to the superior surface of the hyoid bone are transected (see Fig. 9–11B). The tendinous attachments of the digastric muscles to the hyoid are identified. The stylohyoid muscles and the lesser cornua of the hyoid are transected (see Fig. 9–11C). The hyoid bone is transected on each side, separating the body from the greater cornua (see Fig. 9–12A to D). The body of the hyoid bone, the thyroid cartilage, and proximal tracheal segment drop inferiorly, permitting a tracheal anastomosis to be performed without excessive tension on the suture line (see Fig. 9–12E).

An end-to-end anastomosis is performed using either 3-0 Vicryl sutures or No. 28 stainless steel suture material. Fig. 9–14C to E shows the placement of these sutures. All sutures are applied before they are tied. An assistant provides relaxation during suture tying by placing a hook in the trachea below the site of the anastomosis and another in the thyroid notch superiorly.

Oral intubation is performed during this repair. Postoperatively, the chin is kept in flexion for 1 week.

There are two techniques for maintaining an adequate airway during the first few postoperative days. One is to keep an endotracheal tube in place and to keep the patient sedated. The second is to place a tracheotomy tube or a Safe-T-Tube below the area of repair. The author prefers the latter.

TRACHEAL STENOSIS AT THE TRACHEOTOMY LEVEL

Stenosis of the cervical trachea at the level of a tracheotomy orifice is probably the most common type of stenosis. In most cases, it is the result of an infection of the tracheotomy tract that causes polyps and granulation tissue to form and project both external to and into the tracheal lumen. The stenosis usually does not become apparent until attempts at decannulation are made. Stridor may occur immediately on removal of the tracheotomy tube, or, in some instances, it may not become apparent for a few weeks.

A patient with this type of stenosis is best treated by conservative measures if there has been no accompanying chondritis or loss of tracheal support. The polyps and granulation tissue are carefully removed with Takahashi or Brownie forceps. Cultures are taken so that specific local and general antibiotics can be administered. The author has found ciprofloxacin and amoxicillin administered orally for at least 2 weeks to be effective in controlling this infection. A tracheotomy tube is left in place until the infection has resolved.

Sterile precautions should be used in caring for the tracheotomy. The tracheotomy tube should be fully plugged as soon as possible, and the plug should be left in place at all times unless tracheal suctioning is necessary.

A collapse of the upper margin of the tracheal fenestration is a common configuration of tracheal stenosis at the tracheotomy level (Fig. 9–13A). It probably results from either a hurriedly performed tracheotomy or from an H-type incision made in the anterior tracheal wall. This type of stenosis responds well to reconstitution of the tracheal rings or repair of the anterior segment using sternohyoid muscles as has been described. The Safe-T-Tube is inserted (Fig. 9–13B) to support the reconstituted or reconstructed anterior tracheal wall at the upper rim of the tracheotomy orifice.

Occasionally, the stenosis at the tracheotomy site is the result of a prolonged infection with complicating chondritis and necrosis of the cartilaginous rings. Because it usually does not involve more than two or three tracheal rings, a wedge resection, leaving the posterior or membranous wall intact, can be performed with an end-to-end anastomosis (Fig. 9–14). Tracheal-release techniques are not necessary.

Every effort should be made to resolve any existing local infection before surgery. A new tracheotomy is placed at a lower level. The existing tracheotomy tract is excised

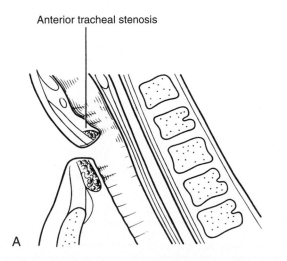

Anterior tracheal stenosis

A

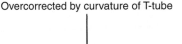
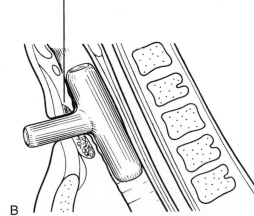

Overcorrected by curvature of T-tube

B

FIGURE 9–13. Repair of anterior tracheal stenosis. *A,* The anterior tracheal stenosis is caused by collapse or buckling-in of the anterior tracheal wall. The scar tissue is removed and the tracheal rings are repositioned or sternohyoid muscles are used to support the anterior wall. *B,* The reconstructed or reconstituted anterior tracheal wall is supported with a tracheal Safe-T-Tube. The anterior tracheal wall is overcorrected by the curvature of the tube at the junction of its intratracheal and external portions.

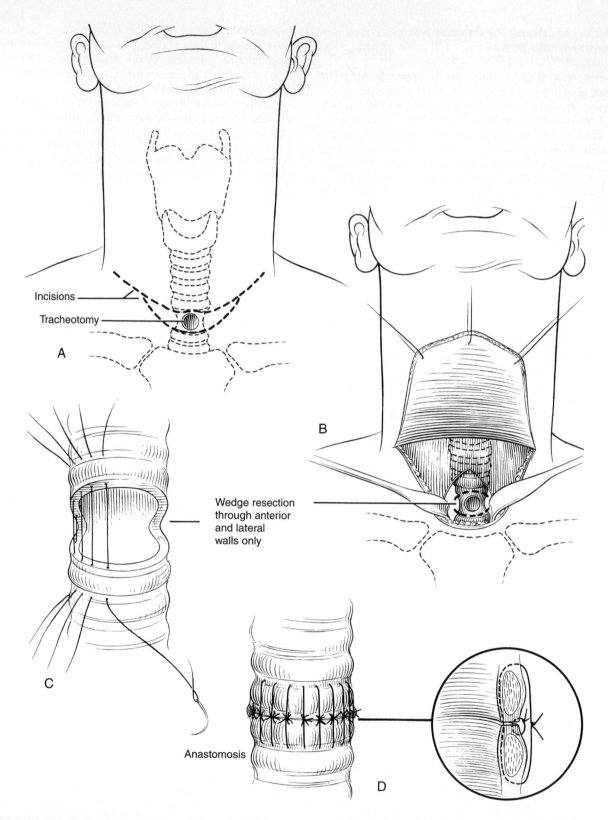

Incisions

Tracheotomy

A

B

Wedge resection through anterior and lateral walls only

C

Anastomosis

D

FIGURE 9–14. Repair of stenosis at the tracheotomy level. *A,* The stenosis is exposed by a horizontal or U-shaped incision that includes the tracheotomy tract. *B,* The flap has been elevated, exposing normal trachea above and below the site of stenosis. A small horizontal incision is made above and below the tracheal fenestration to expose the trachea. The stenosis is gradually resected, and normal trachea is exposed distally and proximally. *C,* The stenosis has been resected with margins of normal trachea above and below the stenotic area. The posterior wall remains intact. *D,* The anastomosis is complete. Internal stenting is not usually necessary when this type of repair is made. A small tracheotomy tube can be inserted in the distal tracheal segment if the surgeon is concerned about the repair. The tracheotomy tube should be plugged as soon as possible after the patient's recovery from anesthesia. For details of anastomosis technique, refer to Figure 9–10.

(see Fig. 9–14*A*). Normal trachea is exposed above and below the site of stenosis (see Fig. 9–14*B*). The posterior wall remains intact. No. 3-0 Vicryl sutures are used for the anastomosis (see Fig. 9–14*C* and *D*). The tracheotomy tube can usually be removed within a couple of weeks.

TRACHEAL STENOSIS BELOW THE TRACHEOTOMY LEVEL

The incidence of stenosis below the site of the tracheotomy has markedly increased in the past decade mainly because intermittent positive-pressure breathing (IPPB) has become accepted for (1) treatment of patients with postoperative disturbance of respiration or circulation after a neurosurgical, thoracic, or abdominal operation; (2) blocking (cuffed tube) the trachea against aspiration or oral secretions, gastric contents, or blood after injury or severe illness; (3) treatment of patients with certain pulmonary diseases, such as atelectasis, emphysema, bronchiectasis, pulmonary fibrosis, or severe asthma; (4) treatment of patients with cardiac disease associated with right-sided congestive heart failure; (5) administration of anesthetics; and (6) resuscitation.

This type of stenosis undoubtedly results from excessive pressure of the inflated cuff against the tracheal mucous membrane along with the motion and friction associated with IPPB (Fig. 9–15*A*). Secondary infection complicates the ulceration of tracheal mucous membrane and exposure of underlying cartilage. Chondritis and necrosis of cartilage and the formation of granulation tissue follows. Proper care of the cuffed tracheotomy tube during IPPB will prevent many of these complications. The longer cuff should be used so that the pressure is exerted over a larger area of tracheal mucosa. The cuff should be inflated only to the point of tracheal obstruction and no further. The complications of overinflation of the cuff should be explained to all personnel involved in the treatment and care of the patient. The cuff should be deflated for at least 10 minutes every hour when IPPB is not being administered unless there is a severe aspiration problem.

Stenosis resulting from a cuffed tracheotomy tube occurs 1.5 to 3 cm below the tracheotomy level. The damage from an overinflated cuffed tracheotomy tube can occur within 48 hours.

TREATMENT

Occasionally, the stenosis at the cuff level will be the result of a granuloma. This can be resected, and a long-lasting steroid preparation (methylprednisolone acetate [Depo-Medrol]) can be injected at its site of origin. As a rule, a patient with circumferential fibrotic stenosis at the cuff level cannot be permanently cured by dilatations with application of steroids and mitomycin-c or prolonged stenting. Conversely, the literature reports satisfactory results obtained by means of frequent dilatations with a bronchoscope or by inserting longer and larger tracheotomy tubes (Moore tubes) extending beyond the site of stenosis. These techniques should be reserved for patients with mild stenosis or those who are too debilitated to permit safe surgical resection.

For the most part, resection of the stenosis and anastomosis are the treatments of choice. These are accomplished as described and illustrated in Figures 9–10 to 9–12. A wedge resection at the level of the stenosis is usually the procedure of choice. A sleeve resection of the stenotic trachea is necessary when the posterior wall is involved. A thoracotomy may be necessary to expose, excise, and repair a tracheal stenosis below the level of the tracheotomy.

STENOSIS OF THE TRACHEA AT THE END OF A TRACHEOTOMY TUBE

Tracheal stenosis resulting from trauma inflicted by the end of a tracheotomy tube (Fig. 9–16*A*) is uncommon. It presumably occurs from pressure erosion of the anterior tracheal lumen, at the end of the tracheotomy tube, and probably as a result of an unsuspected variance between the anatomic structure of the patient's airway and the curvature of the tracheotomy tube. The anterior erosion will result in ulceration, secondary infection, the formation of a granuloma (Fig. 9–16*B*), or loss of tracheal support (Fig. 9–16*C*).

The diagnosis of a granuloma or stenosis occurring at the end of a tracheotomy tube is usually not readily apparent. Respiratory distress may continue even after a change of the tracheotomy tube. This situation can resolve into an acute emergency necessitating immediate lifesaving action. The obstruction at the end of the tracheotomy tube can be visualized with a flexible fiberoptic scope. The tracheotomy tube is removed and a bronchoscope, an endotracheal tube, or a Moore tube is inserted beyond the site of stenosis.

If a granuloma is found, it is resected in the site of its origin injected with a long-lasting steroid preparation to prevent recurrence. The area of stenosis can be bypassed with a Moore tracheostomy tube (Fig. 9–16*D*) after removal of the granuloma (see Fig. 9–16*B*). A Montgomery Thoracic Safe-T-Tube has a long inferior intraluminal limb that can be used to bypass and stent this type of tracheal stenosis (see Fig. 9–16*E*). However, such measures are usually only temporary. In general, the area of stenosis must be resected and the trachea must be anastomosed by way of a thoracotomy.

RECONSTRUCTION OF THE CERVICAL TRACHEA

Successful replacement of the cervical trachea should result in an adequately functioning larynx and a tracheobronchial system without the use of a tracheotomy tube. The objectives of such a procedure should be (1) adequate airway, (2) flexible tracheal support to prevent collapse and stenosis, and (3) complete re-epithelialization lumen.

The principle of the technique presented here is the fashioning of a split-thickness skin graft trough constructed between the upper and lower edges of normal trachea. The trough is closed anteriorly in a second-stage procedure using a "trap door" flap fashioned from a horizontal cervical skin flap. The trap door is supported by struts of rib or septal cartilage.

Biller successfully used this technique along with a silicone tracheal Safe-T-Tube in 23 of 30 patients.

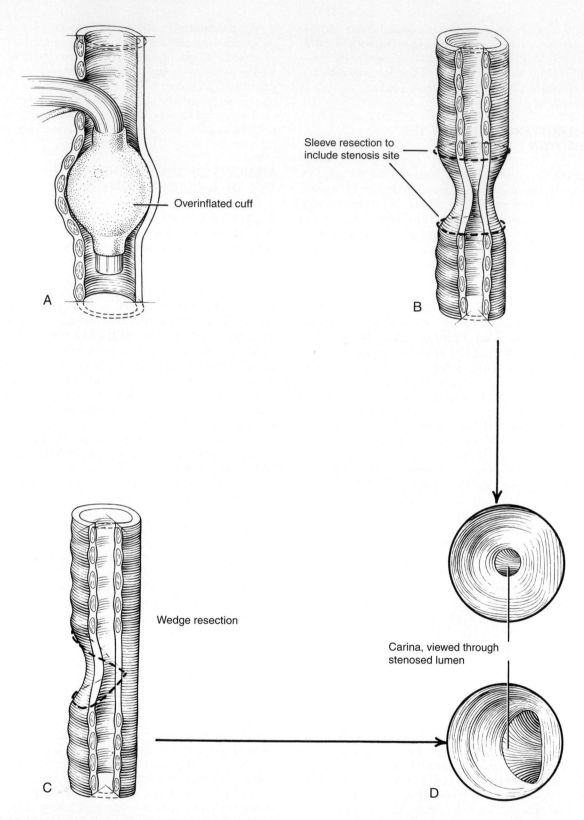

FIGURE 9–15. Stenosis below the tracheotomy level. *A,* Anterior displacement of the tracheal rings by the over-inflated cuff. Lateral displacement occurs simultaneously. *B,* The type of circumferential stenosis that results from loss of tracheal support at the cuff level. A sleeve-type tracheal resection is necessary to repair this defect. *C,* An incomplete stenosis sparing the posterior wall. A wedge resection of the stenotic trachea provides satisfactory treatment for this type of stenosis. *D,* Bronchoscopic comparison of the respective lumina in partial and circumferential stenosis.

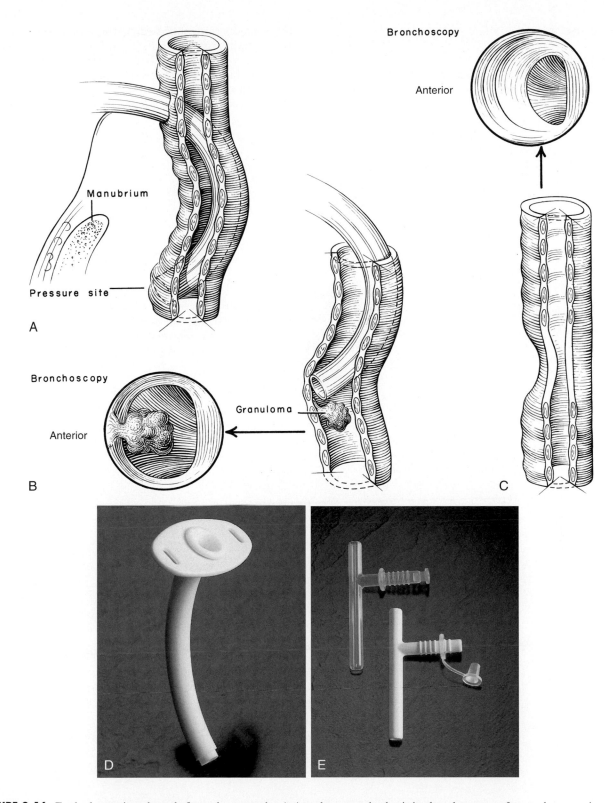

FIGURE 9–16. Tracheal stenosis at the end of a tracheotomy tube. *A,* A tracheotomy tube that is in place does not conform to the anatomic structure of the patient's airway. The end of the tube presses against the anterior tracheal wall. This pressure results in ulceration of the anterior tracheal mucosa. Secondary infection complicates the ulceration, producing either a granuloma or loss of tracheal support. *B,* A granuloma has formed distal to the end of the tracheotomy tube. This can result in a respiratory emergency, necessitating intubation or bronchoscopy to bypass the obstruction. *C,* The configuration of a stenosis at the level of the end of the tracheotomy tube resulting in loss of cartilaginous tracheal support. *D,* A photograph of the Moore tracheotomy tube used to bypass a tracheal stenosis at the end of a tracheotomy tube. *E,* A Thoracic Safe-T-Tube designed especially to bypass and stent a lower tracheal stenosis. The Safe-T-Tube is cared for and changed as described in Chapter 10.

Surgical Technique

First Stage

If the existing tracheotomy is located at the level of the lower end of the tracheal stenosis, it must be lowered to the suprasternal notch.

An anterior horizontal pedicled skin flap (Fig. 9–17A) is fashioned with its base in the right cervical region. Subcutaneous adipose tissue is dissected from the flap to avoid excessive thickness of the "trap door" to be constructed.

A vertical midline incision is made over the area of stenotic trachea. Normal trachea is exposed both superior

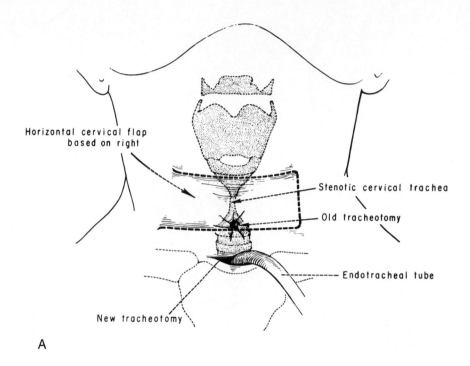

Horizontal cervical flap
based on right

Stenotic cervical trachea

Old tracheotomy

Endotracheal tube

New tracheotomy

A

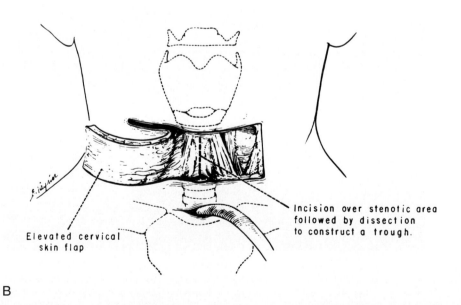

Elevated cervical
skin flap

Incision over stenotic area
followed by dissection
to construct a trough.

B

FIGURE 9–17. Reconstruction of the cervical trachea—first stage. *A,* A horizontal cervical pedicled skin flap is elevated in the anterior cervical region over the area of the absent cervical trachea. The level and width of this flap are determined preoperatively by measurements taken from the lateral-neck radiograph demonstrating the tracheal stenosis. Often, the existing tracheotomy orifice is at the lower margin of the tracheal stenosis. A new tracheotomy fenestration is made in the suprasternal notch. *B,* Subcutaneous adipose tissue is dissected from the flap to avoid excessive thickness of the "trap door" to be used to construct the anterior tracheal wall during the second stage of reconstruction. A vertical midline incision is made in the area of stenotic or absent trachea. The margin of normal trachea is identified proximally and distally by careful dissection. A trough is created between the margins of normal trachea. Remnants of tracheal cartilage are useful in determining the limits of this dissection.

and inferior to the stenosis (Fig. 9–17B). A trough is dissected between the ends of normal trachea. Scattered small fragments of cartilage may aid in determining the limits of this dissection. Fashioning the posterolateral aspect of this trough must be performed with extreme care to avoid injury to the recurrent laryngeal nerves. A 5- × 12-cm, 0.012-inch—thick skin graft is used to line the trough and to cover the defect in the left side of the neck (Fig. 9–18A). The right margin of the skin graft is sutured to the left margin of the cervical pedicled skin flap (Fig. 9–18B).

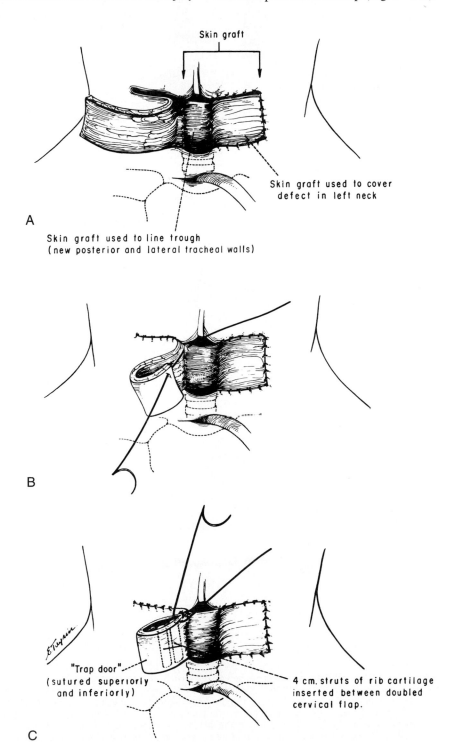

FIGURE 9-18. Reconstruction of the cervical trachea—first stage. A, A split-thickness skin graft is fashioned to line the trough and cover the defect in the left side of the neck. B, The laterally based pedicled skin flap becomes folded as its left margin is sutured to the right margin of the skin graft. C, Two struts of rib or septal cartilage are inserted between the folded pedicles skin flap. The "trap door" is then closed superiorly with dermal sutures. The superior and inferior margins of the skin graft are sutured to the lateral and posterior ends of the distal and proximal tracheal segments. A cylinder-shaped sponge is applied over the skin graft in the trough. The sponge is secured in place with a dressing or several sutures bridged over the stent from the lateral margins of the trough.

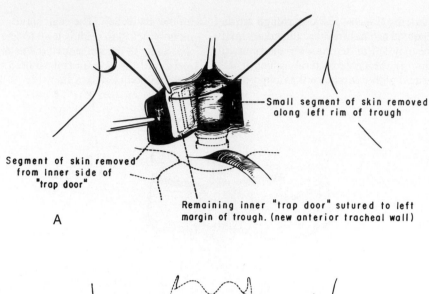

Small segment of skin removed
along left rim of trough

Segment of skin removed
from inner side of
"trap door"

Remaining inner "trap door" sutured to left
margin of trough. (new anterior tracheal wall)

A

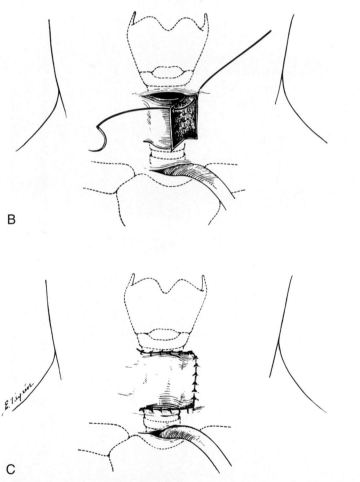

B

C

FIGURE 9–19. Reconstruction of the cervical trachea—-second stage. *A,* The second-stage reconstruction can be performed 6 weeks after the first. A 1.5-cm strip of skin is resected from the inner aspect of the lateral margin of the "trap door." A segment of skin graft is resected from the anterior neck to the left of the trough. The left margin of the "trap door" is sutured to the left margin of the trough as is shown. *B, C,* The left outer margin of the "trap door" is sutured to the left side of the neck, thus filling in a defect created by removal of the skin graft. A narrow strip of skin from the superior and inferior margins of the "trap door" and also the skin over the superior and inferior margins of normal cervical trachea are removed to allow for skin closure superiorly and inferiorly. Suturing the upper margin of the inner aspect of the "trap door" to the anterior margins of the proximal and distal trachea would be extremely difficult and is not necessary for the area is stented with a silicone Safe-T-Tube postoperatively.

Two 4-cm struts of rib or nasal septal cartilage are inserted between the doubled-over cervical pedicled skin flap as pictured in Figure 9–18C. The "trap door" is sutured superiorly and inferiorly.

A Montgomery Safe-T-Tube is selected to support the skin graft.

Second Stage

The second stage operation is performed 3 to 4 weeks after the first. This procedure entails closing the trap door to form the anterior wall of the reconstructed trachea. A strip of skin is removed from the inner surface of the trap door leaving a skin-lined segment 1.5 cm wide that is used to form the anterior tracheal wall (Fig. 9–19A). A narrow, horizontal strip of skin is excised from the upper and lower margins of the inner surface of the trap door.

Vertical parallel incisions, 1.5 cm apart, are made to the left of the trough. The segment of skin between the vertical incisions is removed. The cartilage struts are inspected for viability. The inner aspect of the trap door is sutured to the left margin of the trough to form the anterior wall of the reconstructed trachea (Fig. 9–19B). The outer aspect of the trap door is sutured superiorly, inferiorly, and on the left side, as shown in Figure 9–19C, to complete the operation. A Safe-T-Tube is inserted to stent the reconstructed trachea.

CASE STUDY 9-2

Reconstruction of Cervical Trachea

A 38-year-old woman received multiple injuries during an automobile accident. Her worst injury, to the

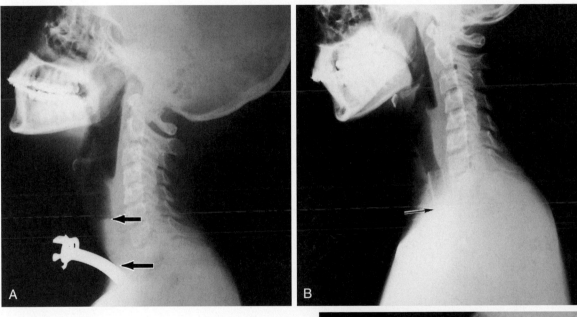

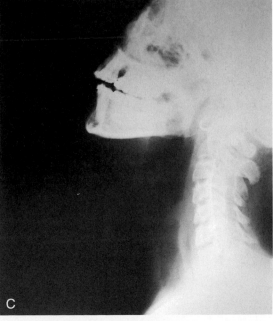

FIGURE 9–20. Tracheal reconstruction. *A,* A lateral-neck radiograph showing loss of almost the entire cervical trachea (*arrows*). When explored, the tracheal cartilage was absent from just below the cricoid to the thoracic inlet. At this time, the first stage of tracheal reconstruction, as described in the text, was performed. *B,* A tracheal Safe-T-Tube (*arrows*) is in place after the second stage of tracheal reconstruction. *C,* A lateral-neck radiograph taken 6 years after two-stage reconstruction of the cricoid trachea. The patient's voice and airway remain normal.

cricoid cartilage and trachea, resulted from striking the steering wheel. The immediate stridor was relieved by a tracheotomy. Radiographs showed a fracture of the cricoid and collapse of the trachea.

Approximately 3 months later, the cricoid fracture was reduced and the tracheal stenosis was repaired with a split-thickness skin graft over a polyethylene stent. This operation, which was performed through a vertical midline incision, was complicated by infection. Consequently, the stent was removed after 2 weeks. Shortly thereafter, complete stenosis of the trachea occurred.

The author first examined the patient 13 months after the tracheal repair described above. The patient had heard of "esophageal voice" and wondered whether she could learn this method of vocal communication with her larynx intact. Several months later, she consented to surgical treatment. The first stage reconstruction was scheduled nearly 2 years after the accident. Preoperative radiographs (Fig. 9–20A) showed the level and length of the cervical tracheal stenosis.

After the second-stage operation, the patient had a normal voice and an adequate airway with and without the Safe-T-Tube in place (Fig. 9–20B). Six years after the reconstruction, the patient's airway and vocal function were normal (Fig. 9–20C). She has been able to participate in such athletic activities as golf and swimming.

Chapter 10
The Montgomery Safe-T-Tube

WILLIAM W. MONTGOMERY   STUART K. MONTGOMERY

The first tracheal T-tube was developed for a patient who had sustained a crushing injury to the cervical trachea, resulting in a complete tracheal stenosis. With the existing technology, her only option was esophageal speech. The first-generation T-tube (1961) was constructed from acrylic plastic. It included an upper and lower intraluminal limb. The external limb was split in half (Fig. 10–1A). The upper and lower intraluminal portions of the T-tube were inserted separately and locked in place with an acrylic washer (Fig. 10–1B). A stopper was inserted into the external limb and, finally, a second washer was applied to stabilize the T-tube (Fig. 10–1C). The acrylic T-tube worked well but was stiff and cumbersome.

The next generation of T-tubes was made using medical-grade silicone. This one-piece design was flexible, soft, and not irritating to the surrounding tissues (Fig. 10–2). The tube was widened at the junction of the external and internal limbs to facilitate suctioning. The ends of the intraluminal portions were tapered to prevent irritation.

In 1984, it became apparent that a method to prevent inward displacement of the T-tube was necessary. At that time, ridges and grooves were added to the external limb. A washer applied to a groove, adjacent to the cervical skin, prevents inward displacement. This most recent version, the Montgomery Safe-T-Tube (Boston Medical Products, Westborough, MA) (Fig. 10–3) is designed to maintain an adequate airway to provide support for a stenotic trachea that has been reconstituted or reconstructed. The Safe-T-Tube can also be used to maintain an airway when the trachea cannot be repaired. Ridges and grooves along the extraluminal limb of the Safe-T-Tube allow a ring washer to be attached to help prevent posterior displacement of the tube. A speaking valve is available for the Safe-T-Tube, eliminating the need for finger occlusion by the patient during phonation.

Pediatric Safe-T-Tubes (Fig. 10–4) feature an angulated extraluminal limb to facilitate suctioning and airway management. These tubes are available in sizes 6 to 9 mm (outside diameter). Shortened limbs can be ordered on a custom basis from Boston Medical Products. The Pediatric Safe-T-Tubes are available in both clear and radiopaque silicone.

Standard Safe-T-Tubes (see Fig. 10–3) are available in sizes 10 to 16 mm (outside diameter) in both clear and radiopaque silicone. The Standard Safe-T-Tube series is based on the original design, which can be used in the majority of cases. Shortened limbs can be ordered on a custom basis from Boston Medical Products.

The Hebeler Safe-T-Tube (Fig. 10–5) features an integral internal balloon to adjust the airflow through the upper end of the tube. The balloon can be inflated for intermittent closure of the upper limb, creating a closed system between the tracheotomy and the lungs. After anesthesia or ventilation, the balloon is deflated and the upper limb becomes open for respiratory access. The Hebeler Safe-T-Tube is available in sizes 12, 15, and 18 mm (outside diameter).

The Thoracic Safe-T-Tubes (Fig. 10–6) feature an extra-long lower limb for thoracic applications. Varying lengths can be ordered from the company. The Thoracic Safe-T-Tube is available in sizes 10 to 16 mm (outside diameter).

The Extra-Long Safe-T-Tube (Fig. 10–7) is available to provide the surgeon total freedom to customize the intraluminal limbs to any desired length. If special lengths are known before surgery, custom length tubes can be ordered through Boston Medical Products. The Extra-Long Safe-T-Tube is available in sizes 10 to 16 mm (outside diameter).

The Tapered Safe-T-Tube (Fig. 10–8) is a unique tube with a dual-diameter design. The superior portion conforms to the contour of the glottis and subglottis, whereas the larger inferior diameter simultaneously acts as a stent for the trachea. The tapered end is designed to project up beyond the true cords to the level of the laryngeal ventricle. The Tapered Safe-T-Tube is available in two sizes: 8 mm/10 mm and 10 mm/13 mm (outside diameters of lower and upper ends).

The HMS System (Healy/Montgomery Stent System) (Fig. 10–9) combines the features of the Pediatric Safe-T-Tube with the advantages of an inner cannula system. It is designed to provide support during repair or reconstruction procedures of the subglottis and trachea. The stent is placed surgically by a laryngofissure and can be removed either endoscopically or by the tracheotomy. After the stent is in position, the inner cannula can be removed for cleaning without disturbing the repaired areas. The HMS System is available is sizes 7, 9, and 12 mm (outside diameter).

Statistically, the most commonly used sizes of the Safe-T-Tube are 10 to 13 mm. The curvature at the junction of the external and internal portions of the Safe-T-Tube is designed to facilitate cleaning and suctioning. The external

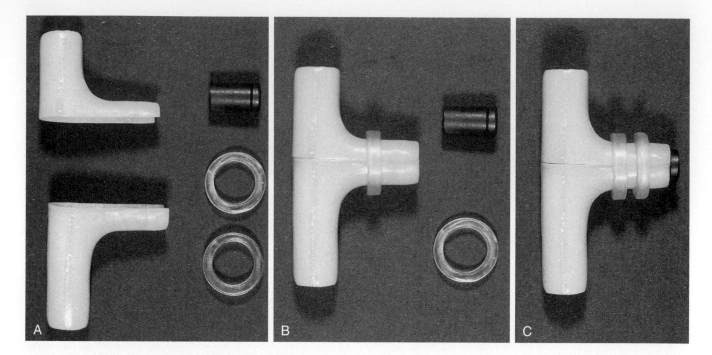

FIGURE 10-1. *A*, Original tracheal T-tube stent constructed from acrylic. Components are: upper and lower halves of the T-tube, two lock washers and a plug. *B*, The two halves have been joined after being inserted into the proximal and distal trachea. The first lock washer is applied to the external limb. *C*, The plug and second lock washer are in place.

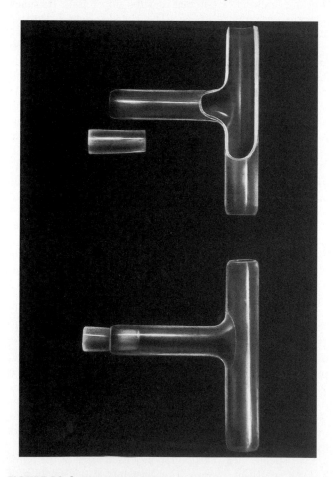

FIGURE 10-2. The original silicone T-tube was designed to serve as both a tracheal stent and a tracheostomy tube. The plug was also made of silicone. The portion of the T-tube that projects from the tracheotomy orifice is of smaller diameter than that of the intraluminal portion.

limb of the Safe-T-Tube can be tilted in an inferior or superior direction to facilitate insertion of suction tubing.

The Safe-T-Tube includes the following features:

1. It serves as both a stent and a tracheostomy tube.

2. Silicone initiates little or no tissue reaction. It does not harden on exposure to body temperature and secretions.

3. The intraluminal portion is sufficient to support a reconstituted or reconstructed trachea.

4. The intraluminal portion is soft enough not to injure the lining or supporting structure of the trachea.

5. The ends of the tube are tapered. Thus, injury does not occur with asynchronous motion between the end of the tube and the tracheal mucosa.

6. Mucus and crusts do not readily adhere to the smooth surfaces of the silicone.

7. The Safe-T-Tube is widened by the curvature at the junction of its intraluminal and extraluminal portions. This supports the anterior tracheal wall at the tracheostomy site and facilitates suctioning and cleaning.

8. The extraluminal portion is long enough to be used in an obese neck. This portion of the Safe-T-Tube can be shortened simply by cutting with scissors.

9. The Safe-T-Tube has ridges and grooves on the extraluminal limb to allow attachment of a ring washer to prevent posterior displacement. The grooves also allow a speaking valve to be attached, when indicated, and permit the Safe-T-Tube to be cut with scissors to a length more acceptable to the patient.

10. Drainage grooves along the superior and inferior aspects (6- and 12-o'clock positions) of the extraluminal limb aid in the drainage of secretions and serve to differentiate the inserted Safe-T-Tube from the inserted Montgomery tracheal cannula, which has only one longitudinal groove (6-o'clock position).

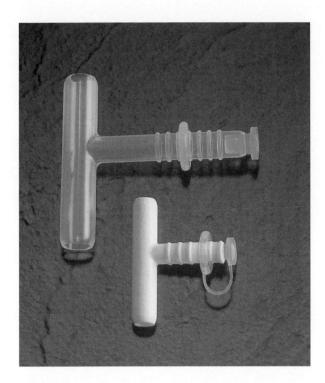

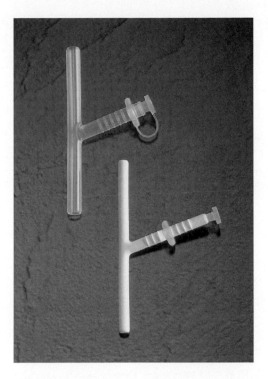

FIGURE 10-3. The Safe-T-Tube is designed to maintain an adequate tracheal airway and provide support to the stenotic trachea that has been reconstructed or reconstituted. The tube is made of nonirritating, flexible medical-grade silicone. The Safe-T-Tube is available in six styles–Pediatric, Standard, Hebeler (internal balloon), Thoracic, Extra-Long, and Tapered—in both clear and radiopaque silicone. The enlarged curvature of the junction of the extraluminal and intraluminal limbs facilitates cleaning and suctioning. Ridges and grooves along the extraluminal limb permit application of a ring washer, which helps prevent posterior displacement of the tube and also secure a speaking valve in place. The ring washer is applied to the groove adjacent to the cervical skin when the tube is in place. Two drainage grooves (at 6 and 12 o'clock) allow drainage of secretions and distinguish the inserted Safe-T-Tube from the Montgomery tracheal cannula, which has a groove at 6 o'clock only. If the distance between the skin and the first ridge is long, two washers can be applied to ensure stability of the tube. The plug is inserted with a twist and will not become dislodged even during forceful coughing. For patient convenience, the plug is attached to the ring washer via a silicone lanyard. The lanyard may be removed using scissors if desired.

FIGURE 10-4. The Montgomery Pediatric Safe-T-Tube.

11. The Safe-T-Tube is supplied with a plug that is secured by friction and will not become dislodged, even with forceful coughing.

12. The Safe-T-Tube does not need frequent changing. In cases when the trachea cannot be reconstructed, the Safe-T-Tube has remained in place and plugged for more than 3 years without a change.

13. The Safe-T-Tube remains plugged most of the time. (In one patient, it remained plugged for 21 years.) This allows for normal respiration and phonation while the tube is in place.

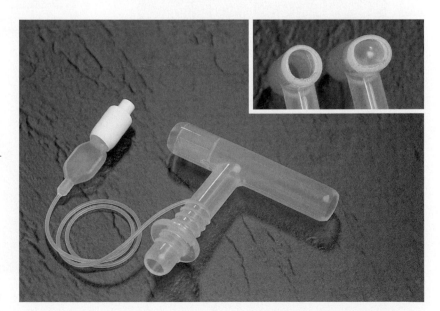

FIGURE 10-5. The Hebeler Safe-T-Tube. Inset: integral internal balloon shown both deflated and inflated.

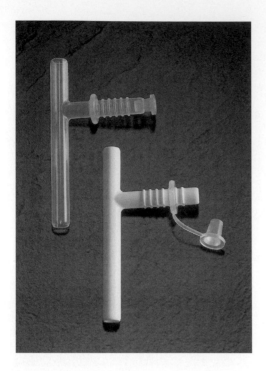

FIGURE 10–6. The Montgomery Thoracic Safe-T-Tube.

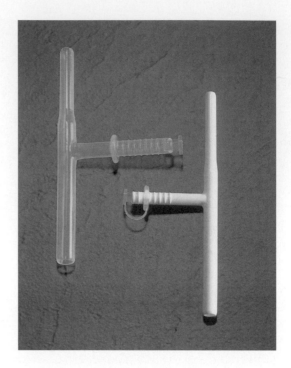

FIGURE 10–8. The Montgomery Tapered Safe-T-Tube.

INDICATIONS FOR USE

The Safe-T-Tube should be used in patients with:

1. acute tracheal injuries;
2. a need to support a reconstituted trachea;
3. a need to support a reconstructed trachea;
4. segmental resection and anastomosis;
5. a need to support intrathoracic tracheal stenosis;

6. tracheal stenosis when the cervical or thoracic trachea cannot be repaired; and
7. a cervical trachea that cannot be reconstructed.

Currently there are a number of patients with tracheas that cannot be reconstructed who have had Safe-T-Tubes in place for periods ranging from 3 to 12 years. A few patients in this group have, over a period of years, regenerated a mucosa-lined trachea supported by scar tissue, which has re-

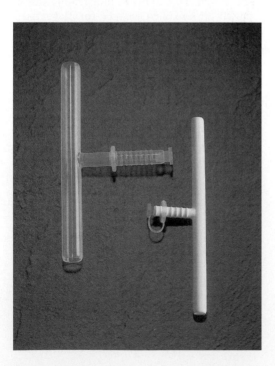

FIGURE 10–7. The Montgomery Extra-Long Safe-T-Tube.

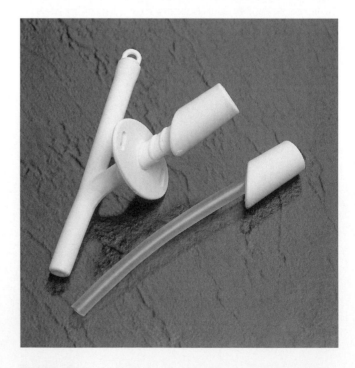

FIGURE 10–9. The HMS System (Healy/Montgomery Stent System).

mained adequately patent so that a Safe-T-Tube or a tracheostomy tube is not necessary.

INSERTION

The Safe-T-Tube should be inserted by a surgeon. Among the necessary equipment are suction apparatus and a large narrow curved hemostat. The Safe-T-Tube is usually in-serted in the operating room with the patient under general anesthesia. However, it can be reinserted in the office or at the bedside in patients who have had the Safe-T-Tube in place for several months.

The end of the intraluminal portion of the Safe-T-Tube, which is inserted inferiorly, is grasped with the index fin-gers and folded on itself (Fig. 10–10A). It is then grasped with the hemostat (Fig. 10–10B) and inserted into the dis-tal trachea by way of the tracheotomy (Fig. 10–10C). The

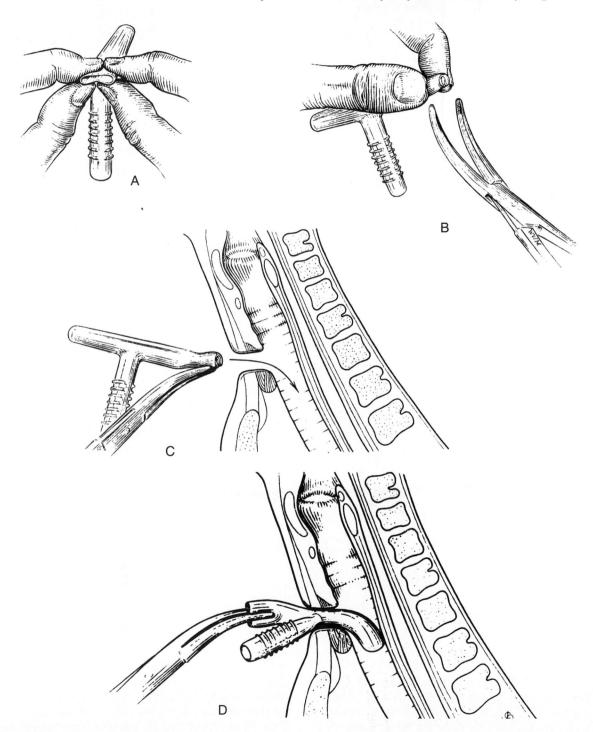

FIGURE 10–10. Insertion. *A*, The end of the intraluminal portion of the Safe-T-Tube, which will be inserted inferiorly, is grasped with index fingers and folded on itself. *B*, The crimped end is grasped with a hemostat. *C*, It is inserted into the distal trachea through the tracheostoma. *D*, The hemostat is released. The upper limb is grasped with the hemostat.

Illustration continued on following page

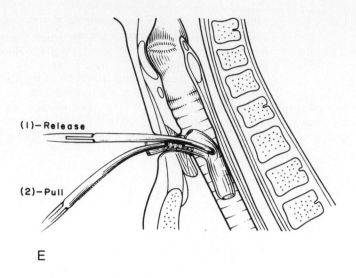

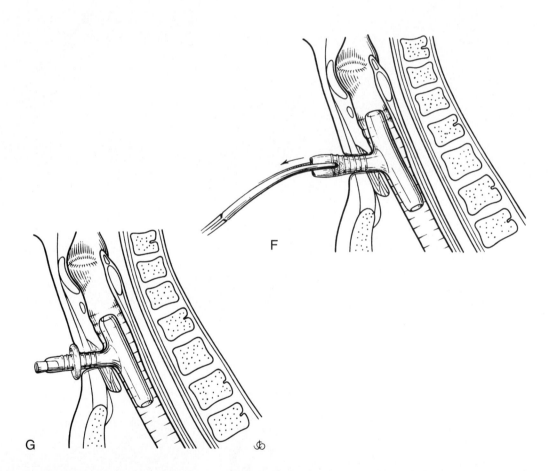

FIGURE 10–10. *Continued E,* The upper intraluminal limb is directed into the trachea until the entire intraluminal portion is in the lower trachea. The hemostat is again released. *F,* An anterior pull on the exterior portion of the Safe-T-Tube will direct the upper limb into proper position. *G,* The ring washer is applied to the groove adjacent to the skin surface.

hemostat is released. The upper intraluminal portion of the Safe-T-Tube is then grasped with the hemostat and directed into the trachea (Fig. 10–10D) until the entire intraluminal portion is within the trachea below the tracheotomy (Fig. 10–10E). The hemostat is again released. An anterior pull on the exterior portion of the Safe-T-Tube will direct the upper limb of the intraluminal portion into place (Fig. 10–10F). A ring washer is applied to the groove adjacent to the skin surface, and the groove is recorded (Fig. 10–10G). If the distance between the anterior tracheal wall and surface of the anterior cervical skin is short, two ring washers can be applied to maintain stability of the Safe-T-Tube.

SUCTIONING

The external portion of the Safe-T-Tube can be tilted superiorly or inferiorly to facilitate suctioning (Fig. 10–11). The junction of the intraluminal and extraluminal portions of the Safe-T-Tube is enlarged to allow for ease of insertion of suction tubing. It is important to select a suction catheter small enough to be inserted easily. In general, most patients require suctioning both superiorly and inferiorly several times a day during the first 10 days after insertion of the Safe-T-Tube. Thereafter, suctioning is usually necessary twice a day.

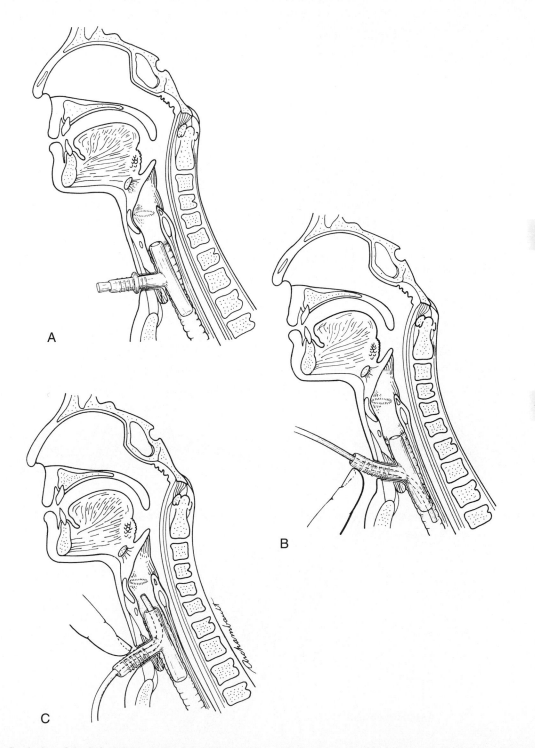

FIGURE 10–11. Suctioning of the Safe-T-Tube. *A,* The Safe-T-Tube in place with the plug inserted into the extraluminal limb. The upper intraluminal limb is usually shorter than the lower, although the tube can be reversed if additional length is needed superiorly. *B,* When suctioning the lower segment of the Safe-T-Tube and trachea, the extraluminal limb is evaluated as the suction tubing is inserted. *C,* The suction tubing is directed superiorly into the upper intraluminal limb of the Safe-T-Tube by bending the extraluminal limb in an inferior direction.

ANESTHESIA WITH THE SAFE-T-TUBE IN PLACE

The loss of anesthetic or air through the upper intraluminal limb of the Safe-T-Tube during surgery can be a problem (Fig. 10–12A). A simple solution to this problem is to use an arterial embolectomy catheter to obstruct the upper intraluminal limb of the Safe-T-Tube. The endotracheal tube attached to the extraluminal portion of the Safe-T-Tube is disconnected. The embolectomy catheter is inserted into the upper intraluminal segment and inflated (Fig. 10–12B). A closed system between the anesthesia apparatus and the distal trachea is established when the endotracheal tube is attached to the Safe-T-Tube (Fig. 10–12C). This technique also permits assisted ventilation with the Safe-T-Tube in place. The Hebeler Safe-T-Tube can also be used for this application (see Fig. 10–5).

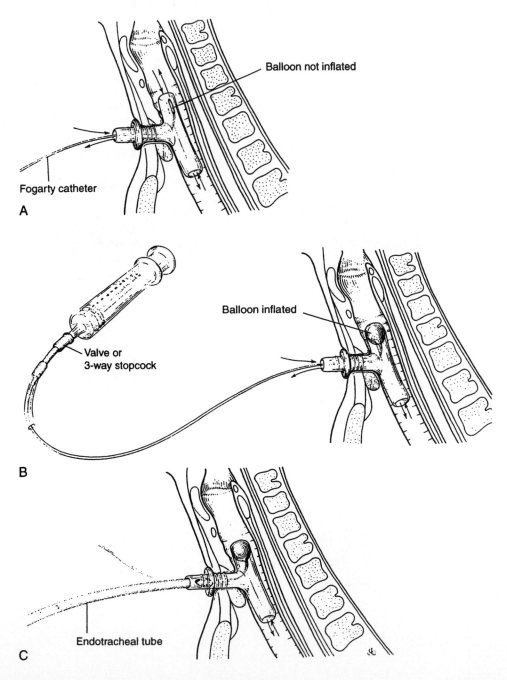

FIGURE 10–12. Anesthesia via the Safe-T-Tube. *A, Arrows:* direction of airflow. A embolectomy catheter is inserted into the upper intraluminal limb of the Safe-T-Tube. *B,* The balloon is inflated to obstruct the lumen of the upper intraluminal limb. *C,* An endotracheal tube is inserted into the extraluminal limb of the Safe-T-Tube to establish a closed system with the distal tracheobronchial system.

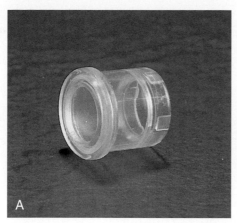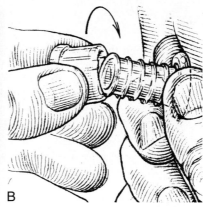

FIGURE 10–13. Speaking valve for the Safe-T-Tube. *A*, A special one-way valve is used when the airway is narrowed above the upper intraluminal limb. A very thin hinged diaphragm opens inward during inspiration and closes against the anterior aspect of the valve housing during expiration. *B*, The valve is easily applied to the shortened Safe-T-Tube and is held in place by four prongs that fit between the rings of the Safe-T-Tube.

SPEAKING VALVE

If the airway is narrowed above the upper intraluminal end of the Safe-T-Tube by edema or vocal fold paralysis in the medial position, a Montgomery speaking valve (Fig. 10–13) can be attached to the extraluminal portion of the Safe-T-Tube. The external limb is shortened to the desired length flush with a ridge using a No. 10 surgical blade. The valve is attached to the Safe-T-Tube and is held in place by four prongs that connect onto the ridge of the external limb of the Safe-T-Tube.

REMOVAL

Most patients do not require a change of the Safe-T-Tube before its final removal. However, occasionally it is necessary to remove and replace the Safe-T-Tube, for example, (1) if the intraluminal portion becomes partially obstructed and cannot be cleaned; (2) if the Safe-T-Tube is not properly positioned; (3) if, when removed, the repair does not appear to be completely healed; or (4) as an emergency procedure (by physician, nurse, or relative) if the Safe-T-Tube becomes obstructed. A tracheostomy tube with an obturator should be kept available to insert immediately after emergency removal of the Safe-T-Tube (Table 10–1).

To remove the Safe-T-Tube, the external limb is grasped with the thumb and index finger of one hand while the index and second finger of the other hand are placed against the skin above and below the external limb, exerting pressure posteriorly (Fig. 10–14*A* and *B*). The Safe-T-Tube is removed with a steady, firm anterior pressure of the extraluminal portion. On rare occasions (e.g., if the Safe-T-Tube has been in place for many months), it may be necessary to make a small vertical incision in the skin above and below the external limb of the Safe-T-Tube to facilitate its removal. The cautery on cutting current is best used for this. The endo-tracheal tube is then inserted during recovery (Fig. 10–14*C*).

POSTOPERATIVE CARE OF THE SAFE-T-TUBE

1. Continue antibiotics administered during surgery for at least 6 days postoperatively.

2. Maintain constant humidity over the Safe-T-Tube if the external limb is not plugged.

3. Keep external limb of the Safe-T-Tube plugged, if possible, when the patient has recovered from anesthesia.

4. Suction tube upward and downward (but not beyond the intraluminal ends) at least four times a day to keep the Safe-T-Tube clean internally.

5. Administer sodium bicarbonate solution (5%, 2 mL) every 4 to 8 hours as needed according to the amount of crusting.

6. Instill and lavage normal saline solution (2 to 5 mL) every 4 hours, or 15 minutes after Step 5.

7. Clean the skin around external portion of the Safe-T-Tube three times daily; remove crusts; apply povidone-iodine solution or 3% Bactroban ointment.

8. Clean the inside of the external limb of the Safe-T-Tube with a cotton-tipped applicator dipped in peroxide. Finish cleaning with dry cotton-tipped applicator.

TABLE 10–1
Corresponding Safe-T-Tube and Standard Tracheostomy Tube Sizes

Safe-T-Tube (mm)	Standard Tracheostomy Tube
6	4 pediatric
7	4 pediatric
8	5 pediatric
9	5 pediatric
10	5 pediatric
11	4 adult
12	4 adult
13	4 adult
14	4 adult
15	6 adult
16	6 adult

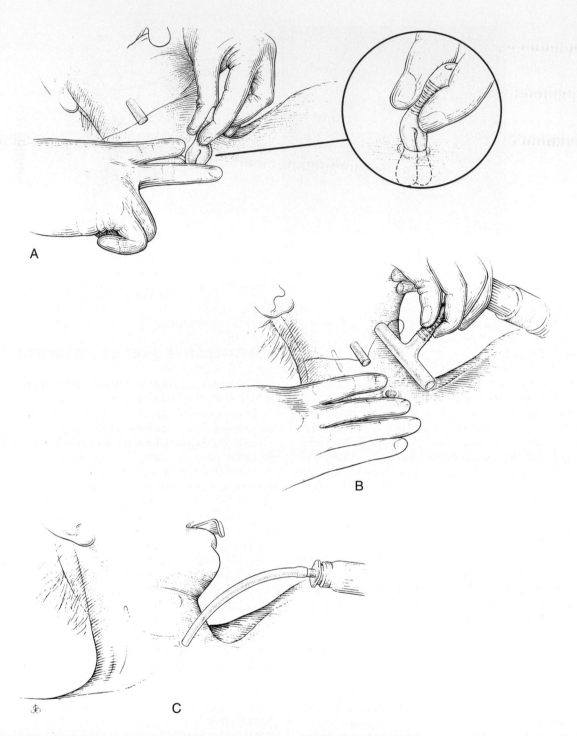

FIGURE 10-14. Removal of the Safe-T-Tube. *A*, A finger is placed above and below the external limb to exert pressure in a posterior direction. As the Safe-T-Tube is pulled from the trachea, the upper and lower intraluminal limbs buckle toward each other *(insert)*. *B*, The Safe-T-Tube springs back to proper shape after the intraluminal limbs part from the tracheotomy fistula. *C*, The endotracheal tube is inserted until the patient has recovered from general anesthesia.

LONG-TERM CARE OF THE SAFE-T-TUBE

1. Continue to use the plug in the external limb of the Safe-T-Tube when possible.

2. Suction upward and downward two to three times daily.

3. If necessary, administer sodium bicarbonate (5%) and saline twice a day.

4. Continue cleaning inside of the Safe-T-Tube twice daily.

5. Continue skin care around the Safe-T-Tube twice daily.

6. If the Safe-T-Tube becomes obstructed, it should be pulled out immediately and a tracheostomy tube inserted. The patient should always have a standard tracheostomy tube available in case emergency removal of the Safe-T-Tube is necessary (see Table 10–1).

Chapter 11
Surgery of the Larynx

WILLIAM W. MONTGOMERY

EXTERNAL APPROACH FOR THE RESECTION OF BENIGN SUBMUCOSAL LARYNGEAL LESIONS

Benign submucosal, supraglottic, and intraglottic neoplasms (including cysts) gradually interfere with phonation and encroach on the laryngeal airway, necessitating their surgical removal. Seen with indirect laryngoscopy, these lesions appear as submucosal swellings involving one side of the larynx. Depending on their position and size, they distort the false vocal cord, laryngeal ventricle, and aryepiglottic fold. In so doing, they extend to or beyond the midline, interfering with the respiratory and phonatory function of the larynx. It is not possible to view the true vocal cord on the side of the lesion with indirect laryngoscopy. However, routine anteroposterior and lateral neck radiographs along with axial computed tomography (CT) scan of the larynx allow the surgeon to locate and differentiate tumors from cysts (Fig. 11–1). If the lesion is solid, it is best to confirm the diagnosis by means of a direct laryngoscopy and biopsy. A biopsy is best obtained by first incising the mucous membrane and then using cupped forceps to bite into the solid lesion. If the lesion is cystic, the surgeon can proceed directly to removal by the external approach. The linear biopsy incision will heal rapidly and not interfere with complete removal of a solid lesion by way of the external approach.

The operation is performed with the patient's head slightly extended and turned to the side opposite the lesion. It is important for the surgeon to have a good knowledge of the anatomic relations in this area (Fig. 11–2). The superior laryngeal nerve may be endangered if the surgeon fails to remember that the internal branch pierces the thyrohyoid membrane at about the level of the notch created by the junction of the superior horn with the lamina of the thyroid cartilage. The external branch of the superior laryngeal nerve is more lateral, passing down over the inferior constrictor to supply the cricothyroid muscle.

Usually a tracheotomy is part of the operation, except when the lesion is small and there is very little reaction. If the lesion is large and the patient is dyspneic, induction of general anesthesia and intubation may be difficult and hazardous. In such cases, local anesthesia is used for the tracheotomy, followed by insertion of an endotracheal tube and general anesthesia.

A horizontal incision is used for this operation. The incision extends from the anterior border of the sternocleidomastoid muscle on the involved side to just beyond the midline, at a level just below the thyroid notch. The incision is made through the platysma to the fascia covering the sternohyoid and omohyoid muscles (Fig. 11–3).

A plane of cleavage is established over the sternohyoid and omohyoid muscles for exposure (Fig. 11–3B). The best exposure is obtained after sectioning these two muscles at the level of the thyroid notch. It is possible to perform this operation by retracting the muscles laterally with a self-retaining retractor. If the muscles are sectioned, chromic catgut sutures (No. 00) are used to retract them (Fig. 11–4). These sutures can be used to reapproximate the muscles during the closure.

The perichondrium over the lateral aspect of the upper half of the thyroid lamina on the uninvolved side is carefully exposed. It is incised on the anterior midline and then along the superior rim, to within 5 to 10 cm of the base of the superior horn (see Fig. 11–4A). It is then elevated from the anterior aspect of the thyroid lamina and reflected inferiorly (Fig. 11–4B). With a slightly curved, sharp periosteal elevator with a round end, the perichondrium is carefully lifted with a straight elevator from the superior margin of the thyroid cartilage. This cartilage is continuous with the perichondrium attached to the posterior side of the thyroid lamina (Fig. 11–4C).

With adequate exposure, the cartilage of the upper half of the thyroid lamina is removed by sharp dissection. If ossification has not occurred, the cartilage can be removed in one segment. Kerrison forceps are used as shown in Figure 11–5A. The oblique line of the cartilage is a useful landmark for the lateral limit of the resection. If the tumor is large, the superior laryngeal vessels and nerves should be identified so that they will not be injured. After the thyroid cartilage has been removed, a bulge produced by the tumor may be seen. A horizontal incision is made through the perichondrium and quadrangular membrane, exposing the lateral aspect of the tumor (Fig. 11–5B and C). The lesion can then be removed.

The cavity created by the removal of the tumor is carefully inspected for both bleeding and dehiscences in the lar-

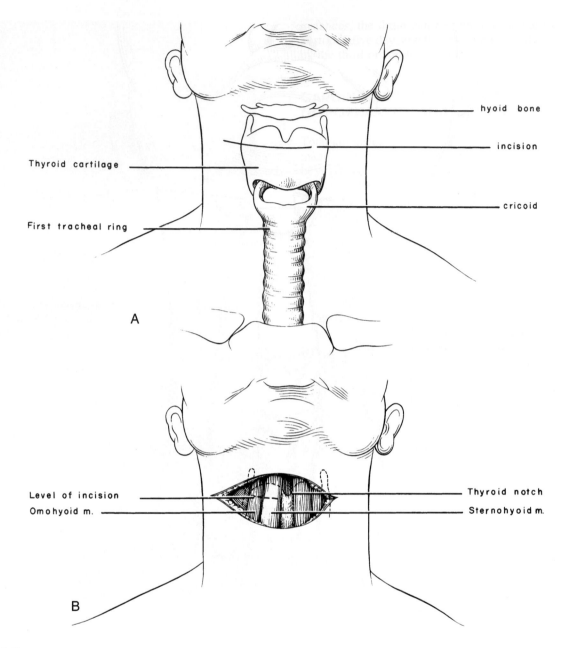

FIGURE 11-3. Resection of a benign submucosal laryngeal lesion by the external approach. *A,* A tracheotomy should be part of this operation if the lesion is large or the patient is dyspneic. It is probably best performed with the use of local anesthesia. Otherwise, an endotracheal tube is inserted, and the tracheotomy is performed before or after the laryngeal procedure, according to the surgeon's choice. *B,* Anterior aspect of the thyroid cartilage and the thyroid notch is exposed. The level for section of the sternohyoid and omohyoid muscles is indicated. Exposure can also be accomplished by retracting the sternohyoid and omohyoid muscles laterally.

TNM CLASSIFICATION

Primary Tumor (T)

TX Minimum requirements to assess the primary tumor cannot be met
T0 No evidence primary tumor

Hypopharynx

T1s Carcinoma in situ
T1 Tumor confined to one site

T2 Extension of tumor to adjacent region or site without fixation of hemilarynx
T3 Extension of tumor to adjacent region or site with fixation of hemilarynx
T4 Massive tumor invading bone or soft tissues of neck

Supraglottis

T1s Carcinoma in situ
T1 Tumor confined to region of origin with normal mobility

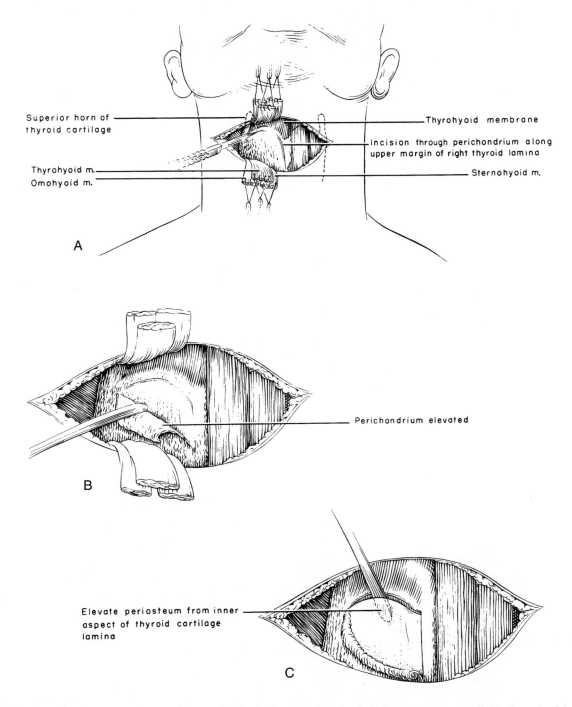

Superior horn of
thyroid cartilage

Thyrohyoid membrane

Incision through perichondrium along
upper margin of right thyroid lamina

Thyrohyoid m.

Omohyoid m.

Sternohyoid m.

A

Perichondrium elevated

B

Elevate periosteum from inner
aspect of thyroid cartilage
lamina

C

FIGURE 11-4. Resection of a benign submucosal laryngeal lesion by the external approach. *A,* Catgut sutures are applied to the ends of the strap muscles. These are left long for traction and can also be used to approximate the muscles during closure. A perichondrial incision is made vertically, in the midline, and along the superior rim of the right thyroid lamina, nearly to the base of the superior horn. *B,* The perichondrium is elevated from the anterior surface of the right thyroid lamina. *C,* The perichondrium is elevated from the inner aspect of the right thyroid lamina.

T2　Tumor involving adjacent supraglottic site(s) or glottis without fixation

T3　Tumor limited to larynx with fixation or extension to involve postcricoid area, medial wall of pyriform sinus, or pre-epiglottic space.

T4　Massive tumor extending beyond the larynx to involve oropharynx or soft issues of neck, or destruction of thyroid cartilage

Glottis

T1s　Carcinoma in situ

T1　Tumor confined to vocal cord(s) with normal mobility (includes involvement of anterior or posterior commissures)

T1b　Lesions in more than one site, same region

T2　Supraglottic or subglottic extension of tumor with normal or impaired cord mobility, or both

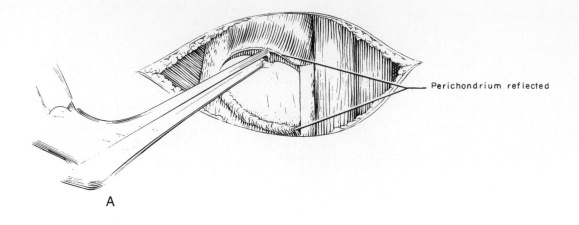

A

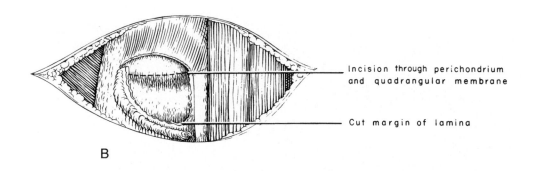

B

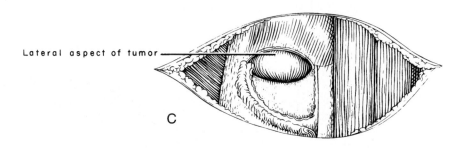

C

FIGURE 11–5. Resection of a benign submucosal laryngeal lesion by the external approach. *A,* In a young patient, the thyroid cartilage can be incised and removed in one segment. However, because any degree of ossification makes this impossible, the cartilage must be removed with Kerrison forceps. If cartilage must be removed lateral to the oblique line, it is best to identify the superior laryngeal vessels and nerve so that they will not be injured. *B,* An incision is made through the inner perichondrium and the quadrangular membrane, varying, of course, according to the presenting dome of the tumor. *C,* Usually the lateral aspect of the tumor becomes immediately apparent. The lesion is a laryngocele, mucous cyst, or solid tumor. The laryngocele is opened, and the surgeon's index finger is inserted into its lumen to facilitate removal. The arytenoid cartilage and true vocal cord can be palpated with the finger for orientation. If the laryngocele ends in a stalk, it is ligated. A cystic lesion is treated in the same manner as a laryngocele after its contents have been aspirated. The solid lesion is most often encapsulated and shells out very easily.

T3   Tumor confined to the larynx with cord fixation
T4   Massive tumor with destruction of thyroid cartilage or extension beyond the confines of the larynx, or both

Subglottis

T1s   Carcinoma in situ
T1   Tumor confined to subglottic region
T2   Tumor extension to vocal cords with normal or impaired cord mobility

T2   Tumor extension to vocal cords with normal or impaired cord mobility
T3   Tumor confined to larynx with cord fixation
T4   Massive tumor with cartilage destruction or extension beyond the confines of the larynx, or both

Nodal Involvement (N)

Cervical Node Classification

In clinical evaluation, the actual size of the nodal mass should be measured and allowance should be made for in-

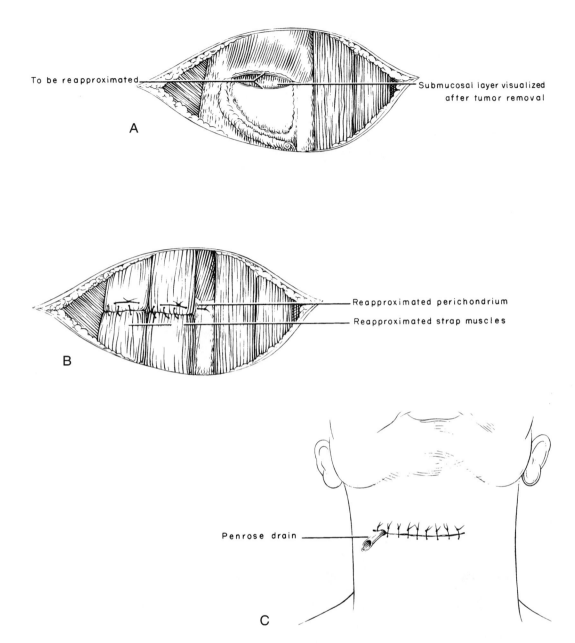

FIGURE 11-6. Resection of a benign submucosal laryngeal lesion by the external approach. *A,* The cavity created by removal of the tumor is demonstrated. This is the submucosal layer of the larynx. If laryngeal mucosal defects occur during resection of the tumor, they should be carefully sutured with a No. 4-0 chromic catgut. *B,* The sternohyoid and the omohyoid muscles have been sutured. Underneath are the reapproximated thyrohyoid muscle, perichondrial layers of the right thyroid lamina, and quadrangle membrane. *C,* A Penrose drain should extend into the space remaining after tumor removal to prevent a hematoma or subcutaneous emphysema resulting from a defect in the laryngeal mucous membrane. Closed suction drainage can also be used.

tervening soft tissues. Most masses over 3 cm in diameter are not single nodes but are either confluent nodes or tumors in the soft tissues of the neck. There are three stages of clinically positive nodes: N1, N2, and N3. The use of subgroups a, b, and c is not required but recommended. Midline nodes are considered homolateral nodes. A CT scan of the neck is valuable when classifying cervical metastases.

NX Minimum requirements to assess the regional node cannot be met
N0 No clinically positive node

N1 Single clinically positive homolateral node 3 cm or less in diameter
N2 Single clinically positive homolateral node more than 3 cm but not more than 6 cm in diameter, or multiple clinically positive homolateral nodes, none more than 6 cm in diameter
N2a Single clinically positive homolateral node more than 3 cm but not more than 6 cm in diameter
N2b Multiple clinically positive homolateral nodes, none more than 6 cm in diameter
N3 Massive homolateral node(s), bilateral nodes, or contralateral node(s)

TABLE 11-1
Anatomic Definitions of the Larynx That Accompany Figure 11-7

Region	Site
Red = Supraglottis	Ventricular bands (false cords)
	Arytenoids
	Epiglottis (both lingual and laryngeal aspects)
	Suprahyoid epiglottis
	Infrahyoid epiglottis
	Arytenoepiglottic folds
Blue = Glottis true vocal cords, including anterior and posterior commissures	
Yellow = Subglottis	Subglottis
(a) T0—No tumor	
T1s—Carcinoma in situ	
Red = Supraglottic	
Blue = Glottic	One site of one region—normal function
Yellow = Subglottic	
(b) T1b—Tumor involving more than one site, same region	
Red = Supraglottic—2 sites	
Blue = Glottic, normal mobility—2 sites	Normal mobility— 2 sides
Yellow = Subglottic	
(c) T2b—Tumor extending to another laryngeal anatomic region	
Red = Supraglottic	Extension to cord
Blue = Glottic	Normal or impaired mobility
Yellow = Subglottic	Extension to cord
(d) T3—Tumor extending to another laryngeal anatomic region with fixation	
Red = Supraglottic	With fixation
	Destruction
	Deep invasion Limited to larynx
Blue = Glottic	Fixation of cord(s)
Yellow = Subglottic	Fixation of cord(s)
(e) T4—Tumor extending beyond larynx	
Red = Supraglottic	1) Vallecula
	2) Base of tongue
	3) Pyriform sinus
	4) Postcricoid
	5) Hypopharynx
Blue = Glottic	1) Pyriform sinus
	2) Postcricoid
	3) Into cartilage
Yellow = Subglottic	1) Trachea
	2) Thyroid gland
	3) Postcricoid

swelling resulting from this procedure may distort the picture. General anesthesia is best used for the laryngoscopy and biopsy, and the smallest possible endotracheal tube should be used (No. 3 to 5.5 endotracheal tube). Sufficient biopsy material should be obtained to make an accurate diagnosis, but not so much as to compromise an already partially obstructed airway. If necessary, the function of the laryngeal structures can be studied by fiberoptic laryngoscopy and fluoroscopy if necessary. Function can also be studied as the patient recovers from general anesthesia.

A careful evaluation of the cervical region is essential. The size and location of enlarged lymph nodes should be carefully recorded. It is important to record whether an enlarged lymph gland is fixed or tender. Evaluation of the thyroid gland is essential, as is a CT scan of the neck, to determine the size and location of metastatic lymph nodes.

Planning the Treatment

Unfortunately, there are no set rules for managing a malignant lesion of the laryngopharynx, even after the lesion has been classified and staged. However, certain generalizations can be made that greatly assist in making the final decision.

Some basic information must be obtained before planning the treatment for any malignant lesion of the laryngopharynx. Each patient must be considered individually after a complete evaluation has been made, taking into account his or her age and life expectancy, personality, mental stability, occupation or profession, economic and family situation, and the distance between the patient's home and the site of treatment. The primary lesion must be evaluated with respect to its exact location, overall size, and duration of symptoms referable to it, as well as whether it is exophytic, ulcerative, infiltrative, or submucosal. Whether the lesion is undifferentiated or well differentiated must also be considered.

The evaluation of cervical metastasis is of utmost importance. Cervical lymph nodes are evaluated by both palpation and CT scan. A small, moveable, nontender lymph node in the middle-anterior jugular chain and an otherwise negative CT scan usually indicate a good prognosis. A lymph node that is tender and that has been present for a short period of time may be inflammatory rather than neoplastic; however, it could be both. In such instances, the possibility of an infection in the primary lesion should be considered and, if present, the infection must be treated. An enlarged, fixed lymph node in the neck usually indicates a poor prognosis. Chemotherapy, radiation, and surgery should be considered. If the CT scan indicates that the carotid artery is involved, the patient should receive work-up for a possible resection of the carotid artery and replacement.

Clinical or radiographic evidence of metastasis, other than in the cervical region, further complicates the therapeutic decision. A single metastasis (e.g., a single pulmonary metastasis), conversely, can often be treated by surgery, radiation, or a combination of the two. This can be accomplished before or after treating the primary lesion.

Methods of Treatment

One way to make the decision about what type of therapy to use is to place yourself in the patient's position. If you were the patient, would you elect treatment by:

1. radiation therapy?
2. radiation therapy, with the possibility of surgery if the response to radiation therapy was not rapid and complete after a total of 4000 rad was administered?
3. surgery?
4. surgery followed by radiation therapy?
5. chemotherapy followed, after a complete response, by radiation therapy? or
6. chemotherapy followed by radiation therapy and surgery?

Treatment—General Rules

Stages I and II
Radiation therapy twice daily and/or conservation surgery.

Stages III and IV
Carcinoma of the larynx at stages III and IV may be best treated with:

1. Radical surgery (total laryngectomy, laryngopharyngectomy, laryngoesophagectomy) combined with unilateral or bilateral radical or modified neck dissection, depending on the extent of the disease. If there is extension to the thyroid gland, thyroidectomy is also included with the surgery.
2. A full course of twice-daily radiation therapy to the primary laryngeal site and both sides of the neck, especially when the tumor extends subglottically, when there is involvement of the laryngeal cartilages, when there is extranodal spread, and when the surgical margins are not free of disease.
3. Three or four cycles of chemotherapy, as per the medical oncologist.

Supraglottic

T1s
Radiation therapy
Resection using laser
Supraglottic partial laryngectomy
T1
Radiation therapy or supraglottic partial laryngectomy
T2
Radiation therapy to primary lesion and both sides of the neck
Supraglottic or suprahemilaryngectomy with ipsilateral neck dissection
Midline lesions with unilateral cervical lymph nodes involved, radiation therapy to primary and both necks, or surgery to resect the primary and bilateral neck dissection.

T3
Extended supraglottic laryngectomy with neck dissection if lesion extends to medial wall of pyriform sinus or pre-epiglottic space without vocal cord fixation
A total laryngectomy is usually indicated if the anterior aspect of the opposite vocal cord is involved, if there is extension to and fixation of the vocal cord, or extension to the posterior commissure, extension to the postcricoid region into the laryngeal cartilages, or if there has been a radiation therapy failure.
T4
Three cycles of chemotherapy, a course of radiation therapy and a total laryngectomy, combined with pharyngectomy or esophagectomy, if these regions are involved, along with a bilateral neck dissection. There is some controversy as to whether the radiation therapy should precede or follow the surgery.

Glottic

T1s or T1a
Microlaryngoscopy and stripping of vocal cord or resection using the CO_2 laser, followed by close monthly observation (strip, observe, rebiopsy if cord is not normal, strip again, radiation therapy if positive)
T1b
As above plus full course of twice-daily radiation therapy
T2
Full course of twice-daily radiation therapy followed by close observation; a hemilaryngectomy can be performed if there is radiation therapy failure
T3
Total laryngectomy
Full course of twice-daily radiation therapy to the larynx and both sides of the neck, if the patient refuses laryngectomy
T4
Chemotherapy
Radiation therapy
Total laryngectomy with bilateral neck dissection

Subglottic

T1 and T2
Twice-daily radiation therapy to the larynx, both sides of the neck, and mediastinum
T3 and T4
Chemotherapy
Total laryngectomy
Ipsilateral thyroidectomy along with isthmus
Lateral neck dissection
Twice-daily radiation therapy to the larynx, both sides of the neck, and mediastinum

Radiation Therapy

Radiation therapy appears to be the treatment of choice for stage I lesions of the vocal cord. Reports indicate a cure rate of up to 92% after this therapy. This high percentage includes the bonus of lesions (carcinoma in situ) that would not have recurred after biopsy if left untreated. Norris and Peale (1966) reported on 16 patients with superficial cordal squamous cell carcinoma that were removed at the time of biopsy. The appearance of the vocal cords rapidly returned to normal within 2 to 3 weeks after the procedure. Eleven of the patients had no recurrence. Five required radiation therapy because of recurrent disease; none had recurrences after this treatment.

Tumors involving both vocal cords with normal mobility (stage 2) respond well to radiation therapy. The response is poor, however, when the anterior commissure is extensively implicated.

Tumors confined to the laryngeal surface of the epiglottis and not extending to the aryepiglottic folds or base of the epiglottis are suitable for radiation therapy. This treatment should also be considered for small tumors confined to one side of the immediate subglottic region.

Advanced lesions that cannot be surgically resected, lesions with fixed high or low cervical metastases, or lesions with distant metastases should receive palliative radiation therapy or should be considered for chemotherapy, surgery, and radiation therapy. The purpose of this therapy is to improve function, relieve pain, and prolong life. Occasionally, there will be a cure.

Surgical Treatment

Surgical treatments can be considered for all lesions of the glottis, except those on one or both cords, without fixation.

Lesions involving the vocal cord with less than 10 mm of subglottic extension, no extension above the undersurface of the false vocal cord, or no involvement of the anterior third of the opposite cord can be considered for a hemilaryngectomy. Hemilaryngectomy is contraindicated if there is extension of disease to or through the thyroid cartilage, metastasis to the precricoid lymph nodes, extension of disease to the posterior commissure, or complete fixation of the vocal cord.

Many laryngeal surgeons prefer to manage stage I lesions with surgery rather than radiation therapy, especially when radiation is a geographic hardship. Numerous surgical procedures have been suggested to improve vocal function after partial resection of the glottis. These procedures are discussed in another section of this chapter.

All glottic lesions mentioned above that are not suitable for partial laryngectomy or hemilaryngectomy must be treated by a wide-field total resection of the larynx.

Combined Chemotherapy, Surgery, and Radiation Therapy

Supraglottic lesions of the laryngopharynx should be considered for treatment by a combination of conservation surgery, total laryngectomy, or total resection of the laryngopharynx and a subsequent course of twice-daily radiation therapy.

Patients Eligible for Conservation Surgery of the Supraglottic Region

1. Supraglottic lesions, which are restricted to an area between the tip of the epiglottis (laryngeal surface) and the false vocal cords.

2. Superior hypopharyngeal lesions or tumors confined to the lingual surface of the epiglottis, vallecula, and base of the tongue posterior to the circumvallate papillae.

3. Pyriform sinus lesions that are limited inferiorly by the apex of the pyriform sinus, superiorly by the lateral glossoepiglottic fold, laterally by the thyroid cartilage, and medially by the aryepiglottic fold and arytenoid cartilage.

4. Posterior pharyngeal tumors that are confined between the lateral margins of the pyriform sinuses and that do not extend below the cricoid inferiorly or the base of the tongue superiorly.

After the evaluation by visualization and CT scan, the surgeon must be certain that the lesion can be resected, with an adequate margin of normal tissue, and also that the patient's respiratory, phonatory, and deglutitory functions are preserved.

Radiation therapy is administered 4 to 6 weeks after the surgery, depending on the progress of healing and whether the patient is swallowing well and underwent decannulation. It is best to perform a radical or functional neck dissection on all patients with supraglottic partial laryngectomies because there is a high incidence (in excess of 30%) of undetectable cervical metastases. Some surgeons and radiotherapists believe that such necks can be treated by radiation therapy, with results as successful as with a neck dissection.

Primary Radiation Therapy, Chemotherapy With Possible Surgery

Certain lesions of the laryngopharynx respond well to radiation therapy and do not recur. To date, no method has been devised to determine which lesions will respond in this manner. To use radiation therapy as the primary method of treatment for all lesions of the laryngopharynx would be unwise and would reduce the incidence of cure, which has gradually increased during the past decade. However, I believe that small lesions (squamous cell carcinoma) of the laryngopharynx that are exophytic, are of short duration, that do not interfere with muscle or joint function, and remain relatively asymptomatic (that is, do not produce symptoms such as odynophonia, odynophagia, or referred discomfort) should be considered individually.

Radiation is the primary treatment for such lesions. The laryngologist and the radiation therapist carefully observe the response of the lesion to this therapy. Twice-daily radiation therapy is preferred. If the tumor appears to be responding well, the therapy is continued to 6000 rad. Conversely, if the response is slow and the lesion is still present after 4000 rad has been administered, surgery is performed 4 to 6 weeks after the completion of a full course of radiation therapy. Many surgeons will disagree with this plan; they believe that a subtotal laryngectomy is always indicated.

Whenever possible, the lesion should be evaluated by both the laryngologist and the radiotherapist before the biopsy is performed. The patient is reevaluated after the first week of radiation therapy (1000 rad). By this time, the response should be definite, with moderate to marked reduction in the size of the lesion. The patient is again examined after the second week (2000 rad). At this time, much of the lesion should be absent, and all functions of the laryngopharynx should remain normal. The final evaluation is made after 4000 rad has been administered. If the lesion is still present, the therapy is continued to 6000 rad. If not, a definitive operation is scheduled for 4 to 6 weeks after the final radiation treatment.

Advanced lesions of the laryngopharynx should be considered for triple therapy, ie, chemotherapy, radiation therapy, and surgery. The three specialists should work together with all of these lesions, treating each patient individually.

TOTAL LARYNGECTOMY

Skin Lesion

The two most popular incisions for total laryngectomy are the T-incision and the U-incision. The latter is preferred because of the decreased incidence of persistent fistulas with its use. The U-incision begins superiorly on each side of the neck at a point corresponding approximately to the tip of the greater horns of the hyoid bone (Fig. 11–8) The incisions are carried inferiorly along the anterior (medial) border of the sternocleidomastoid muscle. They join in the anterior midline 1 cm below the level of the cricoid cartilage. The incision is continued through the platysma muscle. The anterior jugular and communicating veins are divided and ligated. It is best to either cauterize or ligate the bleeders before elevating the apron flap.

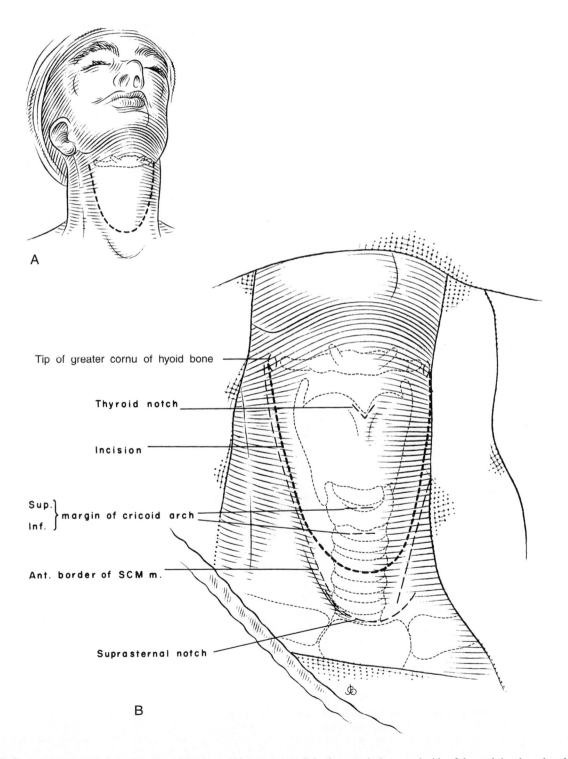

Tip of greater cornu of hyoid bone

Thyroid notch

Incision

Sup.
Inf. } margin of cricoid arch

Ant. border of SCM m.

Suprasternal notch

FIGURE 11–8. *A*, A U-shaped incision is preferred for the total laryngectomy. It begins superiorly on each side of the neck just lateral to the tip of the hyoid bone. It extends inferiorly to below the level of the cricoid cartilage and continues through the platysma muscle. *B*, Note the relationship between the laryngectomy incisions and the surrounding anatomical structures.

Elevation of the Flap

The inferior margin of the apron flap is retraced superiorly with skin hooks. Elevation is accomplished by establishing a plane just superficial to the strap muscles. The platysma muscle and anterior jugular veins are elevated with the flap (Fig. 11–9A). The dissection is continued superiorly until the anterior body of the hyoid bone is palpated. The fascia superior to the hyoid bone is incised exposing the suprahyoid musculature (mylohyoid muscle). Either scissors or a knife may be used for this dissection. The flap may be sutured superiorly to either the drapes or the chin. The suture should be placed through the subcutaneous tissue of the flap rather than through the dermal layer.

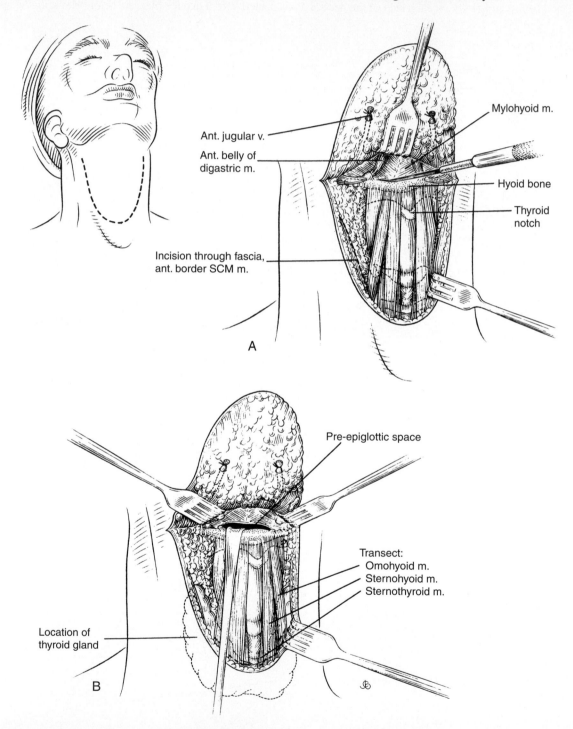

FIGURE 11–9. *A,* After establishing a plane just superficial to the strap muscles, the platysma muscle and the anterior jugular veins are elevated with the flap. The flap is sutured superiorly to the chin. This suture is placed through the subcutaneous tissue of the flap rather than through the dermal layer. The flap should be kept moist throughout the operation. Note the incision of the fascia just anterior and medial to the sternocleidomastoid muscle on the right side. Using a cutting current, the suprahyoid muscles are dissected from the body of the hyoid bone laterally to the lesser cornu on each side. *B,* After a plane of cleavage has been established between the sternohyoid and sternohyoid muscles by blunt dissection, the sternohyoid muscle on each side is transected. The omohyoid muscles are identified on each side and also transected.

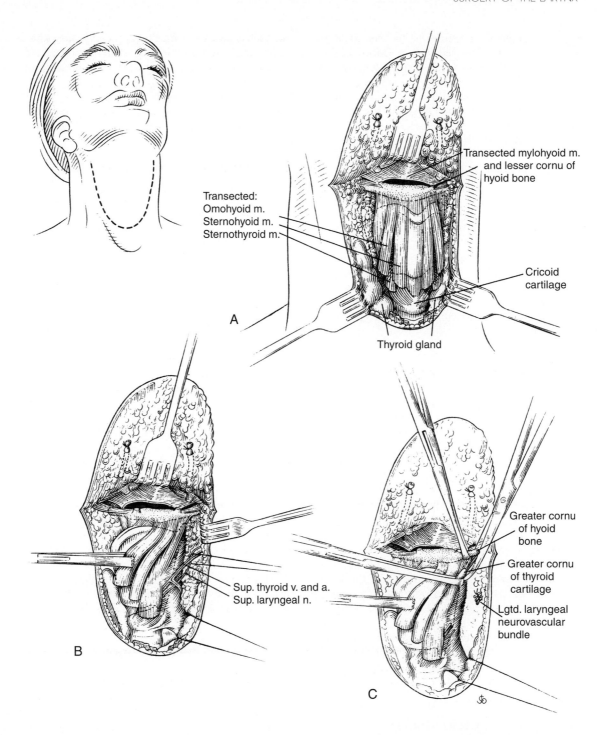

FIGURE 11-10. *A,* The sternohyoid, omohyoid, and sternothyroid muscles have been transected, exposing the thyroid gland on each side, the thyroid isthmus, and, occasionally, the cricoid cartilage. The suprahyoid musculature has been transected along with the lesser cornu of the hyoid bone. *B,* The larynx is rotated to the right by grasping the strap muscles with a Lahey thyroid clamp. The lesser horns of the hyoid bone have been transected. The superior thyroid artery and vein and superior laryngeal nerve are identified by blunt dissection. They are clamped, divided, and ligated. *C,* The tip of the hyoid bone is grasped with Allis forceps and dissected free with scissors. The superior horn of the thyroid cartilage is dissected free after May scissors have been placed behind and along its long axis.

The fascia just anterior or medial to the sternocleidomastoid muscle is carefully incised with a knife (see Fig. 11–9, right side). This allows the fascia surrounding the sternocleidomastoid muscle to be carefully preserved, thus preventing unnecessary postoperative discomfort. The carotid sheath is identified on each side and palpated for evidence of enlarged lymph nodes.

Transection of the sternothyroid muscles must be accomplished with care because of the numerous superficial vessels on the thyroid gland.

Sectioning of the Extrinsic Laryngeal and Suprahyoid Musculature

The body of the hyoid bone is grasped with either an Allis or a thyroid clamp and retracted anteroinferiorly. This tenses the suprahyoid musculature and exposes the superior surface of the body of the hyoid bone. Using a cautery, the suprahyoid musculature is separated from the hyoid bone, staying right on the bone surface (Fig. 11–9).

Superolateral Dissection (FIGURE 11-10)

Dissection is continued laterally along the superior surface of the hyoid bone (Fig. 11–10A). The lesser horns of the hyoid bone are transected. The surgeon dissects the soft tissues along the upper surface of the great horn of the hyoid bone while an assistant retracts the larynx to one side with a gauze sponge or thyroid clamp (Fig. 11–10B).

The greater horn of the hyoid bone on each side is grasped with an Allis clamp, and the tip of the hyoid bone is carefully dissected from the fascia and muscle (Fig. 11–10C). This portion of the dissection must be done with extreme care because of the proximity of most of the major structures in the neck to the tip of the greater horn of the hyoid bone. The remainder of the superior surface of the hyoid bone is then dissected free. The superior horn of the thyroid cartilage is palpated, grasped at its base with an Allis forceps, and pulled forward. The superior horn of the thyroid cartilage is dissected free by placing a male scissors behind and along its long access. The attachment of the inferior constrictor muscle of the thyroid cartilage is dissected free as indicated by the dotted line.

Suture-Ligature of the Thyroid Isthmus
(FIGURE 11-11)

The thyroid isthmus is transected in the anterior midline unless there is a question of breakthrough in the region of the anterior commissure, in which case the entire thyroid isthmus should be included with the specimen to be removed.

A small vertical incision is made through the fascia over the anteroinferior surface of the cricoid cartilage. A hemostat is inserted into the incision (Fig. 11–11A), and a plane of cleavage is established between the thyroid isthmus and the anterior wall of the trachea,

A Kelly clamp, preferably one with longitudinal striations, is used to enlarge the plane between the trachea and the thyroid isthmus and to clamp across the thyroid isthmus

on each side of the midline. The thyroid isthmus is transected in the midline (Fig. 11–11B), and each side is suture ligated with No. 0-0 chromic catgut threaded on a curved noncutting needle.

The thyroid isthmus is dissected away from the trachea and the cricoid cartilage. All bleeding must be controlled before the trachea is entered.

Transection of the Trachea (FIGURES 11-12 and 11-13)

A local anesthetic solution with added epinephrine is infiltrated beneath the fascia covering the trachea to provide hemostasis. The trachea is transected anteriorly between the second and third tracheal rings (see Fig. 11–12A and B), unless the laryngeal lesion extends subglottically.

As soon as the anterior wall of the trachea has been transected, the anesthesiologist removes the endotracheal tube after making certain that the patient is well anesthetized and oxygenated. The upper margin of the trachea is grasped with a thyroid clamp or hook and elevated, exposing the subglottic lumen (Fig. 11–12B). The inferior margin of the cricoid lamina is palpated posteriorly (Fig. 11–12C). The mucous membrane of the trachea is incised on each side and posteriorly. The tracheal transection is beveled in a superior direction as it progresses posteriorly to the inferior margin of the posterior cricoid lamina (Fig. 11–13A and B).

As soon as the trachea has been transected, one suture of No. 0-0 Vicryl is placed in the anterior midline, through the trachea and skin incision inferiorly (see Fig. 11–12C).

The specimen is further elevated superiorly by blunt dissection. This plane develops rapidly, exposing the posterior cricoarytenoid muscle, the anterior wall of the cervical esophagus, and the recurrent laryngeal nerves. The inferior margin of the cricoid lamina is palpated, and the dissection of the posterior wall of the trachea is continued with great care so as not to enter the cervical esophagus (see Fig. 11–13A). Scissors are used to complete the transection on each side along the posterior margin of the thyroid laminae unless it was done earlier (Fig. 11–13C).

Entrance Into the Esophagus (FIGURE 11-14)

Entrance into the cervical esophagus is made in the anterior midline just below the level of the larynx. The fascia at this point is often thick; thus, the dissection must be carried for some distance before the mucous membrane is encountered. The point of entry is through the anterior postcricoid esophagus, just inferior to the arytenoids. It is important to preserve as much of the anterior cervical esophagus as possible in anticipation of the first-stage tracheopharyngeal speech-rehabilitation operation. A right-angle snap hemostat is inserted into the proximal end of the transected trachea (Fig. 11–14A). The end of this hemostat bulges out the superior aspect o the cervical esophagus. An incision is made over the end of the right-angle hemostat so that its end can project through the superior aspect of the cervical esophagus (Fig. 11–14B). This technique facilitates dissection of the cervical esophagus (Fig. 11–14C) and gradually cuts through the layers until the esophagus has been entered. This technique can be difficult and cumbersome. Dissection of

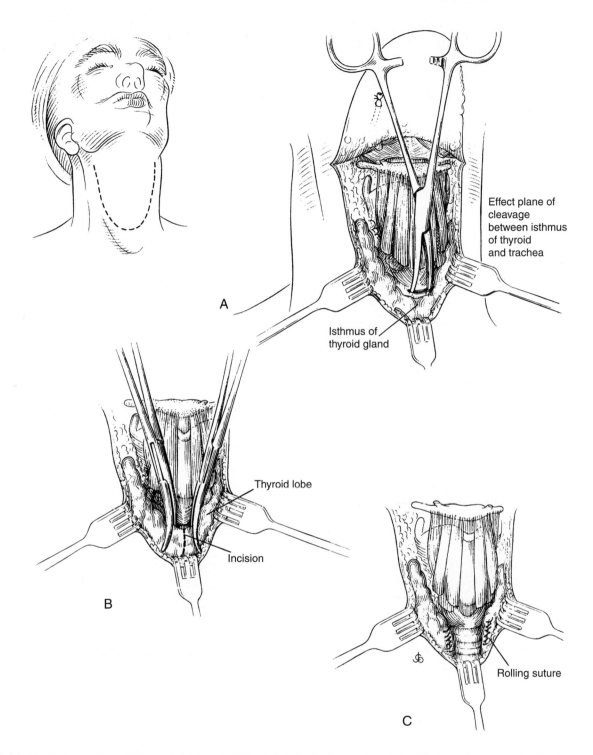

FIGURE 11-11. *A*, A small hemostat is inserted into an incision made in the fascia over the anterior inferior surface of the cricoid cartilage. This is accomplished carefully to avoid excessive bleeding. A Kelly clamp is then used to enlarge the plane between the trachea and the thyroid isthmus. *B*, Kelly clamps are placed on each side of the isthmus before it is incised in the midline. *C*, Each side of the thyroid isthmus is suture ligated using a running suture of No. 3-0 chromic catgut or Dexon suture material.

the cervical esophagus and hypopharynx is continued laterally, first on the side opposite the lesion (Fig. 11–14*D*). After this has been accomplished, the epiglottis is grasped and pulled superiorly, exposing its lingual surface. The opposite side can then be dissected, making certain that an adequate margin is obtained around the lesion. At this point, the vallecula is transected and the laryngeal specimen is removed.

Then a tracheoesophageal shunt can be performed. A hemostat is inserted into the hypopharynx and cervical esophagus, bulging out the posterior wall of the trachea, approximately 1 to 1.5 cm below the posterior cut end of the trachea. An incision in this bulge is made with a No. 15 surgical blade, and the hemostat is inserted into the trachea. A No. 14 nasogastric feeding tube is grasped by the hemostat

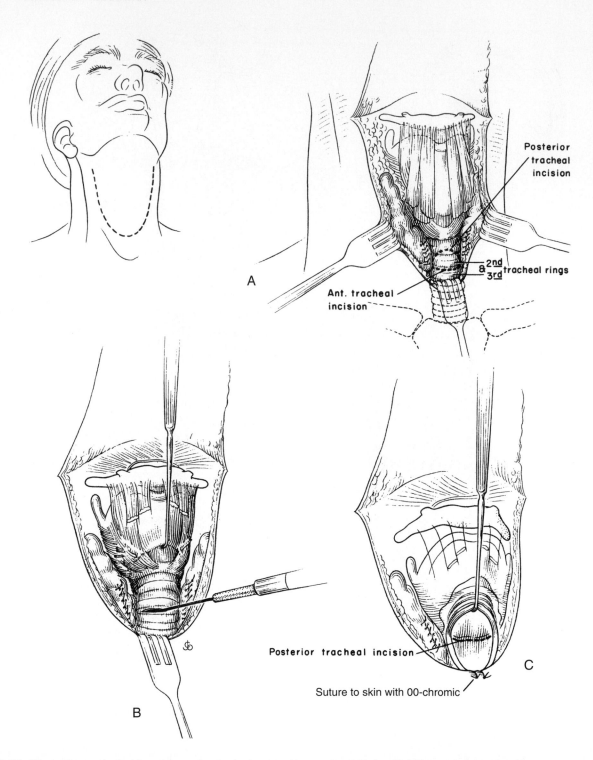

FIGURE 11-12. *A,* The anterior incision of the trachea begins between the second and third tracheal rings unless there is subglottic extension, in which case it is placed at a much lower level. The transection of the trachea is beveled. The posterior tracheal incision is also indicated in this sketch. *B,* A tracheal hook is placed below the cricoid, and the larynx is elevated superiorly. The anterior tracheal incision is made using a cutting current. *C,* The trachea is retracted anteriorly and superiorly, and the lateral and posterior walls of the tracheal mucous membrane are incised with care, exposing the anterior wall of the esophagus.

and pulled through, up into the field. It is then doubled over and inserted down into the stomach. It is good to secure the feeding tube in place with 00 silk sutures to the skin, lateral to the trachea. This ensures that the feeding tube will not become dislodged during the rest of the operation.

Repair of the Cervical Esophagus and Hypopharynx *(FIGURE 11-15)*

Repair of the cervical esophagus and hypopharynx should be performed carefully; a pharyngocutaneous fistula can

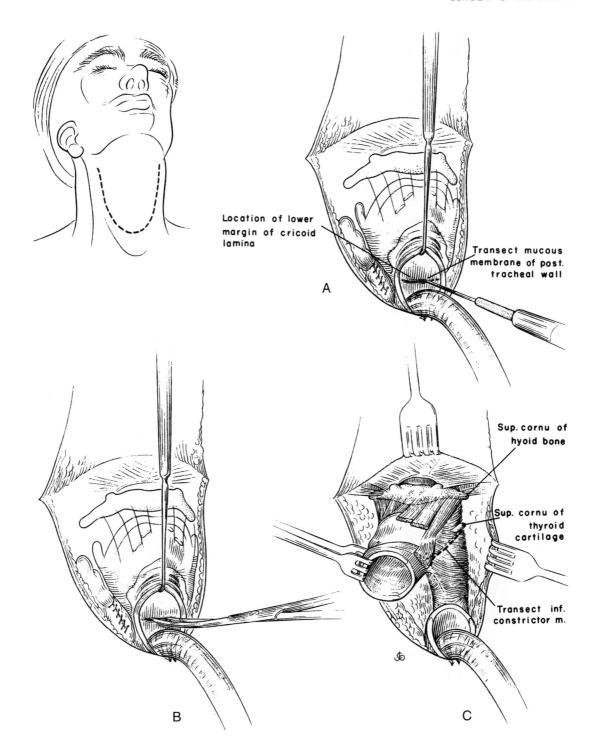

FIGURE 11-13. *A,* The inferior margin of the cricoid lamina is palpated, and the dissection of the posterior wall of the trachea is continued with great care to avoid entering the cervical esophagus. *B,* Scissors are used to complete transection of the trachea. *C,* At this point, the inferior constrictor muscle (dotted line) is transected on each side along the posterior margin of the thyroid lamina.

be a devastating complication. At this time, a primary tracheoesophageal puncture can be accomplished as described previously.

The first layer is closed with interrupted sutures using No. 3-0 Dexon suture material on a taper needle. The needle enters the fascia, approximately 4 mm lateral to the margin of the mucous membrane, and exits in an immediate submucosal layer (Fig. 11–15*A* and *B*). Using this technique

and interrupted sutures only a few millimeters apart ensures a tight closure.

A second layer of closure is accomplished by placing interrupted No. 0-0 chromic catgut or No. 3-0 Dexon in the fascia, immediately lateral to the initial suture line (Fig. 11–15*C*). Only a few of these sutures are necessary. It is important not to compromise the blood supply to the first layer of repair.

The third layer of closure consists of a few sutures approximating the inferior constrictor muscles in the midline (Fig. 11–15D). The second layer of closure is reinforced by a few sutures through the fascia and base of the tongue.

Construction of Tracheostoma and Repair of the Flap *(FIGURE 11-16)*

There are a number of techniques used to ensure that stenosis of the tracheostoma does not develop. The simplest method consists of carefully approximating the skin and mucous membrane of the trachea using No. 2-0 Dexon suture material. The entire cartilaginous portion of the trachea is sutured to the inferior skin margin to widen the diameter of the tracheostoma. This almost invariably eliminates the necessity for a tracheal tube. These sutures are placed with several knots and cut short so that mucus will not adhere to the suture ends. Closed-suction drainage tubing is inserted on each side. This is sutured to the skin, and plastic tape is placed over these sutures and tubing, as shown in Figure 11–16A.

The inferior margin of the U-flap is approximated to the posterior portion of the trachea using No. 3-0 Dexon suture material (Fig. 11–16B).

The platysma and subcutaneous layers are reapproximated with No. 2-0 Dexon suture material. The Hemovac tubing is attached to suction as soon as the subcutaneous closure is airtight so that any accumulated blood can be evacuated. If there is any question of retained blood, saline solution can be instilled beneath the laryngectomy flap. This solution is evacuated by way of the Hemovac tubing. The skin is carefully approximated with interrupted dermal sutures or skin clips (Fig. 11–16C).

Dressing and tracheal tube are unnecessary if the Hemovac apparatus is functioning adequately, a satisfactory repair has been made, and the tracheostoma is of adequate size. Antibiotic ointment is applied to the suture line. A moist sponge is hung anteriorly over the tracheostoma.

Refer to Chapter 5 for use of the salivary bypass tube for treating post laryngectomy fistulae. Refer to Chapter 12 for speech rehabilitation after a laryngectomy.

SUBTOTAL LARYNGECTOMY FOR CARCINOMA OF THE LARYNX *(FIGURE 11-17)*

A malignant lesion involving the true vocal cord, having good mobility and not extending to the anterior commissure, can be resected by laryngofissure and cordectomy (Figs. 11–17 and 11–18). Extension of the disease to the arytenoid cartilage is a contraindication to this operation. In such cases, hemilaryngectomy offers a better chance for cure and allows for repair with approximation of laryngeal mucus membrane. Since the advent of super voltage radiation therapy, the hemilaryngectomy operation can now be used to resect a recurrent lesion after a full course of radiation therapy. If a cordectomy includes the true vocal cord ventricle and false vocal cord and inner perichondrium of the thyroid cartilage, a thyroplasty can be used at a later date to improve on vocal function. If the thyroid cartilage has been altered or partially resected, it is much more difficult to perform a thyroplasty.

Technique of Cordectomy

The endotracheal tube is inserted through a tracheotomy orifice established before initiating the definitive operation. A horizontal skin incision is made at the level of the middle-thyroid cartilage (Fig. 11–17C). A plane is established above and below, just superficial to the fascia overlying the strap muscles.

The thyroid laminae are incised vertically in the anterior midline with a knife or Stryker saw (Fig. 11–17D). The laminae are separated slightly, and a vertical incision is made in the cricothyroid membrane. This incision is continued superiorly with a No. 15 surgical knife or a button knife to the level of the anterior commissure. The vocal cords are separated in the exact midline and under direct vision. The thyroid laminae are widely separated with larger hooks or a self-retaining thyrotomy retractor so that the lesion and the entire endolarynx can be seen (Fig. 11–17E).

Beginning anteriorly, the true and false cords are resected with an electric knife (Fig. 11–18A). The anteroposterior incisions for this resection are made just above the false vocal cord and below the true vocal cord. The vocal process of one arytenoid cartilage is transected as the specimen is resected. All tissue to the level of the inner aspect of the thyroid lamina is included with the specimen.

The mucous membrane is undermined superiorly and inferiorly so that its margin can be approximated with No. 3-0 chromic catgut sutures (Fig. 11–18B). Some surgeons make no attempt at this repair and allow the wound to heal by secondary intention. The thyroid laminae are approximated with No. 3-0 chromic catgut (Fig. 11–18C and D). The soft tissues are repaired and drained (Fig. 11–18E).

Hemilaryngectomy

Certain glottic lesions that are unsuitable for radiation therapy or persist after a full course of radiation therapy, and are not significantly extensive to warrant a total laryngectomy, are amenable to hemilaryngectomy. Included in this group is a vocal cord carcinoma that is recurrent after a therapeutic dose of radiation therapy.

Axial CT scan is valuable in determining the extent of the carcinoma and whether it can be totally encompassed using a hemilaryngectomy. When one is making a decision to perform a hemilaryngectomy, it is important to ascertain that the lesion can be completely removed, without sacrifice of the primary respiratory and sphincteric functions of the larynx. The allowable extent of such a lesion would be the anterior commissure, the anterior third of the opposite cord, and the vocal process of the arytenoid cartilage, but not the posterior commissure, and not more than 10 mm of subglottic extension (Fig. 11–19A and B). The involved cord may have limited mobility. A complete fixation of the vocal cord is usually a definite contraindication to hemilaryngectomy.

Consent for a total laryngectomy should be obtained before a hemilaryngectomy is performed because it is possible that total removal of the larynx will be indicated after the tumor is viewed directly. A preliminary tracheotomy is performed, and an endotracheal tube is inserted through the tracheotomy orifice for general anesthesia.

Text continued on page 285

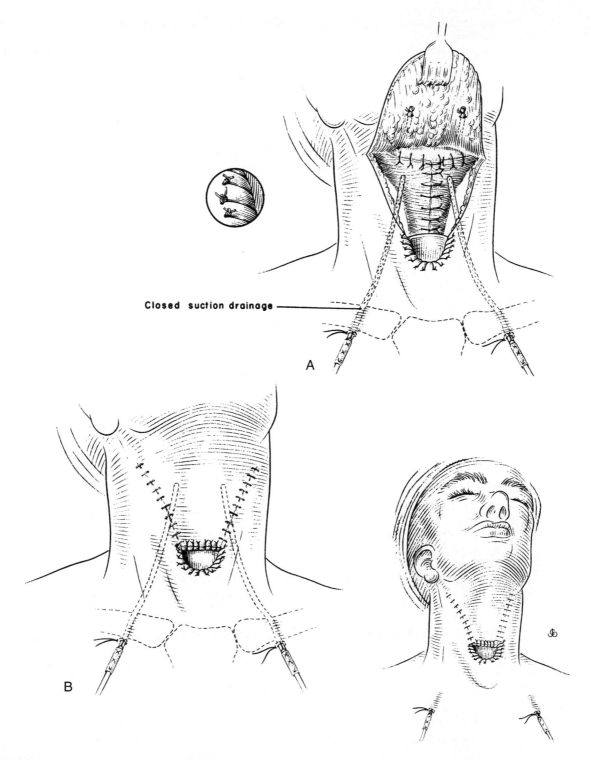

Closed suction drainage

A

B

FIGURE 11-16. *A,* The skin and mucous membrane of the trachea are carefully approximated using No. 2-0 Dexon suture material. The entire carti-laginous portion of the trachea is sutured to the inferior skin margin to widen the diameter of the tracheostoma. This almost invariably eliminates the need for a tracheal tube. These sutures are placed with several knots and cut short so that mucus will not adhere to the suture ends (insert). Closed-suc-tion drainage tubing is inserted on each side. This is sutured to the skin as shown. Plastic tape is placed over the sutures on the tubing, as shown in *B.* The inferior margin of the U-flap is approximated to the posterior portion of the trachea using No. 2-0 Dexon suture material. It is important to approx-imate the platysma before applying skin sutures or clips.

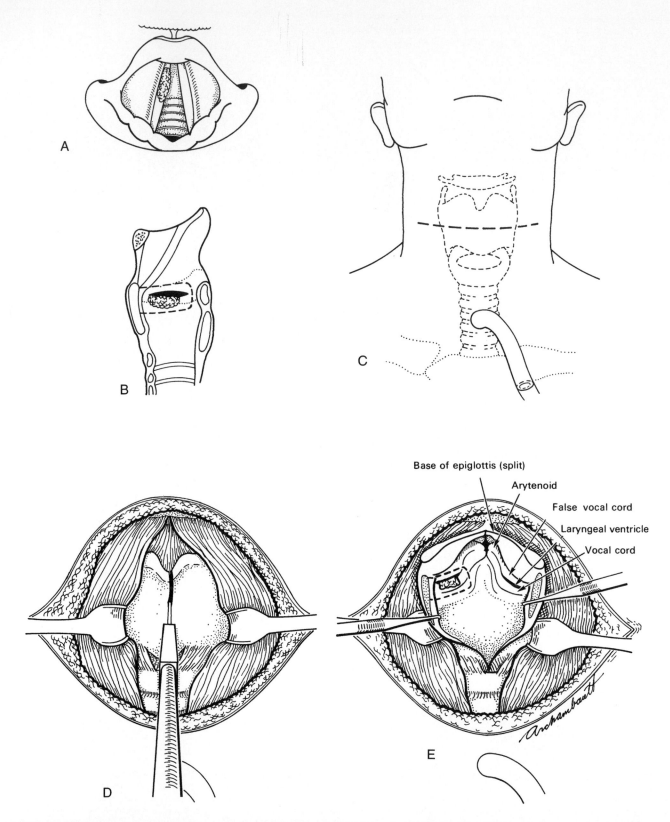

Base of epiglottis (split)

Arytenoid

False vocal cord

Laryngeal ventricle

Vocal cord

FIGURE 11-17. Subtotal laryngectomy for carcinoma of the larynx—laryngofissure and cordectomy. *A,* An indirect laryngoscopic view of a true vocal cord lesion that does not extend to the anterior commissure or the vocal process of the arytenoid cartilage. This side of the larynx is not fixed. *B,* The right larynx, viewed from the left side, showing the anterior and posterior limits of the lesion. The lesion does not extend either into the laryngeal ventricles or subglottically. There, lesions can be removed by way of suspended laryngoscopy with laser resection or by a laryngofissure as described here. *C,* A horizontal incision is made at the level of the middle-thyroid cartilage for exposure after a preliminary tracheotomy. A plane of cleavage is established superiorly and inferiorly between the platysma muscle and the infrahyoid musculature. *D,* The thyroid laminae are separated with a knife or Stryker saw, care being taken not to incise the underlying soft tissues. A vertical incision made in the cricothyroid membrane is continued superiorly with a No. 15 surgical knife or button knife, as the thyroid laminae are separated slightly with small skin hooks. *E,* As the thyroid laminae are retracted with large hooks or a self-retaining retractor, the endolarynx can be seen. The outline for cordectomy is shown above the false vocal cord, below the true vocal cord, and across the vocal process of the arytenoid cartilage.

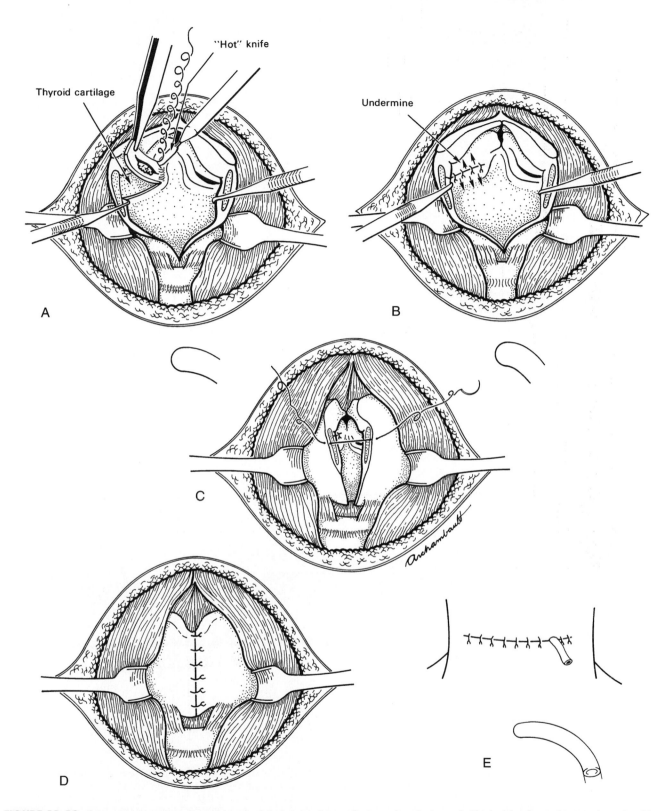

FIGURE 11-18. Subtotal laryngectomy for carcinoma of the larynx—laryngofissure and cordectomy. *A,* The incision for cordectomy is made with an electric knife. The specimen is grasped anteriorly, and all tissue medial to the thyroid laminae, including the inner perichondrium, is resected. *B,* Mucous membrane is undermined above and below the area of resection. The margins of mucous membrane are approximated with No. 3-0 chromic catgut interrupted sutures. Some surgeons prefer to let the defect heal by secondary intention. *C,* The thyroid laminae are approximated anteriorly. A silicone keel is not necessary with this operation. *D,* The thyrotomy incision has been repaired with No. 2-0 or 3-0 chromic catgut sutures. The thyrohyoid membrane above and the cricothyroid membrane below are carefully approximated to prevent an air leak into the tissues of the neck. *E,* The infrahyoid muscles are approximated in the midline. The remainder of the wound is repaired in layers and drained.

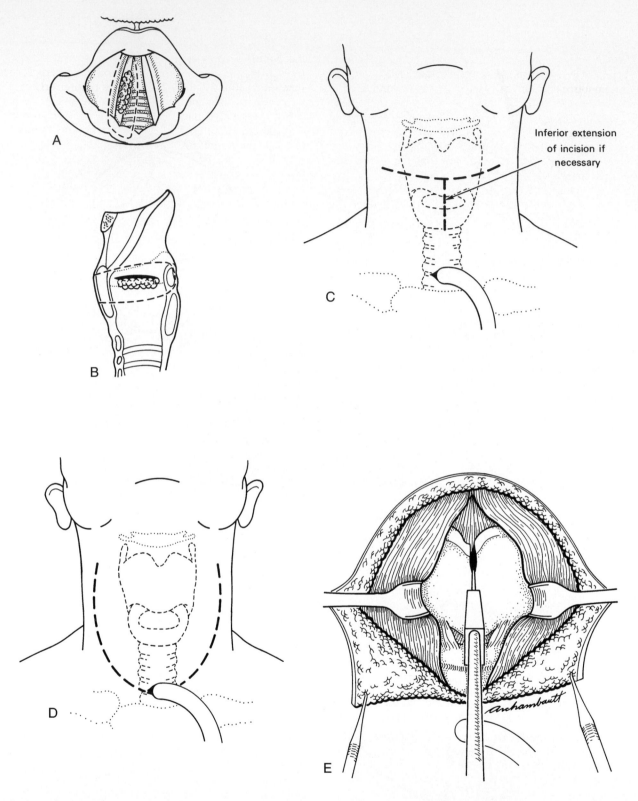

FIGURE 11-19. Subtotal laryngectomy for carcinoma of the larynx—hemilaryngectomy. *A,* An indirect laryngoscopic view of a carcinoma of the right vocal cord that is too extensive for cordectomy and not extensive enough for total laryngectomy. This lesion may extend to the anterior commissure and anterior one third of the opposite cord. It may extend to the vocal process of the arytenoid cartilage, but not to the posterior commissure. There should be not more than 10 mm of subglottic extension. There may be limited motion on the involved side, but complete fixation is a contraindication to hemilaryngectomy. *B,* The right larynx is viewed from the left side. The resection can include the anterior commissure, true and false vocal cords, and the arytenoid cartilage. *C,* A horizontal skin incision over the lower thyroid cartilage is used to provide exposure. This may be extended inferiorly in the midline if the operation is to be converted to a total laryngectomy. *D,* U-shaped anterior cervical incision can be used for exposure. This includes the tracheotomy incision. With this exposure the operation is much more easily converted to a total laryngectomy. *E,* The incision for the thyrotomy is made in the anterior midline, provided the anterior commissure is free of disease. If the anterior commissure or the anterior third of the opposite vocal cord is involved, this incision is made 0.5 cm from the midline on the opposite thyroid lamina (side of disease extension).

Technique

A tracheotomy is performed with the use of local anesthesia. An endotracheal tube is inserted for the administration of a general anesthetic. A horizontal cervical incision is made over the thyroid cartilage just above the cricothyroid membrane (Fig. 11–19C). Flaps are elevated superiorly and inferiorly over the fascia covering the strap muscles. The strap muscles are divided in the midline, and the thyroid cartilage is exposed.

The strap muscles are separated in the midline, from the level of the hyoid bone, to below the cricoid cartilage. The anterior vertical incision is made through the thyroid lamina with a tangential Stryker saw (Fig. 11–19E). The site of the lesion determines the point of this incision through the thyroid lamina. The incision is made in the anterior midline, equally dividing the thyroid laminae, if the lesion does not involve the anterior commissure. If the lesion does extend to the anterior commissure or extends to the anterior one third of the opposite vocal cord, the initial thyroid lamina vertical incision must be fashioned 0.5 cm from the midline, on the side of the extension.

Self-retaining retractors are extremely valuable for separating the strap muscles and the margins of the horizontal skin incision.

If the lesion extends to the subglottic area, the vertical incision is made dividing the anterior cricoid arch. The intraluminal exposure is widened carefully with hooks, retracting the thyroid laminae and allowing the anterior commissure of both vocal cords to be viewed. An incision is made through the anterior commissure, or contralateral vocal cord, under direct vision, as the margins of the thyroid cartilage are retracted laterally. This can be accomplished with a knife or cautery. The thyroid laminae are widely retracted, bringing into full view the endolarynx and the lesion. It is at this point that a decision must be made whether to proceed with the hemilaryngectomy or perform a total laryngectomy.

If a hemilaryngectomy is to be continued, an anteroposterior mucosal incision is made in the subglottic region with a Bovie. A vertical incision is made in the posterior midline and an anteroposterior incision, parallel to the incision below the vocal cord, is made above the false vocal cord (Fig. 11–20A). Usually an arytenoidectomy is necessary and is easily performed after the interarytenoid muscle is severed and the cricoarytenoid joint is entered.

Some surgeons prefer to remove the entire thyroid cartilage on the side of the lesion. For the most part, this is not necessary, and leaving a thin strip of cartilage above and below should not jeopardize any chance for total excision.

The lateral aspect to the posterior margin of the thyroid cartilage is dissected free to provide exposure (Fig. 11–20B). Horizontal incisions, which correspond to the mucosal incisions below the true vocal cord and above the false vocal cord, are made through the thyroid cartilage (Fig. 11–20C). The cartilaginous incisions are continued through the posterior border of the thyroid cartilage. The entire specimen is removed (Fig. 11–20D). Two small holes are drilled through the margins of the remnants of the thyroid cartilage (Fig. 11–21A). Two nonabsorbable sutures are placed through these holes so that the margins of the thyroid cartilage can be united or more closely approximated (Fig. 11–21B). This will facilitate the internal repair, slightly buckled in this side of the larynx, producing an excellent ridge against which

the opposite vocal cord can approximate for good phonation. After bleeding has been controlled, a large mucous membrane flap (Fig. 11–21C) advances inferiorly to cover the defect and is sutured to the inferior mucosal margin with 3-0 Vicryl or chromic catgut (Fig. 11–21D). It is important that the anterior aspect of the remaining vocal cord is sutured to the perichondrium of the thyroid cartilage anteriorly. If a portion of the opposite cord has been resected anteriorly, a silicone keel is inserted (Figs. 11–21E and 11–23B and C). The strap muscles are carefully approximated in the midline. The wound should be drained for at least 48 hours (Fig. 11–21F). A nasogastric feeding tube and tracheotomy are inserted.

Postoperative Care

The patient is nourished by nasogastric feedings for 5 or 6 days postoperatively, after which time he or she can usually tolerate a soft diet. The tracheotomy is removed after $1\frac{1}{2}$ or 2 weeks, unless insertion of a silicone keel has been necessary, in which case, the patient does not undergo decannulation until 1 week after removal of the keel (3 weeks).

Anterior Commissure Resection

Occasionally, the anterior commissure of the larynx will be involved at the vocal cord level with a squamous cell carcinoma, and radiation therapy is not the treatment of choice, or the lesion may recur after radiation therapy. Such a lesion may be amenable to resection of the anterior commissure if the site of the greatest involvement does not include the vocal process of the arytenoid cartilage and the lesion on the opposite side does not extend to the middle-cord position (Fig. 11–22A and B). An axial CT scan of the larynx will demonstrate that the cartilage anterior to the anterior commissure is not involved. Fixation of one side of the larynx is a contraindication for this operation; however, slight limited motion is not. There may be subglottic involvement up to 1 cm.

Technique

A tracheotomy is performed with the use of local anesthesia. An endotracheal tube is inserted by way of the tracheotomy for administration of general anesthesia. A horizontal incision is made over the thyroid laminae, just above the cricothyroid membrane (Fig. 11–22C). The flaps are elevated superiorly and inferiorly over the fascia covering the strap muscles. The strap muscles are divided in the midline, exposing the thyroid cartilage.

Bilateral vertical thyrotomy incisions are made on each side with a tangential Stryker saw (see Fig. 11–22B). These should correspond to the posterior limits of the lesion, as determined by CT scan and also by flexible fiberoptic laryngoscopy. The inferior incision is made through the cricothyroid membrane, unless there is significant subglottic involvement. In such cases, a vertical incision is used to divide the cricoid arch anteriorly. This incision extends superiorly to the thyrotomy incisions. The cricoid incision is retracted with skin hooks as the patient is placed in hyperextension. Proper illumination with a headlight is essential to view the true and false cords on each side. Vertical incisions are made in the thyroid laminae, posterior to the level of the lesion.

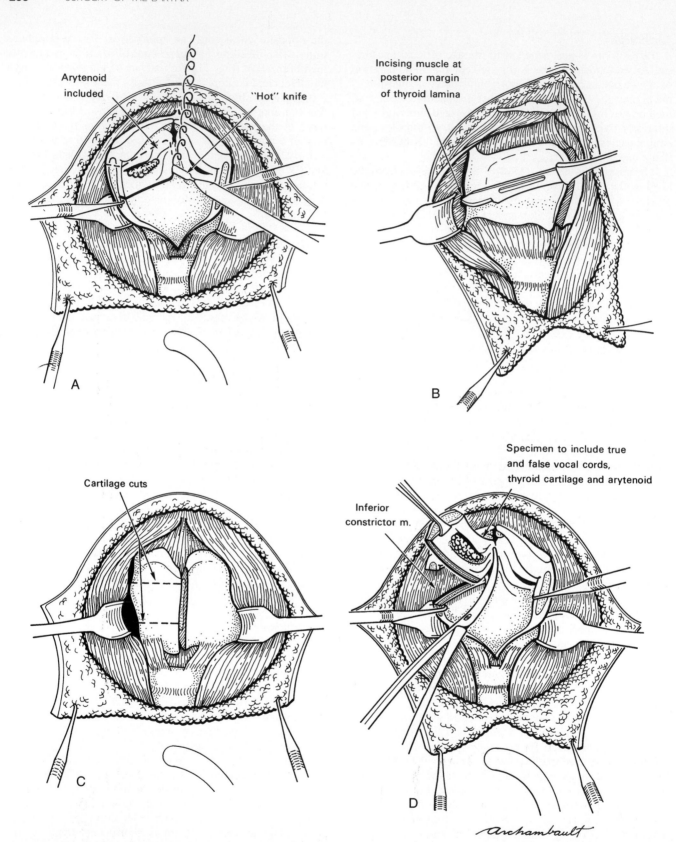

FIGURE 11-20. Subtotal laryngectomy for carcinoma of the larynx—hemilaryngectomy. *A,* The mucosal incisions are made with an electric knife, as outlined. The posterior vertical incision is made in the posterior commissure. An arytenoidectomy is usually included with the operation. *B,* The lateral surface and posterior margin of the thyroid cartilage on the involved side are dissected free. *C,* Horizontal incisions, corresponding to the mucosal incision, are made through the thyroid lamina. *D,* The specimen, which includes true and false cords, the arytenoid, and a portion of the thyroid lamina, is resected en bloc.

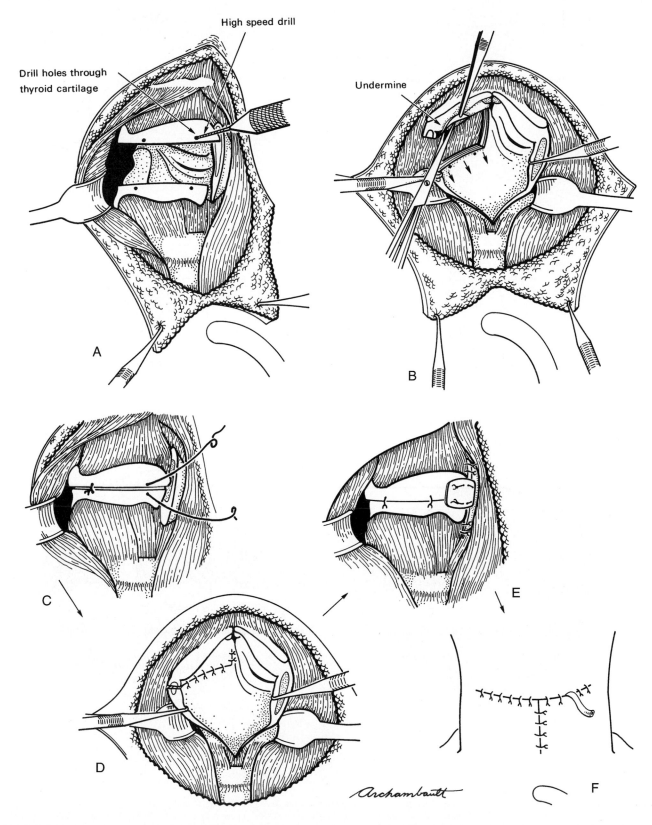

FIGURE 11-21. Subtotal laryngectomy for carcinoma of the larynx—hemilaryngectomy. *A,* Two small holes are drilled adjacent to the margins of the remaining thyroid cartilage. *B,* A large mucosal flap is elevated superiorly over the arytenoid region, aryepiglottic fold, and the medial wall of the pyriform sinus. A margin of mucous membrane is elevated below. *C,* Either wire or nonabsorbable sutures are placed through the holes in the margins of the thyroid cartilage. *D,* The cartilage margins are either united or more closely approximated. The mucous membrane is repaired internally with No. 2-0 interrupted chromic catgut sutures. *E,* A silicone keel is inserted and fixed in place. *F,* The remainder of the thyrotomy incision and wound are repaired in layers and drained.

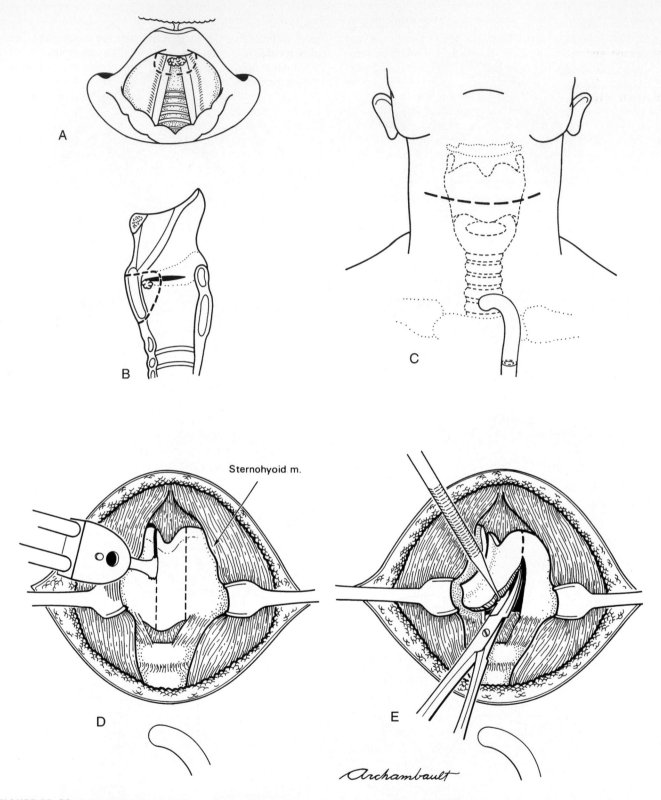

FIGURE 11-22. Subtotal laryngectomy for carcinoma of the larynx—anterior commissure resection. *A,* A malignant lesion of the anterior commissure is seen by indirect laryngoscopy. The anterior half of each vocal cord is resected with the anterior commissure. *B,* The right side of the larynx is viewed from the left. The resection includes a section of the thyroid cartilage, the false cord, laryngeal ventricle, and true vocal cord. The anterior subglottic region is automatically included with this resection. *C,* After a preliminary tracheotomy and administration of an anesthetic through an endotracheal tube, a horizontal anterior cervical incision is made to provide exposure. A plane is established above and below, between the platysma and fascia covering the infrahyoid muscles. The infrahyoid muscles are retracted laterally, exposing the thyroid cartilage. *D,* Bilateral vertical thyrotomy incisions are made. These conform to the extent of tissue to be resected. The dissection is continued inferiorly across the cricothyroid membrane. The subglottic region is thus entered on each side. From here, the dissection of soft tissue is continued superiorly with great care, under good illumination, and with the patient's neck in hyperextension. *E,* A horizontal incision is made across the thyrohyoid membrane, and the specimen is removed.

It is best to start on the site of least involvement (Fig. 11–22D). Horizontal incision is made across the thyrohyoid membrane, and the specimen is removed. The posterior commissure, outline of the arytenoids, and the remaining portion of the true and false vocal cords can be seen after this resection (Fig. 11–23A). Usually it is not possible to make any repair by advancing or rotating mucosal flaps. Instead, a silicone keel is inserted to prevent anterior glottic stenosis (Fig. 11–23B and C). The thyroid laminae above and below the laryngeal keel, the thyrohyoid, and cricoid are approximated with 3-0 Vicryl sutures, and the subcutaneous tissues are repaired with 3-0 chromic catgut sutures (Fig. 11–23D). The wound is drained. The keels should remain in place for 3 or 4 weeks, depending on the appearance of the larynx, when viewed by flexible fiberoptic laryngoscopy. The tracheotomy tube remains in place for 1 week after removal of this silicone keel.

Supraglottic Partial Laryngectomy Indications

Because the lymphatics of the larynx are situated above the true vocal cords and drain laterally to the neck rather than inferiorly to the glottis, certain supraglottic lesions can be dissected with preservation of the glottis. However, the selection of patients for treatment with supraglottic partial laryngectomy must be done with care, for the diagnostic workup, surgical technique, and postoperative care are much more complicated for this operation than for a total laryngectomy.

Small exophytic lesions in the supraglottic area that do not disturb laryngeal function are best treated with a full course of radiation therapy. This is especially true of lesions involving the free margins of the epiglottis. Other more extensive or ulcerative lesions involving the valleculae, base of tongue, epiglottis, aryepiglottic folds, and all walls of the pyriform sinus to a level 1 cm above its apex should be considered for a supraglottic partial laryngectomy. The lesion should not extend into the base of the tongue, the lateral hypopharyngeal wall, or the anterior commissure, below the superior surface of the false vocal cord, or into the interarytenoid space.

The true vocal cords and arytenoids should function normally. With conservation surgery, respiratory sphincteric and phonatory function of the glottis should be preserved. If this is not possible, a total laryngectomy is indicated. Some laryngeal surgeons will remove one arytenoid cartilage and fix the vocal cord on that side to the midline, and at the same time preserve laryngeal function, believing that this is worth a try and that if it fails, a total laryngectomy can be performed subsequently.

Selected lesions of the posterior hypopharyngeal wall can be resected by way of the transhyoid approach, with preservation of the larynx.

Indications for a Radical Neck Dissection

Because the lymphatics of the larynx that are situated above the true vocal cords drain laterally to the neck rather than inferiorly into the glottis, certain supraglottic lesions can be dissected with preservation of the glottis. However, the selection of patients for treatment with supraglottic partial laryngec-

tomy must be done with care, for the diagnostic workup, surgical technique, and postoperative care are much more complex for this operation than for a total laryngectomy.

Small exophytic lesions in the supraglottic area that do not disturb laryngeal function are best treated with a full course of radiation therapy. This is especially true of lesions involving the free margin of the epiglottis. Other more extensive or ulcerative lesions involving the vallecula, base of the tongue, epiglottis, aryepiglottic folds, and all walls of the pyriform sinus to the level of 1 cm above its apex should be considered for a supraglottic partial laryngectomy. The lesion should not extend into the base of the tongue, the lateral hypopharyngeal wall, or the anterior commissure, below the superior surface of the false vocal cord, or into the interarytenoid space.

The true vocal cords and arytenoids should function normally. Invasion of cartilage, other than extension of a lesion to the region of one arytenoid, is a contraindication for supraglottic, and phonatory function of the glottis should be preserved. If this is not possible, a total laryngectomy is indicated. It is possible to remove one arytenoid cartilage and fix the vocal cord on that side to the midline and at the same time preserve laryngeal function.

Selected lesions of the posterior hypopharyngeal wall can be resected by way of the transhyoid approach with preservation of the larynx.

Indications for radical neck dissection with supraglottic laryngectomy are the subject of much controversy. Biller and associates believe that a radical neck dissection is indicated in all patients with supraglottic carcinoma; 32% of their patients had lymph node involvement, some of the nodes being palpable and others nonpalpable. Ogura and Biller state that radical neck dissections are indicated for all supraglottic carcinomas except those involving the free epiglottis. Certainly a radical neck dissection is indicated in the presence of:

1. enlarged cervical lymph nodes (bilateral neck dissection for bilateral cervical metastases);
2. pyriform sinus lesions;
3. lesions of the vallecula and base of the tongue; or
4. lesions of the epiglottis that extend to the aryepiglottic folds.

In general, a radical neck dissection is not indicated for lesions of the free epiglottis or for midline lesions without palpably enlarged cervical lymph nodes and a negative cervical CT scan.

Some surgeons believe a functional neck dissection is suitable for patients without palpably enlarged lymph nodes. Others suggest that a functional neck dissection should be considered when all involved lymph nodes are mobile, especially when a simultaneous bilateral neck dissection spares the internal jugular vein, the sternocleidomastoid muscle, and the spinal accessory nerve. This deserves further study and evaluation for, when compared with the radical neck dissection, functional neck dissection is attended with a definite decrease in mortality and morbidity, and also with a much better cosmetic result. Muscle function is preserved, eliminating the disabling and often painful shoulder drop. The carotid artery is, of course, well protected when a functional neck dissection is performed. Before a supraglottic partial laryngectomy is performed, consent for a total laryngectomy should be obtained because subtotal removal may be contraindicated after the tumor has been viewed directly.

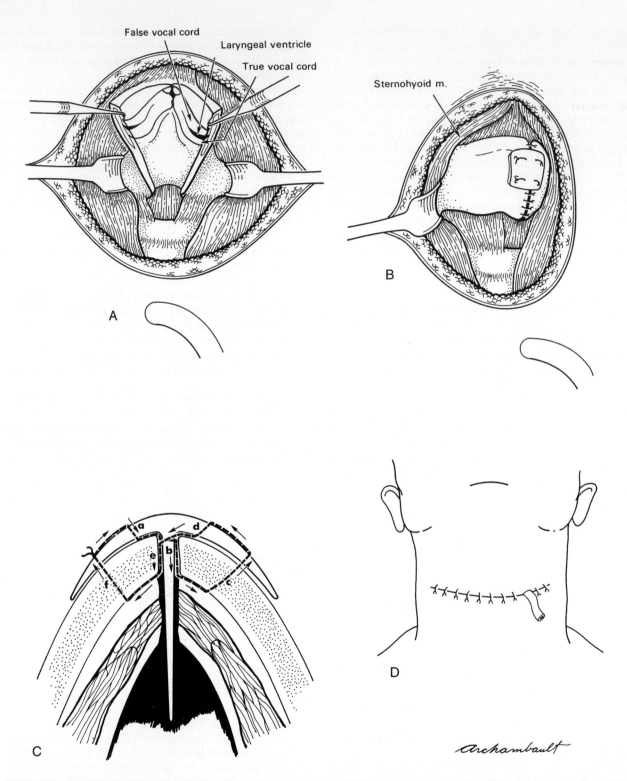

FIGURE 11-23. Subtotal laryngectomy for carcinoma of the larynx—anterior commissure resection. *A,* The posterior commissure, outline of the ary-tenoids, and remaining portion of the true and false vocal cords can be seen as the thyroid laminae are retracted laterally. *B,* A silicone keel is inserted and fixed in place to prevent anterior glottic stenosis. The keel remains in place for 3 to 4 weeks. It can be removed as an office procedure by reopen-ing the central portion of the horizontal skin incision. *C,* A figure-eight suture of No. 3-0 polyethylene material is used to secure the keel in place. This suture tightly approximates the thyroid laminae. It also compresses the extralaryngeal portion of the keel against the thyroid laminae to prevent postop-erative leakage of air and secretions. It is first passed down through the medial aspect of the extralaryngeal portion of the keel (a), and then through the base of the intralaryngeal portion (b). From here, it is passed through the thyroid cartilage and back through the opposite extralaryngeal portion of the keel (c). The figure-eight suture is completed by continuing in a similar fashion, returning the suture through the extralaryngeal keel to meet its oppo-site end (d, e, and f). *D,* The remainder of the thyrotomy wound, the thyrohyoid and cricothyroid membranes, and the subcutaneous tissues are repaired with No. 3-0 chromic catgut sutures.

Preliminary Studies

The general medical evaluation should include chest radiograph to exclude the possibility of pulmonary metastasis and detect possible evidence of chronic lung disease. Preoperative evaluation is essential to determine whether the patient will reestablish swallowing postoperatively and to ensure that the patient will not develop pulmonary complications. Preoperative pulmonary function tests are used to determine whether the patient has a proper exchange of gases, function sufficient for deep inspiration, and a suitable cough.

The glottic lesions should be repeatedly and carefully studied by way of indirect laryngoscopy (Fig. 11–24A). Often this is the best means for observing lesions in the supraglottic region. The lesion is described (exophytic, ulcerative, and so on), and its exact location and extent are recorded. The status of the mucous membrane surrounding the lesion should be noted.

Laminagrams and CT scan of the larynx are of value in determining the exact status of the true vocal cords, laryngeal ventricles, and anterior commissure as well as in outlining the surface of the lesion. (Refer to Chapter 1 for details of the studies.) If possible, these studies should be conducted before direct laryngoscopy and biopsy.

The larynx is carefully evaluated by direct laryngoscopy. The findings are the same as those mentioned for indirect laryngoscopy. Areas not clearly observed by indirect laryngoscopy are noted. An adequate, but not extensive, biopsy specimen is obtained for pathologic diagnosis. The specimen is taken with extreme care when the lesion partially obstructs the airway. A tracheotomy should be avoided before a definitive surgical procedure because of the increased risk of wound infection. The vocal cord and arytenoid function are again evaluated as the effects of general anesthesia lighten.

Technique

The skin incision begins at the tip of the hyoid bone on the side opposite the lesion. It continues horizontally across the anterior neck, at the level of the thyrohyoid membrane, to the tip of the hyoid bone on the ipsilateral side, unless a neck dissection is to be included with the operation (Fig. 11–24C). If a neck dissection is to be included, the incision is extended to the mastoid tip, curving below the submandibular triangle. The radical neck incision is continued inferiorly as with the Conley modification of the Schobinger incision. The incision permits an adequate blood supply to the skin flap and proper covering of the carotid artery system. The flap is elevated in a subplatysmal plane.

The radical or functional neck dissection is performed as a preliminary procedure. The supraglottic partial laryngectomy can be more easily executed after the neck dissection, which, when completed, remains attached only to the thyrohyoid membrane. The operation can be further simplified by detaching the neck dissection from the thyrohyoid membrane and removing the entire hyoid bone as a separate specimen. I believe that these two maneuvers do not jeopardize the patient's chance for cure.

The sternohyoid, omohyoid, and thyrohyoid muscles are sectioned at their insertion into the hyoid bone, thereby exposing the thyrohyoid membrane and the thyroid cartilage (Fig. 11–24D). The muscle attachments to the superior surface of the hyoid bones are sectioned and the hyoid bone is removed (Fig. 11–24E).

A perichondrial incision is made across the superior border to the thyroid cartilage to the base of each superior cornu, and then inferiorly to a point midway down the lateral surface of the thyroid cartilage (Fig. 11–25A). The perichondrium on the anterolateral surface of the thyroid cartilage is carefully elevated and reflected inferiorly (Fig. 11–25B). The perichondrium is also elevated from the posterior surface of the portion of the thyroid cartilage to be removed. The thyroid perichondrium will be used to repair after the supraglottic partial laryngectomy.

A horizontal incision is made across the thyroid cartilage, midway between the thyroid notch and its inferior border, with a tangential Stryker saw (Fig. 11–25C). The cartilage incision is continued superiorly on each side along lines corresponding to the perichondrial incision. The thyroid cartilage above the horizontal incision is resected (Fig. 11–26A).

Entrance into the pharynx is gained by way of the lateral wall of the pyriform sinus, unless the lesion extends to this region. Entry into the pharynx can be made by way of the vallecula unless the tumor involves the lingual surface of the epiglottis, vallecula, or base of the tongue (Fig. 11–26B). The completed pharyngotomy incision extends across the vallecula or base of the tongue inferiorly through the lateral wall of the pyriform sinuses (Fig. 11–26C). If a tracheotomy has not already been performed, it is executed at this time so that the endotracheal tube for administration of an anesthetic can be redirected through the orifice.

Once the tumor is in view, the surgeon should adjust position so that he or she is standing facing the top of the patient's head. Excellent illumination is mandatory and is best secured with a headlight. The epiglottis is grasped with a tenaculum and retracted anteriorly and inferiorly (Fig. 11–27A). Placing a hook in the interarytenoid space can stretch the larynx. If the tumor extends to the aryepiglottic fold or to the region of the false vocal cord, the anterior aspect of the arytenoid cartilage is carefully palpated to detect extension of the disease. The pyriform sinus on the side opposite the lesion comes into direct view as the epiglottis is retracted forward. An incision made through its lateral wall permits a clear view of the entire supraglottic region as the epiglottis is retracted further anteriorly and inferiorly. The aryepiglottic fold is transected on each side by placing one blade of the dissecting scissors in the laryngeal ventricle and the other in the pyriform sinus (Fig. 11–27B). The dissection is continued anteriorly on each side, above the true vocal cords, to the anterior commissure and then across the base of the epiglottis. At this point, the specimen is removed (Fig. 11–27C).

It may be necessary to perform an arytenoidectomy if the disease process extends to the arytenoid to ensure proper laryngeal sphincteric function postoperatively.

The arytenoid cartilage is resected with the specimen if the lesion extends to this region. If possible, the vocal process is preserved. It is of utmost importance to suture the vocal process, or muscle remaining after arytenoidectomy, to the cricoid cartilage in the midline. Otherwise, proper sphincteric action of the glottis may not be possible.

Lesions involving the pyriform sinus but not involving

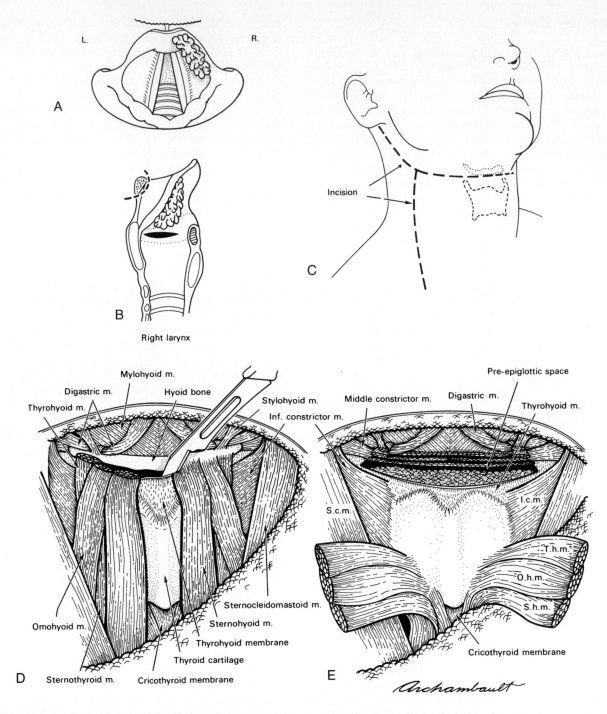

FIGURE 11-24. Supraglottic partial laryngectomy. *A,* Often the supraglottic lesion can be accurately outlined when viewed by indirect laryngoscopy. The lesion shown here, as viewed by direct laryngoscopy, involves the right laryngeal surface of the epiglottis, medial aspect of the right aryepiglottic fold, and extends to the right false vocal cord. The medial surface of the right false vocal cord and the laryngeal ventricle are normal. *B,* A midsagittal section of the larynx is used to show the extent of the lesion shown in *A. C,* The skin incision begins at the tip of the hyoid bone on the side opposite the lesion. It is continued anteriorly across the neck at the level of the thyrohyoid membrane to the ipsilateral hyoid tip. If a radical neck dissection is to be included with the operation, the incision is continued posteriorly to the tip of the mastoid bone and then inferiorly. The flaps are elevated in a subplatysmal plane, exposing the underlying strap muscles and the hyoid bone. *D,* Some surgeons prefer to remove the radical neck dissection specimen and the hyoid bone as separate specimens. These two maneuvers facilitate the remainder of the operation and most likely do not jeopardize the patient's chance for cure. The sternohyoid, omohyoid, and thyrohyoid muscles are sectioned at their insertion along the margin of the hyoid bone at this time. *E,* After removal of the hyoid bone, the thyrohyoid membrane and the thyroid cartilage are exposed by reflecting the sternohyoid, omohyoid, and thyrohyoid muscles inferiorly.

its apex can be resected during supraglottic laryngectomy if laryngeal function remains normal. Such a resection should include the epiglottis, aryepiglottic fold, false vocal cord, arytenoid cartilage, and involved portions of the pyriform sinus. The approach to these lesions is gained by extending the thyroid cartilage incision, on the side of the lesion, from the midline inferiorly to the origin of the inferior cornua. Entrance into the pharynx is gained by way of the vallecula

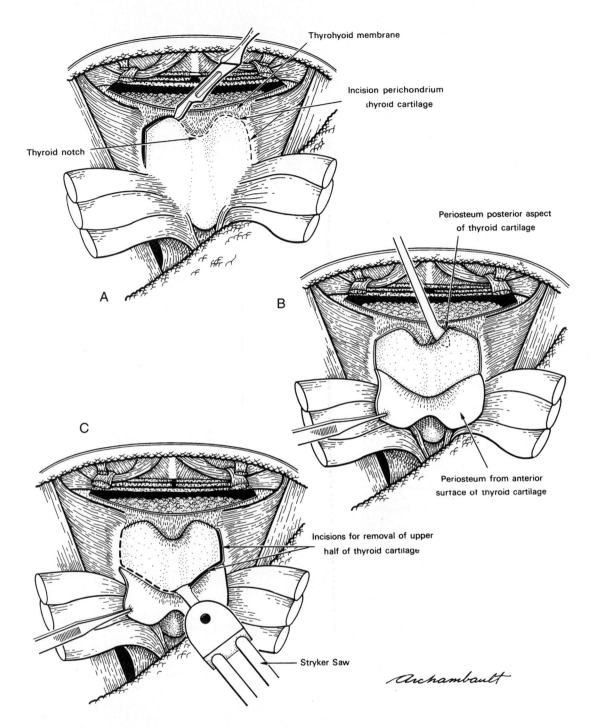

FIGURE 11–25. Supraglottic partial laryngectomy. *A,* An incision is made across the superior border of the thyroid cartilage to the base of each superior cornu. A vertical incision is extended inferiorly at each end of the horizontal incision to the level of the middle thyroid cartilage. *B,* The perichondrium is carefully elevated from the anterolateral surface of the thyroid cartilage and reflected inferiorly. A plane of cleavage is established between the thyroid cartilage to be resected and the underlying perichondrium. *C,* With a Stryker saw, horizontal incisions are made across the thyroid cartilage midway between the notch and the inferior border. The cartilage incision is continued superiorly at each side along lines corresponding to the perichondrial incisions.

and lateral wall of the pyriform sinus opposite the lesion. Although more of the laryngopharynx is resected when a pyriform sinus lesion is excised, repair is appreciably more difficult.

A cricopharyngeal myotomy is an essential part of the supraglottic partial laryngectomy (Fig. 11–28*A*). If it is not performed, rehabilitation of deglutition is either delayed or impossible. The myotomy is accomplished by inserting the index finger of one hand into the cervical esophagus while a vertical incision is made in the inferior constrictor muscle with a No. 15 surgical blade. The vertical incision is posteriorly placed to avoid injury to the recurrent laryngeal nerve. All muscle fibers should be carefully incised until the submucosal layer is clearly in view.

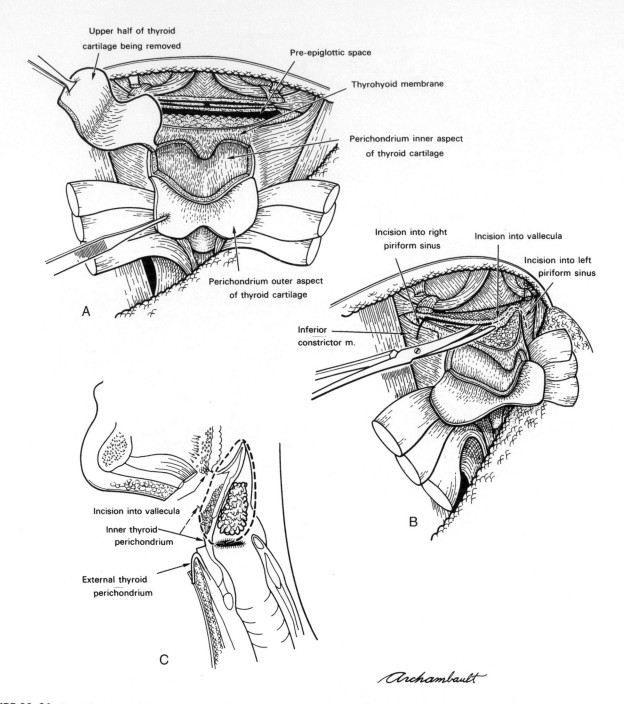

Upper half of thyroid
cartilage being removed

Pre-epiglottic space

Thyrohyoid membrane

Perichondrium inner aspect
of thyroid cartilage

Perichondrium outer aspect
of thyroid cartilage

A

Incision into right
piriform sinus

Incision into vallecula

Incision into left
piriform sinus

Inferior
constrictor m.

B

Incision into vallecula

Inner thyroid
perichondrium

External thyroid
perichondrium

C

Archambault

FIGURE 11–26. Supraglottic partial laryngectomy. *A,* The thyroid cartilage above the horizontal incision is resected, exposing the underlying perichondrium. *B,* Entrance into the pharynx is gained through the lateral wall of the pyriform sinus unless the lesion extends to this region. Entry to the pharynx is made by way of the vallecula, if the lesion approaches the lateral wall of the pyriform sinus. Regardless of the point of entry into the pharynx, an incision across the vallecula (or base of tongue), extending down into the pyriform sinus on each side, is necessary for adequate exposure of the supraglottic larynx. *C,* A midsagittal section of the larynx and pharynx is used to show the incision and extent of tissue removal necessary for proper resection of this particular lesion (Fig. 11–24*A* and *B*). The exact incisions for resection cannot be determined until the lesion and surrounding structures are in clear view.

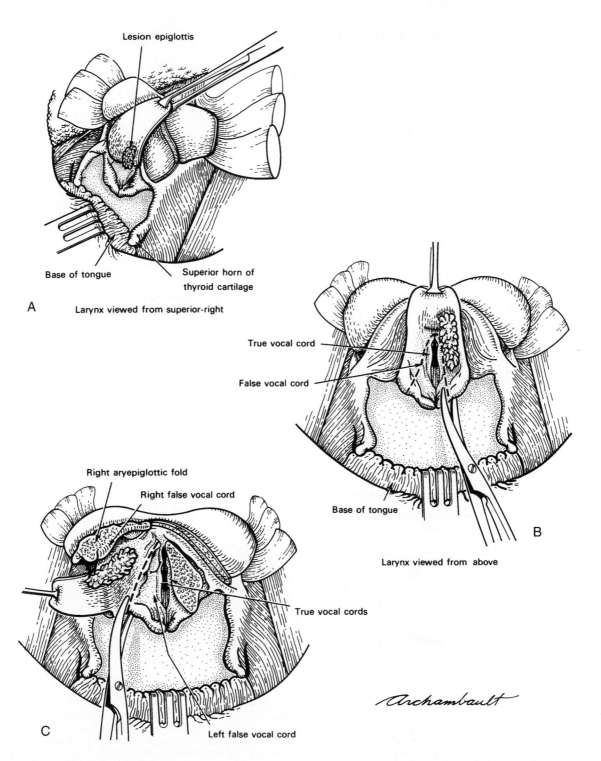

Lesion epiglottis

Base of tongue

Superior horn of
thyroid cartilage

A   Larynx viewed from superior-right

True vocal cord

False vocal cord

Base of tongue

B

Larynx viewed from above

Right aryepiglottic fold

Right false vocal cord

True vocal cords

C

Left false vocal cord

Archambault

FIGURE 11-27. Supraglottic partial laryngectomy. *A,* Once the pharynx has been exposed, surgeons should continue the operation while standing at the head of the table, using a headlight for illumination. In this figure, the tip of the epiglottis has been grasped with a tenaculum and retracted anteriorly and inferiorly. The larynx is viewed from the superior and right side of the patient. Occasionally, it is necessary to place a hook in the interarytenoid space and stretch the larynx to outline the margins of the tumor accurately. The suprahyoid musculature and base of the tongue are retracted superiorly. *B,* The larynx is viewed from the midline as seen by the surgeon standing at the head of the operating table. Unless the lesion extends posteriorly to the arytenoid, the aryepiglottic fold is transected on each side by placing the blade of the dissecting scissors into the laryngeal ventricle or above the false vocal cord and the other blade in the pyriform sinus. The arytenoid on each side can be resected if the tumor extends posteriorly to involve this structure. *C,* The dissection is continued anteriorly towards the base of the epiglottis in or above the laryngeal ventricle. The right aryepiglottic fold, laryngeal ventricle, and right base of epiglottis have been transected. The epiglottis is pulled to the left and anteriorly giving better exposure of the left endolarynx. In this particular instance, with the lesion confined to the right epiglottis and medial aspect of the right aryepiglottic fold, the dissection of the left side is continued across the aryepiglottic fold and above the false vocal cord to the base of the epiglottis anteriorly.

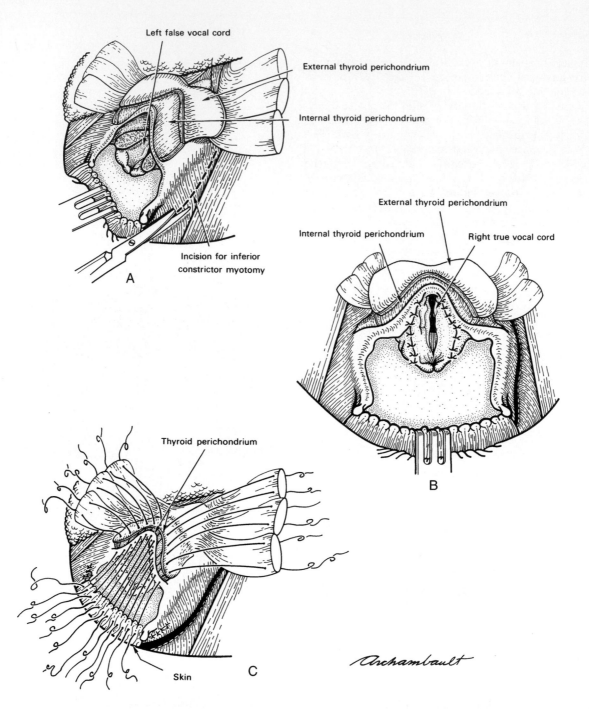

Left false vocal cord

External thyroid perichondrium

Internal thyroid perichondrium

Incision for inferior
constrictor myotomy

A

External thyroid perichondrium

Internal thyroid perichondrium

Right true vocal cord

B

Thyroid perichondrium

Skin

C

Archambault

FIGURE 11–28. Supraglottic partial laryngectomy. *A,* An inferior constrictor myotomy is an essential part of the supraglottic laryngectomy. The tissue is easily cut over the surgeon's left index finger, which has been placed in the cervical esophagus. The muscle can be incised with a No. 15 surgical blade or with scissors as shown. The myotomy incision is extended inferiorly to include the cricopharyngeal portion of the inferior constrictor muscle. The myotomy is performed as far posteriorly as possible to avoid injury to the recurrent laryngeal nerve. *B,* The repair after supraglottic partial laryngectomy begins by carefully approximating the margin of the mucous membrane of the pyriform sinus to the lateral margin of the laryngeal ventricle (right) or to the margin of resection above the false vocal cord (left). There is usually some distortion of the true vocal cord when the repair is accomplished as is shown on the patient's right side. The repair is continued anteriorly by placing multiple interrupted No. 3-0 chromic catgut sutures. *C,* Proper closure of the pharyngotomy incision is imperative. This is accomplished suspending the larynx to the base of the tongue. Laterally, the base of the tongue is sutured to the inferior constrictor musculature and underlying mucous membrane. Anteriorly, the sutures are placed through the base of the tongue, the internal and external perichondrium of the thyroid cartilage, and the "strap" muscles. An attempt is made to approximate the mucous membrane of the larynx to that of the base of the tongue. All sutures (No. 2-0 chromic catgut) for closure of the pharyngotomy incision are placed in holding clamps and tied one after the other with the patient's neck in flexion. The remainder of the wound is closed in layers. A Penrose drain or closed-suction drainage should also be included.

Wound Closure

The first step in repair consists of suturing the mucosal margin of the laryngeal ventricle to that of the pyriform sinus laterally with No. 3-0 Vicryl sutures (Fig. 11–28*B*).

The larynx is suspended to the base of the tongue by suturing the thyroid cartilage perichondrium and infrahyoid muscles directly to the muscles of the base of the tongue (Fig. 11–28*C*). It is unnecessary and inadvisable to attempt approximation of the perichondrium to the mucous membrane of the base of the tongue. The repair is made with No. 2-0 Dexon sutures. First-layer sutures are also placed between the base of the tongue and the inferior constrictor muscle. All sutures are placed and held with hemostats. The patient's head is flexed and air removed from the bag beneath his or her shoulders before the first layer of sutures is tied, one after the other. The remainder of the closure is accomplished

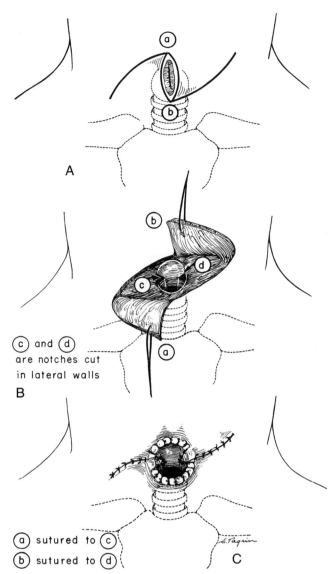

FIGURE 11-30. Repair of a vertical-slit stenosis. *A,* This operation is a variation of that shown in Figure 11–29. *B,* After the flaps have been elevated and excess tissue has been resected, a triangular section of each lateral tracheal wall is removed. *C,* The tip of each flap is sutured into the apex of the triangle. This gives the stomal orifice a funnel shape.

with No. 3-0 Dexon interrupted sutures and No. 5-0 dermal sutures. A rubber drain is inserted, or closed-suction drainage is used. A nasogastric feeding tube, tracheotomy tube, and cervical dressing complete the operation.

Postoperative Management

The tracheotomy tube can be removed when the laryngeal edema has subsided, usually between 1 and 2 weeks after the operation. The patient is fed by way of a nasogastric feeding tube until the tracheotomy fenestration has closed. Swallowing practice can be started several days before the nasogastric feeding tube is removed. The patient is instructed to take a deep breath, hold it, swallow, and then inhale. Foods easiest to swallow are semisolids such as junket, gelatin, custard, and ice cream. When these are well tolerated, the patient is grad-

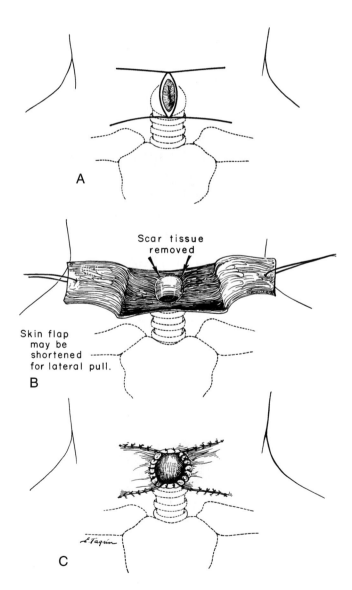

FIGURE 11-29. Repair of a vertical-slit stenosis. *A,* Skin flaps are elevated on each side of the stenosed stoma. *B,* Scar tissue and fat are excised around the stomal orifice. *C,* If necessary, the skin flaps may be shortened to effect a lateral pull.

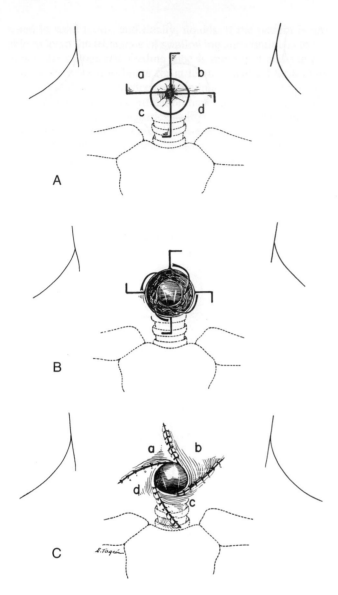

FIGURE 11–34. Repair of a concentrically stenosed stoma. *A,* Incisions for flaps and peristomal skin excision. *B,* Method for rotation of flaps. *C,* Advancement of these flaps provides a radial pull in all quadrants.

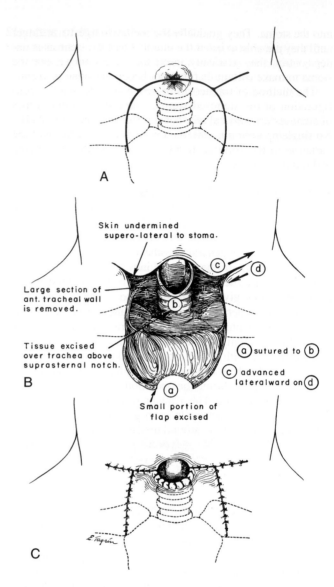

FIGURE 11–35. Repair of an interior-shelf stenosis. *A,* The inverted-U incision and its relationship to the underlying trachea, clavicles, and manubrium. *B,* The flap is reflected inferiorly. It is important to advance the skin flaps, as indicated by the arrows to effect lateral pull on the stoma. *C,* The repaired stoma and suture lines.

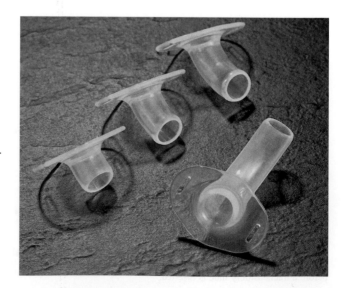

FIGURE 11–36. Singer Laryngectomy Tube.

performed with the patient under local and topical anesthesia, as outlined above, or general anesthesia. The flap is elevated to the level of the sternoclavicular joints. Fascia and adipose tissue are excised anteriorly to the trachea above the suprasternal notch. The periosteum over the manubrium and sternoclavicular joints should be avoided. It is frequently necessary to ligate the inferior thyroid veins. A section of the anterior tracheal wall is removed as shown. The skin superior and lateral to the stoma is undermined. A small portion of the flap "a" is excised. Flap "a" is sutured to flap "b." By advancing flap "c" laterally onto flap "d," two effects are accomplished: Lateral pull is exerted on the revised stoma, and the width of the defect below the stoma is decreased so that the flap becomes more adequate for closure.

The patient wears a No. 8 to 12 Singer Laryngectomy Tube (Fig. 11–36) for about 2 weeks or until healing is complete. Incomplete healing will result in crusting, which can cause obstruction and predisposes the tissues to infections.

Chapter 12
Alaryngeal Speech

WILLIAM W. MONTGOMERY

After a total laryngectomy, the patient has three alternatives for developing alaryngeal communication. Esophageal speech is by far the best form of speech after a laryngectomy because it requires no equipment and is "hands free." Unfortunately, it requires considerable motivation on the part of the patient as well as a teacher with good esophageal speech who has had a laryngectomy. Currently such a teacher is not in my geographic area, and only 10% of patients are learning good esophageal speech. From 1945 to 1994, there were good laryngectomized speech teachers in this area, and overall, more than 60% of my patients learned good esophageal speech.

For a short period after laryngectomy, the patient can communicate using a Cooper-Rand type of intraoral vibrator or a neck vibrator. Use of these vibrators requires instruction by a speech pathologist or a laryngologist. The Servox, Durex, and Western Electric electrolarynx are currently available.

The majority of laryngologists today rehabilitate the speech of patients who have undergone laryngectomy by either a primary or a secondary tracheoesophageal puncture procedure. I prefer primary tracheoesophageal puncture because it allows the patient to avoid more anesthesia and surgery. The feeding tube is inserted into the tracheoesophageal puncture site and down into the stomach. When it is time for the patient to start oral feeding after laryngectomy, the feeding tube is removed and a valve is inserted into the tracheoesophageal puncture. It is best to wait another week before starting tracheoesophageal speech.

PREOPERATIVE SESSION

Most patients are traumatized by being informed of the loss of the larynx and voice and by the possibility of not being cured. During the immediate postoperative period, they are unable to swallow or smell and have no voice. Thus, preoperatively, the patient and the family should be told by the surgeon and speech pathologist that the patient will most likely be able to have speech by one of three methods: (1) the artificial larynx voice (electronic voice device); (2) the esophageal voice; and (3) the tracheoesophageal voice. If at all possible, the patient should meet someone who has had a laryngectomy and who is experienced using all three types of communication.

I recommend a preoperative consultation by a speech-language pathologist. Ideally, this consultation is conducted with the patient and family and should include a full description of alaryngeal voice alternatives and a demonstration of an artificial larynx and esophageal voice. The patient can learn to use an intraoral artificial larynx preoperatively and will be able to use this device during the immediate postoperative period when it will be the patient's only method of communication other than writing.

The American Cancer Society sponsors a laryngectomy visitation program. A trained "laryngectomy visitor" should visit the patient and demonstrate an esophageal voice or other means of speaking. It is important for patients to see someone who has been rehabilitated. Most laryngectomy patients report that learning about alternatives for communication before surgery is very beneficial psychologically. The Society has published several pamphlets describing the anatomic and physiologic changes that occur as the result of laryngectomy. This literature can be provided to the patient and the family during the preoperative session.

ELECTRONIC VOICE DEVICES

The speech-language pathologist teaches the patient use of the intraoral artificial (electronic) larynx as soon as possible after surgery if teaching did not occur preoperatively. Most often, the patient can be discharged from the hospital with a "loaner" electronic device to use until the best type of vocal rehabilitation is determined. This is done whether the choice is esophageal speech or primary or secondary tracheal esophageal puncture. There are two types of these artificial larynges: (1) the intraoral device and (2) the neck-vibrating device.

The electronic intraoral artificial larynx is the one most often used during the immediate postoperative period. Some patients also use it as a permanent method of communication. The most commonly used electronic intraoral larynx is the Cooper-Rand (Fig. 12–1). This prosthesis generates a good-sounding voice and is equipped with both volume and pitch controls. This battery-powered prosthesis is available with both soft and rigid tubes. The Servox and Aurex electronic neck-vibrating devices can be equipped with an in-

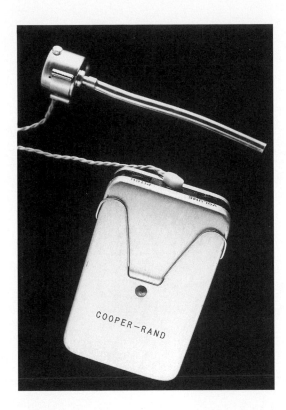

FIGURE 12-1. The Cooper-Rand intraoral artificial laryngeal device.

The neck-vibrating devices for voice rehabilitation are widely used by patients who have not developed acceptable esophageal or tracheoesophageal speech. These devices are battery powered; some units offer convenient rechargeable battery packs.

The Western Electric (Fig. 12–3) artificial voice device is lightweight and less expensive than most devices. It may be ordered through AT&T.

The Aurex artificial voice device offers more features than the one made by Western Electric (Fig. 12–4). It comes with a rechargeable battery. The pitch and volume control are of high quality. The Servox artificial voice device is an excellent prosthesis (Fig. 12–5). It is equipped with a rechargeable battery, volume control, pitch control, and quality control.

Selecting an Artificial Voice Device

Selection of an artificial voice device should be a joint decision between the speech-language pathologist and the patient. Patients should be loaned various devices to use before determining the most appropriate type for them. Generally, the intraoral device is used for a short period, after which the patient is offered a neck-vibrating device. Good speech is more often acquired with a neck-vibrating device because the patient must have excellent articulation skills to produce intelligible speech with an intraoral device.

Instructions to the Patient

Instruction with an artificial device is centered on teaching the patient to:

1. Achieve appropriate placement of the device for optimal sound generation.

traoral tube that is placed on top of the vibrating head (Fig. 12–2A and B). These prostheses offer the alternative of converting to a neck-vibrating artificial voice device, eliminating the need to purchase another. The Western Electric neck-vibrating device, the most economical, can be permanently converted to an intraoral device (Fig. 12–2C).

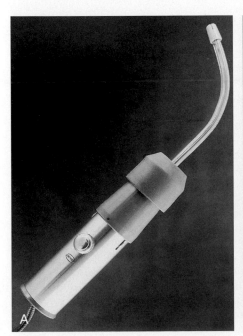
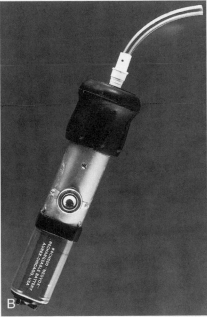
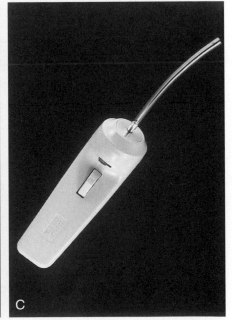

FIGURE 12-2. A, The Servox device with intraoral tube. B, The Aurex device with intraoral tube. C, The Western Electric device with intraoral tube.

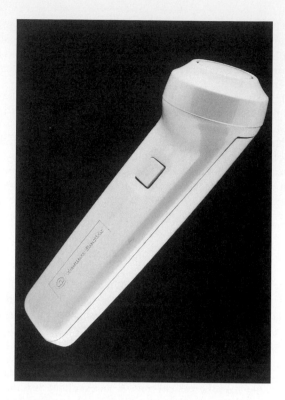

FIGURE 12-3. The Western Electric artificial voice device.

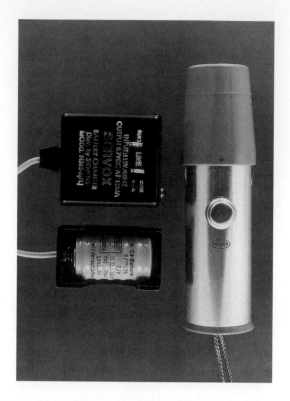

FIGURE 12-5. The Servox artificial voice device.

2. Learn voicing and devoicing.
3. Produce excellent articulation.
4. Phrase normally.
5. Use with the telephone.

6. Make pitch, volume, and quality adjustments when needed.
7. Minimize stoma noise.

Most patients who learn to produce artificial voice preoperatively succeed in producing acceptable artificial voice postoperatively within a relatively short period of time.

ESOPHAGEAL VOICE

Esophageal voice is by far the best form of vocal communication in a patient who has undergone laryngectomy. The esophageal speech therapist (preferably one who has also undergone laryngectomy) and the surgeon should demonstrate esophageal voice to the laryngectomy patient preoperatively. Every effort should be made to have the patient preoperatively visit a laryngectomy patient with good esophageal speech. If the patient has the opportunity to hear and discuss the principles of esophageal voice production preoperatively, it is often easier to begin actual esophageal voice therapy.

Generally, esophageal voice therapy begins immediately after discharge from the hospital. Patients should be seen for a minimum of two 1-hour sessions per week. Eventually, the patient should be considered for participation in group therapy in addition to individual therapy sessions.

Esophageal voice is taught with three traditional approaches: injection, inhalation, and explosion. Esophageal voice therapy typically lasts between 3 and 9 months. Patients who have not developed acceptable esophageal voice after 9 months of therapy should be considered for the tracheoesophageal shunt or an electronic voice device.

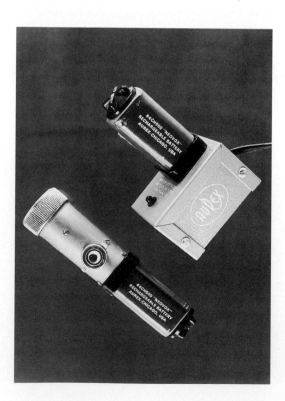

FIGURE 12-4. The Aurex artificial voice device.

The disadvantage of a primary tracheoesophageal shunt is that the patient does not have ample time to learn esophageal speech.

ONE-STAGE (POSTLARYNGECTOMY) OPERATION FOR VOICE REHABILITATION

For my patients, the best form of speech rehabilitation has been accomplished by a one-stage operation after a laryngectomy. Many of these patients can simulate a sneeze and cough, can blow their nose, and can have more than one octave singing range. The disadvantage of this procedure is that it adds approximately 1 hour to the laryngectomy surgery and also requires a second operation after the first healing has taken place.

A mucosal tube connects communication between the hypopharynx and anterior cervical cutaneous trephine incision and is constructed during the hypopharyngeal repair after a laryngectomy. The feeding tube can be inserted by way of this mucosal tube rather than the nose. Once the patient has healed and is not learning adequate esophageal speech, and has no leakage by way of the mucosal tube, then the second stage is performed, which consists of a skin tube communication between the pharyngostoma and the tracheostoma.

CONSTRUCTION OF SKIN TUBE COMMUNICATION DURING TOTAL LARYNGECTOMY

Constructing the mucosal communication between the lower hypopharynx and anterior cervical region begins after the trachea has been transected and the larynx has been elevated in preparation for removal of the larynx. As much hypopharyngeal mucous membrane as possible is dissected away from the larynx in the postcricoid region before the hypopharynx is entered. If possible, the mucous membrane is preserved to the level of the cricoarytenoid joint. In so doing, sufficient mucous membrane is obtained to construct a 2.5-cm-long tube, allowing the hypopharynx to communicate with a trephine opening in the anterior cervical skin.

Delicate scissors, forceps, and a needle holder are necessary for this procedure, which is performed as shown in Figures 12–6 and 12–7. A trephine opening, 4.5 to 5.0 mm in diameter, is made with either a corneal-transplant or a hair-transplant knife. It should be placed at least 0.5 cm below the beard line. If this is not possible, depilation can be accomplished during the postoperative period.

No dressing is required when closed-suction drainage is used. Antibiotic ointment can be applied to the line of skin repair and to the pharyngostoma. A tracheal tube is usually not necessary. Debris and crusts are carefully removed from all suture lines at least once daily. There should be little or no salivary leakage from the pharyngostoma because of the downward and posterior direction of the mucous membrane tube. Conversely, any pressure against or edema of the esophagus below the entrance of the mucosal tube will result in some transient salivary leakage. In such instances, the mucosal tube serves nicely for the escape of saliva and seems to prevent undermining of the skin flaps by salivary leakage and fistula formation.

This operation has been successfully performed during the repair of 87 consecutive total laryngectomies at the Massachusetts Eye and Ear Infirmary. A few of the patients underwent a full course of radiation therapy before this procedure. In none of the 87 patients did a postlaryngectomy pharyngocutaneous fistula occur. It has been suggested that the pharyngostoma serves as a pressure-release valve, preventing fistula formation.

The pharyngostoma can be excised in the surgeon's office if the patient has learned esophageal speech and has decided against a second-stage reconstruction.

COMPLETION OF SKIN TUBE COMMUNICATION AFTER TOTAL LARYNGECTOMY

The external portion of the tracheopharyngeal communication can be completed as a planned procedure 3 to 4 weeks after total laryngectomy or after sufficient time has elapsed to determine that the patient is not developing esophageal speech. The operation consists of constructing a skin tube communication in the anterior cervical region between the pharyngostoma and the tracheostoma. Contraindications for completion of the tracheopharyngeal communication are good esophageal voice, low level of intelligence, advanced age, and emotional instability.

Hair is not usually a problem because the trephine opening in the middle anterior cervical region can be placed below the beard line. If hair is present around the pharyngostoma or between the pharyngostoma and the tracheostoma, it should be removed by depilation. This can be satisfactorily accomplished with the aid of the Hyfrecator and a depilation needle. The Hyfrecator cord is inserted into the low-voltage outlet and the dial is set at about 30. Magnification is necessary and can be obtained with either loupes or the surgical microscope. The needle is inserted along the hair to the region of its root and current is applied. Usually satisfactory depilation requires several sessions at 10-day intervals.

A step-by-step technique for the construction of the dermal tube between the pharyngostoma and the tracheostoma is shown in Figures 12–8 and 12–9.

A closed suction drainage is used rather than a dressing. A No. 8 or 10 laryngectomy tube is inserted at the end of the operation so that the patient can become accustomed to the presence of a foreign object in the trachea. After a few weeks, a modified cervical tracheal T-tube is inserted until the patient has mastered this form of speech. During this period, the assistance of a speech pathologist is a luxury. Most patients produce speech by placing a finger or thumb over the tracheostoma or by pressing against a necktie or scarf.

The speech using this technique has remained good to excellent in these patients for over 20 years without complications.

TRACHEOESOPHAGEAL (PHARYNGEAL) VOICE REHABILITATION

Approximately one half of patients who undergo total laryngectomy are unable to master the art of esophageal speech and will not use an electronic artificial voice device. Many

Text continued on page 310

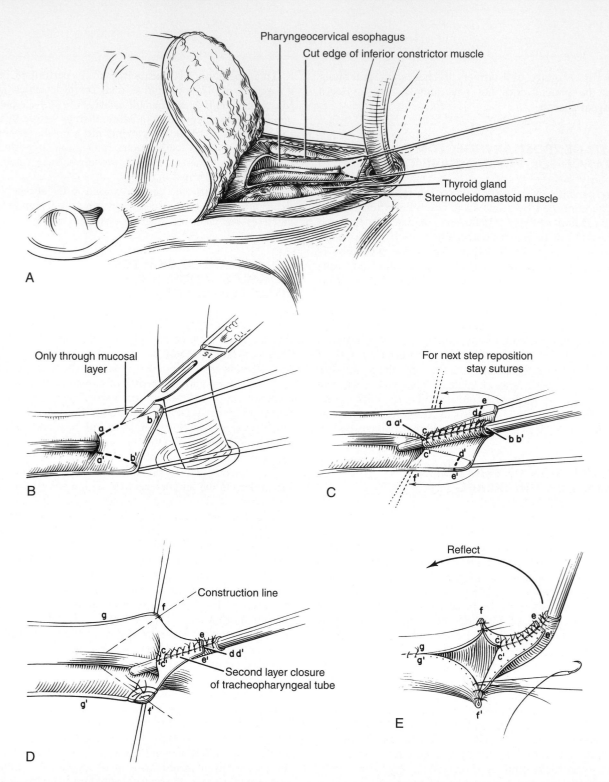

FIGURE 12–6. Construction of skin tube communication during total laryngectomy. *A,* The postlaryngectomy defect in the anterior wall of the hypopharynx is shown along with the margin of the inferior constrictor muscles. One traction suture of No. 4-0 chromic catgut is placed on each side of the excessive mucous membrane inferiorly. These sutures are placed approximately 24 mm apart. *B,* A – b and a′ − b′ indicate the mucous membrane incisions for the construction of the tube. These incisions can be made with either a sharp knife, as shown, or with delicate scissors. It is most important to include only mucous membrane in the incision. B and b′ are 15 mm apart. The incisions are angled slightly toward each other so that a and a′ are 10 mm apart. The incisions should be equal and about 25 mm long. *C,* The mucous membrane is slightly elevated on each side in a medial direction. Its elevated edges are sutured together with interrupted No. 4-0 chromic catgut on a noncutting, curved needle. In so doing, a is sutured to a′ and b is sutured to b′. An ophthalmologic needle holder, forceps, and magnifying glasses are helpful in placing these sutures. A few millimeters of mucous membrane are resected on each side as indicated by incisions d – e and d′ − e′. Mucous membrane edges c – d and c′ − d′ are very slightly elevated so that they may be sutured together over the mucous membrane tube. Interrupted No. 4-0 chromic catgut is also used for this suturing. *D,* Mucous membrane margins c – d and c′ − d′ have been sutured together. A few of these sutures should also include the anterior aspect of the mucosal tube so that the two layers will remain in contact. The No. 4-0 chromic catgut traction sutures are removed and replaced in a position approximating f and f′. Closure of the postlaryngectomy hypopharyngeal defect begins at these two points. *E,* Closure of the hypopharyngeal defect has been started at f and f′ with No. 3-0 or No. 4-0 chromic catgut. A nasogastric feeding tube is inserted at this time. Points e and e′ are sutured together. As repair progresses, these points are sutured to the mucous membrane just inferior to the angle created by the junctions of mucous membrane points g and g′. At the termination of this repair, the orifice of the mucosal tube should point superiorly.

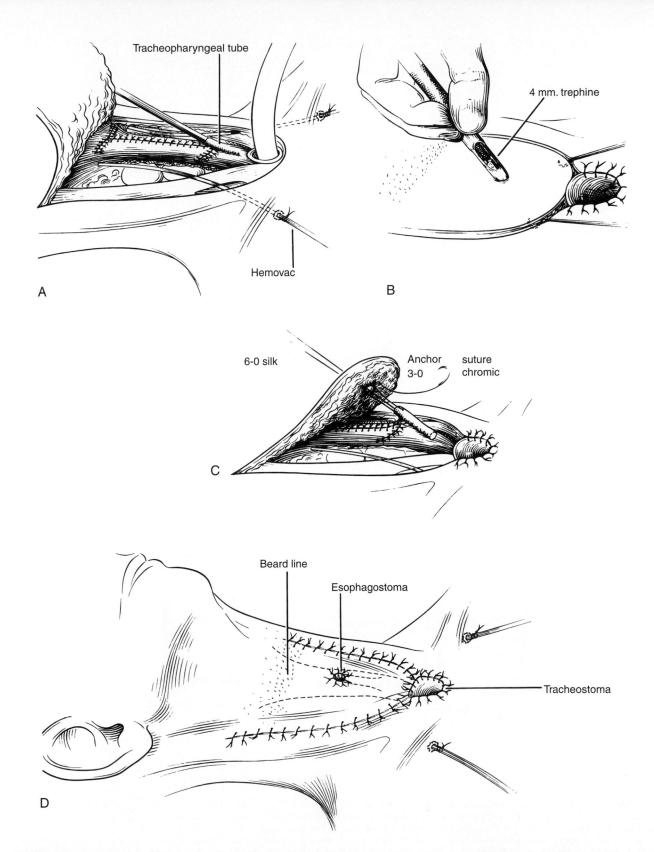

FIGURE 12-7. Construction of skin tube communication during total laryngectomy. *A,* The construction of the mucous membrane tube has been completed as well as the repair of the hypopharyngeal defect. The latter is repaired in three layers as is usually done after a total laryngectomy. Closed-suction drainage tubing is inserted at this time. *B,* The superiorly based laryngectomy flap is reflected inferiorly after the inferior and lateral aspects of the tracheostoma have been constructed. A mark is made in the midline of this flap at the level of the upper end of the mucous membrane tube. If possible, this point should be below the beard line. Folded gauze sponges are placed beneath the flap, and a circular incision is made through the skin, subcutaneous tissue, and platysmal muscle with a 4.5 or 5.0 trephine knife. Transected vessels can be ligated by elevating the skin flap. *C,* A suture of No. 4-0 chromic catgut is placed in each quadrant of the superior rim of the mucous membrane tube. These sutures are passed through the trephine opening with the needles intact and tagged. Four No. 3-0 chromic catgut sutures are used to anchor the mucous membrane tube to the undersurface of the skin flap. *D,* The superior rim of the mucous membrane tube is pulled through the trephine opening by gentle traction of the No. 4-0 chromic catgut sutures. The mucous membrane is approximated to the skin edge, care being taken not to rotate the skin tube. Four additional sutures of No. 6-0 silk are necessary to complete the pharyngostoma (esophagostoma).

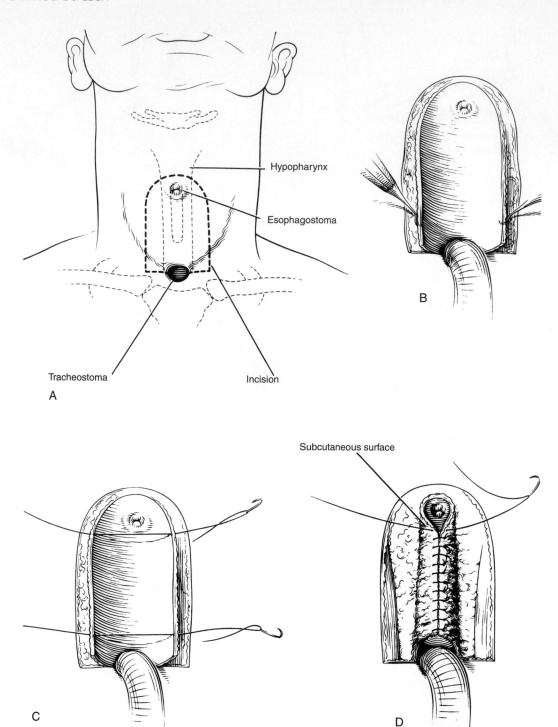

FIGURE 12–8. Completion of skin tube communication after total laryngectomy—second-stage procedure. *A,* Vertical incisions are made in the anterior cervical region on each side of the pharyngostoma (esophagostoma) and the tracheostoma, 5 cm apart. The superior aspects of these incisions are extended medially and joined 1 cm above the pharyngostoma (esophagostoma). The lower ends of the vertical incisions are directed medially so that they incise the lateral rims of the tracheostoma in the 3 o'clock and 9 o'clock positions. *B,* The medial margins of the vertical incisions are carefully elevated by means of skin hooks and sharp dissection. Forceps should not be used on these skin edges. A subcutaneous plane is also established superior to the pharyngostoma (esophagostoma). *C,* Sutures of No. 3-0 chromic catgut on a cutting needle are placed to, but not through, the skin edges, as shown. The vertical margins are sutured together, creating a skin tube. *D,* The skin tube is nearly completed with the exception of that portion anterior to the pharyngostoma (esophagostoma). A single-layer closure is sufficient. Additional sutures only jeopardize the blood supply to the skin margins.

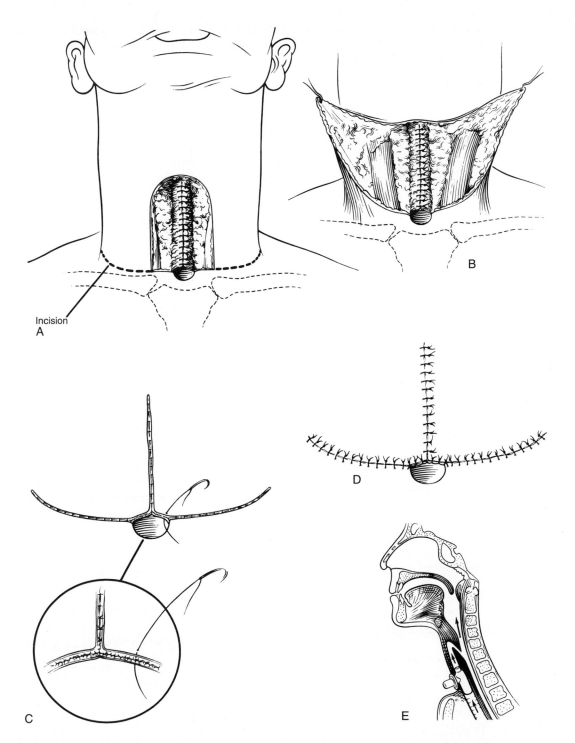

FIGURE 12-9. Completion of skin tube communication after total laryngectomy—second-stage procedure. *A,* The construction of the skin tube connecting the pharyngostoma (esophagostoma) with the tracheostoma is complete. An incision is made inferiorly on each side, in the supraclavicular region, much as that used for a thyroidectomy. *B,* A flap is elevated on each side, exposing the sternocleidomastoid muscles. These flaps must be sufficiently elevated and based posterosuperiorly so that there will be no undue tension when they are approximated in the midline. *C,* The pedicled flaps have been mobilized and sutured together in the midline. It may be necessary to remove a small triangle of skin superiorly to make a straight-line closure without creating a "dog ear." Inferiorly, the medial aspect of the cervical flaps and the inferior aspect of the anterior wall of the skin tube are sutured together, forming the upper half of the tracheostoma. *D,* The repair has been completed. As a rule, the endotracheal tube may remain in place during this operation, except when those sutures necessary to reconstruct the upper half of the tracheostoma rim are applied. Closed suction drainage is used rather than a dressing. *E,* This sketch demonstrates the flow of air through the silicone tracheal T-tube, through the skin tube between the tracheostoma and the pharyngostoma (esophagostoma), and through the mucosal tube and on top to the upper phonatory system.

of these patients become withdrawn from society and lost to follow-up by their physicians. To remedy this, a number of procedures have been introduced that allow a communication between the tracheostoma and the esophagus that produces intelligible speech.

Tracheoesophageal Shunt

The tracheoesophageal shunt procedure, popularized by Drs. Mark Singer and Eric Blom, has been used widely during the past few years as a simple method to restore speech after total laryngectomy. In many surgical procedures today, a tracheoesophageal approach is constructed at the time of total laryngectomy. If this for some reason is not successful, then it can be allowed to heal and a secondary puncture is performed at a later date.

The tracheoesophageal shunt procedure is indicated after a total laryngectomy when the patient cannot learn good esophageal speech and is not satisfied with the speech obtained by an electronic vibrating device. There are a number of prerequisites that must be present before this procedure is attempted:

1. A competent speech pathologist who is experienced with this technique should be available.
2. The patient should be intelligent and highly motivated.
3. Good pulmonary status should be present.
4. The patient should have adequate manual dexterity to manage the prosthesis.
5. The stoma should be of adequate size so that the prosthesis may be easily inserted (1.5 cm) and not so large that it cannot be easily occluded to create positive pressure for speech formation.
6. If preoperative or postoperative radiation therapy has been administered, 3 to 6 months should elapse before performing this procedure.
7. The patient should be free of inferior constrictor spasm.

Tracheoesophageal Preoperative Assessment

The tracheoesophageal shunt procedure should be thoroughly discussed with the patient who cannot learn intelligible esophageal speech. If patients have not had adequate instruction in esophageal speech, then they are encouraged to do so.

The patient is tested for the presence of inferior constrictor muscle spasm. A No. 14 French catheter is inserted by way of the nasal cavity to a level approximating the site for creating a tracheoesophageal fistula or about the level of the thoracic inlet. The rough measurement for this distance is 25 cm from the nostril. Air is blown into the catheter by the examiner and the voice tested. If patients demonstrate a spasm and are unable to produce speech when air is blown into the catheter, they are considered poor candidates for a tracheoesophageal shunt procedure, unless an inferior constrictor myotomy is performed or the inferior constrictor is injected with botulism toxin. Before either of these is accomplished, a parapharyngeal nerve block using 1% lidocaine solution can be injected into the level C2-C3 to relax the inferior constrictor muscle. Speech should improve almost immediately.

Technique for Constructing a Tracheoesophageal Fistula

An esophagoscopy is performed under general anesthesia with complete neuromuscular relaxation. The hypopharynx and esophagus should be examined for evidence of recurrent disease, narrowing, or strictures.

A 7 × 1.3 × 30 cm esophagoscope is inserted into the hypopharynx and rotated 180 degrees so that the bevel faces forward. It is inserted to a point where the light can be viewed by way of the tracheostoma behind the posterior tracheal wall. The beveled opening of the scope, which faces anteriorly, can be palpated with a finger placed in the tracheostoma.

The site for the tracheoesophageal puncture is determined and marked. This mark is made approximately 10 to 15 mm below the superior mucocutaneous junction in the midline posterior wall of the trachea. A No. 14 gauge angiocatheter needle is used to make the puncture (Fig. 12–10). The angiocatheter needle is inserted through the posterior tracheal wall and into the perforation in the esophagoscope or into the beveled end of the esophagoscope.

A No. 16 angiocatheter is threaded through the angiocatheter needle (see Fig. 12–10). If there is any problem with pulling the catheter through the tracheoesophageal puncture, the site is enlarged with a fine curved hemostat. The puncture can also be enlarged with a No. 11 surgical blade. It is grasped with forceps inside the esophagoscope and pulled out through the oral cavity. The end of the angiocatheter protruding from the tracheostoma is tied to the end of a No. 14 French catheter, and the end of the French catheter is pulled from the mouth or the esophagoscope is removed.

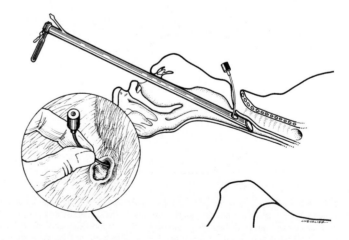

FIGURE 12–10. A 7 × 1.3 esophagoscope is introduced into the esophagus to the level of the tracheostoma and rotated so that the bevel faces anteriorly. The light transmitted through the mucous membrane and palpation will serve to determine the site of the end of the esophagoscope. A No. 14 intravenous catheter needle is bent to a curve and inserted through the posterior tracheal wall and into the perforation in the esophagoscope (shown here) or in the beveled end of the esophagus. A No. 16 angiocatheter is threaded through the needle, grasped by the endoscopist with alligator forceps, and pulled out the oral cavity. A catheter is inserted in to the nasal cavity and out the mouth. The angiocatheter is tied to this catheter and pulled out of the nasal cavity.

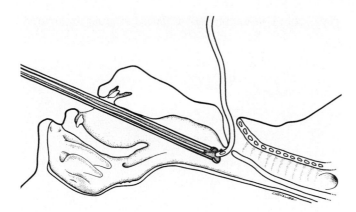

FIGURE 12–11. The end of the angiocatheter protruding from the tracheostoma is tied to a No. 14 French catheter. The opening in the posterior wall of the trachea is enlarged with a fine hemostat or a No. 11 surgical blade.

A catheter is inserted into the nasal cavity, through the nasopharynx and oropharynx, and out the mouth. The end of the angiocatheter is secured to the end of the French catheter, and it is pulled out the nasal cavity (Fig. 12–11). The two ends of the catheter are tied together to make a loop that enters the nasal cavity and exits the tracheoesophageal puncture, or the end of the catheter is directed down the esophagus into the stomach. I usually secure this catheter in place with a skin suture. The patient is discharged from the hospital the same day and advised to return to the surgeon and speech pathologist in about 2 weeks. During this visit, the catheter is removed and a prosthesis of the proper length and diameter is inserted. The speech pathologist demonstrates to the patient the technique for removal and replacement of this prosthesis. Usually good speech is obtained at the time of this visit; however, several sessions are sometimes necessary before intelligible speech is mastered.

The tracheoesophageal shunt may be constructed at the time of laryngectomy if it is the decision of the patient and surgeon, with the understanding that esophageal speech will not be an option. The technique is quite simple. After the larynx has been removed, a sharp curved hemostat is inserted into the esophagus. This will outdent the posterior wall of the trachea below the site of its transection. This point should be about 1½ cm inferior to the cut end of the trachea. The tines of the hemostat are opened slightly, and an incision is made into the esophagus with a No. 11 surgical blade. As the end of the opened hemostat projects into the trachea, it grasps the end of a No. 14 feeding tube. The feeding tube is pulled up into the surgical field and then directed into the stomach. The feeding tube is securely fastened to the peritracheostoma skin with silk sutures. When the feeding tube is removed after 7 or 8 days, a tracheoesophageal valve is inserted. It is best to wait one additional week to start speech.

The Middle and Inferior Constrictor Myotomy

If the preoperative air insufflation test has demonstrated pharyngoesophageal spasm, preventing airflow for speech, a middle and inferior constrictor myotomy is performed at

the time of the puncture. This operation is also used in patients who have undergone the tracheoesophageal shunt procedure and have failed to accomplish speech. Again, these patients demonstrate poor pharyngoesophageal airflow when air is insufflated by way of the shunt.

The operation is performed using general anesthesia. A No. 36 or No. 38 mercury esophageal bougie or a large endotracheal tube is inserted into the cervical esophagus. An incision is made along the vertical limb of the U-shaped scar, and the anterior border of the sternocleidomastoid muscle is delineated. The carotid sheath is identified and retracted laterally. The prevertebral fascia is dissected free so that the inferior constrictor muscle can be clearly visualized. Allis clamps are placed on the pharynx, and the tissues are rotated so that the posterior aspect of the pharyngeal constrictors is clearly seen. A posterior midline incision is made through the muscle from the level of the base of the tongue to the tracheostoma. It is important to sever all muscle fibers so that the mucous membrane can be visualized. This technique is discussed in detail in Chapter 4. Closed-suction drainage is inserted before the wound is closed.

Tracheoesophageal shunt speech can be attempted 2 days after this operation unless the pharynx or esophageal membrane has been inadvertently incised and repaired. In such cases, 10 days of healing should pass before speech is attempted.

Complicating Factors With the Tracheoesophageal Shunt

Some patients are unable or unwilling to care for the vocal prosthesis owing to such factors as poor general health, disinterest, visual problems, and depression.

There is a risk of aspiration of saliva or of the vocal prosthesis. Repeated application of electrocautery to the tracheoesophageal puncture will stimulate stenosis and improve or prevent leakage. If the leakage is severe, the prosthesis must be removed and the tracheopharyngeal puncture must be closed. The incidence of aspiration has markedly decreased with the advent of the inner phalange on the prosthesis (esophageal side).

Marked inflammatory reactions have occurred in and around the tracheostoma, especially in patients who have received radiation therapy. This reaction usually subsides rapidly with the use of antibiotics (erythromycin) and local measures.

Some patients are unable to produce fluent speech even after an inferior constrictor myotomy is performed and after trying various types of prostheses.

An external tracheostoma valve has been used in some patients. It provides tracheoesophageal voice without the necessity for finger occlusion of the stoma. Candidates for this valve are patients whose speech is characterized by low effort and minimal resistance to the tracheoesophageal airflow.

A buildup of fungal debris, which inactivates valve function and causes leakage, has become an increasing problem with tracheoesophageal speech. It is managed by Mycostatin orally and by frequent changes of the valve.

Dr. Panje performs the tracheoesophageal shunt procedure with local anesthesia as an outpatient procedure. Codeine is used to reduce the cough reflex. The pharynx is

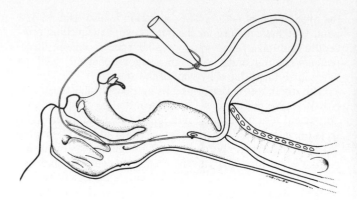

FIGURE 12-12. The end of the No. 14 French catheter is pulled out through the nasal cavity. The ends are tied together forming a loop, or the distal end of the catheter is pushed down the esophagus into the stomach.

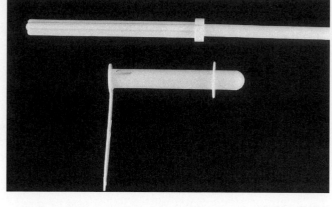

FIGURE 12-13. Blom-Singer voice prostheses.

anesthetized with 15 mL of viscous lidocaine (Xylocaine), and the trachea is anesthetized with 4% cocaine solution. Again, the diameter of the tracheostoma must be at least 1.5 cm. An esophageal tube is passed until it can be seen bulging the posterior wall of the trachea just below the upper margin of the tracheostoma. This site is anesthetized with a small amount of 1% lidocaine (Xylocaine) solution with epinephrine. A No. 20 needle is inserted through the posterior wall of the trachea and anterior wall of the esophagus and into the rubber esophageal tube (see Fig. 12–10). The puncture is made in the posterior midline $1\frac{1}{2}$–2 cm below the upper margin of the tracheostoma. A vertical incision approximately 7 mm long is made using a No. 11 surgical blade. The incision is carried to the esophageal tube. It must be remembered that the tracheoesophageal wall is $\frac{1}{2}$ cm to 1 cm thick. The esophageal tube is removed gradually to a point just above the site of the puncture, and a No. 14 feeding tube (Fig. 12–11) is inserted toward the stomach through the tracheoesophageal fistula. The feeding tube can also exit via the nose, as shown in Figure 12–12. The catheter is sutured to the skin lateral to the tracheostoma with 3-0 silk sutures. The proximal end of the feeding tube is plugged. The patient is sent home and is instructed not to remove the catheter. If the catheter comes out, it should be replaced immediately. The patient returns to the office in 2 weeks, at which time the voice prosthesis is inserted. Figure 12–13 shows the original Blom-Singer voice prosthesis, which I have used in patients. Today, new voice prosthesis designs are being developed, which will hopefully reduce some of the current problems associated with leakage and longevity.

Chapter 13
Laryngeal Paralysis

WILLIAM W. MONTGOMERY   STUART K. MONTGOMERY   MARK A. VARVARES

Physicians must have a comprehensive knowledge of the anatomy and physiology of the larynx to diagnose and treat the abnormalities that occur when laryngeal innervation is disrupted. The symptoms that result from a disturbance in laryngeal innervation are variable. Vocal function can range from slight hoarseness or loss of singing ability to severe hoarseness and, occasionally, complete aphonia. The airway can be altered from a slight degree of dyspnea on exertion, which may be noticed only in the presence of an upper respiratory infection, to severe dyspnea necessitating a tracheotomy. Dysphagia associated with recurrent laryngeal nerve paralysis varies from minimal (an occasional cough due to aspiration) to severe (the patient is unable to swallow without aspirating).

The purpose of this chapter is to aid surgeons with the diagnosis and management of patients afflicted with alterations in motor and sensory innervation of the larynx.

ANATOMY AND FUNCTION OF THE LARYNX

The basic structures of the larynx are the thyroid, cricoid, and paired arytenoid cartilages held together by muscle and fibroelastic tissue. The larynx is lined with mucous membrane. The basic function of the larynx is accomplished by the intrinsic musculature and supported by the extrinsic musculature. The external laryngeal muscles include the thyrohyoid, sternothyroid, omohyoid, inferior constrictor, stylohyoid, geniohyoid, mylohyoid, hyoglossus and posterior, and anterior bellies of the digastric.

The arytenoid cartilages articulate with the superolateral aspect of the posterior lamina of the cricoid cartilage. The articulation forms a shallow, elongated arthroidial (ball-and-socket) joint with joint cavity, synovial lining, joint capsule, and supporting posterior cricoarytenoid ligament.

The arytenoid cartilage is shaped like an irregular three-sided pyramid. The three surfaces face posteriorly, anterolaterally, and medially. The base has angles facing medially, laterally, and anteriorly. The lateral angle is the muscular process to which the posterior and lateral cricoarytenoid muscles are attached. The anterior process projects forward and inserts into the vocal fold as the vocal process. The apex of this pyramid-shaped arytenoid cartilage projects medially

and posteriorly as the corniculate cartilage. The epiglottis and cuneiform cartilages have a lesser role in the function of the larynx.

The cricoarytenoid joint has three types of movement: a rocking or rotary movement around the joint axis, a linear glide parallel to the joint axis, and a pivotal motion around the strong posterior cricoarytenoid ligament.

A brief review of the anatomy and action of the intrinsic muscles of the larynx is necessary to comprehend fully the signs and symptoms associated with cricoarytenoid arthritis, as well as those associated with bilateral laryngeal paralysis with the vocal cords in the midline position.

The cricothyroid muscle (Fig. 13–1A) must be included in this review because it indirectly influences the function of the cricoarytenoid joint. This muscle arises from the external surface of the arch of the cricoid cartilage. It has a straight and an oblique portion. The straight portion inserts into the border of the thyroid cartilage. The oblique portion inserts into the inferior horn, inferior border, and inner surface of the thyroid cartilage. The cricothyroid muscle is innervated by the external branch of the superior laryngeal nerve. As it contracts, the posterior cricoid lamina tilts downward and backward. The fulcrum for the action is the cricothyroid joint. The tilting of the cricoid cartilage increases the distance between the anterior commissure and the vocal processes of the arytenoid cartilage and thus lengthens, or stretches, the vocal folds. The strong posterior cricoarytenoid ligament prevents anterior displacement of the arytenoid cartilage as the cricothyroid muscle contracts.

The external thyroarytenoid muscle (Fig. 13–1B) extends from the anterior aspect of the thyroid cartilage to the lateral surface of the arytenoid cartilage. It rotates the arytenoid cartilage medially and pulls it forward. The first action adducts the vocal cords, and the second action is antagonistic to the action of the cricothyroid muscle.

The internal thyroarytenoid muscle (Fig. 13–1B) also arises from the anterior aspect of the thyroid cartilage. Some of its fibers insert on the vocal process of the arytenoid cartilage, whereas others insert directly into the vocal cord. Disagreement as to the exact function of this muscle still exists. The muscle fibers attached to the vocal process adduct and shorten the anterior aspect of the vocal fold. The fibers attached directly to the vocal fold are said to abduct this segment of the fold. Pressman (1942), when studying the mechanism of phonation by high-speed motion pictures, noted that during the formation of high notes, the posterior part of each vocal fold is held in tight adduction, while the anterior part is abducted and then thrown into vibration by expired air. The abducting ability of the internal thyroarytenoid muscle may explain Pressman's observation. The thyroarytenoid muscle is innervated by the recurrent laryngeal nerve.

The posterior cricoarytenoid muscle (Fig. 13–1C) arises from the posterior surface of the cricoid lamina and inserts into the muscular process of the arytenoid cartilage. It is innervated by the recurrent laryngeal nerve. The posterior cricoarytenoid muscle is the only true abductor of the vocal folds. It swings the muscular process posteriorly, and by this action, the vocal process of the arytenoid cartilage is displaced laterally.

The lateral cricoarytenoid muscle (Fig. 13–1D) arises from the upper border and outer surface of the arch of the cricoid cartilage. It inserts into the anterior aspect of the muscular process of the arytenoid cartilage. As it contracts, the muscular process is pulled downward and forward, thus adducting the vocal fold. It is the antagonist of the posterior cricoarytenoid muscle and is also innervated by the recurrent laryngeal nerve.

The arytenoid muscle (Fig. 13–1E) has an oblique and a transverse portion, extending from the posteromedial aspect of one arytenoid to the corresponding aspect of the other arytenoid. The oblique muscle receives its motor nerve supply from the recurrent laryngeal nerve. It is also innervated by the internal branch of the superior laryngeal nerve. Experimental evidence indicates that these branches from the superior laryngeal nerve are not voluntary motor fibers. Contraction of the arytenoid muscle brings the two arytenoid cartilages together, thus closing the posterior commissure.

The innervation of the larynx is very complex. Normal laryngeal function requires fine coordination between the sensory innervation and antagonistic abductor and adductor muscle contractions.

The larynx is supplied by paired recurrent and superior laryngeal nerves. The recurrent laryngeal nerve innervates the intrinsic muscles of the larynx, with the exception of the cricothyroid muscle. Its point of origin and course differ on each side of the body. On the right side, it leaves the vagus nerve anterior to the subclavian artery, behind which it winds, and then ascends to the side of the trachea posterior to the common carotid artery. On the left side, it departs from the vagus to the left of the aortic arch. It winds below the arch immediately behind the attachment of the ligamentum arte-

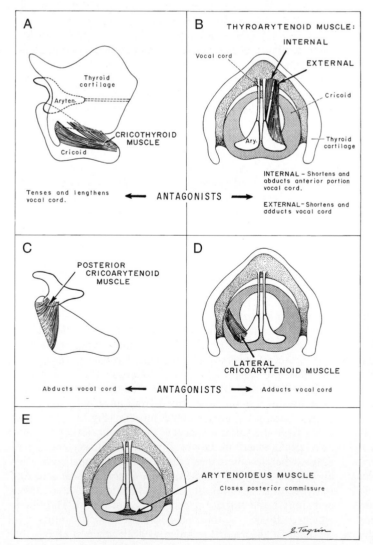

FIGURE 13–1. *A,* Cricothyroid muscle. Origin: external surface of cricoid arch. Insertion: inferior horn, inferior border, and inner surface of thyroid cartilage. Action: tilts the posterior cricoid lamina downward and backward on the cricothyroid joint. This action lengthens and tenses the vocal folds. *B,* Thyroarytenoid muscle. External portion. Origin: anterior inner surface of thyroid cartilage. Insertion: anterior and lateral surface of the muscular process of the arytenoid cartilage. Action: rotates the arytenoid cartilage medially and pulls it forward, thus shortening and adducting the vocal folds. Internal portion. Origin: anterior inner surface of the thyroid cartilage. Insertion: vocal process of arytenoid cartilage and directly to the vocal folds. Action: shortens and abducts the vocal cords anterior to the vocal process. *C,* Posterior cricoarytenoid muscle. Origin: posterior surface of the cricoid lamina. Insertion: posterior and lateral surface of the arytenoid muscular process. Action: abducts the vocal folds. *D,* Lateral cricoarytenoid muscle. Origin: arch of the cricoid. Insertion: anterior surface of an arytenoid muscular process. Action: adducts the vocal folds. *E,* Arytenoid muscle. Origin and Insertion: the muscle bridges between the two arytenoids. Action: closes the posterior commissure.

riosum and then ascends to the side of the trachea. The nerves on each side course upward in the tracheal esophageal groove. Each nerve enters the larynx just posterior to the cricothyroid articulation, where it divides. There are three components of the recurrent laryngeal nerve: (1) fibers that supply the adductor muscles of the larynx; (2) fibers that supply the abductor muscles; and (3) sensory and secretory fibers to the larynx and subglottic region. The anterior branch of the recurrent laryngeal nerve, or adductor branch, runs anterosuperiorly on the lateral surface of the lateral cricoarytenoid and thyroarytenoid muscles, which it innervates along with the vocalis and aryepiglottic muscles. The posterior, or abductor branch, innervates the posterior cricoarytenoid and transverse and oblique arytenoid muscles.

The superior laryngeal nerve originates from the inferior ganglion of the vagus nerve and descends medial to the internal and external carotid arteries. As it curves anteroinferiorly toward the larynx, it divides into a small external laryngeal and a large internal branch. The external branch, or external laryngeal nerve, descends under the sternothyroid muscle along with the superior laryngeal artery, but on a deeper plane. It winds closely around the inferior thyroid tubercle and terminates in the cricothyroid muscle, which it innervates. The internal branch, or internal laryngeal nerve, innervates (sensory) the mucous membrane of the larynx down to the level of the vocal folds. It descends to the thyrohyoid membrane, which it penetrates with the superior laryngeal artery, and divides into an upper and a lower branch. The upper branch courses horizontally and innervates the mucous membrane of the pharynx, epiglottis, vallecula, and vestibule of the larynx. The lower branch passes inferiorly on the medial wall of the pyriform recess and innervates the aryepiglottic fold and mucous membrane on the posterior surface of the arytenoid cartilage and arytenoideus muscle. It ends by penetrating the inferior constrictor muscle and anatomizing with an ascending branch of the recurring laryngeal nerve.

CLASSIFICATION OF LARYNGEAL PARALYSIS

Laryngeal paralysis is best classified according to the result of the particular denervation. For example, unilateral paralysis of the recurrent laryngeal nerve should be identified according to the resultant position of the paralyzed vocal fold (e.g., a unilateral recurrent laryngeal nerve paralysis in the position of abduction). A classification of the various types of laryngeal paralysis is outlined in Tables 13–1, 13–2, and 13–3.

TABLE 13–1
Laryngeal Paralysis: Recurrent Laryngeal Nerve (RLN)

Unilateral		
Position	Adduction	
	Paramedian	
	Abduction	
Bilateral		
Position	Adduction	
	Paramedian	
	Abduction	

TABLE 13–2
Laryngeal Paralysis: Superior Laryngeal Nerve (SLN)

Motor (external branch)	
Unilateral	
Bilateral	
Sensory and Motor	
Unilateral	
Bilateral	

Unilateral Recurrent Laryngeal Nerve Paralysis

The unilaterally paralyzed recurrent laryngeal nerve may paralyze the vocal cord in the position of adduction, the paramedian position, or the position of abduction.

When the unilaterally paralyzed vocal cord assumes the position of adduction, the voice is almost invariably normal. However, patients may notice some alteration in their singing voice.

In patients with recurrent laryngeal nerve paralysis and the vocal cord in the paramedian position, the symptoms are variable. Some patients can compensate quite well and note only slight alterations in their voices. However, they do have difficulty changing pitch and are usually unable to sing. The compensation is accomplished by the unparalyzed cord adducting beyond the midline; the cricothyroid muscle can still lengthen and tense the paralyzed cord, and some posterior medial motion is achieved by the action of the bilaterally innervated interarytenoid muscle. Other patients cannot compensate and present with a breathy type of hoarseness and considerable monotony to their voice. Some patients can improve their voice quality by working with a voice therapist, but most patients require a medialization thyroplasty or some other procedure to mobilize the paralyzed cord medially.

Recurrent laryngeal nerve paralysis that results in the cord assuming the position of abduction is much more serious clinically. The patient has a whispered voice or may be aphonic. There is a poor cough reflex. The patient is unable to laugh and complains of frequent aspiration.

Bilateral Recurrent Laryngeal Nerve Paralysis

Paralysis of both recurrent laryngeal nerves resulting in the vocal cords assuming the position of adduction can present

TABLE 13–3
Laryngeal Paralysis: Combined Recurrent and Superior Laryngeal Nerve

Unilateral—SLN and RLN		
Position	Adduction	
	Paramedian	
	Abduction	
Unilateral SLN and bilateral RLN		
Position	Adduction	
	Paramedian	
	Abduction	
Bilateral SLN and unilateral or bilateral RLN		

TABLE 13-4
Symptoms of Unilateral Recurrent Laryngeal Nerve Paralysis

Position	Symptoms
Adduction	None +/−loss of singing quality
Paramedian	Hoarseness (air escape)
	Aspiration
	+/−loss of cough, laugh
Abduction	Hoarseness
	Aspiration
	+/−loss of cough, laugh

TABLE 13-6
Symptoms of Superior Laryngeal Nerve Paralysis

Motor (External Branch)	
Type of Paralysis	**Symptoms**
Unilateral	Slight hoarseness
	Vocal cord bowed on paralyzed side
	Vocal chink not straight
	Vocal cord at lower level
Bilateral	Hoarseness
	Singing quality down
	Cords bowed
	No cricoid tilt

as a life-threatening situation. However, section of both recurrent laryngeal nerves may leave the patient with an adequate vocal chink, and the cords may not migrate to the complete adduction position for days, weeks, months, and sometimes years after the original injury. The patient with paralyzed vocal cords in the adducted position most often has a good strong voice but a poor airway. After performing a tracheotomy to relieve the inspiratory stridor, it is often apparent that the voice has a monotone quality and there is a definite change in the singing voice.

Some patients can compensate for bilateral recurrent laryngeal nerve paralysis with the cords in the paramedian position. Patients with this type of paralysis have varying degrees of hoarseness caused by air escape. Aspiration may be present as well as loss of the cough reflex and the ability to laugh.

Paralysis of the recurrent laryngeal nerves that results in the cords assuming the position of abduction is a very serious medical problem. The patient has no voice, aspirates freely, and is without a cough reflex or the ability to laugh (Table 13-5). Most patients with this type of paralysis present to the otolaryngologist with a cuffed tracheotomy tube in place.

Superior Laryngeal Nerve Paralysis

Unilateral Superior Laryngeal Nerve Paralysis (External Motor Branch)

Unilateral paralysis of the external branch of the superior laryngeal nerve is often overlooked clinically. In some patients, paralysis of the cricothyroid muscle can produce a sensation of pressure on the affected side of the throat. Frequent clearing of the throat, a mild hoarseness that is especially noted by the patient, a weak voice, and an inability to make a high-pitched sound may be present (Table 13-6).

The latter disability may interfere with the patient's singing voice. A paralyzed cricothyroid muscle may be difficult to detect. The posterior commissure may be pulled toward the side of the paralyzed cricothyroid muscle. At rest, the larynx appears to be symmetrical. With phonation, however, the opposite aryepiglottic fold is elongated and the aryepiglottic fold on the side of the cricothyroid muscle paralysis is shortened. The vocal cord on the side of the cricothyroid muscle paralysis is shorter, somewhat bowed, and wrinkled or wavy in appearance. It may be at a different level than the opposite cord.

Bilateral Superior Laryngeal Nerve Paralysis (External Motor Branch)

Bilateral paralysis of the external branch of the superior laryngeal nerve is difficult to recognize clinically because of the symmetry of the larynx at rest. However, by palpating the neck, it can easily be detected that the cricoid cartilage does not tilt to lengthen and tense the vocal cords. Indirect laryngoscopy shows subtle changes, such as flaccidity, bowing, and hyperemia of both vocal cords. Shortly after onset of the paralysis, the voice is at a lower pitch, weaker, and breathy. It lacks inflection, and whereas the speaking voice is often normal, the singing voice is abnormal.

Unilateral Superior Laryngeal Nerve Paralysis (Sensory and Motor)

Complete paralysis of the superior laryngeal nerve on one side can result in aspiration due to a sensory deficit. However, it is not severe (Table 13-7), and the patient can usually learn to compensate for it in a few weeks or months. The appearance of the larynx is similar to that described under unilateral superior laryngeal nerve paralysis (motor branch).

TABLE 13-5
Symptoms of Bilateral RLN Paralysis

Position	Symptoms
Median	Inspiratory stridor, most often normal voice
Paramedian	Hoarseness (air escape)
	Some aspiration
	Loss of cough, laugh
Abduction	No voice
	Aspiration
	No cough
	No laugh

TABLE 13-7
Superior Laryngeal Nerve Paralysis: Sensory and Motor

Type of Paralysis	Symptoms
Unilateral	Some hoarseness
	Hoarseness
	Cord lower level
	Asymmetry cords
Bilateral	Aspiration
	Hoarseness
	No tilt cricoid
	Cords bowed

Bilateral Superior Laryngeal Nerve Paralysis (Sensory and Motor)

Bilateral paralysis of the superior laryngeal nerves results in aspiration. The appearance of the larynx is the same as that described for bilateral paralysis of the cricothyroid muscles. The literature contains reports of patients compensating for this aspiration; however, this has not been our experience. Most patients require a cuffed tracheotomy and nasogastric feeding tubes as a temporary procedure, followed by an operative procedure to relieve the aspiration.

Combined Recurrent and Superior Laryngeal Nerve Paralysis

Combined Unilateral Recurrent and Unilateral Superior Laryngeal Nerve Paralysis

The signs and symptoms of combined unilateral recurrent and unilateral superior laryngeal nerve paralysis (Table 13–8) are not too different from those described for unilateral paralysis of the recurrent laryngeal nerve. The subtle changes resulting from paralysis of the cricothyroid muscle in addition to the muscles supplied by the recurrent laryngeal nerves are difficult to detect but can be recognized. When the vocal cord remains in the position of adduction, unilateral combined paralysis causes a greater degree of hoarseness. When the vocal cord assumes the paramedian position, there is a greater degree of hoarseness and aspiration. When the paralyzed vocal cord assumes the position of abduction, the symptomatology is severe. Aspiration is the greatest problem. The patient is usually without a voice and loses the cough reflex. Surgical intervention is required.

Combined Unilateral Superior Laryngeal Nerve Paralysis and Bilateral Recurrent Laryngeal Nerve Paralysis *(TABLE 13-9)*

A patient with bilateral recurrent laryngeal nerve paralysis with the vocal folds in the position of adduction and the additional problem of aspiration from unilateral superior laryngeal nerve paralysis can have severe complications. If the patient is not aspirating, a regular tracheotomy tube can be used. If the patient is aspirating, then a cuffed tracheotomy tube is necessary. The presence of a tracheotomy often increases the degree of aspiration. Some patients can compensate for this and live with a tracheotomy. If the aspiration is completely compensated for, the surgeon can consider an operative procedure to improve the airway.

TABLE 13-8
Combined Recurrent and Superior Laryngeal Nerve Paralysis: Unilateral RLN and SLN Paralysis

Position	Symptoms
Adduction	None +/−hoarseness
Paramedian	Hoarseness
	Aspiration
Abduction	Hoarseness (severe)
	Aspiration (severe)
	Loss of cough
	Loss of laugh

TABLE 13-9
Combined Recurrent and Superior Laryngeal Nerve Paralysis: Unilateral SLN and Bilateral RLN

Position	Symptoms
Adduction	Inspiratory stridor
Paramedian	Hoarseness
	Aspiration
	Loss of cough, laugh +/−laryngeal insufficiency
Abduction	Laryngeal insufficiency

Combined bilateral recurrent laryngeal nerve paralysis with the vocal cords in the paramedian position and added unilateral superior laryngeal nerve paralysis result in severe hoarseness, aspiration, and loss of cough reflex. Very few patients can compensate for this, and most require a tracheotomy with a cuffed tube and nasogastric or gastrostomy feeding tube and then an operative procedure for control of aspiration.

Bilateral recurrent laryngeal nerve paralysis in the position of abduction combined with unilateral superior laryngeal nerve paralysis results in complete laryngeal insufficiency. It can be temporized with a cuffed tracheotomy tube, but surgical intervention must be implemented to prevent pulmonary complications and establish a means of nutrition.

Combined Bilateral Superior and Bilateral Recurrent Laryngeal Nerve Paralysis *(TABLE 13-10)*

Combined bilateral superior and bilateral recurrent laryngeal nerve paralysis is a very rare but serious situation. Regardless of the position of the vocal cords, there is severe aspiration, and operative procedures are indicated to control pulmonary complications.

DIAGNOSIS AND WORK-UP

Evaluation of laryngeal paralysis is sometimes very simple; the diagnosis may be apparent after taking the patient's history of the present illness and reviewing the symptoms. For example, the patient may have a history of a viral or bacterial infection, a neck injury, or a thyroid, cervical, or thoracic operation before the onset of vocal cord paralysis. However, a more extensive investigation is usually necessary to uncover the cause for the paralysis and even then the etiology may remain obscure.

TABLE 13-10
Combined Recurrent and Superior Laryngeal Nerve Paralysis: Bilateral, SLN, and Unilateral or Bilateral RLN Paralysis

Position	Symptoms
Adduction	Laryngeal insufficiency
Paramedian	Functionless larynx
Abduction	Functionless larynx

Work-Up

Past history: operations (thyroid, chest, intracranial, cervical); trauma (laryngeal internal and external); head injury; chest injury.

Present illness: first symptom(s): duration (constant or intermittent); severity (increasing or decreasing); any history of upper respiratory infection during onset.

Hoarseness: raspy, breathy, high or low pitched.

Dysphagia: constant or intermittent; with liquids or solids; any weight loss.

Aspiration: minimal, moderate, or severe (with repeated aspiration pneumonias).

Ability to cough: slight or moderate ability, or inability to cough.

Odynophonia: duration and severity; intermittent or constant.

Odynophagia: degree; associated with weight loss; pain radiating to ear; sensation of lump in throat.

Dyspnea: slight, moderate, or severe (requiring a tracheotomy).

Examination

On examination of the neck, all extrinsic laryngeal muscles and the laryngeal cartilages should be palpated. Is there any widening of the thyroid laminae? Palpate for cricoarytenoid joint tenderness. Note the motion of the cricoid and thyroid cartilages as the patient phonates.

INDIRECT LARYNGOSCOPY AND NASOPHARYNGOSCOPY

Does the patient have a normal gag reflex on each side? Is there any inflammatory process of the larynx? Is the paralysis unilateral or bilateral? Note the position of the paralyzed cord or cords (abduction, adduction, or paramedian). Test the inspiratory laryngeal airway as the patient sniffs in through the nose. Describe the position of the cords during phonation. Is there any shortening, change in color, or wrinkling of the vocal cords? The arytenoid should be carefully observed for dislocation or malposition.

Radiologic Work-Up

The best way to evaluate a patient with vocal cord paralysis is to have an axial computed tomography scan taken from the base of the skull through the chest. This demonstrates any etiologic factors and also gives a good evaluation of the airway. Cinefluoroscopy is of value for studying laryngeal function. A magnetic resonance image from the skull through the chest may be necessary to demonstrate a central, cervical, or thoracic lesion causing a vocal fold paralysis.

Direct Laryngoscopy

During direct laryngoscopy, any abnormalities of the epiglottis, aryepiglottic folds, pyriform sinus, arytenoids, and postcricoid region are noted. The position of the arytenoids is visualized, and a passive mobility test (spatula test) of the arytenoids is performed. Inspect the ventricular bands, ventricles, and subglottic region as well as the vocal folds. Note any evidence of inflammation, web, or stenosis of the posterior commissure.

TREATMENT

Unilateral Recurrent Laryngeal Nerve Paralysis in the Position of Adduction *(TABLE 13-11)*

Attempts to repair an injured or divided recurrent laryngeal nerve are pointless. Axonal confusion occurs as the nerve regenerates, with random reinnervation of the antagonistic laryngeal muscles resulting in synkinesis of the abductor and adductor muscles similar to that after facial-nerve paralysis. This, of course, results in ineffective vocal cord function. Results of repair to the sensory innervation to the larynx were not found in the literature. However, it should be successful.

Unilateral recurrent laryngeal nerve paralysis in the position of adduction is ideal for both speaking and breathing. There is an adequate airway and no change in the patient's vocal function other than some disturbance in the pitch range and singing voice. No treatment is indicated other than voice therapy, if the patient so desires. It must be remembered that unless the cause for this paralysis is obvious, the diagnostic evaluation should be pursued.

Unilateral Recurrent Laryngeal Nerve Paralysis in the Paramedian Position

A unilateral recurrent laryngeal nerve paralysis in the partially abducted (paramedian) position results in hoarseness and air loss during phonation. The two vocal folds do not approximate during phonation. This incomplete vocal fold adduction results in interference with coughing and laughing and can result in aspiration.

There is controversy as to when to treat this paralysis other than with vocal therapy. In general, if the function has not returned by 6 months, it is time to consider intervention. Rare cases of good functional return occur up to 1 year after onset of paralysis.

The patient should be referred to a voice laboratory for evaluation by video laryngoscopy and video laryngostroboscopy. The parameters of this evaluation include amplitude, range, functional frequency, jitter, and maximum phonation time. If possible, photographs are taken during maximum adduction and maximum abduction and kept in the patient's record.

TABLE 13-11
Treatment: Unilateral RLN Paralysis

Position	Treatment
Adduction	No treatment
	+/−Vocal therapy
Paramedian	Vocal therapy
	Augmentation by injection of Teflon, adipose, or Gelfoam paste
	Medialization thyroplasty
Abduction	Medialization thyroplasty

INJECTION TECHNIQUE

In 1911, Brüning, a German laryngologist, devised a technique of injecting the paralyzed vocal cord with paraffin using a specially designed syringe. The technique was very successful, but was later abandoned because the paraffin implant frequently extruded and produced a well-known complication, paraffinoma. In 1955, Arnold revived Brüning's technique using autogenous and homogeneous cartilage particles. Subsequently, a number of materials were used: autogenous cartilage, heterogeneous bovine bone paste, tantalum oxide, Teflon, tantalum powder, and silicone.

Teflon paste (polytef PTFE), a polymer of tetrafluoroethylene, is one of the most inert of all known plastic materials; it has a density of 2.4. The Teflon powder is mixed with glycerin as a vehicle, using equal volumes of each substance. The Teflon powder, with its small particle size, fulfills all of the criteria for the ideal substance for injection to displace the vocal cord medially: It is well tolerated by tissues; it is not reabsorbed; and it is finely dispersed in a harmless vehicle so that it may be injected through a long needle using the Brüning syringe.

In the decade before its use in the larynx, Teflon was proven to be well tolerated by human tissues in thousands of cases of stapedectomy and in its use as an arterial substitute. In 1962, Arnold published his results from laboratory experimentation with the Teflon-glycerin mixture and also its clinical use for the rehabilitation of paralytic dysphonia. Kirchner and colleagues performed experimental studies using Teflon on the canine larynx. They demonstrated that there were no carcinogenic effects of Teflon, that Teflon was inert and well tolerated by the tissues, that Teflon had no necrosing effect on cartilage, and that the implant became surrounded by a fibrous capsule.

In 1963, Lewy published a comparative analysis of tantalum-glycerin and Teflon-glycerin mixtures. He found that both mixtures were well tolerated by the tissues with minimal reaction, that there was no drift of the injected material, and that the result of the injection was not altered with the passage of time. He also concluded that the Teflon-glycerin mixture was preferred because it was easier to use and could be prepared in advance.

After performing histologic studies following Teflon injection in human beings, Stone and Arnold stated that Teflon was definitely not carcinogenic, that there was a minimal foreign-body reaction with Teflon, that there was no reaction in the surrounding tissues (both muscle and cartilage), and that the Teflon was surrounded by a fibrous capsule. Thus, by 1966, polytef had proven to be safe for clinical use. At that time, however, its use was limited to a relatively small number of laryngologists because the injection technique was considered difficult and the selection of cases was believed to require the judgment of an accomplished laryngologist.

We compiled the results of patients having had a Teflon injection for unilateral vocal cord paralysis in this group and found that 81% of the patients had a good voice. Teflon was accepted for general use in 1972. After 2 decades' experience with Teflon paste and further evaluation of patients, we found that only 60% had good voices and that there were an increasing number of patients with Teflon granulomas. At this time, we discontinued the use of Teflon injection for treatment of unilateral vocal cord paralysis and began using Dr. Isshiki's thyroplasty Type I operation. The technique for Teflon injection is included in this chapter because Teflon is still used by a few otolaryngologists in the country; additionally, other agents such as Gelfoam paste and adipose tissue can be used for short-term therapy.

Preoperative Information for the Patient

Preoperatively, the patient should be told the reasons for his or her breathy hoarseness, aspiration, and ineffective cough. The patient should be informed that the procedure involves a direct laryngoscopy, that is, the introduction of an illuminated metal tube into the throat. During the procedure, a needle attached to a pressure syringe similar to a "caulking gun" is introduced through the laryngoscope and into the tissues outside the paralyzed vocal cord. The bulk of the implant causes the paralyzed vocal cord to be moved in the direction of the opposite functioning cord. This enables the functioning cord to strike against the paralyzed cord, thereby improving the voice and cough and preventing aspiration.

The patient must understand that there is approximately an 80% chance for improvement and a slight chance that the condition might worsen. The main reason for failure is the difficulty of controlling the exact positioning of the Teflon paste in the tissues and the fact that, in some cases, the Teflon drifts to adjacent tissues as it is being injected. The patient should also be informed that there is a possibility of failure necessitating tracheotomy as well as the risks attendant with any operation and anesthesia.

Technique of Anesthesia

The patient is sedated with fentanyl and Versed intravenously. The anterior floor of the mouth, pharynx, and larynx are anesthetized topically using 4% cocaine or 4% Xylocaine spray. The patient is then titrated with an agent such as intravenous propofol and encouraged to take deep breaths.

Technique of Injection

The patient is placed in the position for direct laryngoscopy, and an anterior commissure laryngoscope is introduced. If elevation of the epiglottis is painful or produces gagging or laryngospasm, additional 4% cocaine solution is sprayed directly through the laryngoscope. A No. 19 or 20 laryngeal needle is used along with a Brüning syringe (Fig. 13–2).

The Brüning syringe must be loaded promptly and tested immediately before injection to ensure that the Teflon flow is smooth (Figs. 13–3 and 13–4). Teflon paste must not be introduced into the syringe the day before it is used. Both the needle and the Brüning syringe must be carefully cleaned with ethyl alcohol after their use.

Some practice is required to gain expertise with the Brüning syringe. Teflon continues to flow from the needle tip after each click, and there is no method for determining the exact amount being injected other than keeping a careful eye on the cord being injected. It is also essential that the site of the injection be clearly visible as the Teflon paste is be-

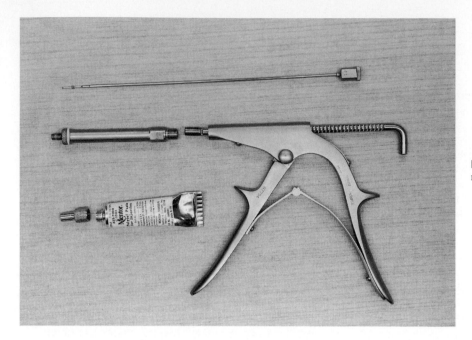

FIGURE 13–2. The Arnold-Brüning intralaryngeal Teflon injection set.

ing injected. The patient should phonate gently on command so that the proper amount of voice return can be established. The injection should be ceased as soon as the end of good voice return is reached.

The laryngeal needle is introduced through the anterior commissure laryngoscope so that its tip is at the level of the true vocal fold. The bevel of the needle tip should be facing medially (Fig. 13–5A). The tip of the needle is moved laterally over the superior surface of the paralyzed vocal fold until it displaces the false cord slightly in a lateral direction (Fig. 13–5B). With the needle in an oblique lateral direction, it is advanced through the floor of the ventricle and into the substance of the lateral thyroarytenoid muscle (Fig. 13–5C). The first injection is made at a point midway be-

tween the anterior commissure and the vocal process of the arytenoid. This injection is continued until the patient can approximate the opposite cord against the side being injected while phonating (Fig. 13–5D).

Some authors advocate the use of the needle guard to prevent advancing the needle beyond a depth of 4.5 mm. The ideal depth in any particular case, however, will vary with the size of the larynx. Also, the needle guard may give a false sense of security in that injections far beyond the depth of 4.5 mm can result as the needle guard indents the mucous membrane of the laryngeal ventricle (Fig. 13–6A).

The amount of Teflon paste necessary will vary with the size of the larynx and the degree of lateral displacement of the paralyzed fold. It is best to err on the side of underin-

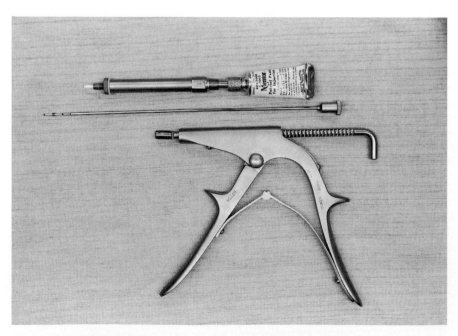

FIGURE 13–3. The cap is removed from the tube, which contains 7 mL of Teflon paste. After the seal of the tube is punctured, the loading adapter is screwed onto the tip of the Teflon paste tube. The loading adapter is inserted into the proximal end of the loading chamber. The end of the Teflon paste tube is rolled up and the tubes are squeezed with the one hand as the loading chamber is held in the other. It takes considerable pressure and a few minutes to fill the loading chamber.

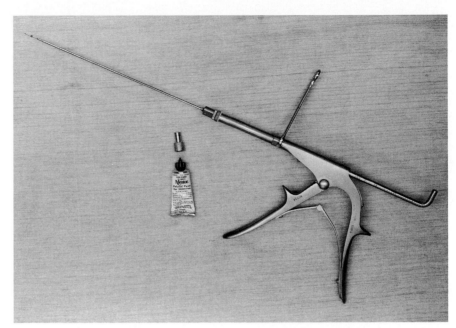

FIGURE 13-4. The loading chamber is attached to the handle of the syringe and tightened with a wrench. The needle is attached to the loading chamber.

jection rather than overinjection because Teflon, once injected, is difficult to remove. The needle should remain in place as long as possible after the injection. This will minimize the amount of Teflon paste lost because some Teflon paste exudes from the puncture site after the needle is removed.

Occasionally, one injection is sufficient to restore good phonatory function. However, a second injection is usually necessary. This is accomplished just lateral to the anterior aspect of the vocal process of the arytenoid and serves to close the posterior commissure.

Again, it is difficult to estimate the amount of Teflon needed in any given case because the Brüning syringe is not calibrated, some Teflon continues to flow from the tip of the needle after it is removed, and a varying amount of Teflon paste exudes from the puncture site after the needle is removed.

In the past, it was believed that a Teflon injection remained as an encapsulated mass restricted to the region of the lateral thyroarytenoideus muscle. However, a number of histopathologic studies have demonstrated that Teflon paste often extends into the lateral cricoarytenoideus muscle, through the cricothyroid space, and even extralaryngeally. For the most part, this situation has not been clinically significant in that there was very good rehabilitation of the laryngeal disorder in each case and there were no complicating signs and symptoms, except in one case in which the extralaryngeal mass was misinterpreted as a thyroid nodule. This could have been diagnosed preoperatively by a computed tomography scan. It is thus obvious that a certain amount of drift and misplacement of the Teflon paste will occur regardless of the technique and skill of the surgeon.

As mentioned previously, an increasing number of Teflon granulomas are appearing in our patients, and a number of good voices as a result of Teflon injection have been reduced from 81% to 60%. Ten to 12 mg of Decadron administered intravenously will reduce the amount of edema and postoperative discomfort. The authors usually send the patient home with a Medtrol dose pack (4 mg).

Postoperative Care

The patient may report postoperative pain localized on the side of the larynx injected. This is especially true when it has been necessary to inject lateral to the vocal process of the arytenoid to close the posterior commissure. This is much reduced if Decadron is used. Postoperative vocal function will gradually improve over a 2- to 4-week period.

Complications

Local swelling in the larynx may occur as a reaction to Teflon injection. Again, the use of dexamethasone sodium phosphate (Decadron) intraoperatively and at the end of an 8-hour period will do much to reduce the swelling. A number of surgeons have reported respiratory distress and stridor occurring within 24 hours after a Teflon injection. These patients were successfully treated with intravenous cortisone, ampicillin, and steam inhalations. A few cases have been reported with severe edema necessitating a tracheotomy. In all cases, the edema gradually subsided and the tracheotomy was removed. The authors believe that this complication can be avoided with the use of steroids intraoperatively.

Pain, which usually subsides in about a week, may persist for many weeks. Expectoration of Teflon particles or blood-tinged saliva may occur during the first 1 to 2 postoperative days.

Teflon granuloma may occur at any time after a Teflon injection, even many years later. Several techniques have been presented to remove a Teflon granuloma. The authors prefer evaporating the Teflon using a CO_2 laser by way of

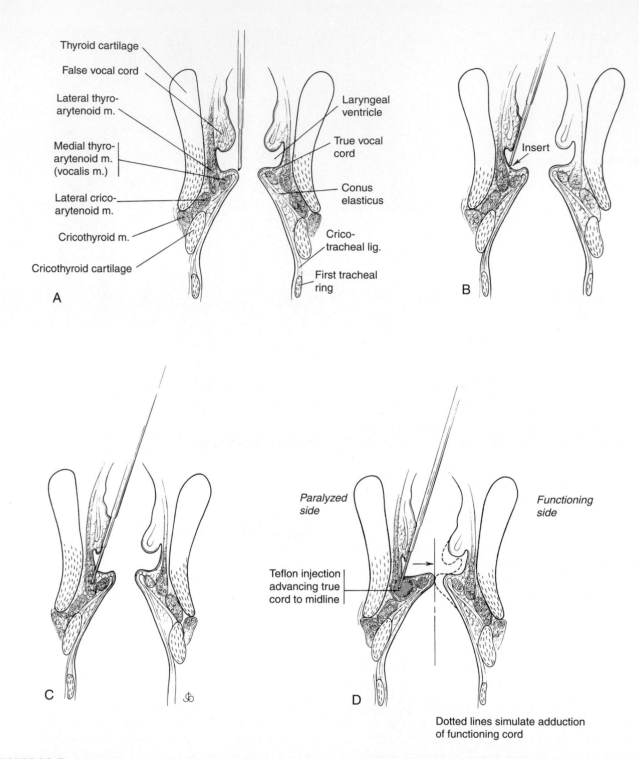

FIGURE 13–5. *A*, The needle is introduced through an anterior commissure laryngoscope to the upper medial margin of the mid-ligamentous vocal fold. *B*, The tip of the needle is then moved laterally to displace the false vocal fold and advanced to the lateral aspect of the laryngeal ventricle. *C*, The needle (No. 18 or No. 19) is introduced into the lateral aspect of the lateral thyroarytenoid muscle. The depth of this injection depends on the size of the larynx, i.e., the depth in a small female larynx may be 3 mm and in a large male larynx 5 mm. The depth can be estimated by remembering that the total length of the needle tip is 14 mm. *D*, Approximately 0.3 to 1.0 mL of Teflon paste is needed to reach the end point, the approximation of the ligamentous folds during phonation. Each click of the Brüning syringe delivers about 0.2 mL of Teflon paste as long as time is allowed for compression and dissipation of the paste. There should thus be a delay of about 15 seconds between clicks. It is possible to deliver about 1.6 mL of Teflon paste with one loading of the Brüning syringe. The actual amount of Teflon retained in the tissue, of course, depends on the amount that exudes from the mucosal puncture site after the needle is removed. A second injection is usually required, into the lateral thyroarytenoideus muscle at a point identified by the tip of the vocal process medially, so that the posterior commissure can be closed during phonation.

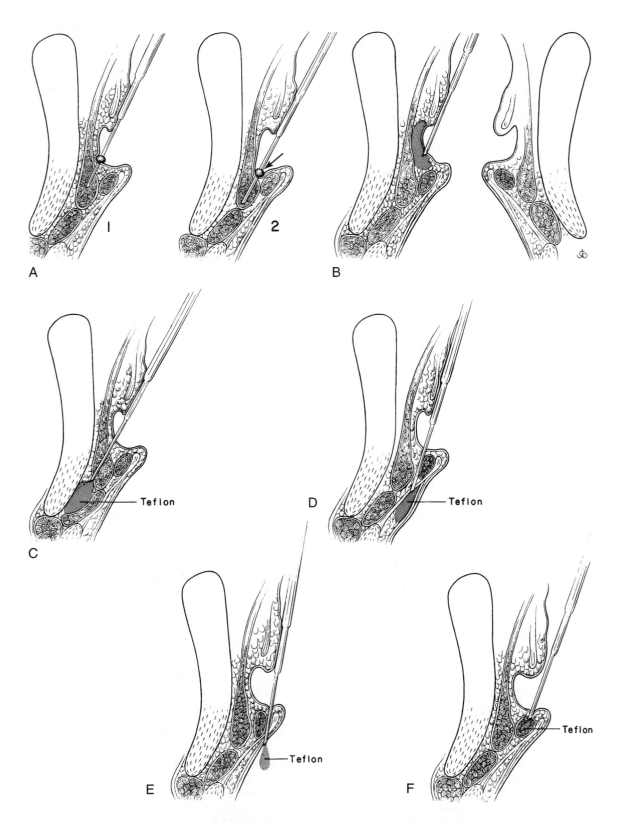

FIGURE 13–6. *A,* Some Teflon injection needles come with a cuff or guard placed 4.5 mm from the end of the needle tip (see text for details). *B,* Coronal incision of the larynx through the mid-ligamentous portion of the vocal fold. The needle injection is shallow. Teflon will be deposited submucosally, and the result is obliteration of the laryngeal ventricle with no medial displacement of the vocal fold. *C,* Injection is in the proper direction but too deep. Teflon paste will be deposited in the lateral cricothyroid muscle or through the cricothyroid space and outside the larynx. In such cases, a mass may be palpated in the neck. *D,* The needle is placed too medially and deeply between the mucosa and the conus elasticus. This injection will result in a subglottic bulge. *E,* The needle is directed too medially and deeply, and the tip penetrates the subglottic mucous membrane. As Teflon paste is injected, it can be seen entering the subglottic lumen. *F,* The needle is introduced into the medial thyroarytenoideus. This infiltrates the vocalis portion of the thyroarytenoideus muscle and serves only to immobilize this area rather than displace the vocal fold medially.

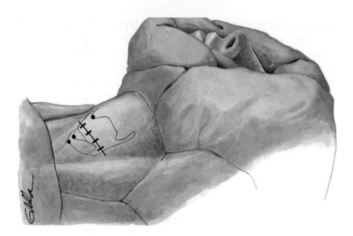

FIGURE 13-8. Draping and incision. The patient's anterior neck is prepared and draped to expose the ipsilateral and contralateral sides; the face remains exposed. Oxygen can be administered by placing tubing under the head drapes. The thyroid notch, cricothyroid membrane, and inferior margin of cricoid cartilage (dots) are marked. A horizontal incision is marked approximately 0.5 cm above the inferior margin of the thyroid cartilage. The area for incision, as well as deep tissues, is infiltrated with 1% Xylocaine with 1:100,000 epinephrine. The incision begins 2 cm from midline on contralateral side and is extended on the ipsilateral side of the neck to the anterior border of the sternocleidomastoid muscle. Hatch marks are made so that accurate approximation of incision can be accomplished.

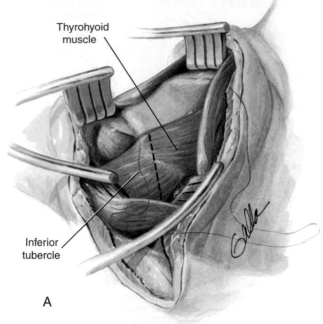

A

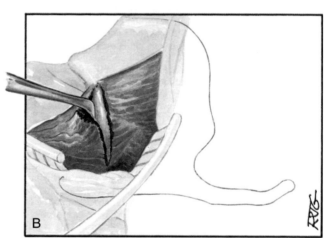

B

FIGURE 13-10. Exposure. *A,* Strap muscles are retracted laterally to expose thyrohyoid muscle on the surface of the thyroid lamina. Muscle is transected just above the inferior border of the thyroid lamina. *B,* Thyrohyoid muscle is detached from its inferior attachment by means of sharp dissection or cutting current on cautery. Thyroid lamina, its inferior border, and inferior thyroid tubercle are exposed.

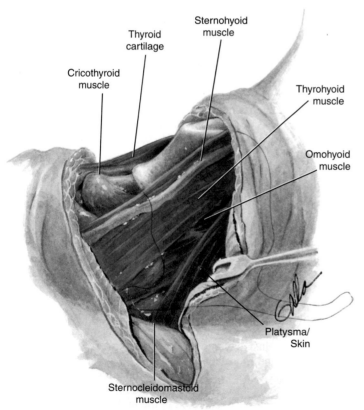

FIGURE 13-9. The skin incision is extended through the platysma layer to expose the sternohyoid and omohyoid muscles. Flaps are established superiorly and inferiorly in the plane superficial to the fascia covering these strap muscles. Flaps are separated with a self-retaining retractor. Midline (medial raphe) is identified, and two sternohyoid muscles are separated to expose the thyroid notch, anterior aspect of thyroid cartilage, cricothyroid membrane, and cricoid cartilage. Undersurfaces of the ipsilateral sternohyoid and omohyoid muscles are dissected so that they can be retracted laterally (Gelpi retractor). If there has been much scarring from previous surgery, it may be necessary to transect these muscles to obtain adequate exposure.

tractors, or a Weitlaner for vertical exposure and a Gelpi self-retractor for horizontal exposure. Most often, it is not necessary to transect the strap muscles.

The thyrohyoid muscle is transected (Fig. 13–10*B*) to expose the thyroid lamina. The inferior thyroid tubercle is palpated, and midway along the inferior border of the thyroid lamina, it is exposed by sharp and blunt dissection.

Surgical instruments have been designed to aid the surgeon in performing the procedure (Fig. 13–11). Included are instruments used to accurately locate and outline the window in the thyroid lamina (Figs. 13–12 and 13–13). The first instrument, called the Window Caliper, is used to locate the superior border of the thyroplasty window and the anterosuperior corner (key point of the window). There is a caliper designed specifically for male patients and one specifically

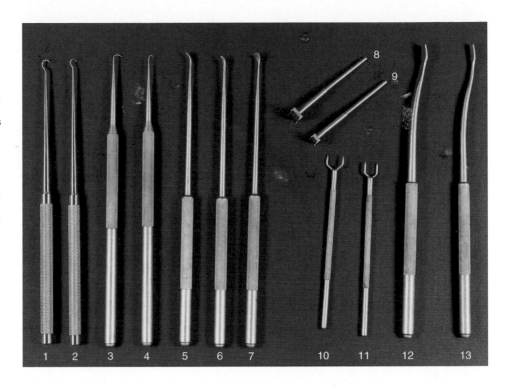

FIGURE 13–11. Instruments used for medialization laryngoplasty. Instruments 1 and 2—Curved hooks: hooks used for traction on thyroid cartilage. Instruments 3 and 4—Sharp hooks: small and large hooks used to elevate cartilage from the thyroplasty window. Instruments 5 and 6—Duckbill elevators: male and female instruments to elevate inner perichondrium from thyroid cartilage. Instrument 7—Chisel elevator: sharp chisel used to separate inner perichondrium from cartilage. Instruments 8 and 9—Window Outline Instruments, male and female. Instruments 10 and 11—Window calipers, male and female. Instruments 12 and 13—Implant inserters: instruments for final insertion of implant (male and female).

for female patients. After the inferior thyroid tubercle has been exposed and defined, the inferior border of the thyroid lamina is exposed anterior and posterior to this structure. One point of the caliper touches the inferior border of the thyroid lamina, anterior to the thyroid tubercle, and the other, a point directly superior. As the inferior point is lifted free, a Bovic cautery is applied to the tip of the measuring device, and a cautery mark will appear at the superior point (Fig. 13–13A). A similar cautery point is made beginning on the inferior border, posterior to the inferior thyroid tubercle (Fig. 13–13B). Anterior and posterior cautery marks are connected with a marking pen. This line is extended to the anterior aspect of the thyroid lamina. With the same

caliper, a mark is made along this line, beginning at the anterior midline and extending posteriorly. This cautery mark is the point of the anterosuperior corner (key point) of the thyroid lamina window (Figs. 13–12A and 13–13C). The distance is 7 mm in the female and 9 mm in the male larynx.

Outline of Thyroplasty Window

The instrument for making the outline of the window is a specially designed attachment for a standard cautery handle called the Window Outline Instrument (Fig. 13–14A). This instrument is first inserted into the Bovie handle with the

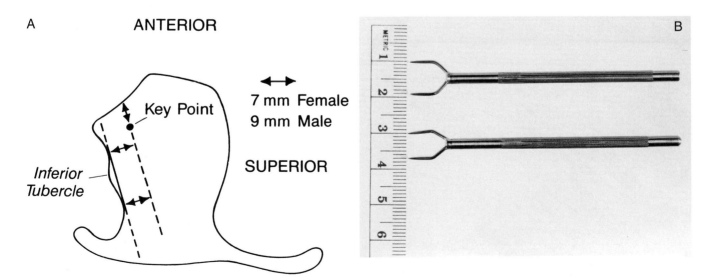

FIGURE 13–12. Window caliper. *A,* Orientation of window in thyroid lamina. The window caliper is used to measure from the inferior border of thyroid cartilage, anterior and posterior to inferior thyroid tubercle, to superior border of thyroplasty window. It also measures distance from the anterior midline of thyroid cartilage to anterior-superior angle (key point) of the thyroplasty window. *B,* Photograph of the window caliper. Distance between the tines of the window caliper is 7 mm in the female instrument and 9 mm in the male instrument.

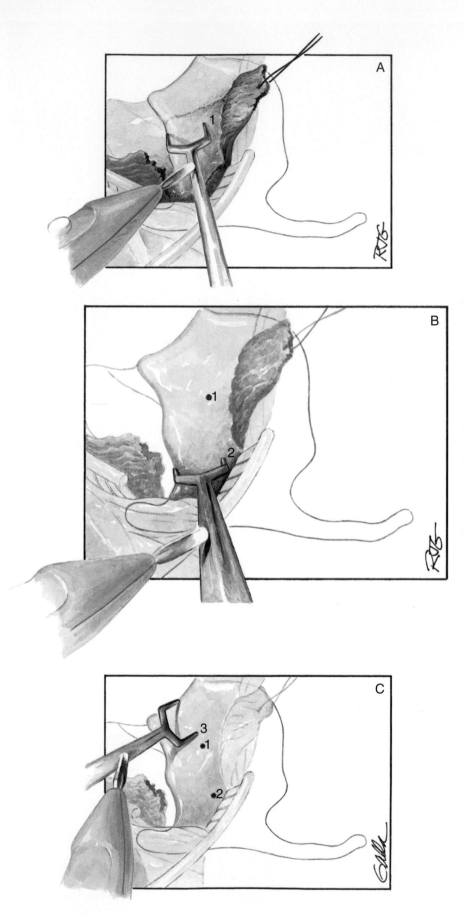

FIGURE 13–13. Window caliper. *A,* Measuring from the inferior border of the thyroid lamina, anterior to inferior thyroid tubercle, to the point (1) that is to be the superior margin of the thyroplasty window. *B,* Measuring from the inferior border of the thyroid lamina posterior to the inferior thyroid tubercle. (2) Points 1 and 2 are connected with a surgical marker to identify the superior margin of the thyroplasty window and also the direction of the vocal fold. *C,* Measuring from anterior midline, along line 1–2, to find the key point (3) that represents the anterior superior angle of the thyroplasty window.

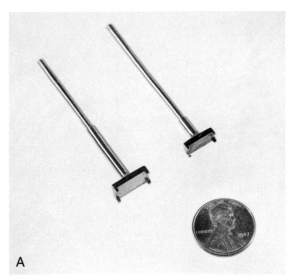

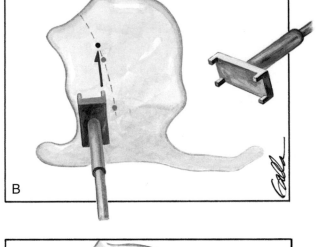

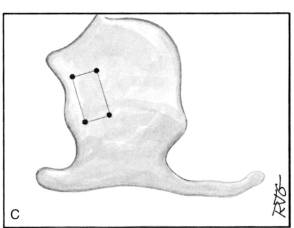

FIGURE 13–14. Window Outline Instrument. *A,* Photograph of the Window Outline Instrument used to outline the thyroplasty window. Male device measures 7 × 12 mm, and female 5 × 10 mm. *B,* Anterior-superior point of the Window Outline Instrument is placed on the key point. Posterior-superior point of Window Outline Instrument is placed along the line indicating the superior border of the thyroplasty window. Cautery current is applied, making four marks that locate the four corners of the thyroplasty window. *C,* Four corners of thyroplasty window are connected with a surgical marking pen.

tip placed so that the anterosuperior corner and superior border correspond to the key point mark and line on the thyroid lamina (Fig. 13–14*B*). Current is applied, and four marks appear on the cartilage surface (Fig. 13–14*C*). These marks are connected with a marking pen to complete the outline of the window.

Method for Cutting Window

A small tangential electric saw and blade (Fig. 13–15) have been specially designed for the thyroplasty type I operation and other laryngeal framework surgery. The outer perichondrium is not disturbed. This saw can be used in all cases re-

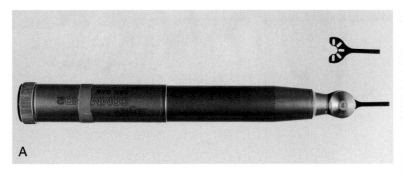

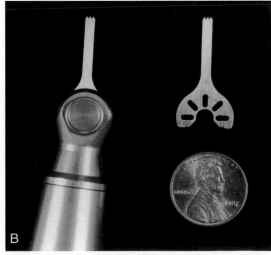

FIGURE 13–15. Thyroplasty saw handle and blade. *A,* Photograph of whole handle and blade. *B,* Small size of handle and blade is specially designed for laryngeal framework surgery.

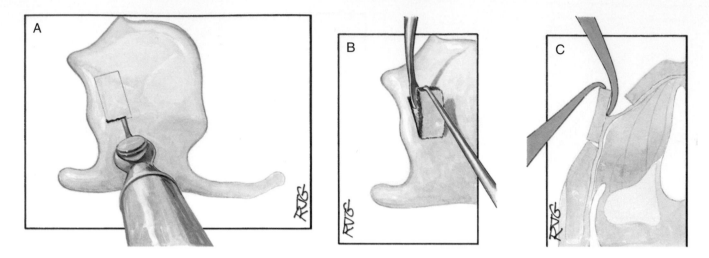

FIGURE 13–16. Thyroplasty window. *A,* Cutting thyroplasty window is done with care to avoid injuring underlying soft tissue. It is best to start cutting the window posteriorly in case bleeding is encountered. As soon as four sides of the window are completely cut, a piece of cartilage in the window will become loose. *B,* When the piece of cartilage in the window becomes loose, its anterior margin is grasped and elevated with a small or large sharp hook. *C,* Underlying perichondrium is separated from cartilage.

gardless of whether the cartilage has undergone ossification. Cutting the window (Fig. 13–16) is accomplished with great care to avoid injuring the underlying soft tissue. It is best to make the posterior cut first because occasionally there is troublesome bleeding. Once the four sides of the rectangular window have been cut and the cartilage moves freely, it is grasped anteriorly with the sharp hook (small or large) and is carefully separated from the underlying perichondrium with the chisel elevator specially designed for this purpose (Fig. 13–16*B* and *C*). The rectangular piece of cartilage is removed.

The Window Outline Instrument is then inserted into the thyroplasty window to confirm that the correct-size window has been created (Fig. 13–17*A* and *B*). If not, the window can be altered with the thyroplasty saw. A tight fit of the Window Outline Instrument into the window is ideal.

Incision of Inner Perichondrium

After removal of the cartilage from the window, the inner perichondrium is elevated from the underlying cartilage in all directions (Fig. 13–17*C*). It is most important to elevate the perichondrium posteriorly to the level of the vocal process of the arytenoid.

Measuring for Implant

At this point, a fiberoptic laryngoscope is inserted by way of the nasal cavity, which has been anesthetized (Fig. 13–18*A*).

A measuring device (Fig. 13–18*D*) is inserted through the window in the thyroid lamina. There are five sizes for

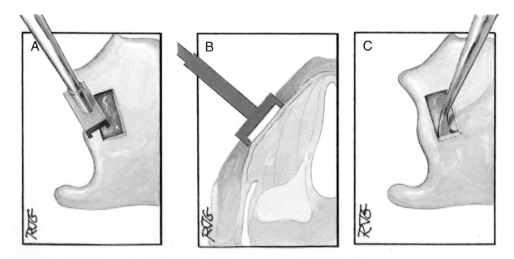

FIGURE 13–17. Thyroplasty window. *A, B,* Window Outline Instrument is inserted into the thyroplasty window to make certain it is large enough to admit the implant. If the window is too small, it can be easily adjusted with a thyroplasty saw. Tight fit is ideal. Occasionally, there is bleeding from the medullary layer of cartilage. This can be controlled with cautery or bone wax. *C,* Once the cartilage piece has been removed from the thyroplasty window, the inner perichondrium is elevated from cartilage in all directions. Perichondrium must be elevated posteriorly to the level of the vocal process of arytenoid.

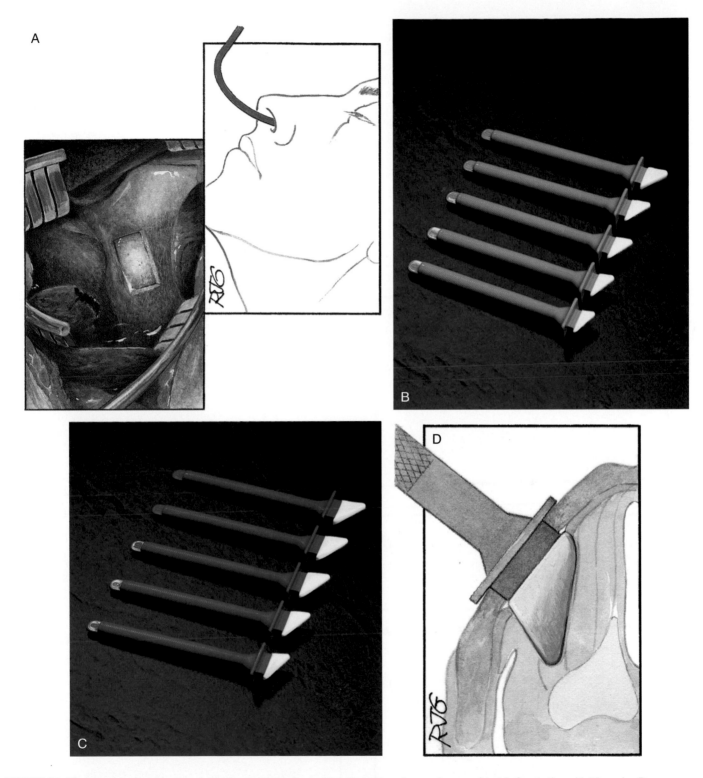

FIGURE 13–18. Measuring implant size. *A,* The larynx is visualized with a fiberoptic endoscope by an assistant before testing with Measuring Device. Soft tissues in the window will light up. It may be necessary to cover the window while the endoscopist becomes oriented. *B,* The female Implant Measuring Devices are green in color. On each handle is imprinted size and gender. Female Implant Measuring Device sizes are 6, 7, 8, 9, and 10 mm. *C,* The male Implant Measuring Devices are blue in color and include sizes 8, 9, 10, 11, and 12 mm. *D,* Measuring Device is inserted while vocal folds are being observed. Complete closure during adduction and good voice are the end points. Ideal measurement is recorded so that the correct size of implant can be selected.

the male and female larynges (Fig. 13–18*B* and *C*). When inserted, the measuring device accurately simulates the corresponding implant. The vocal folds are observed with a fiberoptic laryngoscope as the measuring device is inserted. The end point is complete closure of the vocal chink from the anterior commissure to the posterior commissure and a good voice when the patient is asked to vocalize. The ideal measurement is noted, and the corresponding implant is selected. The size of the implant is noted in the patient's record at this time.

Insertion of Implant

Additional anesthesia is administered at the time of implant insertion. The thyroplasty implant is grasped with broad forceps (Fig. 13–19*A*), and the posterior tip of the medial triangular portion of the implant is inserted through the window. The posterior slot in the tiered base of the implant is engaged in the posterior rim of the window in the thyroid lamina. A specially designed spatula, the implant inserter, is inserted into the slot anteriorly, as a finger applies pressure against the pos-

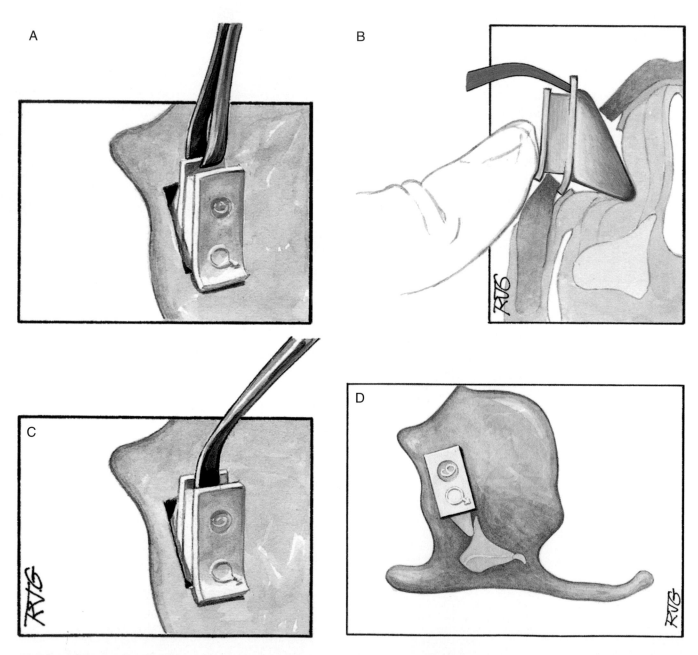

FIGURE 13–19. Insertion of implant. *A*, Lidocaine hydrochloride, 50 to 100 mg, is administered intravenously before insertion of the implant. Implant is grasped with forceps, and the posterior tip of the triangular portion is inserted through the window in the direction of the vocal process of arytenoid. *B*, The tiered base of the implant is engaged in the cartilage rim posteriorly and held there with the index finger of the nondominant hand. *C*, Implant Inserter (male or female) is placed in the slot anteriorly, and the implant is snapped into place. An extra bit of intravenous anesthesia is given before this last step because it can be painful. Vocal folds are again observed during adduction, and voice quality is evaluated. *D*, Implant in place with its posterior tip against vocal process of arytenoid. Male No. 9 implant is in place.

terior aspect of the implant as shown in Figure 13–19*B*. The thyroplasty implant is snapped into place with the implant inserter (Fig. 13–19*C*). The three-tiered base locks the implant securely in the window. The size of the implant is visible and should be noted in the patient's record at this time (Fig. 13–19*D*). If the implant requires change at the time of surgery or change or removal at a later date as a secondary procedure, the anterior end of the external portion of the implant (lateral tier) is grasped with forceps or a hemostat. With lateral pull, the implant snaps out as easily as it was inserted.

Repair

The sternohyoid muscles are reapproximated in the midline (Fig. 13–20*A*) with 3-0 or 4-0 chromic catgut. The platysma and subcutaneous layers are reapproximated with 4-0 chromic catgut, and the skin is repaired with a running suture of 6-0 mild chromic catgut (Fig. 13–20*B*). Butterfly-closed suction drainage is used along with red-top vacuum tube (Fig. 13–20*C*). To place a butterfly drain, one passes a mosquito hemostat over the sternocleidomastoid muscle to a point 1.5 cm lateral and inferior to the lateral aspect of the incision. The skin is tented out, and with a No. 15 blade, one slightly opens the hemostat and makes a small incision over the tip of the hemostat. The tip is then pushed through the skin opening and grasps the end of the butterfly drainage tubing. The drainage tubing is secured in place with a 4-0 silk suture. Steri-Strips are applied over the entire suture line after applying Mastosol liquid adhesive or tincture of benzoin to the skin (Fig. 13–20*C*).

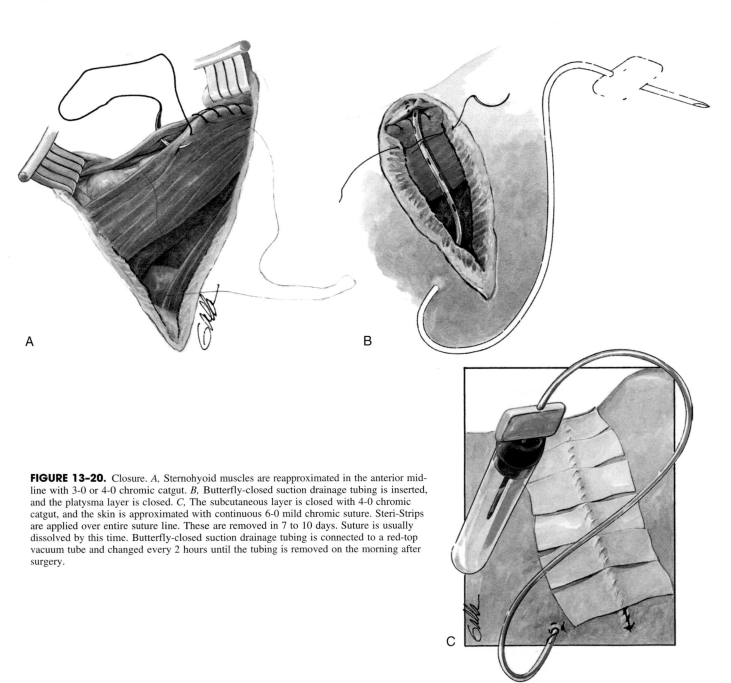

A

B

C

FIGURE 13-20. Closure. *A,* Sternohyoid muscles are reapproximated in the anterior midline with 3-0 or 4-0 chromic catgut. *B,* Butterfly-closed suction drainage tubing is inserted, and the platysma layer is closed. *C,* The subcutaneous layer is closed with 4-0 chromic catgut, and the skin is approximated with continuous 6-0 mild chromic suture. Steri-Strips are applied over entire suture line. These are removed in 7 to 10 days. Suture is usually dissolved by this time. Butterfly-closed suction drainage tubing is connected to a red-top vacuum tube and changed every 2 hours until the tubing is removed on the morning after surgery.

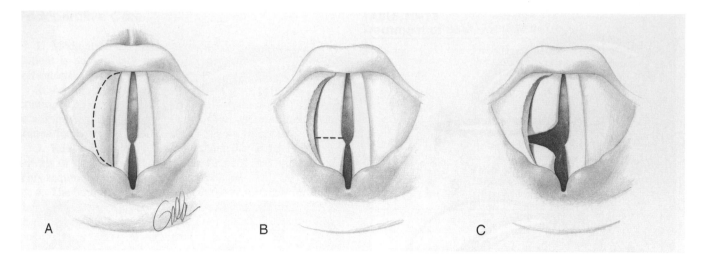

A   B   C

FIGURE 13–24. Kashima Cordotomy Procedure. *A,* Using CO_2 laser, the left vestibular band (false cord) is resected as outlined. This gives a good view of the lateral aspect of the left vocal cord. *B,* A horizontal cut is made just anterior to the vocal process of the arytenoid to the lateral aspect of the vocal cord. *C,* The completed operation.

goscope stretches and fixes the vocal fold, making the procedure much easier to perform. The arytenoid is palpated to make certain that there is no fixation of the cricoarytenoid joint. Using microcautery, or laser, an incision is made along the lateral aspect of the vocal ligament. This incision parallels the free edge of the vocal fold (Fig. 13–25). The thyroarytenoid muscle is resected using cautery or laser, thus creating a defect, or pocket, between the conus elasticus and the cartilage laterally. This compartment is closed when the cord is lateralized by sutures.

To lateralize the vocal fold, two sutures are introduced through No. 19 needles that have been passed externally through the thyroid lamina. The first needle is introduced at the mid-cord position below the level of the vocal fold. The second needle is introduced above the true vocal fold (Fig. 13–26). The sutures are pulled out through the laryngoscope, tied, and then pulled back to the level of the vocal fold. On the external surface of the neck, the two sutures are passed through silicone sheeting and crimped in place using lead sinkers (Fig. 13–27). The sutures remain in place for 2 weeks, at which time they are removed after the airway is reassessed. If the procedure is successful, the patient can undergo decannulation.

We prefer the Kashima cordotomy because it is simple and effective most of the time. If it is not effective, we perform an open arytenoidectomy by way of a thyrotomy.

Arytenoidectomy by Thyrotomy

We prefer the thyrotomy approach for an arytenoidectomy because of its simplicity. Bleeding can be more easily controlled and the result can be visualized. Approximately 80% of patients will have successful decannulation with only a minimal alteration in their phonatory function with the first operation. If the first operation fails, then we believe that a contralateral arytenoidectomy is not indicated. Instead, an ipsilateral arytenoid is revised, and a conforming laryngeal stent inserted for 3 weeks.

Usually a tracheotomy has been necessary long before an arytenoidectomy is contemplated. If not, it is performed as a preliminary procedure either with the patient under general anesthesia with an endotracheal tube in place or with the use of local and topical anesthesia. The endotracheal tube is inserted by way of the tracheotomy fenestration so that it will not be in the way during the endolaryngeal procedure.

Technique
A horizontal skin incision is made midway between the thyroid notch and the cricothyroid membrane as an approach

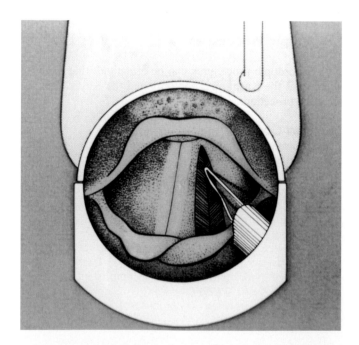

FIGURE 13–25. Vocal cord lateralization. An incision is made along the lateral aspect of the vocal fold and, using microcautery, the thyroarytenoid muscle is resected. This can also be accomplished using the CO_2 laser.

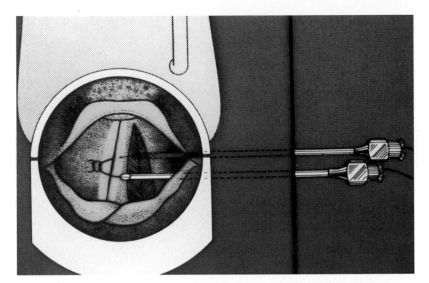

FIGURE 13-26. The sutures are introduced above and below the vocal fold from outside and through the thyroid lamina using No. 18 needles. The sutures are tied together and the needles are removed.

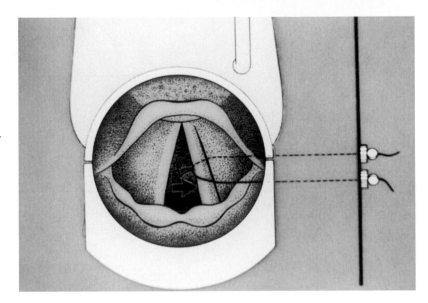

FIGURE 13-27. The vocal fold has been displaced laterally and the defect created by resecting the thyroarytenoid muscle closed as the sutures are pulled laterally and fixed in place.

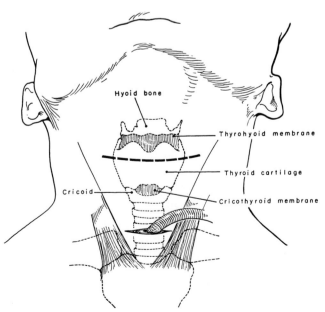

FIGURE 13-28. A horizontal skin incision is made midway between the thyroid notch and the cricothyroid membrane as an approach to the anterior aspect of the thyroid cartilage.

to the anterior aspect of the thyroid cartilage (Fig. 13–28). The fascial layers over the sternohyoid and omohyoid muscles are separated in the midline, exposing the thyroid notch, the anterior aspect of the thyroid cartilage, and the cricothyroid membrane (Fig. 13–29A).

We no longer perform the laryngeal scissors technique for executing a thyrotomy. Instead, a layered technique is used to prevent deviation from the anterior commissure. The thyroid cartilage is incised at the anterior vertical midline using a No. 10 surgical blade if the cartilage has not undergone ossification. An electric oscillating saw is used to accomplish this incision if ossification has occurred (Fig. 13–29B).

Using small skin hooks, the two thyroid laminae are

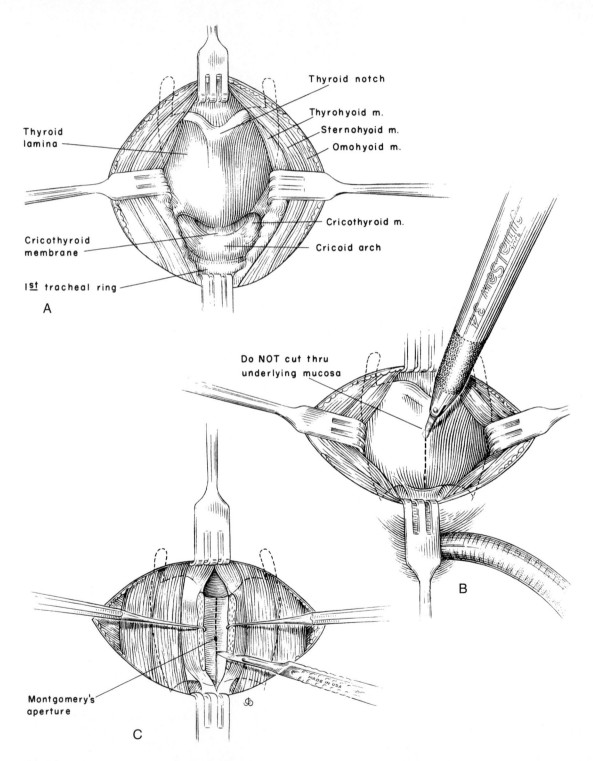

FIGURE 13–29. *A,* The thyroid laminae are exposed. *B,* A midline thyrotomy is performed with a tangential saw. *C,* The two thyroid laminae are separated with hooks, exposing the underlying soft tissue. A midline incision is made, increasing the depth until a small aperture is encountered. This almost invariably represents a point just below the anterior commissure.

slightly separated after the thyroid cartilage incision has been completed. The airway is entered through a vertical incision in the cricothyroid membrane. This incision is continued superiorly in the anterior midline under direct vision of the vocal folds. Using this technique, the anterior commissure can be accurately incised in the midline (Fig. 13–29C). At this point, the transoral endotracheal tube is removed and a sterile endotracheal tube is inserted into the trachea through the tracheostoma. The endotracheal tube is connected to sterile tubing that is directed to the anesthesiologist.

Before the self-retaining thyrotomy retractor is inserted, additional exposure is obtained by extending the incision above the thyroid notch with a button knife, incising a small portion of the thyroid membrane and base of the epiglottis. The self-retaining thyrotomy retractor is then inserted, exposing the larynx (Fig. 13–30A). The larynx is packed with gauze stripping that has been impregnated with 4% cocaine solution.

A 1.5-cm vertical incision is made through the epithelium just anterior to the vocal process of the arytenoid (Fig. 13–30A). The vocal process is easily identified by virtue of its being made prominent as the thyroid laminae are spread apart anteriorly with the thyrotomy retractor. The vocal process is dissected free (Fig. 13–30B).

The arytenoid, posterior cricoarytenoid, lateral cricoarytenoid, and thyroarytenoid muscles are sectioned with a No. 15 Bard-Parker blade (Fig. 13–31A and B). The blade is also used to cut across the cricoarytenoid joint (Fig. 13–32A). It is important not to grasp the arytenoid with any instrument other than an arytenoid hook or fixation forceps because it is easily crumbled. The mucous membrane incision is loosely approximated with one or two No. 4-0 chromic catgut sutures (Fig. 13–32B).

The self-retaining retractor is removed, and a plane of cleavage is established lateral to the thyroid laminae, on the side of the arytenoidectomy. A No. 5-0 braided steel or No. 3-0 nylon suture on a large, heavy, curved cutting needle is passed above the vocal fold in the mid-cord position and through the thyroid lamina (Fig. 13–33A). With the exposure obtained by using an orbital retractor, the needle is easily pulled through the lateral surface of the thyroid cartilage. It is then removed and rethreaded on the other, or intralaryngeal, end of the suture and passed, by a similar route, below the vocal fold (Fig. 13–33B). It is

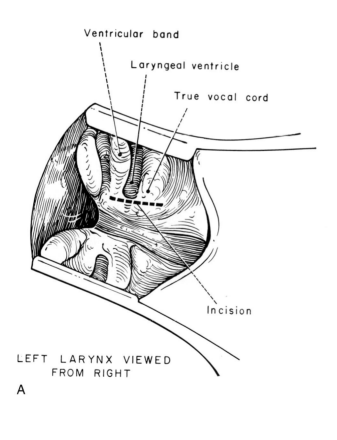

Ventricular band

Laryngeal ventricle

True vocal cord

Incision

LEFT LARYNX VIEWED
FROM RIGHT

A

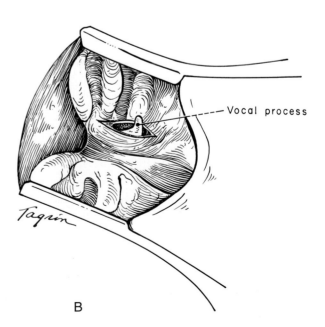

Vocal process

B

FIGURE 13–30. *A,* A self-retaining thyrotomy retractor is inserted, exposing the larynx. A 1.5-cm vertical incision is made through the epithelium just anterior to the vocal process of the arytenoid. *B,* The vocal process is dissected free.

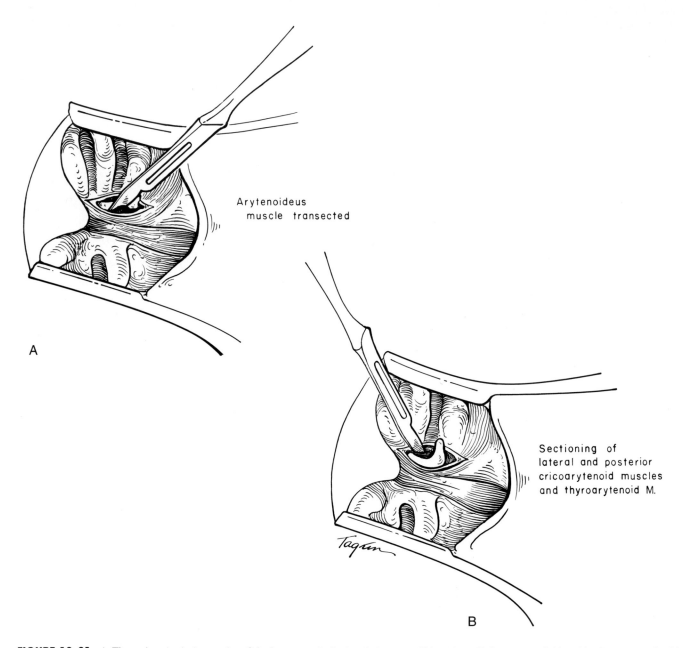

A

Arytenoideus
muscle transected

Sectioning of
lateral and posterior
cricoarytenoid muscles
and thyroarytenoid M.

B

FIGURE 13–31. *A,* The various intrinsic muscles of the larynx are incised at their arytenoid insertions. Before accomplishing this, the surgeon should be familiar with the detailed anatomy of both the arytenoid and the intrinsic laryngeal muscles. The arytenoid muscle is being sectioned medial to the body of the arytenoid cartilage. *B,* The lateral and posterior cricoarytenoid muscles are sectioned with a No. 15 surgical blade or fine curved scissors.

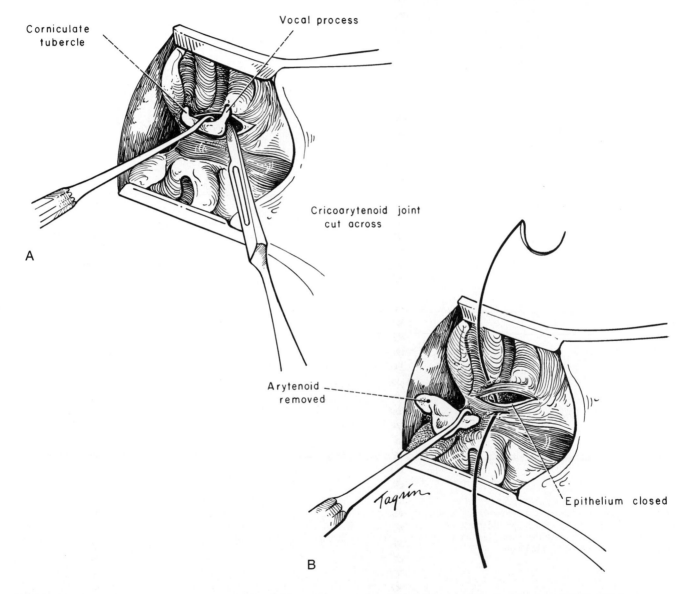

FIGURE 13-32. *A,* The cornicular process has been dissected, and the arytenoid cartilage is free except for the cricoarytenoid joint. This is transected, and the arytenoid cartilage is removed. *B,* The arytenoid cartilage is removed. The incision is loosely approximated with one or two No. 4-0 chromic catgut sutures.

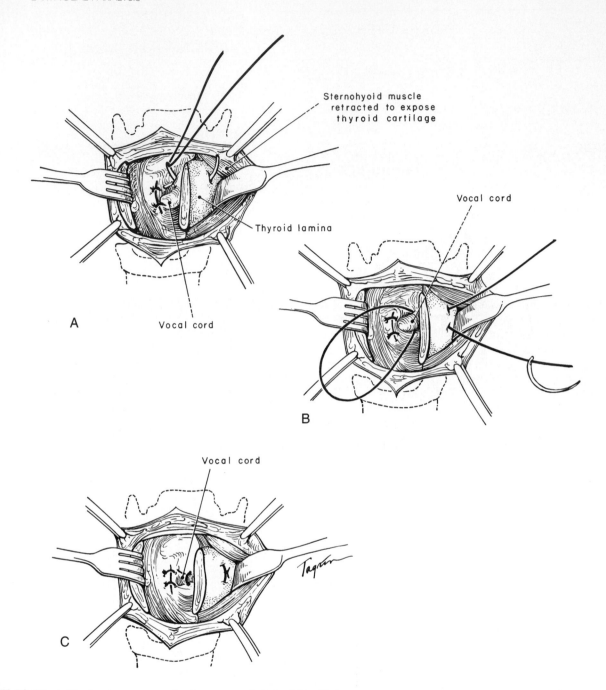

FIGURE 13–33. *A,* The thyrotomy retractor has been removed. A No. 5-0 braided prolene or nylon suture is inserted above the vocal fold, in the mid-cord position, and through the thyroid lamina. *B,* The needle is reinserted, after being threaded to the other or intralaryngeal end of the suture, below the vocal fold and through the thyroid lamina. *C,* The vocal fold has been displaced laterally with only moderate tension, and the suture is tied on the external surface of the thyroid lamina.

important that the suture is not so tight that it will cut through the vocal fold during the postoperative period. Several knots are tied on the lateral surface of the thyroid lamina (Fig. 13–33C).

The thyrotomy incision is closed with subcutaneous and dermal sutures. The thyroid laminae are sutured an-

teriorly. A drain is inserted and left in place for 48 hours. A dressing, exerting moderate pressure, should be used during the first few postoperative days. As soon as indirect laryngoscopy shows the laryngeal airways to be adequate, the tracheotomy is plugged for a few days and is then closed.

Chapter 14
Surgery for Chronic Aspiration

WILLIAM W. MONTGOMERY

Stroke is the third most common cause of death in the United States today. In 1999, there were 750,000 full-fledged strokes in this country. It is estimated that 40,000 to 50,000 patients die each year as a result of complications from chronic laryngeal aspiration after a stroke. Deaths result from repeated aspiration pneumonia rather than the first episode. This is a very important health issue when we are attempting to reduce the cost of medical care. Patients aspirate everything, including their own saliva, are voiceless, and have an ineffective cough. Chronic aspiration accompanies other neurologic diseases such as amyotrophic lateral sclerosis.

Chronic aspiration with a functionless larynx remains a problem even with a gastrostomy and a cuffed tracheotomy tube in place. Most of these patients will have required a cuffed tracheotomy tube by the time they are first seen by an otolaryngologist. If a tracheotomy has not been performed, this should be the initial therapeutic measure. A tracheostomy tube with a soft cuff is essential to prevent irreversible damage to the trachea. It is not uncommon that a cuffed tracheotomy tube left in place long enough will devitalize a segment of the trachea and lead to tracheal stenosis and leakage of saliva into the lungs. Vigilant care of the patient with dysphagia and chronic aspiration after stroke can prevent pneumonia and death. It should be the goal of the physician to make certain the patient recovers from the initial stroke because the prognosis is often much better than first anticipated.

The only effective treatments for chronic aspiration are to block off the larynx, remove it, or re-route it into the trachea. In the past, the only treatment for a functionless larynx has been a laryngectomy.

There are three operative procedures designed to control severe aspiration by blocking the airway. All three are difficult to perform and difficult to reverse if function returns. Placing a Montgomery Laryngeal Stent (Boston Medical Products, Inc., Westborough, MA) has provided recent success in controlling chronic aspiration. The diversion operation also has been successful.

EPIGLOTTIS SEW-DOWN OPERATION

In 1972, Habal and Murray introduced a technique using the epiglottis as a flap to close the larynx at a supraglottic level. The operation is performed by way of a horizontal incision

at the level of the hyoid bone (Fig. 14–1A). After the platysma is divided, the hyoid bone is retracted superiorly, and the sternohyoid muscles are sectioned. The thyrohyoid is separated from its attachment to the posterior surface of the hyoid bone, thus entering the hypopharynx above the epiglottis (Fig. 14–1B). The epiglottis is retracted anteriorly and an incision is made around the border of the epiglottis, aryepiglottic folds, and arytenoids (Fig. 14–1C). After margins are created by dissection, the epiglottis is sutured to the aryepiglottic folds and arytenoids (Fig. 14–1D). Bilateral rotation flaps of mucous membrane from the adjacent pyriform sinuses are used to cover the raw surfaces of the epiglottis (Fig. 14–1E). This operation is difficult to perform; leakage often occurs, and the operation itself is most difficult to reverse.

LARYNGEAL CLOSURE OPERATION

I have used the laryngeal closure operation for the past 19 years to treat patients with chronic aspiration. The operation eliminates aspiration and reestablishes deglutition. Phonatory function is lost, and the patient must communicate with one of the various vibratory speech devices. (Patients and their families should be informed that the operation eliminates phonatory function.) The operation has been successfully used for a number of neuromuscular disorders involving the laryngopharynx. Only one patient thus far recovered sufficiently so that a successful reversal of the laryngeal closure operation could be accomplished. The types of disorders with the laryngeal closure include primary brain tumors, vascular disorders of the central nervous system, metastatic carcinoma of the medulla, progressive cerebellar atrophy, amyotrophic lateral sclerosis, axial Parkinson's disease, and bilateral laryngeal paralysis in abduction.

Technique

Anesthesia is administered by way of a transoral endotracheal tube rather than through the existing tracheotomy. An endotracheal tube between the vocal folds simplifies the thyrotomy (laryngofissure) approach to the glottis and allows the surgeon to convert the tracheotomy to a tracheostomy.

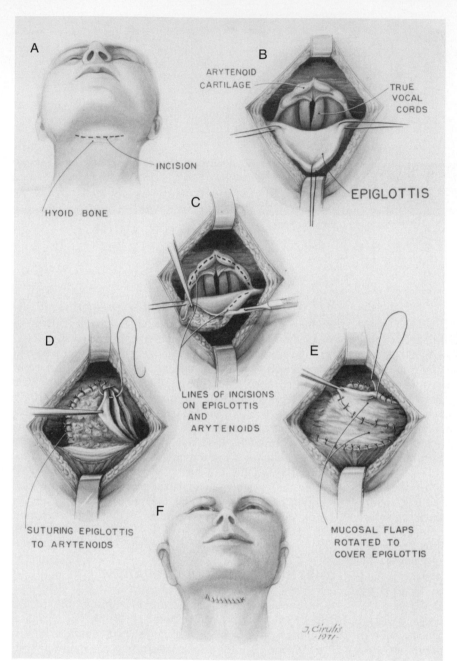

FIGURE 14–1. *A,* The horizontal skin incision at the level of the hyoid bone. *B,* The larynx is exposed by transecting the platysma, elevating the hyoid bone, and transecting the sternohyoid muscles and thyroid membrane. *C,* Incisions are shown around the margin of the epiglottis, aryepiglottic folds, and arytenoids. *D,* The epiglottis is sutured to the arytenoids and aryepiglottic folds. *E,* Bilateral rotational mucous membrane flaps are obtained from the pyriform sinus. These are used to cover the denuded surface of the epiglottis and also create a second layer of closure. *F,* The incision is closed.

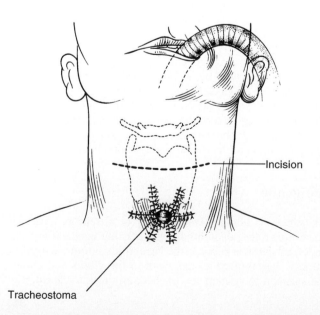

FIGURE 14–2. The tracheotomy is converted to a tracheostomy. The thyroid cartilage is exposed using a horizontal cervical incision.

The latter is an attempt to eliminate the need for a tracheotomy tube and to reduce the need for tracheal care. The multiple-flap technique has been used in this instance to convert the tracheotomy to a tracheostomy (Fig. 14–2). The skin flaps are elevated and advanced, and their margins are sutured to the tracheal mucous membrane.

The technique for thyrotomy has been described and illustrated in the section on arytenoidectomy. The thyroid lamina are retracted laterally using a self-retaining thyrot-

omy retractor or large skin hooks. An incision is made with an electrical knife along the medial convexities of the true and false folds. These incisions are continued across the posterior commissure (Fig. 14–3A). The glottis is denuded of epithelium circumferentially by resecting a strip of mucous membrane between the two parallel incisions (Fig. 14–3B).

A No. 2-0 nylon suture is passed through the anterior aspect of an ipsilateral thyroid lamina and true vocal fold (Fig.

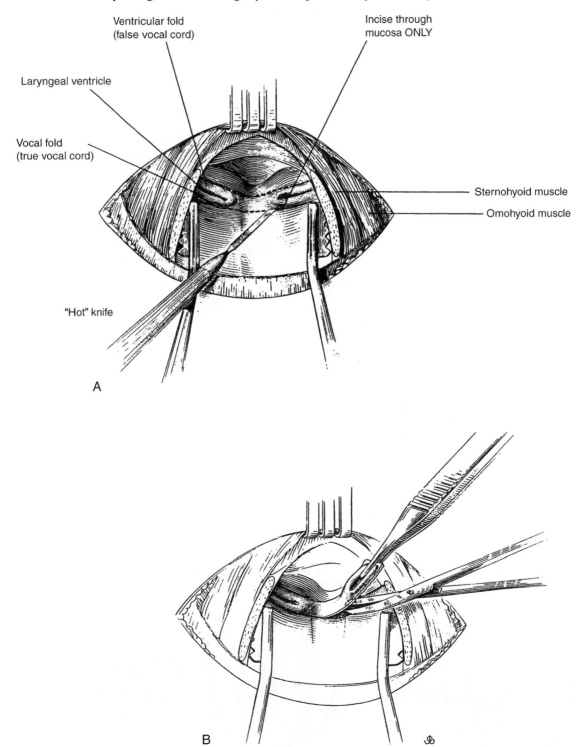

FIGURE 14-3. *A,* Mucosal incisions are made to outline mucous membrane removal. *B,* Mucous membrane is being removed from the true and false vocal folds, laryngeal ventricle, and posterior commissure.

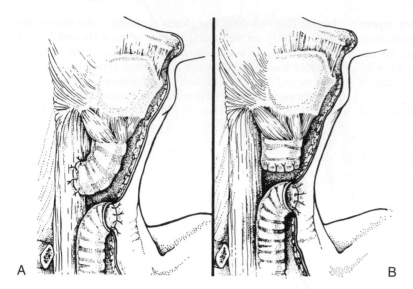

FIGURE 14-7. *A*, Standard diversion procedure as originally described. *B*, Modified diversion with blind-end closure of proximal trachea when a high tracheotomy precludes tracheoesophageal anastomosis.

drained as illustrated in Figure 14–6*B* and *C*. A cuffed tracheotomy tube remains in place for 8 to 10 days after this surgery.

DIVERSION OPERATION FOR CHRONIC ASPIRATION

In 1973, Lindeman presented a procedure for treatment of intractable aspiration. During this operation, the trachea is exposed for a distance of 4 to 5 cm and, by careful dissection, is freed from the surrounding structures. The recurrent laryngeal nerves are identified and preserved. The trachea is completely severed (Fig. 14–7) between the third and fourth rings. The upper segment of trachea is retracted superiorly while an esophageal dilator is inserted to facilitate this procedure.

A vertical incision is made in the cervical esophagus somewhat larger than the diameter of the trachea. An end-to-side anastomosis is accomplished using No. 3-0 nylon suture material. The strap muscles are re-approximated in the midline over the anastomosis. The distal trachea is brought directly to the skin as a tracheostomy. Dr. Lindeman reports that this operation also has been successfully reversed.

LARYNGEAL STENT PROCEDURE

In 1991, Dr. Edward Wiseberger presented 25 patients with chronic aspiration treated with insertion of the Montgomery laryngeal stent. In 24 of the 25 patients, inserting the stent reduced the aspiration to the point that the pneumonia cleared. Eight of the patients were able to establish adequate deglutition by mouth after the stent was removed, which is a good demonstration of the procedure's reversibility. Wiseberger concluded that the stent used as the laryngeal obtu-

rator is a very effective temporary solution to the problem of intractable aspiration with secondary pneumonia. He inserted the stents endoscopically.

I have found it necessary to insert the laryngeal stent by way of a laryngofissure to more adequately obtain a good fit. There are four sizes of the laryngeal stent. If one does not fit tightly, the anterior thyroid lamina can be reduced anteriorly so that the fit is more adequate. The stent is sutured to the thyroid lamina with two No. 2-0 prolene sutures. Thus, there are no external holding devices.

The above technique offers the patient a number of advantages: (1) It shortens the hospital stay, (2) it markedly reduces the cost of care, (3) it helps patients to control their saliva, and (4) it eliminates repeated aspiration pneumonia.

FUTURE DEVELOPMENT OF AN ASPIRATION STENT

Research is under way to develop a stent that would prevent any aspiration and also allow for some form of vocalization. The goal was to develop a new type of laryngeal stent, which is intended to control laryngeal aspiration and reestablish swallowing. A successful stent must be anatomically correct to ensure a proper fit and seal and constructed using a flexible and biocompatible material. Prototype laryngeal stents have been developed from wax using both male and female cadaveric larynges, thereby gaining experience as to what the optimal anatomically shaped stent should look like.

The future goal of this research will be to refine and further develop stent prototypes using a more sophisticated technology of spiral computed tomography imaging for laryngeal measurement and computer-aided, design-driven three-dimensional modeling. Further improvements and enhancements will be made to the stent design to allow for airflow and restored speech functions.

Chapter 15
Laryngeal Stenosis

WILLIAM W. MONTGOMERY

ACUTE LARYGEAL STENOSIS

Acute laryngeal stenosis most commonly results from external trauma. It may also occur after endoscopy, intubation, or any surgical procedure involved with the intrinsic larynx or its supporting cartilaginous structures. The various mechanisms devised for moving about on the surface of the earth undoubtedly account for the majority of laryngeal injuries. During the sudden deceleration at the instant a vehicle accident takes place, the driver (whose seatbelt is fastened) is first thrown into cervical hypertension. A fraction of a second later, the body is thrust forward, and the anterior larynx strikes either the steering wheel or dashboard, thereby inflicting varying degrees of damage on any one or all of the driver's laryngeal structures and cervical trachea. The addition of the shoulder strap to the seat belt prevents many of these injuries. An apparent increase in the number of laryngeal injuries is the result of more efficient and rapid transfer of the patient from the accident scene to well-equipped emergency facilities where life-saving intubation can be performed. These injuries are much worse when seatbelts are not worn. Many people still do not wear seatbelts.

Emergency Measures

Proper management of acute laryngeal injuries is of utmost importance because the respiratory, phonatory, and deglutitory disabilities after laryngeal trauma frequently persist to the chronic stage. If radiographs of the cervical spine cannot be obtained before a tracheotomy is performed, any manipulation of the neck should be accomplished with extreme care. Because fracture of the cervical vertebrae is commonly associated with laryngeal injuries, the neck must be splinted until these radiographs can be obtained.

Initial Assessment and Treatment

The status of the airway determines the first treatment. The necessity for an immediate tracheotomy should be obvious. Rapid evaluation of the patient will distinguish between obstruction at the larynx and obstruction above the larynx. With obstruction above the larynx, the stridor is of low pitch and the patient's cheeks are sucked in during attempted inspiration and blown out during expiration. The stridor at the laryngeal level is high-pitched. Suprasternal retraction during inspiration may be present. The airway is reestablished by inserting an endotracheal tube or performing a tracheotomy. Artificial breathing may be required. There may be decreased stimulation for respiration such as with a head injury, breathing may be painful with chest or abdominal injury, or atelectasis may be present due to aspiration of blood or a chest injury. Cerebral circulation needs oxygen and not carbon dioxide for stimulating respiration. Bleeding from the neck is of secondary priority. Rarely is it of such severity that it must be controlled simultaneously with the establishment of an airway. Surface bleeding can be controlled by pressure or with hemostats. Bleeding into the airway is controlled by inflating a cuffed endotracheal or tracheotomy tube.

Shock controls are initiated by intravenous fluid replacement. A large-caliber intravenous needle is inserted. Blood samples are obtained at this time for typing, crossmatching, and evaluation of blood loss and physiologic functions.

If patients are conscious, a history can be obtained while attending to their immediate needs. All events, beginning with the time of the accident, and all the complaints reported by the patients and those who accompany them should be listened to, recorded, and investigated.

Antibiotic and steroid therapy is indicated to reduce edema and control infection. Usually an intravenous access is available; we use Kefzol (cefazolin), 0.5 to 1.5 g intravenously every 8 hours and Decadron (defam ethasone) 8 to 12 mg intravenously every 8 hours.

Symptoms and External Findings

The diagnosis of laryngeal injury is not difficult to make unless the patient is unconscious or the laryngeal injury is overshadowed by other injuries. Any one or all of the laryngeal functions can be disturbed. Usually respiratory and phonatory functions are disturbed simultaneously. Deglutitory complications are manifested by aspiration, dysphagia, or odynophagia. Local pain may occur with laryngeal injury, especially during speaking or swallowing. This pain can be referred to the region of the ears. If possible, the time interval between the injury and onset of these signs and symptoms should be determined. Early symptoms do not necessarily correlate with the severity of the injury.

The classic external findings of acute laryngeal injury are subcutaneous emphysema and a flattening of the contour of the anterior cervical region. Most often, laryngeal injuries are not compounded externally, and thus, the external appearance may give little evidence of the underlying damage. Subcutaneous emphysema can be readily palpated. Anterior cervical flattening is noticed when the convexity of the thyroid cartilage, as viewed from the side, is lost. In these cases, it is often difficult or impossible to palpate the thyroid notch. Other findings with external examination include:

- Fracture of the hyoid bone
- Widening of the thyrohyoid membrane
- Fracture displacements of the thyroid cartilage
- Fracture of the cricoid cartilage
- Separation of the cricoid cartilage from the larynx or trachea

An accurate assessment of the phonatory and respiratory functions of the larynx can be accomplished readily by simply listening to the patient's speech and quiet respiration with the mouth open. Laryngeal edema may cause the patient to swallow frequently. Observation of the patient will disclose disturbances with deglutition and the presence of aspiration.

Indirect Laryngoscopy

If the patient is conscious and in no immediate respiratory distress, an indirect laryngoscopy may be possible. A flexible fiberoptic examination of the larynx by way of a nasal cavity is the best way to evaluate the larynx. During these examinations, the following are assessed:

1. The amount and location of laryngeal edema
2. Whether the anteroposterior dimension of the glottis is shortened; shortening is caused by
    a. the posterior displacement of the base of the epiglottis
    b. depressed fractures of the thyroid cartilage
    c. anterior displacement of the arytenoids or
    d. separation of the intrinsic muscles or hematoma
3. The amount and degree of ecchymosis or hematoma
4. Whether the laryngeal mucosa is lacerated and, if so, whether cartilage fragments are present in the lacerations
5. Narrowing of the subglottic airway
6. Decrease in or loss of laryngeal function caused by trauma to or sectioning of the recurrent laryngeal nerve(s), hemorrhage into the muscles, or disturbed origin or insertion of the intrinsic laryngeal musculature
7. Asymmetry or a deviation of the vocal chink from its normal anteroposterior direction.

Radiographic Examination

With external trauma, radiographic evaluation of the larynx and cervical spine is essential before any definite investigation or therapy is performed. The cervical spine is not unlike a coil spring that absorbs the shock of the forces that caused the laryngeal injury. It is not surprising, then, that fractures of the cervical spine are commonly associated with laryngeal injury.

Routine anteroposterior and lateral neck radiographs with copper filtration are often very useful. Fluoroscopy can be used in evaluating laryngeal function. Computed tomography scans are essential to accurately outline the type and degree of damage to the hyoid bone and the thyroid and cricoid cartilages. Laminograms of the larynx can also accurately outline the type and degree of damage to the hyoid bone and the thyroid and cricoid cartilages.

Direct Laryngoscopy

Direct laryngoscopy performed in the immediate period after the injury is hazardous and usually adds little to the information obtained from indirect laryngoscopy, fiberoptic examination, and radiographic evaluation. If a direct laryngoscopy is performed, it should be conducted with extreme care because it may further damage the airway, necessitating an immediate tracheotomy.

Tracheotomy

At times, the decision as to whether to perform a tracheotomy can be difficult to make, especially when subcutaneous emphysema is present and laryngeal functions appear to be normal. Careful observation is certainly not out of order, provided that the emphysema is not increasing rapidly and the patient is not coughing frequently. A tracheotomy should be performed when subcutaneous emphysema is rapidly increasing or a large laceration within the larynx is present, especially if cartilage can be seen in the laceration.

Systemic Examination

The cervical region should be carefully examined for tenderness, signs of cervical vertebral fracture, and subcutaneous emphysema. The neck is immobilized until it is certain that a fracture of the spine does not exist. Examination of the chest may show open or closed injuries. The chest is palpated for evidence of tenderness, and auscultation is performed to determine the heart action, character of the breath sounds, and signs of atelectasis. The abdomen is examined for tenderness, rigidity, and tympany. The upper abdominal quadrants are examined for evidence of liver and spleen injury. Tympany probably denotes gastric dilation. Repeated small emeses are characteristic of a dilated stomach. Pneumogastrium can be a complication of a tracheotomy after a laryngeal injury. This condition should be treated by inserting a nasogastric tube because if pneumogastrium is severe and prolonged, it can be fatal. The extremities are examined for loss of, or abnormal, function and evidence of fractures. Finally, a rapid but complete assessment of cranial nerve function is made.

Medical Treatment

Whether a tracheotomy is performed, the patient is placed in bed with the head elevated and on voice rest in a room with high humidity. Oxygen is administered as needed. Antibiotic therapy is usually indicated; however, if internal and external lacerations, subcutaneous emphysema, displaced fractures, or hematomas are not present, antibiotics may not be needed. Steroid therapy in maximum dosage should be instituted immediately. This has been shown to be of great value for rapid resolution of hematoma and of edema, which is at its maximum 6 hours after injury. The steroids slow granulation tissue formation, reduce the degree of fibrosis, and are said to reverse neuromuscular complications more rapidly in patients in whom they are administered.

Thyrotomy

Is a thyrotomy necessary, and if so, when? The need for a ·racheotomy does not necessarily indicate that a thyroidectomy should be performed. The disturbance of the laryngeal airway can be caused by ecchymosis, edema, or subcutaneous emphysema resulting from a small laceration of the mucous membrane associated with a nondisplaced fracture. The subcutaneous emphysema present in these circumstances develops rapidly when the patient, whose larynx is narrowed by edema, coughs.

In general, it is best to wait 3 to 5 days after the injury occurs before performing a thyrotomy to allow time for the acute reaction to subside.

After the acute reaction has subsided, the degree of damage and status of laryngeal function can be more readily assessed. At this time, repairs can be made more easily and accurately, and the internal structures will more readily tolerate internal splinting. If possible, open reduction should not be deferred beyond 10 days after the injury.

What is to be accomplished during thyrotomy?

1. Fractures of the hyoid bone, thyroid, and cricoid cartilages can be plated or wired after being replaced to their anatomical positions.

2. When the cricoid has separated from the larynx or trachea, repair can be made. This should be done as soon as possible after the injury.

3. All lacerations can be repaired. This is accomplished with No. 4-0 chromic catgut applied with a noncutting ophthalmic needle. Fragments of cartilage should be removed from lacerations before closure of the wounds. Often, the lacerated tissues cannot be completely approximated. The gaps will be bridged rapidly when a laryngeal stent is used. As a general rule, epithelial grafts are not indicated in patients with acute laryngeal injuries. Hematomas, unless very small, should be evaluated.

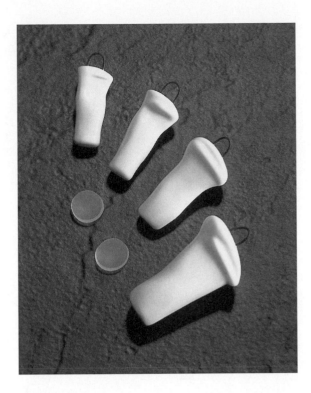

FIGURE 15–1. The Montgomery Laryngeal Stent is a molded silicone prosthesis designed to conform to the normal endolaryngeal surface. It is available in four sizes: the adult small, the adult medium, the adult large, and the pediatric (*left*). The stent is constructed from medical-grade silicone material, which is firm enough to ensure a conforming fit while minimizing injury to soft tissues. The silicone material produces no tissue reaction and allows re-epithelialization of the endolaryngeal mucosa.

4. Posterior displacement of the base of the epiglottis may not be resolved even after other injuries have been repaired. It is a positive indication for laryngeal stenting. A definitive procedure for correction of this defect should be deferred pending the result obtained from internal stenting.

5. Dislocation of an arytenoid can be very difficult to correct. If the arytenoid can be replaced to its anatomic position and maintained there with an internal stent, no further treatment is indicated. If the arytenoid cannot be replaced to its anatomic position, it should be resected.

Internal splinting with a conforming silicone laryngeal stent is indicated with any condition that could possibly lead to chronic stenosis. The technique for inserting and securing in place the Montgomery Laryngeal Stent (Boston Medical Products, Westborough, MA) is shown in Figures 15–1 and 15–2 and described in the accompanying legends.

Much controversy exists concerning the length of time that a laryngeal stent should be left in place. Certainly 3 weeks is the minimum period, and 6 weeks is usual. The value of stenting beyond 3 months is questionable. Indications for stenting for up to 3 months are (1) posterior displacement of the base of the epiglottis; (2) dislocation of the arytenoids(s); (3) depressed fractures of the cricoid cartilage; and (4) markedly displaced fractures of the thyroid cartilage. The surgeon must, at the time of repair, estimate the length of time that stenting will be needed according to the type and degree of injury.

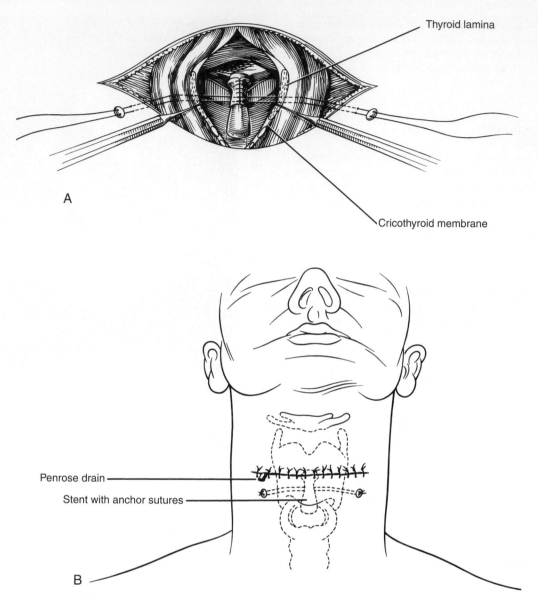

Thyroid lamina

Cricothyroid membrane

A

Penrose drain

Stent with anchor sutures

B

FIGURE 15–2. *A,* The laryngeal stent is secured in place by two sutures placed through the skin, thyroid lamina, subglottic space and out the opposite side through the thyroid lamina and skin. The sutures are tied loosely over silicone buttons (included with stent) on each side of the neck. In this case, the mucosal or skin graft–covered laryngeal stent has been inserted into the larynx and is secured in place with two No. 3-0 nylon sutures. *B,* The completed operation. No. 3-0 nylon suture material is supported externally by silicone buttons. A Penrose or closed suction drain is inserted. This will be removed on the second postoperative day.

CASE STUDY 15–1

Acute Laryngeal Trauma

A 17-year-old girl sustained severe laryngeal injury while skiing. An emergency tracheotomy was performed by an otolaryngologist, who was also skiing at the time, because of a rapidly decreasing laryngeal airway. She was placed on antibiotics and steroids and referred to Massachusetts Eye and Ear Infirmary. Her fiberoptic evaluation showed extensive laryngeal edema and lacerations with exposed cartilages. Her laryngeal airway was absent, and she was unable to phonate.

Preoperative soft tissue radiographs of the larynx demonstrated glottic and subglottic edema, a 2-cm traumatic separation between the true and false vocal cords, and retrodisplacement of the epiglottis (Fig. 15–3).

At the time of surgical exploration, the thyroid cartilage was found to be fractured and displaced (Fig. 15–4). After laryngofissure, the larynx was visualized as separated at the ventricular level. The arytenoids were exposed, and there was a 2-cm inferior displacement of the larynx below the level (i.e., 2-cm space between true and false cords). Both recurrent laryngeal nerves were intact.

After a repair using 4-0 chromic suture material on

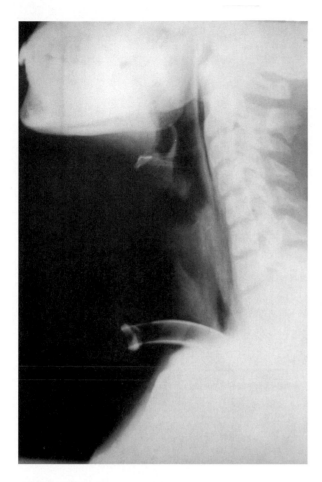

FIGURE 15-3. Preoperative soft tissue radiograph of the larynx demonstrating glottic and subglottic edema and a 2-cm traumatic separation between the true and false vocal cords.

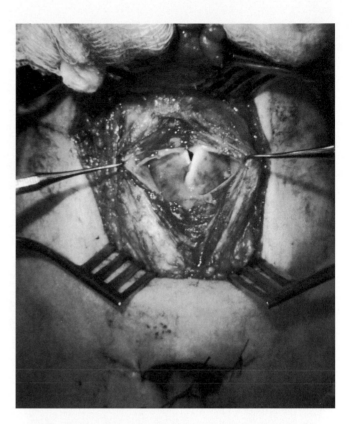

FIGURE 15-4. At the time of surgical exploration, the thyroid cartilage was found to be fractured and displaced.

an ophthalmic taper needle, the larynx was stented with a Montgomery Laryngeal Stent (Fig. 15–5), which has the following advantages: (1) It is made of nonreactive soft silicone to decrease granulation and cicatrix; (2) it has a preformed contour to maintain the proper relations of the vocal cords and supraglottic and subglottic structures; (3) four sizes are available, specific for both children and adults; (4) it provides a superior ligature loop to aid the endoscopic removal 3 to 6 weeks after its insertion.

A lateral neck radiograph (Fig. 15–6) shows the stent in place; it was removed after 3 weeks. Figure 15–7 shows a normal larynx 1 year after the injury.

LARYNGEAL INLET STENOSIS

Inlet stenosis results from either posterior displacement of the base of the epiglottis or anterior displacement of one or both arytenoid cartilages. It is caused by direct trauma to the anterior neck in the region of the thyrohyoid membrane at the thyroid cartilage notch (Fig. 15–8). The base of the epiglottis is displaced posteriorly, narrowing the laryngeal inlet. There is usually an associated fracture of the thyroid cartilage in the region of the thyroid notch. The superior as-

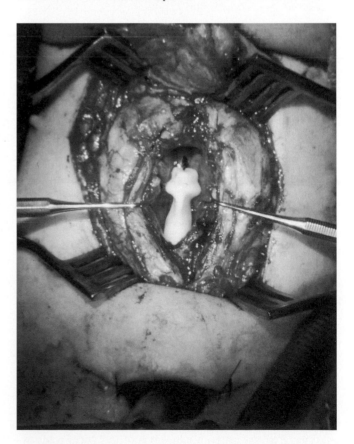

FIGURE 15-5. After repair, the larynx was stented with the Montgomery Laryngeal Stent.

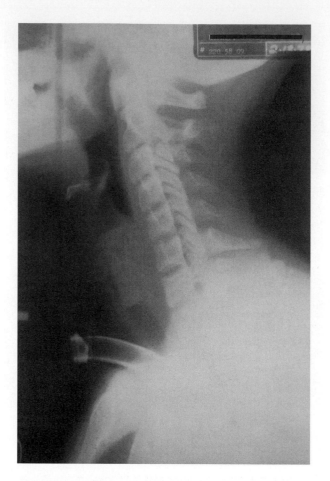

FIGURE 15–6. Lateral neck radiograph showing the stent in place.

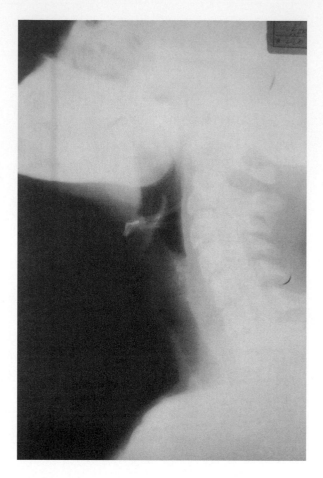

FIGURE 15–7. Radiograph taken 1 year postoperatively, showing a normal larynx.

pect of each thyroid lamina in this region may be depressed so that the notch can no longer be palpated. During the acute stage of this injury, ecchymosis and edema about the arytenoids may be present, and one or both arytenoids may be displaced anteriorly.

The diagnosis can be made using indirect laryngoscopy and fiberoptic flexible laryngoscopy. Anteroposterior and lateral radiographs of the larynx using a copper filter usually are sufficient to confirm this diagnosis. An axial computed tomography scan of the larynx adds detail.

Treatment

The laryngeal inlet is best approached by way of a high anterior horizontal cervical incision (Fig. 15–8A), or just below the level of the thyroid notch. A plane is established anterior to the fascia covering the strap muscles. The dissection is continued in this plane until the anterior larynx is exposed from the level of the thyrohyoid membrane to the cricothyroid membrane (Fig. 15–8D). A vertical midline incision is made through the fascia and periosteum over the thyroid cartilage. After a laryngofissure, the cricothyroid membrane is carefully split in the anterior midline. Because anterior adhesions of the vocal folds often accompany this type of lesion, it is very important to divide the cords carefully in the anterior midline. Thyrotomy scissors, or a button knife, seems best suited for this dissection.

Exposure is maintained with a self-retaining thyrotomy retractor or heavy skin hooks. The base of the epiglottis is widely exposed (Fig. 15–9A). An incision is made through the fascia and perichondrium around the anterior surface of the base of the epiglottis. Care should be taken not to disturb the cartilage (Fig. 15–9B). This segment of fascia and perichondrium is removed, and the anterior aspect of the base of the cartilaginous epiglottis is exposed. With a small posterior elevator, a plane is established between the cartilaginous base of the epiglottis and the mucoperichondrium on the posterior surface of the epiglottis (Fig. 15–9C). The exposed cartilage is removed, revealing the posterior mucoperichondrium (Fig. 15–10A). This is incised in the midline. With no. 3-0 chromic catgut, the flaps of the posterior surface of the mucoperichondrium are sutured to the cut edges of the fascia and anterior perichondrium on each side (Fig. 15–10B).

Because, as mentioned above, anterior adhesions of the vocal folds often accompany this type of injury, a silicone keel is inserted before the thyrotomy incision is closed (Fig. 15–11). The wound is repaired in layers with no. 00 chromic catgut and skin sutures, and a Penrose or rubber-band drain is fixed in place subcutaneously.

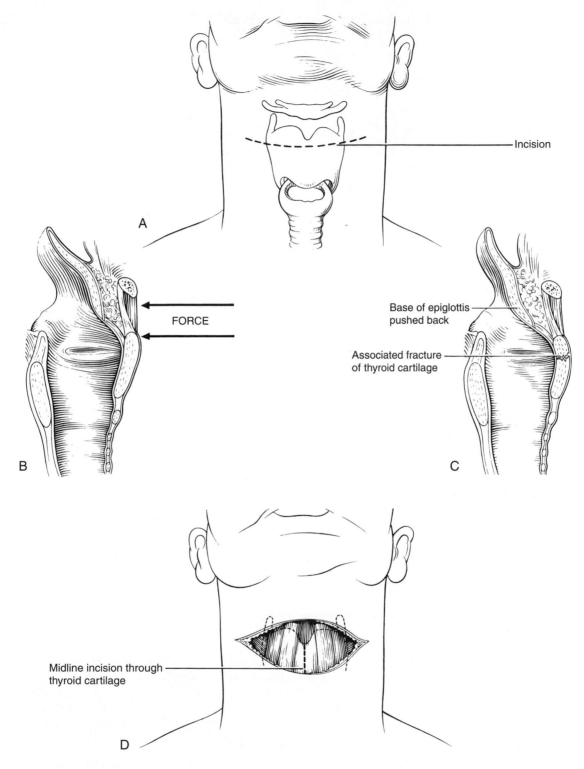

FIGURE 15–8. Laryngeal inlet stenosis. *A,* The horizontal anterior cervical incision is used for repair of inlet stenosis. *B,* The force producing the injury responsible for laryngeal inlet stenosis is directed posteriorly, in the region of the thyrohyoid membrane and superior aspect of the thyroid cartilage. *C,* The base of the epiglottis, the hyoid bone, and a fragment of the thyroid cartilage are displaced posteriorly by the injuring force. Note the associated fracture of the thyroid cartilage. *D,* A plane has been established anterior to the fascia covering the strap muscles. The anterior thyroid cartilage is exposed from the thyrohyoid membrane to the cricothyroid membrane. The thyrotomy incision is made in the anterior midline of the thyroid cartilage with either thyrotomy scissors or a saw.

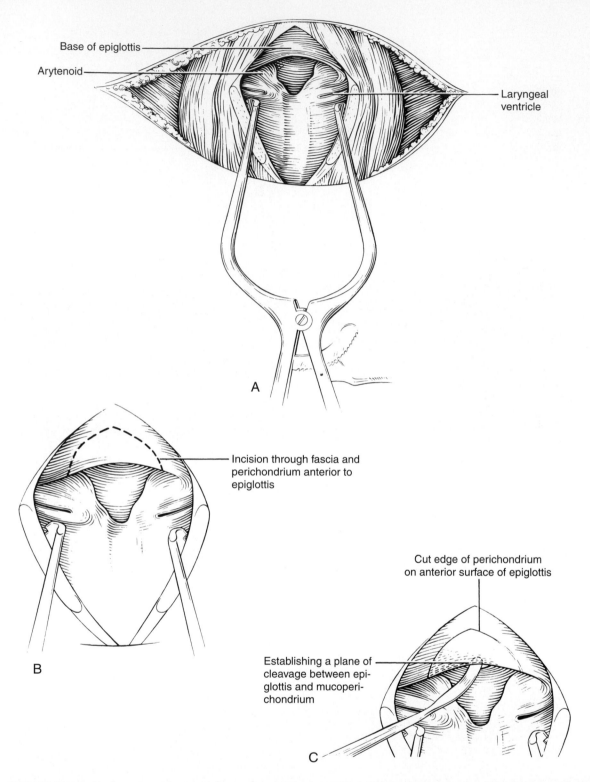

FIGURE 15-9. Laryngeal inlet stenosis. *A,* The thyrotomy incision is completed. The laryngeal lumen is exposed with a self-retaining retractor or by using hooks that are carefully inserted in the plane of the thyrotomy incision and rotated 90 degrees before lateral traction is applied. The base of the epiglottis is carefully dissected anteriorly in preparation for reconstruction of the laryngeal inlet. *B,* An incision, as indicated by the broken lines, is made through the fascia and perichondrium anterior to the base of the epiglottis. The epiglottic cartilage is not disturbed. A plane is established anterior to the epiglottic cartilage, and the fascia and perichondrium are removed. *C,* With a small periosteal elevator, a plane of cleavage is established between the cartilaginous epiglottis and the underlying mucoperichondrium on the posterior surface of the epiglottis.

Case Study 15–2

Laryngeal Inlet Stenosis

A 23-year-old woman presented for treatment 4 months after being thrown through the windshield of an automobile. She had sustained multiple facial lacerations, concussion, and a laryngeal injury. An emergency tracheotomy had been performed shortly after the accident. The patient had an inspiratory airway when the tracheotomy tube was occluded. The volume of her voice was barely above a whisper. The superior aspect of the thyroid cartilage was depressed, and the thyroid notch could not be palpated. Visualization by indirect laryngoscopy was difficult because of the posterior displacement of the base of the epiglottis (Fig. 15–10C). A marked decrease in the anteroposterior dimension of the larynx was evident. The right

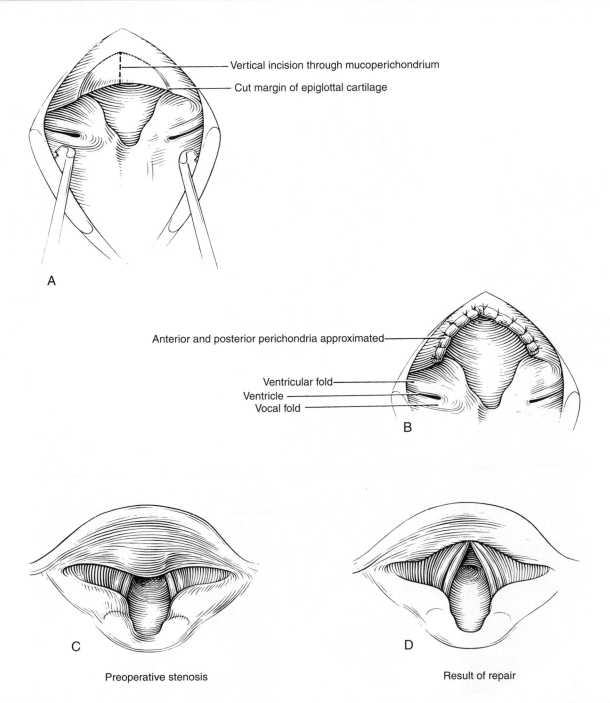

Vertical incision through mucoperichondrium

Cut margin of epiglottal cartilage

A

Anterior and posterior perichondria approximated

Ventricular fold

Ventricle

Vocal fold

B

C

Preoperative stenosis

D

Result of repair

FIGURE 15–10. Laryngeal inlet stenosis. *A,* A segment of the cartilaginous base of the epiglottis has been removed, and a vertical midline incision is made through the posterior mucoperichondrium. *B,* The posterior mucoperichondrium flaps are reflected laterally on each side and sutured to the fascia and anterior perichondrium with No. 3-0 chromic catgut. *C,* The appearance of the larynx with an inlet stenosis. Because of the posterior displacement of the base of the epiglottis, the larynx is difficult to view by either indirect or direct laryngoscopy. *D,* The appearance of the larynx after repair of the inlet stenosis.

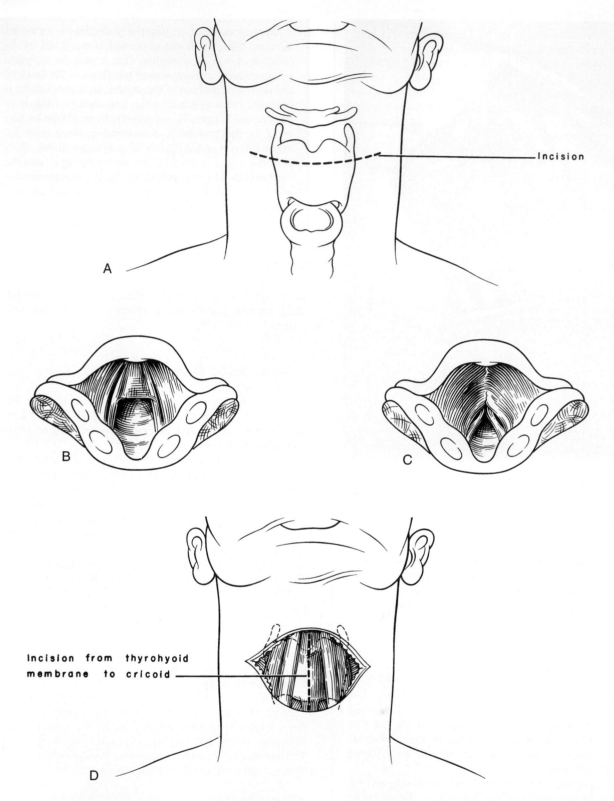

FIGURE 15-13. Anterior glottic stenosis. *A,* A horizontal anterior cervical skin incision is made approximately 2 cm below the thyroid notch. This is carried through the platysma to the fascia overlying the sternohyoid and omohyoid muscles. Flaps are elevated superiorly and inferiorly. A plane of cleavage is established in a median raphe between the two sternohyoid muscles to expose the anterior thyroid cartilage. *B,* Anterior glottic stenosis (laryngeal web) involving the vocal folds. This is usually congenital, but it may follow an intralaryngeal operation or external trauma. *C,* Anterior glottic stenosis involving the true vocal cords, false cords, and laryngeal ventricle. This is the type of stenosis most often caused by external trauma. *D,* An anterior vertical midline incision is made through the thyroid laminae. This is accomplished by using a knife if the cartilage has not undergone ossification; if it has become ossified, use of a saw is necessary. The incision should extend from the thyrohyoid membrane to the cricoid cartilage for adequate exposure. The underlying soft tissue is not disturbed at this point.

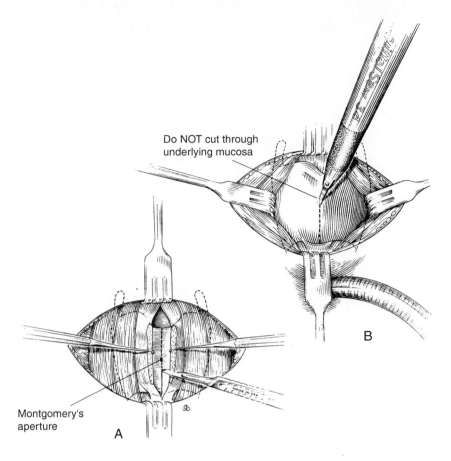

FIGURE 15-14. *A,* The thyroid lamina has been incised in the midline. *B,* The underlying tissue is gradually incised using a vertical stroke. Almost invariably a small opening will appear just below the anterior commissure.

Do NOT cut through underlying mucosa

Montgomery's aperture

cheal tube is inserted through the glottis to keep the vocal cords apart, even if a tracheotomy is present. This technique facilitates the laryngofissure procedure.

An anterior horizontal cervical skin incision is made at the level of the mid-thyroid cartilage (Fig. 15–13*A*). A plane is established anterior to the fascia covering the strap muscles, both superiorly and inferiorly.

The thyrohyoid membrane, thyroid cartilage, and cricothyroid membranes are exposed after the sternohyoid muscles have been carefully separated in the midline (median raphe).

The anterior midline thyrotomy is performed either with a knife or a saw, depending on the degree of ossification of the thyroid cartilage. The underlying soft tissues are not disturbed at this time.

The thyroid laminae are held apart with small hooks. The underlying soft tissues are gradually incised using a vertical stroke with a no.15 surgical knife. Almost invariably a small opening (Figs. 15–14*B* and 15–15) will appear just below the anterior commissure. This opening indicates the anterior midline. The remainder of the laryngofissure can be

FIGURE 15-15. The thyroid laminae are being retracted with small hooks, giving a view of the underlying soft tissues. A small opening will appear just below the anterior commissure as these tissues are incised vertically.

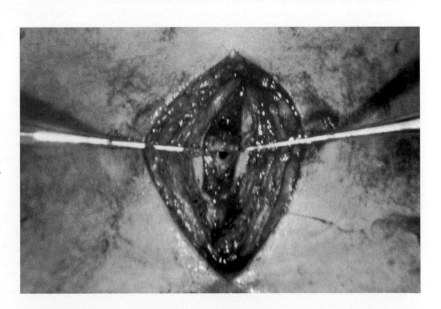

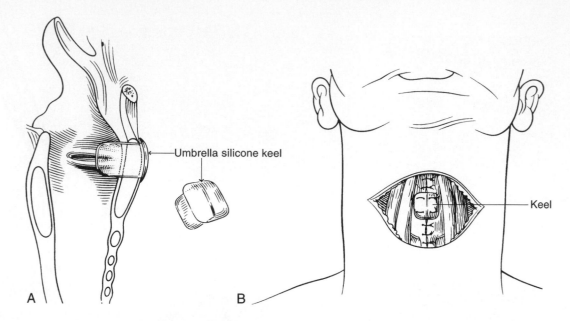

FIGURE 15–16. Anterior glottic stenosis. *A,* Midsagittal sketch showing the umbrella-like silicone keel in place. The thin intralaryngeal portion does not extend to the level of the vocal process. The extralaryngeal portion will conform snugly to the contour of the exterior thyroid lamina. A sketch of the silicone keel is shown to the right of this drawing. *B,* The silicone keel has been fixed in place with two figure-eight sutures of no. 3-0 nylon suture material (Fig. 15–17*B*). The thyroid laminae, thyrohyoid membrane, and cricothyroid membrane are approximated above and below the keel. The sternohyoid muscles are sutured together over the extralaryngeal portion of the keel.

accomplished with either a knife or scissors, without being misdirected.

When the laryngofissure has been complete, the thyroid cartilages are retracted laterally and the larynx is inspected. If the stenosis or web is thick, it may be necessary to remove excessive scar tissue to ensure against irregularities or excessive thickness of the vocal cords.

A series of experiments conducted on canine larynges has shown that a silicone keel (Figs. 15–16 and 15–17*A*) is best suited for application after the repair of an anterior glottic stenosis. Other metallic and plastic keels were studied. This silicone keel did not cause granulation tissue to form in the region of the anterior commissure until at least 3 weeks after insertion of the keel (Fig. 15–17*C* and *D*). The length of time necessary for complete regrowth of vocal cord epithelium following simulated anterior glottic stenosis and the insertion of the silicone keel was found to be between 9 and 12 days. It was thus concluded that granulation tissue formation in the anterior commissure and recurrent stenosis could be avoided and complete re-epithelialization of the vocal cords could be expected when the silicone keel remained in place no longer than 2 or 3 weeks (Fig. 15–18*C*).

The Montgomery Laryngeal Keel is available in three sizes, either clear or radiopaque. The intralaryngeal portion of the keel is available in Nos. 12-, 14-, and 16-mm dimensions. The intralaryngeal portion of the keel should not extend to the posterior commissure. The keel is sutured to the thyroid laminae and is shown in Figs. 15–16 and 15–17*B*, with two figure-eight no. 3-0 nylon sutures. These sutures tightly approximate the thyroid laminae and fix the keel firmly in place. The thyroid laminae are carefully approximated above and below the keel with 3-0 Vicryl suture material. The sternohyoid muscles are approximated, and the skin incision is closed in layers.

Drainage is accomplished with either closed suction or a Penrose drain.

If a midline anterior stenosis or web is present along with bilateral vocal cord paralysis, correction of the stenosis, as outlined above, will not improve the airway. An arytenoidectomy is necessary in addition to repair of the anterior glottic stenosis. A Montgomery Laryngeal Stent (Boston Medical Products, Westborough, MA) (see Fig. 15–22*B*), rather than a silicone keel, is inserted. The laryngeal stent remains in place for approximately 1 month and is removed by way of a laryngofissure. Granulation tissue is carefully resected from the anterior commissure, and a silicone keel is inserted as described above. It is removed after 2 weeks.

Postoperative Care

The postoperative course after repair of an anterior glottic stenosis is usually uneventful unless the thyrotomy closure is not sufficiently tight. In such cases, subcutaneous emphysema or an air pocket can develop between the strap muscles and the skin flaps. The diagnosis can be made by palpation or a lateral neck radiograph. When this condition exists, the wound should be drained at once.

The tracheotomy stoma should remain open for approximately 1 week after the operation. This helps prevent escape of laryngeal secretions into the extralaryngeal space by way of the thyrotomy wound and allows for more rapid re-epithelialization of the vocal cords.

Unless the operation has been complicated by infection, the keel can be removed, as an office procedure, 2 to 3 weeks after the repair. The central portion of the skin incision is infiltrated with a local anesthetic. An incision (no longer than 1 inch) is necessary for exposure. The blue nylon sutures are easily visible against the translucent keel. The skin incision is closed with two vertical mattress sutures after removal of the keel.

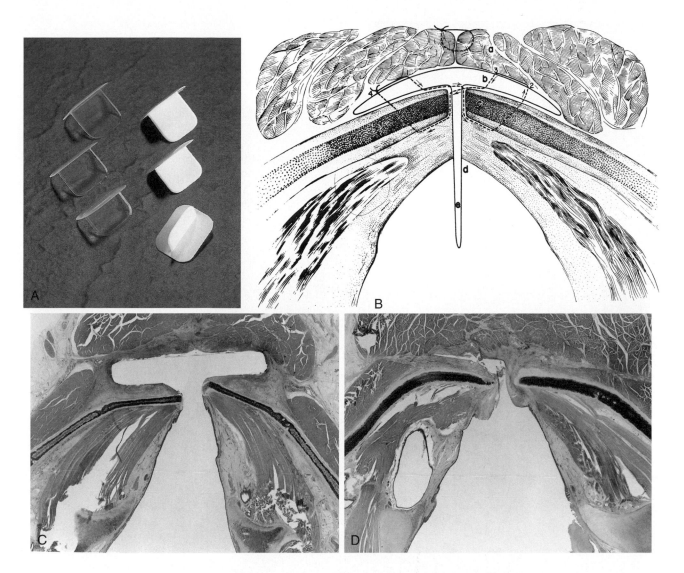

FIGURE 15–17. Anterior glottic stenosis. *A,* The Montgomery Laryngeal Keel, with its unique umbrella shape, is used in the repair of anterior glottic stenosis. It is made of soft medical-grade silicone and is one piece, specifically designed to conform to the anatomy of the anterior commissure to prevent restenosis or the formation of granulation tissue. *B,* Tight closure of the thyroid laminae and fixation of the laryngeal keel are best accomplished by using two figure-eight sutures (No. 3-0 nylon). This suture is first placed through the extralaryngeal portion of the keel (1) and then through the base of the intralaryngeal extension. It is continued through the thyroid laminae and extralaryngeal portion of the keel on the opposite side (2). The second half of the suture (3 and 4) is placed in a direction reverse to that of the first half. The figure-of-eight sutures must be completed before insertion of the keel. Sutures are placed through the thyroid laminae above and below the keel, and the sternohyoid muscles are approximated in the midline over the keel. a = sternohyoid muscles; b = extralaryngeal portion of the keel; c = thyroid laminae; d = anterior commissure; e = intralaryngeal portion of the keel. It is available in sizes 12, 14, and 16 (anteroposterior intralaryngeal), radio-clear, and radiopaque. *C,* Canine larynx with simulated anterior glottic stenosis 2 weeks after insertion of an umbrella silicone keel. Granulation tissue is not present, and epithelium extends to the anterior commissure. *D,* Silicone keel experiment of 3 weeks' duration with a very slight amount of granulation tissue in the region of the anterior commissure. Epithelium extends nearly to the anterior commissure. The degree of recurrent stenosis in this experiment would be negligible. Experiments of 4 or more weeks' duration all demonstrated a significant amount of granulation tissue.

CASE STUDY 15–3

Anterior Glottic Stenosis

The patient, a 24-year-old woman with anterior glottic stenosis secondary to a dashboard injury to the larynx, was admitted to the hospital. Two previous procedures had been successful in stabilizing the cartilaginous framework of the larynx. An anterior glottic stenosis persisted after repair with the tantalum keel. The stenosis was sufficient to interfere with vocal function and to limit the airway to the extent that a tracheotomy was necessary.

In a third procedure, the thick anterior glottic stenosis was resected through an anterior thyrotomy incision, and a silicone keel was inserted. The keel was removed 2½ weeks postoperatively. The tracheotomy tube was removed 2 weeks later. Six weeks after the operation, the patient's airway was normal and her vocal function was excellent (Fig. 15–18*B*).

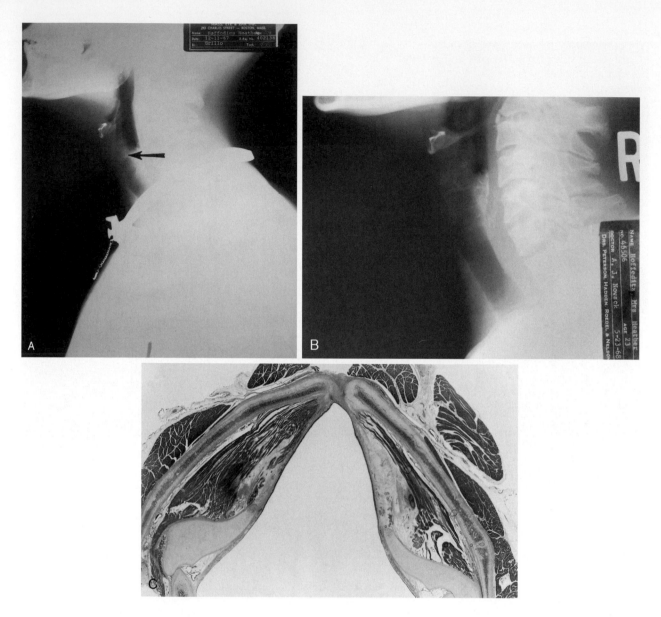

FIGURE 15–18. Anterior glottic stenosis. *A,* Lateral-neck radiograph of a 24-year-old woman who had an inadequate laryngeal airway and voice impairment. Indirect laryngoscopy clearly demonstrated an anterior glottic stenosis. The defect resulted from an injury occurring as the patient was thrust forward against the steering wheel. On the film, a decreased air shadow can be seen at the glottic level. *B,* Lateral neck radiograph taken less than 1 month after repair of the anterior glottic stenosis demonstrates a normal glottic air shadow. A keel remained in place for 2 weeks after the operation. The tracheotomy stoma was no longer needed after 1 additional week. The results of the technique used have been documented by experimental evidence. Re-epithelialization of the vocal cords occurs within 1 week after repair of simulated anterior glottic stenosis in the canine larynx. *C,* Horizontal section through a canine larynx. The laryngectomy was performed 1 month after the keel was removed. The keel had remained in place 2 weeks after repair of simulated glottic stenosis. Epithelium extends to the anterior commissure, which is well formed.

Posterior Glottic Stenosis

The posterior commissure can be involved with a stenosis as a result of external or internal trauma or of infection (eg, tuberculosis or diphtheria). Posterior stenosis may also be present as a part of complete laryngeal stenosis. Posterior glottic stenosis is also present as part of a complete laryngeal stenosis.

Diagnosis

The diagnosis of posterior glottic stenosis by indirect laryngoscopy and by radiographic studies can be elusive (Fig.

15–19*A*). The process may not be immediately apparent on laryngeal examination (Fig. 15–20*B*). The vocal folds will not abduct during inspiration and will not meet during phonation. Close observation of the arytenoids and the interarytenoid space may show a limited adduction, abduction, or rotation of the arytenoids. Posterior glottic stenosis is often not readily apparent until it is viewed by way of a laryngofissure (Figs. 15–19*C* and 15–20*B*).

Treatment

The posterior web is easily disrupted by making a vertical midline incision (Fig. 15–19*C*); however, it will recur if the denuded posterior commissure (Figs. 15–19*D* and 15–20*D*) is not covered by mucous membrane. The interarytenoideus muscle is usually involved with fibrosis and is nonfunctioning, thereby preventing lateral excursion and limiting adduction of the interarytenoids. If this is the case, the fibrous tissue and the interarytenoideus muscle must be resected (Fig. 15–19*D*).

A superiorly based mucous membrane flap is obtained from the interarytenoid space above the area of posterior stenosis. It is fashioned by making a vertical mucosal incision on each side of the interarytenoid space. The flap is elevated in the submucosal plane (Fig. 15–20*D*). Bleeding is controlled using bipolar cautery. The mucosal flap is re-

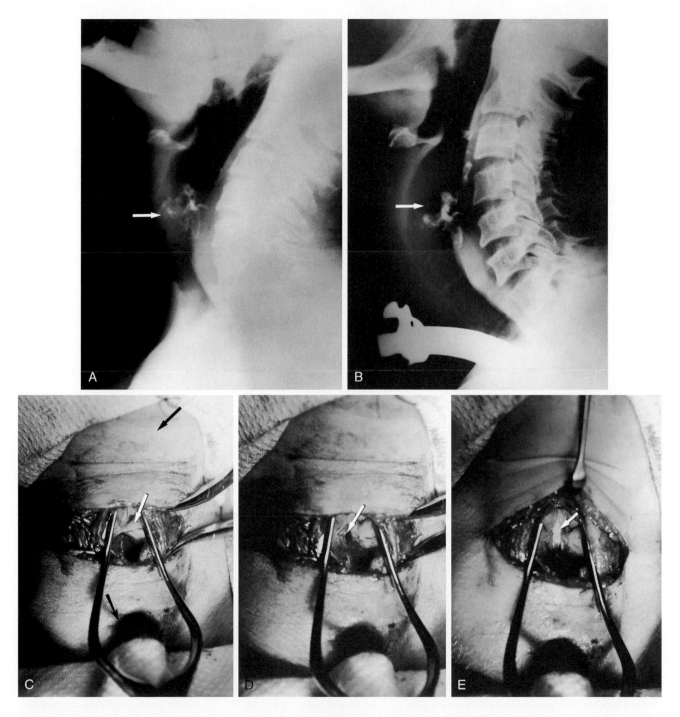

FIGURE 15–19. Posterior glottic stenosis. *A,* Lateral neck radiograph demonstrating a narrowing of the glottic airway. The posterior glottic stenosis, a complication of laryngeal tuberculosis, was not fully appreciated on either laryngoscopy or radiographic examination. At the time of the operation, interarytenoid scar tissue was found. This interferes with both adduction and abduction of the arytenoids with a resulting hoarseness and limited airway. The *arrow* points to the area of stenosis. *B,* Postoperative radiograph demonstrating an adequate airway and the absence of a tracheotomy tube. The posterior stenosis was repaired by resecting the interarytenoid scar tissue and using a superiorly based mucosal flap. Since the time of the operation, the patient has had a normal airway (*arrow*) without hoarseness. *C,* Thyrotomy showed the posterior glottic stenosis that interfered with adduction and abduction of the arytenoids (*upper arrow,* chin; *middle arrow,* posterior stenosis; *lower arrow,* tracheotomy). *D,* The web has been incised (*arrow*), scar tissue resected, and the interarytenoideus muscle incised and resected. *E,* Repair has been accomplished by using a superiorly based mucosal flap.

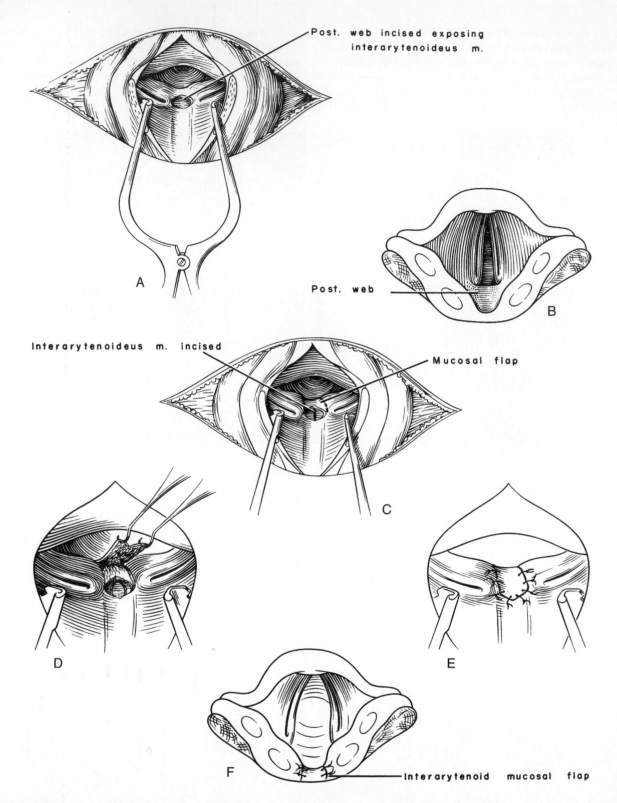

Post. web incised exposing
interarytenoideus m.

A

Post. web

B

Interarytenoideus m. incised

Mucosal flap

C

D

E

F

Interarytenoid mucosal flap

FIGURE 15–20. Posterior glottic stenosis. *A,* The posterior commissure is seen through a laryngofissure. The web has been incised by making a vertical midline incision, exposing the interarytenoid muscle. This muscle is divided in the midline and resected, for it is usually fibrotic, nonfunctioning, and prevents lateral as well as medial excursion of the arytenoids. *B,* The posterior web as seen on indirect laryngoscopy. The degree of pathologic change is often not appreciated by this examination. However, limited excursion of the arytenoids is apparent. *C,* A vertical mucosal incision is made on each side of the interarytenoid space. Additional length for the flap can be obtained by extending its base to the superior surface of the interarytenoid space. *D,* The mucosal flap has been elevated. Bleeding is controlled by cautery. *E,* The flap has been advanced over the area of stenosis. The inferior sutures (No. 4-0 chromic catgut) are secured before applying those along each side. *F,* The repaired posterior stenosis is viewed by means of indirect laryngoscopy.

flected inferiorly over the area void of mucous membrane and sutured in place with No. 4-0 chromic catgut or 4-0 Vicryl suture material (Figs. 15–19E and 15–20E and F).

If the larynx functions well bilaterally and the mucous membrane flap fits snugly in place, internal support is not necessary.

When a unilateral or bilateral laryngeal paralysis is present, or if there is fixation of the cricoarytenoid joint, an arytenoidectomy is performed and a conforming laryngeal stent is inserted and secured in place as shown in Figure 15–23. The stent should remain in place for at least 3 weeks, until healing is complete.

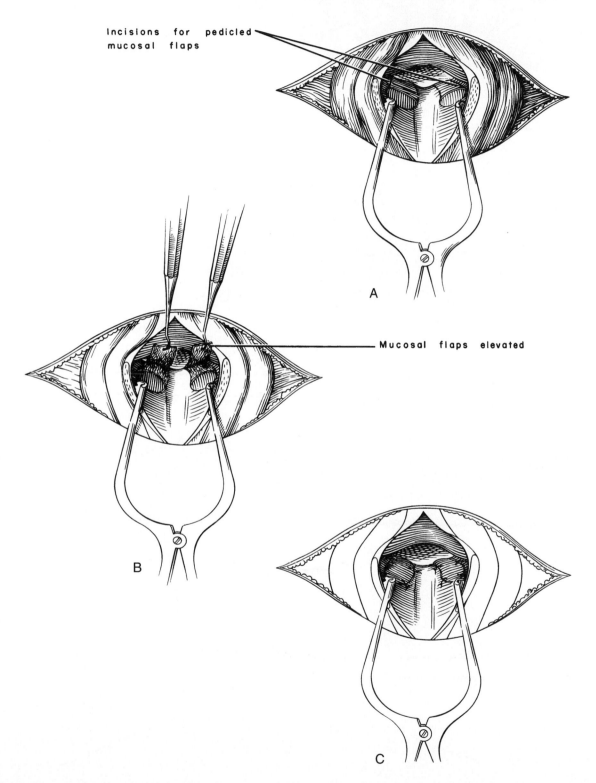

FIGURE 15–21. Complete glottic stenosis. *A,* The thyroid laminae have been retracted laterally, and a nearly complete stenosis of the larynx is exposed. However, the posterior commissure remains free. The scar tissue has been resected. Incisions for the construction of superiorly based mucosal flaps, which will be used to cover the areas void of mucous membrane, are outlined. *B,* The flaps have been elevated superiorly by sharp dissection carefully executed. Long, delicate, pointed scissors aid in this dissection. *C,* The flaps have been advanced inferiorly and sutured in place. A contoured silicone laryngeal stent is necessary after this type of repair.

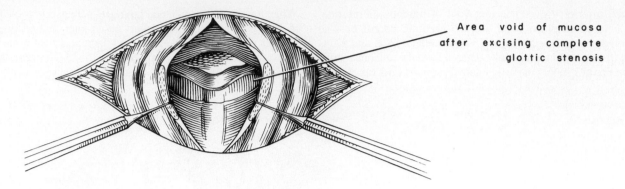

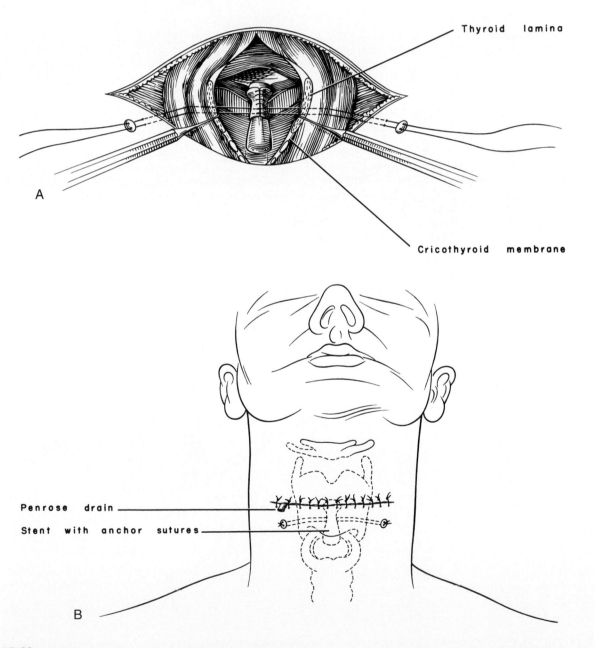

FIGURE 15–22. Complete laryngeal stenosis. Complete stenosis of the larynx at the level of the glottis, too extensive for the repair by pedicled mucosal flaps, is shown.

FIGURE 15–23. Complete laryngeal stenosis. *A,* The mucosal or skin graft–covered silicone stent has been inserted into the larynx and is secured in place with two No. 3-0 nylon sutures. It is best to suture the grafts to the patient rather than to the stent. *B,* The completed operation. The No. 3-0 nylon suture material is supported externally by silicone buttons. A drain has been inserted. This will be removed on the second postoperative day.

Complete Glottic Stenosis

Complete glottic stenosis can result from extralaryngeal trauma (crushing), intralaryngeal trauma, and severe laryngeal infection. The diagnosis is obvious by indirect or flexible fiberoptic laryngoscopy. Computed tomography scans are very valuable in denoting the superior inferior extent of the stenosis.

Treatment

A direct laryngoscopy is performed, and a search of an airway is made. Most often, a small passage through the larynx can be found. This is gradually increased in size with bougies, and as large a bougie as possible is left in place while a laryngocricotracheal fissure approaches the stenosis.

An anterior horizontal cervical skin incision can be made at the level of the mid-thyroid cartilage. We prefer an anterior vertical midline skin incision to approach a complete glottic stenosis. It is important that the sectioning of the thyroid cartilage be exactly in the midline to avoid creating a false passage or injuring the laryngeal musculature. The stenotic larynx is usually best approached from below but occasionally from above.

Once the endolarynx is encountered, the scar tissue is carefully resected, preserving all identifiable landmarks. The arytenoids should be palpated to determine whether they are fixed. If they are fixed, it may be necessary to remove one arytenoid to establish an airway.

If the stenosis is high in the larynx, it can be repaired using superiorly based pedicle flaps, which are pulled down from the interarytenoid space (Fig. 15–20) and the aryepiglottic folds (Fig. 15–21A). The superiorly based mucosal flaps are carefully dissected in the submucosal plane (Fig. 15–21B). They must be very thin and are advanced inferiorly and sutured in place with 4-0 chromic or 4-0 Vicryl suture material (Fig. 15–21C). Small ophthalmic needles are helpful in performing this delicate suturing.

Occasionally, the area devoid of mucous membrane is too extensive to be covered by pedicled mucosal flaps; in such instances, a mucosal graft may be obtained from the buccal region. When the buccal graft is obtained, the orifice of Stensen's duct is identified before the graft is obtained. The postoperative discomfort from the donor site is remarkably slight as the results and defect are closed primarily in a horizontal line with 3-0 chromic catgut. A 2 × 4 cm mucosal graft may be obtained from one side of the nasal septum. The submucosal layer of the nasal septum is dense, and subsequent graft shrinkage is minimal. A split-thickness skin graft can be used but can result in dryness and occasionally the growth of hair in the larynx. The skin graft is best obtained from the supraclavicular region because of the proximity to the field of surgery and its lack of hair.

The Montgomery Laryngeal Stent (Fig. 15–1) has been developed to help support the endolaryngeal grafts (Fig. 15–22). The silicone is of a precise hardness to offer support without injuring the surrounding tissues. It bends with ease, is compressible, and conforms exactly to the inner contour of the larynx. In the past, the graft has been sutured to the stent (Fig. 15–23A), inserted into the larynx, and fixed in place with 3-0 nylon or prolene suture material. More recently, tacking the grafts to the denuded surface of the larynx seems to give a better result because there is no movement of the graft when the patient swallows as there is when the graft is attached to the stent. The stents are available in one size suitable for children, and three sizes for adults. The 3-0 nylon sutures are supported externally by silicone buttons (Fig. 15–23A and B). Closed suction drainage is applied, and the wound is closed in layers.

Chapter 16
Subglottic Stenosis

WILLIAM W. MONTGOMERY

Subglottic stenosis can be a simple surgical problem or it can be a most difficult airway stenosis to repair. The incidence of severe glottic stenosis has increased with the increase in megasurgery, requiring prolonged postoperative intubation. Lesser degrees of subglottic stenosis can be managed by endoscopic procedures, such as bougienage, injection of long-lasting steroids (Aristocort), laser procedures, and application of mitomycin C.

ETIOLOGY

Subglottic stenosis can result from external trauma to the larynx, most commonly in the form of a blunt injury rather than a penetrating wound. Cricothyrotomy and high tracheotomy can be complicated by subglottic stenosis. The recent increase in these operations has definitely caused an increase in the incidence of subglottic stenosis. An overinflated endotracheal tube cuff, especially when associated with assisted respiration, can injure the subglottic stenosis. Thermal injury to the subglottic region is common and often severe. A traumatic intubation or endoscopy can result in subglottic stenosis.

Subglottic stenosis may occur after radiation therapy to the larynx, either shortly after or as long as 20 years after the radiation therapy. It is extremely difficult to treat, and frequently the disease process cannot be reversed. Diseases such as Wegener's granulomatosis and relapsing polychondritis are often complicated by subglottic stenosis. There is currently a treatment protocol for these diseases by the National Institutes of Health consisting of injection of long-lasting steroids into the subglottic region by way of the laryngeal ventricles, followed by bougienage.

Congenital webs or strictures of the subglottic region are usually diagnosed in the neonatal period but, occasionally, may not become symptomatic until adulthood. Neoplasms, both malignant and benign, can occur in the subglottic region and cause stenosis. In our experience, the most common benign lesions are hemangioma, chondroma, and fibroma. The most common malignant tumors are squamous cell carcinoma and adenocarcinoma.

There is an idiopathic type of subglottic stenosis that develops over a number of years and usually becomes clinically significant during the second and third decades of life. With this disease, a gradual increase occurs in the thickness of the tissue between the mucous membrane of the cricoid perichondrium (Fig. 16–1).

SYMPTOMS

The symptoms associated with slowly progressive subglottic stenosis may be minimal. The disease may remain undiagnosed for a number of years. Many of our cases have been previously misdiagnosed and treated as lower pulmonary disease, such as asthma. When the subglottic stenosis becomes moderate to severe, symptoms such as a subtle voice change, hoarseness, frequent coughing and expectoration of crusts, wheezing, and finally dyspnea on exertion will alarm the patient sufficiently to seek medical care.

DIAGNOSIS

The diagnosis of subglottic stenosis can usually be made by indirect laryngoscopy using a mirror, or by a flexible fiberoptic laryngoscope. However, it is impossible to determine the level of stenosis by this examination.

It is important to study the status of the laryngeal airway and vocal cord function during this examination. A subglottic stenosis extending to the cord level can interfere with cord function and also narrow the airway at the cord level. If the larynx cannot be properly evaluated by indirect laryngoscopy, it is imperative to perform a fiberoptic examination while the patient is awake because it is impossible to properly evaluate vocal cord function during direct laryngoscopy under general anesthesia.

Soft tissue radiographs of the larynx and trachea, including the anteroposterior copper filter view, will satisfactorily outline the level and degree of the subglottic stenosis (see Fig. 16–1A–D). Computed tomography scan and magnetic resonance imaging may or may not add additional information to the plane radiographs. Vocal cord function can be evaluated by fluoroscopy.

Direct laryngoscopy and bronchoscopy are usually delayed until the time of definitive surgery to avoid exposing the patient to an extra general anesthesia.

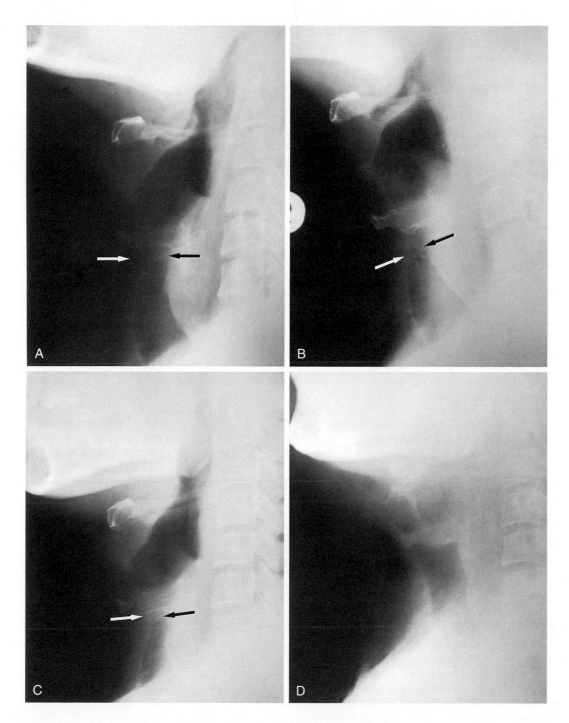

FIGURE 16–1. Idiopathic subglottic stenosis. *A,* Radiograph of a 38-year-old man with gradually increasing dyspnea on exertion that lasted for 3 years. The narrowing of the subglottic region (*arrows*) is minimal. *B,* A repeat study 2 years later demonstrated increased narrowing of the subglottic airway (*arrows*). *C,* One year later the subglottic airway is narrowed sufficiently to cause marked dyspnea (*arrows*). *D,* A radiograph 1 month after repair and removal of Montgomery Safe-T-Tube. The subglottic air pocket persisted for 2 weeks; his subglottic airway remained unchanged for the next 12 years when he died of other causes.

TREATMENT

Acute and subacute subglottic stenosis is approached by way of direct laryngoscopy and bronchoscopy if possible. If an inflammatory process is present, cultures are obtained for diagnosis and antibiotic selection. When granulation tissue is encountered, the site or sites of its origin are first injected with a steroid, either methylprednisolone acetate (Depo-Medrol) 40 mg/mL or dexamethasone sodium phosphate (Decadron) 4 mg/mL. The granulation tissue is carefully removed, and the site of its origin is cauterized or treated with mitomycin C, 0.4% saturated to a cotton pledget, for 3 minutes. This type of subglottic stenosis can also be treated using laser surgery. If the mucous membrane is intact and the subglottic stenosis is caused by submucosal thickening, the subglottic region is infiltrated with steroids by inserting the needles through the laryngeal ventricles on both sides lateral to the vocal cords and through the conus elasticus. After this, the subglottic region is bougied up to normal size if possible. Adjuvant therapy with systemic steroids in high doses and topical therapy using dexamethasone sodium phosphate Respihaler two puffs twice a day are valuable. A tracheotomy should be avoided if at all possible, although one should not procrastinate if the subglottic stenosis is severe, if the patient is obviously dyspneic, and if the blood gases are abnormal. Internal stenting is necessary when the subglottic stenosis results from blunt trauma and fracture of the cricoid arch.

CHRONIC SUBGLOTTIS STENOSIS

The operation for chronic subglottic stenosis should begin with a direct laryngoscopy. The exact degree and location of the stenosis can be determined. If the stenosis is not severe and the mucous membrane is intact, the technique of steroid injection followed by bougienage, as described above, can be tried.

Another technique when the stenosis is not severe is to make radial incisions with the CO_2 laser and treat the area of stenosis by leaving a cotton pledget saturated with 5 mg/mL of mitomycin C for 5 minutes. Usually, however, after bougienage, the bougie remains in place or is replaced by an endotracheal tube, followed by a definitive surgical repair, by way of a laryngofissure.

Anesthesia is administered by way of an endotracheal tube inserted through the stenosis or by way of the existing tracheotomy. Regardless of the route of anesthesia, it is important that an endotracheal tube, bougie, or bronchoscope be inserted through the area of the stenosis to facilitate staying in the midline and obtaining exposure during a laryngocricofissure.

The subglottic region can be exposed using either a horizontal skin incision at the lower aspect of the thyroid cartilage or, as we prefer, a vertical midline incision.

The fascia over the sternohyoid and omohyoid muscles is exposed by dissecting superiorly and inferiorly; the field is exposed using two large self-retaining retractors. The sternohyoid muscles are separated in the midline exposing the thyroid notch, the anterior aspect of the thyroid cartilage, cricoid arch, and first and second tracheal rings. The thyroid laminae are exposed by retracting the sternohyoid, thyrohyoid, and omohyoid muscles laterally (Fig. 16–2A).

The laryngeal scissors and button-knife techniques for executing a thyrotomy have been abandoned, and a layered technique that prevents deviation from the midline and anterior commissure is preferred. The thyroid cartilage is incised in the vertical midline using a No. 10 surgical blade if the cartilage has not undergone ossification. An electric oscillating saw is used if ossification has occurred (see Fig. 16–2B). It is important to carry this incision through the cartilage only and not the underlying tissue.

After the cartilage incision has been completed, the two thyroid laminae are slightly separated with small skin hooks. The airway is entered through a vertical incision in the midline. Unless the stenosis extends up to the level of the anterior commissure, a small opening will almost invariably appear just below the anterior commissure (Fig. 16–2C). If this opening does not appear, it can be assumed that the stenosis extends to the level of the true vocal cords. In such cases, the airway is entered through a vertical incision in the cricothyroid membrane. If the stenosis is present at the cricothyroid membrane level, the surgeon must enter the airway by splitting the trachea in the anterior midline above the level of the existing tracheotomy. This incision is carried superiorly through the cricoid arch and cricothyroid membrane before completing the laryngofissure.

A very narrow area of stenosis, such as a subglottic web (Fig. 16–3), is removed with ring punches or sharp dissection, leaving only a narrow mucosal defect (Fig. 16–3B). A very narrow mucosal defect does not require stenting. However, this is usually not the case, and it is best to insert a Montgomery laryngeal stent (Fig. 16–3C) to prevent reformation of the web before the mucous membrane has bridged the defect gap. The stent is inserted into the larynx so that its ventricular projections fit into the laryngeal ventricles. If a graft is needed, it is preferable to apply the graft to the patient rather than to the stent. Buccal mucous membrane or split thickness skin graft can be attached to the subglottic region using 5-0 Vicryl suture material. If the web is low in the subglottic area, a Montgomery Safe-T-Tube (Chapter 10) can be used for stenting (see Fig. 9–36C). The T-tube will not interfere with vocal function and will provide the patient with a normal airway while healing takes place. The stent or T-tube should remain in place for 2 to 4 weeks.

Occasionally, a subglottic stenosis will result from the formation of dense fibrous tissue between the mucous membrane and the perichondrium of the cricoid cartilage. After a laryngocricotracheal fissure is performed, the mucous membrane is carefully elevated on each side of the subglottic region, beginning inferiorly. The fibrous tissue is resected to the level of the cricoid perichondrium. The mucosal flaps are replaced and sutured in place with No. 5-0 or 6-0 Vicryl suture material. It is most often necessary to use a laryngeal stent after this type of repair, unless the stenosis is low in the subglottic region and a Safe-T-Tube will secure the mucosal flaps against the cricoid perichondrium. This repair should be stented for at least 2 weeks with a laryngeal stent or T-tube, and usually not longer than 4 weeks, depending on the severity of the stenosis.

A severe circumferential subglottic stenosis in which the mucous membrane has been replaced by a fibrous tissue must be treated aggressively. All fibrous tissue is resected to the level of the cricoid perichondrium (Fig. 16–4). If, after accomplishing this, the subglottic lumen appears ample, the cricoid perichondrium may be resurfaced using buccal mucous membrane or nasal septal mucosa (Fig. 16–5) using 5-0 or 6-0 Vicryl suture material. The graft can be attached to either the stent (Fig. 16–5B and C) or the subglottic tissue. The author prefers the latter. The stent should remain in place for approximately 4 weeks (see Fig. 16–4).

Occasionally, a severe subglottic stenosis will extend to the level of the vocal cords. In such cases, the stenotic tissue must be resected over the conus elasticus on each side, as well as from the perichondrium over the cricoid cartilage. The mucosal grafts are secured in place with 5-0 or 6-0

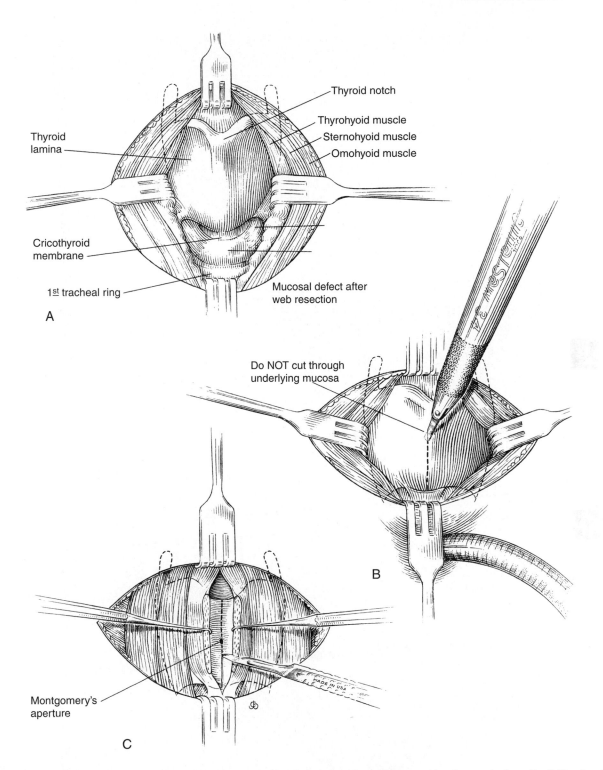

FIGURE 16-2. *A,* The thyroid laminae, cricoid, and first and second tracheal rings are exposed by retracting the muscles laterally. *B,* The thyroid lamina is incised in the vertical midline with a surgical blade or an electric oscillating saw (Stryker "sagittal 34" with frontal sinus saw blade). *C,* The two thyroid laminae are separated with hooks, exposing the underlying soft tissue. A midline incision is made, increasing the depth until a small aperture is encountered. This almost invariably represents a point just below the anterior commissure.

Vicryl suture material. Often this repair cannot be properly stented with a laryngeal stent or a regular Safe-T-Tube. In such cases, we have found an extra-long Safe-T-Tube to be valuable (Fig. 16–6). If aspiration is a problem, a Hebeler Safe-T-Tube, with integral internal balloon, can be used

(Fig. 16–7). Again, the tube should be placed so that the upper end projects through the glottis to the level of the laryngeal ventricles. This is ideal because proper stenting will be accomplished, and there is usually not a problem with aspiration. If the T-tube projects up above the ventricle or

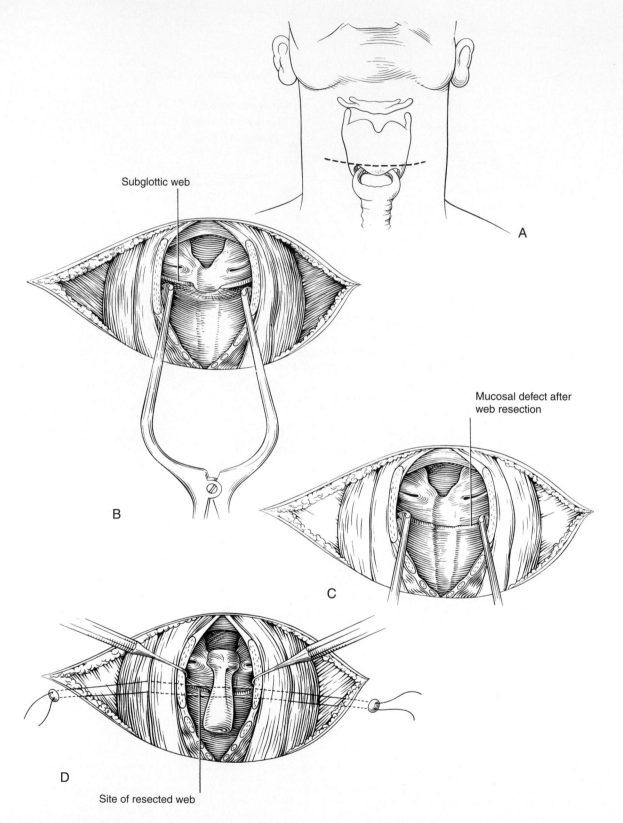

Subglottic web

Mucosal defect after web resection

Site of resected web

FIGURE 16–3. *A,* A horizontal incision is made at the lower edge of the thyroid lamina—a vertical incision can also be used. *B,* The larynx and subglottic trachea are exposed. A narrow web is shown. *C,* The narrow web has been resected, leaving a narrow, linear, horizontal mucosal defect. No grafting is necessary. *D,* The conforming silicone stent is secured in place by sutures placed through the thyroid laminae, under the sternohyoid muscles, and externally through the skin. The sutures are tied over silicone buttons on each side of the neck.

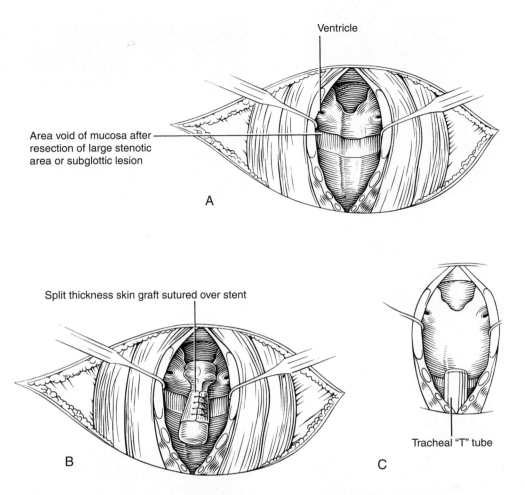

Ventricle

Area void of mucosa after resection of large stenotic area or subglottic lesion

A

Split thickness skin graft sutured over stent

B

Tracheal "T" tube

C

FIGURE 16–4. *A,* A more extensive subglottic stenosis than that shown in Fig. 9–35*C* has been resected, leaving a larger area devoid of mucous membrane. Either a skin or mucous membrane graft is necessary. *B,* The mucous membrane graft has been sutured to the laryngeal stent. The authors prefer that the mucosal graft be sutured to the patient rather than the stent. *C,* The Safe-T-Tube is used for stenting after repair of a stenosis in the low subglottic region. This allows the patient to enjoy normal respiration and phonation immediately after the operation. The upper end of the Safe-T-Tube can be shortened so that it remains 1 cm below the level of the vocal cords. If the stenosis is high and the Safe-T-Tube is used, the upper end should extend just above the vocal cords, at the level of the laryngeal ventricles.

ventricular bands, then aspiration can be a problem. The T-tube should remain in place for 4 weeks and then removed under general anesthesia, and the patient's subglottic region should be evaluated. If the subglottic appears to be adequately reconstructed, the T-tube is replaced with a silicone tracheal cannula or a regular tracheotomy tube for an additional week or two as a trial.

A severe subglottic stenosis may be caused by a structural alteration of the cricoid cartilage (Fig. 16–8). We suspect that this is caused either by internal trauma to the subglottic region that has been complicated by secondary infection or external blunt trauma to the cricoid arch. The structural defect is often not detected until after a number of repairs have failed. If mucous membrane is present, an excellent way to repair this severe defect is by incising the posterior cricoid lamina in the midline posteriorly and widening the posterior cricoid lamina with a cartilage graft. To accomplish this, the subglottic region is exposed with a laryngocricoid tracheal fissure. The vertical dimension of the posterior cricoid lamina is palpated. An incision is made through the mucous membrane in a vertical midline from

the interarytenoid muscle to the inferior aspect of the posterior cricoid lamina (Fig. 16–9*A*). The posterior thyroid lamina can usually be incised with a surgical blade. An oscillating saw is used when ossification has occurred. The halves of the posterior cricoid lamina are separated by expanding with a hemostat. This exposes the postcricoid cervical esophagus (Fig. 16–9*B*). Retraction of the thyroid laminae (laryngofissure) is relaxed so that a full-thickness segment of thyroid lamina can be obtained. The thyroid cartilage graft should include both the inner and outer perichondrium. A very large graft (enough to widen both the anterior and posterior cricoid) can be taken from both thyroid laminae without damage to the support structures (Fig. 16–9*C*).

The grafts are secured in place by passing a No. 3-0 Vicryl suture through the mucous membrane, the cricoid lamina, and again through the mucous membrane (Fig. 16–10*A*). A piece of muscle fascia is obtained to cover margins of the posterior cricoid lamina (Fig. 16–10*B*). The fascia graft is tucked underneath the cartilage grafts superiorly and inferiorly and secured in place with No. 3-0 Vicryl su-

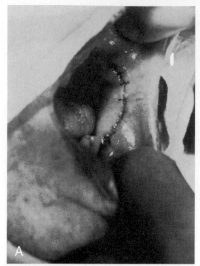

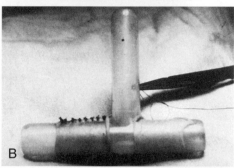

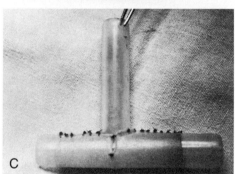

FIGURE 16-5. *A,* A photograph of the repair after resection of a large buccal mucosal graft. The incisions should avoid the parotid duct pupilla and orifice. A 2- × 4-cm mucous membrane graft can be obtained from the nasal septum. There is very little shrinkage with this graft because of its dense submucosal fibrous layer. *B,* Grafting material (refer to text), preferably mucous membrane, is fashioned so that it may be sutured to the silicone laryngeal stent or directly to the patient. *C,* The graft has been sutured to the silicone stent with no. 4-0 chromic catgut material. The sutures are applied directly to the silicone stent so that the graft is not inadvertently displaced as the stent is inserted into the larynx. Again, the authors prefer suturing the graft directly to the patient rather than to the stent.

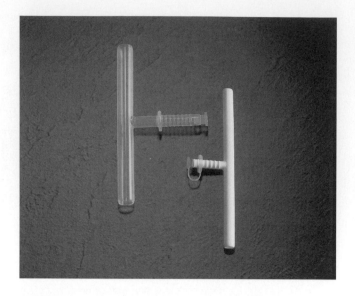

FIGURE 16-6. The Montgomery Extra-Long Safe-T-Tube.

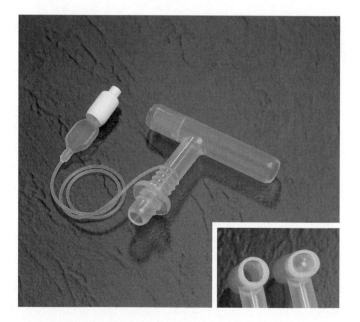

FIGURE 16-7. The Hebeler Safe-T-Tube. *Inset:* Integral internal balloon shown deflated and inflated.

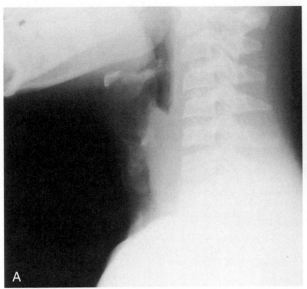

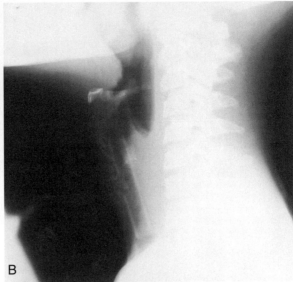

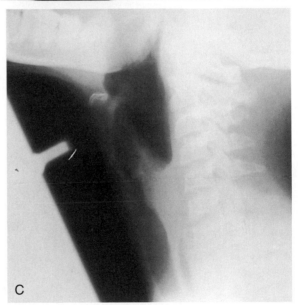

FIGURE 16-8. *A,* A lateral radiograph showing complete stenosis of the subglottis in a 13-year-old patient. *B,* The subglottic stenosis was repaired by widening the cricoid anteriorly and posteriorly and grafting with thyroid cartilage and buccal mucosa. A silicone Safe-T-Tube is inserted to a level just above the true vocal cords to support the repair. *C,* The Safe-T-Tube was removed in 4 weeks. A Montgomery Long-Term Cannula was inserted for 2 weeks and then removed. The patient's airway has remained adequate without a tracheotomy.

ture material (Fig. 16–10C). The entire posterior defect can then be covered with a buccal mucosal graft if the surgeon believes that it is necessary. A laryngeal stent or T-tube is inserted and secured in place.

For the past 14 years, we used two pins to secure one posterior cricoid cartilage graft in place. These two pins can be made by cutting a straight needle 4 mm wider than the graft. We use pins made from medical implant grade surgical stainless steel. They are 1 mm in diameter, sharpened at both ends, and then sand blasted to obtain roughness to hold them in place. We have used pins 8, 9, and 10 mm in length (Fig. 16–11).

An elliptical-shaped cartilage graft (Fig. 16–12) is obtained from the contralateral thyroid lamina. This is used to widen the anterior cricoid arch. The graft is secured in place with one nonabsorbable suture, such as No. 3-0 nylon suture material (Fig. 16–12). The remainder of the repair is accomplished with 3-0 Vicryl suture material. The operation is closed in layers, and a drain is placed to prevent subcutaneous emphysema.

When all other methods fail, a partial resection of the cricoid cartilage and upper trachea may be accomplished in an attempt to correct subglottic stenosis. The larynx, cricoid, and trachea are exposed as described above. A horizontal incision is made between the tracheal rings below the estimated lower limit of the stenosis. If the lumen at this level is not adequate, another horizontal incision is made at a lower level to find a normal and stable tracheal lumen. The cricothyroid membrane is incised in the anterior midline to inspect the subglottic region. The anterior thyroid laminae can be excised, from the immediate subglottic region anteriorly to the lower limits of the cricothyroid joints posteriorly. This resection can include the entire anterior cricoid arch and the posterior cricoid lamina up to the level of the cricothyroid joint. The dissection must be performed very carefully posteriorly because the recurrent laryngeal nerves are near the cricothyroid joint. A nerve stimulator is useful to identify the recurrent laryngeal nerves in the lateral tracheoesophageal grooves and as they pass behind the cricothyroid joints. If the tracheal

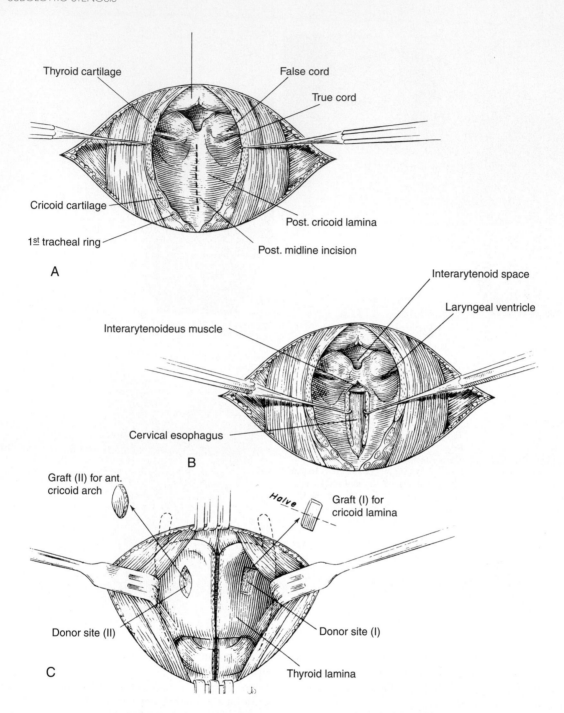

FIGURE 16–9. *A,* An incision is made through the mucous membrane in the vertical midline from the interarytenoideus muscle to the inferior aspect of the posterior cricoid lamina. *B,* The posterior lamina is then incised. This can usually be accomplished with a no. 10 surgical blade; however, if necessary, an oscillating saw is used. The halves of the posterior cricoid laminae are separated using hooks or a hemostat. *C,* Retraction of the thyroid laminae is relaxed so that a full-thickness segment of thyroid lamina can be obtained. The thyroid cartilage graft should include both inner and outer perichondrium. A very large graft can be taken from both thyroid laminae without damage to the support structures.

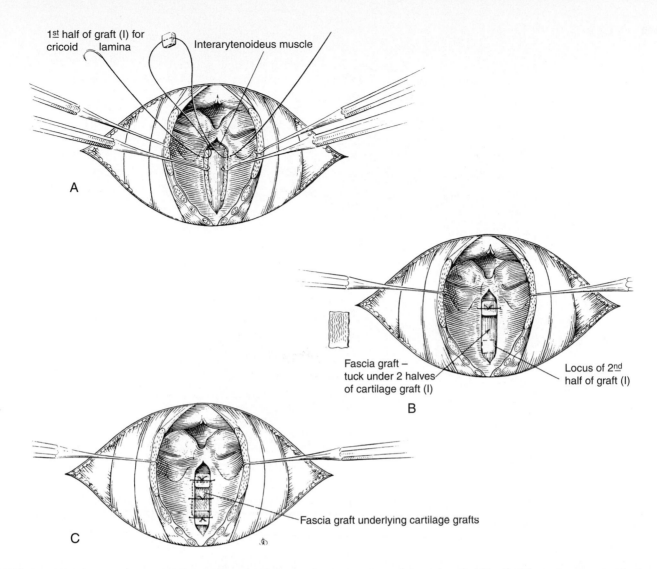

FIGURE 16-10. *A,* The thyroid lamina graft is then halved and placed to separate the halved posterior cricoid lamina. The grafts are secured in place by passing a No. 3-0 Vicryl suture through the mucous membrane, the cricoid lamina, cartilage graft, and finally, the contralateral cricoid lamina and mucous membrane. *B,* A piece of muscle fascia is obtained to cover the anterior wall of the postcricoid cervical esophagus and margins of the posterior cricoid lamina between the two grafts. *C,* The fascia graft is tucked underneath the cartilage grafts superiorly and inferiorly and secured in place with No. 3-0 Vicryl suture material.

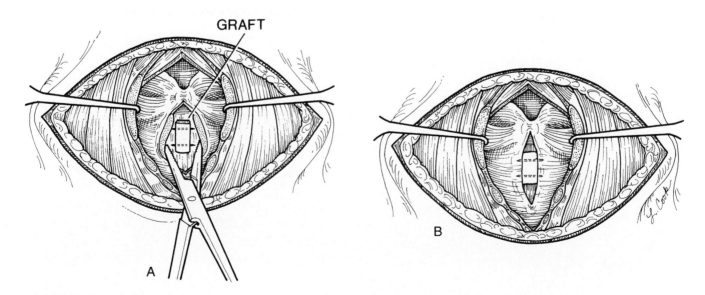

FIGURE 16-11. *A,* Two pins are inserted through the cartilage graft. A hemostat is used to separate the posterior cricoid laminae. *B,* The cartilage secured in place with two stainless steel pins.

379

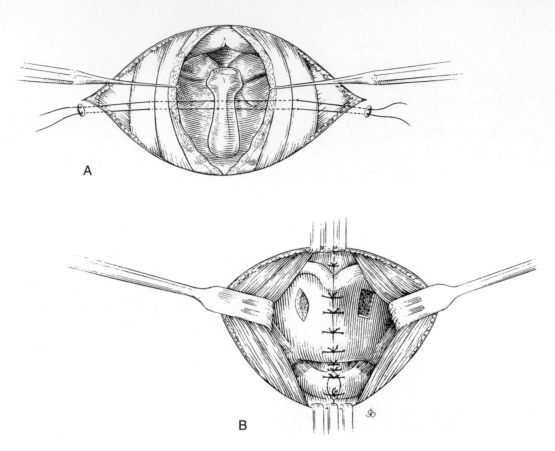

FIGURE 16–12. *A,* A Montgomery laryngeal stent is inserted and secured in place. *B,* An elliptical-shaped cartilage graft is obtained from the contralateral thyroid lamina. This is used to widen the anterior cricoid arch. The graft is secured in place with one nonabsorbable suture, such as No. 3-0 nylon. The remainder of the repair is accomplished with 3-0 Vicryl suture material.

mucous membrane is intact posteriorly, it should not be disturbed. The repair is accomplished by anastomosing the transected trachea to the transected subglottis. No. 3-0 Vicryl suture material is suitable for this repair. If the two ends cannot be brought together easily or if there is any tension on the suture line, a suprahyoid laryngeal release procedure is performed. Stenting is usually not required with this type of repair. The tracheotomy should remain in place for several weeks until it is certain that the stenosis will not recur.

Chapter 17
Obstructive Sleep Apnea and Snoring

JOHN B. LAZOR

OBSTRUCTIVE SLEEP APNEA

Overview and Epidemiology

Obstructive sleep apnea (OSA) is defined by the occurrence of episodic partial or complete obstruction of the upper airway during sleep. This may lead to the development of various mental or physical sequelae that characterize obstructive sleep apnea syndrome (OSAS). Accurate determination of the prevalence of OSA has been hindered by the lack of a consistent definition of the degree of nocturnal respiratory disturbance that constitutes OSA. The concepts of the apnea index (number of apneic events per hour), apnea/hypopnea index (AHI = number of apneas and hypopneas per hour), and respiratory disturbance index (RDI = number of respiratory disturbances per hour), have been developed in an attempt to quantify the level of respiratory disturbance of individuals subjected to diagnostic polysomnography. Although no consensus has been reached on this point, an AHI or RDI greater than 5 is generally viewed as abnormal in an adult population.

On this basis, OSAS has been shown to be the most common organically based cause of excessive daytime sleepiness with estimates ranging from 1% to 16% among adult men. Although in the past, many have viewed OSAS primarily as a disease found in men, recent investigation has demonstrated a prevalence from 1% to 5% among adult women.

Risk factors for the disease include male gender, obesity (particularly obesity of the upper body), age between 40 and 65 years, various craniofacial anomalies, the use of cigarettes or alcohol, poor physical fitness, certain endocrinopathies (especially hypothyroidism and acromegaly), and genetic predisposition to OSAS. The latter includes, among others, individuals with Down syndrome, Prader-Willi syndrome (a congenital syndrome involving mental retardation, sexual infantilism, polyphagia with obesity, and muscular hypotonia), and congenital craniofacial abnormalities such as Pierre Robin syndrome.

Obstructive sleep apnea syndrome is linked with a wide variety of physical disorders and mental deficits. The excessive daytime somnolence from OSAS may increase the risk of work-related and motor vehicle accidents. Particularly strong is the association between OSAS and cardiovascular disease. Whereas about half of the patients with OSA have hypertension, more than 25% of those with essential hypertension are believed to have OSAS. In addition, some form of cardiac arrhythmia can be detected in 48% to 75% of OSAS patients. An increase in adjusted risk for coronary heart disease and myocardial infarction among patients with OSA has been documented. Finally, an increased risk of cerebrovascular disease among those with OSAS has also been reported. It has been more difficult to estimate the mortality of OSAS since the use of various treatment modalities, including nasal continuous positive airway pressure (CPAP), tracheotomy, and multiple upper airway surgical procedures, has had a positive impact on survival. However, in a study of 385 patients, He and colleagues reported a significantly increased mortality among those with an apnea index greater than 20 as compared with OSAS patients with less severe disease (10.6 versus 2.1 among untreated patients). Evidence for the importance of treatment in altering the mortality associated with OSAS comes from the Stanford experience with this disease. Here, patients treated conservatively for OSAS were found to have an overall 5-year mortality of 11% as compared with 0% for a group that underwent tracheotomy despite the fact that the conservatively managed group had lower mean apnea indexes than the tracheotomized group (43 versus 69). After 11 years of follow-up, a statistically significant difference in survival favoring the tracheotomized group has been reported. Thus, there exists considerable evidence that untreated OSA is associated with increased mortality rates.

Anatomy

The aerodigestive tract is composed of both rigid and compliant structures. Abnormal anatomic and physiologic function of the structures from the nose to the larynx can result in suboptimal aerodigestive function and OSAS. Anatomic abnormalities at the nasal level may include obstruction secondary to turbinate hypertrophy, septal deviation, or mucosal edema. The nasopharynx may be compromised by adenoid tissue, benign or malignant masses, or scarring from surgical trauma. With nasal obstruction, there is a large inspiratory pressure decrease across the nose, leading to a high subatmospheric pressure at locations within the potentially collapsible pharynx.

The oropharynx extends from the plane of the hard and soft palate superiorly to the plane of the hyoid bone inferiorly and communicates with the nasopharynx above and the hypopharynx below. Hypertrophy or redundancy of the soft palate, uvula, anterior and posterior pillars, or palatine tonsils may result in obstruction at the oropharynx level. In addition, macroglossia, retrognathia, and obesity contribute to obstruction at the oropharyngeal level. Palatal motion is mediated through contraction of the levator veli palatini and tensor veli palatini muscles. The palatopharyngeus and palatoglossus muscles activate phasically during the inspiratory portion of the breathing cycle, dilating the oropharynx. Also during inspiration, intraluminal pressure is negative (subatmospheric) and tends to produce pharyngeal collapse. Assuming constant flow, narrow airways would result in even more negative intraluminal pressure through forces related to Bernoulli's principle. This is opposed by the distending action of the pharyngeal muscles whose tone can decrease during sleep.

The hypopharynx extends from the level of the hyoid bone to the lower border of the cricoid cartilage and includes the pyriform sinuses, the post-cricoid area, and the posterior pharyngeal wall. Although infrequent, lesions or masses in the hypopharynx may cause obstruction at this level. Laryngeal abnormalities afflicting the supraglottic structures or the vocal folds may potentiate OSAS.

Cardiovascular Pathophysiology

As mentioned, OSAS is associated with multiple forms of cardiovascular disease. Although the pathophysiology explaining the causal relationship that may exist between OSA and various forms of cardiovascular disease has not yet been fully elucidated, many studies have begun to explore the possible etiologic link between OSA and hypertension, myocardial infarction, cerebrovascular disease, and various cardiac arrhythmias

Among patients with OSAS, a specific cyclic pattern of blood pressure elevation has been demonstrated. After initial decreases in blood pressure were noted early in an apneic event, steady increases in blood pressure began to occur during apneic episodes with a peak reached just after termination of the apnea; that is, during arousal from sleep. Shepard demonstrated a 25% increase in systolic and diastolic blood pressure associated with these apneic events. Also demonstrated was a correlation between the degree of oxyhemoglobin desaturation and the level of increase in blood pressure; how this might relate to sustained daytime hypertension among those with OSAS is unclear. Several possibilities have been explored, including a hypothesized role of excessive activity of the sympathetic nervous system among patients with OSAS. Although the data to date have been inconsistent, it appears that patients with OSAS do have sympathetic nervous system activity as reflected by elevated levels of norepinephrine or epinephrine, which could cause hypertension on the basis of vasoconstriction or increased cardiac output. The fact that nasal CPAP seems to lower catecholamine levels in some subjects serves as further evidence for this possible link.

Several other hypotheses regarding the relationship between OSAS and hypertension have been examined. The potential role of prostanoids in blood pressure elevation in OSAS patients has been studied with initial results that suggest a relative increase in the ratio of vasoconstricting to vasodilating prostanoids in untreated OSAS patients who improved with nasal CPAP therapy. The association of OSA and hypertension has been hypothesized to contribute to abnormal renal function. Nephrotic syndrome, proteinuria, and increased urinary sodium excretion in patients with OSAS have been reported by various authors. In addition, it is believed that increased urinary sodium levels are linked to elevations in blood pressure. Baruzzi demonstrated elevated urine sodium levels in a study of patients with OSAS. Exactly how OSAS might cause renal impairment is unclear.

Support for a causal link between OSAS and hypertension comes from a recent report that demonstrated that systolic, diastolic, and mean arterial blood pressures were significantly related to the AHI. Noteworthy is the fact that the body mass index did not contribute to this apparent causal association.

Regarding myocardial ischemia, it has been reported that an apnea index of greater than 5.3 is predictive of myocardial infarction. Although possibly a nonspecific finding, ST segment depressions on electrocardiographic examination, which are generally suggestive of decreased cardiac blood flow, have recently been reported in association with OSA. This lends further support for the hypothesized link between respiratory disturbance during sleep and an increased risk of myocardial infarction. The oxygen demand during an apneic event is increased due to increases in preload (as evidenced by increased venous return) and afterload (as evidenced by elevated transmyocardial pressure) on the basis of negative intrathoracic pressure. This occurs at a time when the patient is relatively hypoxemic due to the disrupted breathing involved with an apneic event. This disruption of the normal balance of myocardial oxygen supply and demand could lead to ischemia and infarction.

The mechanism by which OSA may contribute to the development of cerebrovascular accidents is unknown. Although some have suggested that the loss of autoregulation of cerebral blood flow may be important in OSA patients, recent studies have not supported this hypothesis.

Another theory involves an elevated hematocrit, which can be seen in patients with OSA. This increased blood viscosity could, in turn, predispose the patient to a cerebrovascular accident. Others have hypothesized that increases in intracranial pressure could be an important factor in causing cerebrovascular accidents in patients with OSAS. Cyclic increases in intracranial pressure have been documented in association with elevation in blood pressure, and, as noted previously, apneic episodes are known to increase systemic blood pressure. Additional studies are needed to test these various hypotheses.

Multiple cardiac arrhythmias including sinoatrial block, atrial and ventricular ectopy, second-degree atrioventricular block, and ventricular tachycardia are very common in patients with OSAS. The most common arrhythmia in this group is a sinus bradytachyarrhythmia. Heart rate slows during an apneic episode because of increased vagal output. As the apnea terminates with arousal, elevated sympathetic nervous system activity and decreased parasympathetic activity cause a rapid heart rate. In addition to altered autonomic nervous system activity, hypoxemia is also believed to play a role in the development of certain cardiac arrhythmias, including an increased incidence of ventricular ectopy in patients with OSAS. Again, however, although the association between OSAS and cardiac arrhythmias is strong, the possible etiologic mechanism is unproved.

Obstructive sleep apnea often involves hypoxemia leading to pulmonary hypertension and strain on the right side of the heart. Thus, the respiratory acidosis–based pulmonary vasoconstriction, the systemic hypertension related to apneas, and the cardiac arrhythmias may all contribute to the poor ejection fractions sometimes noted in patients with OSAS. The significant improvement in right-sided ejection fraction among the subjects of a recent study examining OSAS patients after uvulopalatopharyngoplasty (UPPP) once again underscores the potential importance of OSA in contributing to cardiovascular derangements in this patient population.

Pediatric Obstructive Sleep Apnea

Obstructive sleep apnea is also common among children. However, although some aspects of the disorder are similar to those of adult OSAS, there are features of pediatric sleep apnea in terms of presentation and subsequent treatment that are unique to this group. In addition, diagnostic criteria for OSA have not yet been established for pediatric patients. Recent evidence suggests that the pathophysiology of OSA in children is sufficiently different from that of adults and that the commonly used AHI is inappropriate as a diagnostic tool in children. Noteworthy in the presentation of pediatric OSAS is the very common finding of other concurrent disorders or anatomic defects. That is, a large percentage of pediatric OSAS patients have significant craniofacial deformities often on the basis of various syndromic conditions. Furthermore, conditions including Down syndrome and Prader-Willi syndrome also predispose children to OSA in part because of neuromuscular deficits frequently found in some children with these syndromes. Neuromuscular disorders are fairly common among children with OSAS. This is believed to contribute to the development of disordered breathing during sleep caused by excessive pharyngeal hypotonia. Interestingly, contrary to the well-known Pickwickian stereotype, a smaller percentage of children with OSAS are obese as compared with the very high prevalence of obesity in adults with sleep apnea. In fact, many children with OSAS are underweight because of failure to thrive or other underlying illnesses. Finally, adenotonsillar size can be an important cause of narrowing of the upper airway due to the relatively small pharyngeal size in children.

Whereas the symptoms of OSA in adults are well described, children with OSA may manifest symptoms of irritability, learning disabilities, and hyperactive behavior. Also commonly noted are snoring and nocturnal enuresis. Eventually, cardiovascular sequelae including polycythemia, systemic hypertension, and cor pulmonale are possible.

Regarding diagnosis, particular attention must be made to exclusion of central apnea in children. The current gold standard for evaluation of apnea continues to be polysomnography. However, as previously mentioned, diagnostic criteria have only been established for the adult population, and there is reason to believe that these criteria may miss the diagnosis in many cases of pediatric OSAS. Rosen and coworkers reported that the majority of children with disordered sleep and significant oxyhemoglobin desaturation did not actually have complete obstructive events. Rather, the children believed to have OSAS experienced a pattern of "continuous partial obstructive hypoventilation with cyclic decreases in oxyhemoglobin saturation, hypercarbia, labored paradoxical respiratory efforts, and snoring." This is clearly a different pattern than the intermittent complete obstruction often detected in adults with OSAS, and it suggests the need for further elaboration of the pathophysiology of pediatric OSAS. It would seem that further study is required to definitively determine appropriate parameters for polysomnographic diagnosis of OSA in children.

Beyond polysomnography, additional tests including airway imaging techniques, electrocardiography, echocardiography, chest radiographs, a complete blood count, and blood gas analysis may also be helpful both for diagnostic purposes and to assess the severity of disease. Finally, a family history of OSAS and snoring may be a useful diagnostic clue because OSA is believed to cluster in some families.

Although the treatment of OSAS in general is discussed elsewhere, it is important to note that many cases of childhood OSAS are successfully treated with adenotonsillectomy—a procedure that is rarely useful on its own in adults with OSA. This underscores the fact that some cases of pediatric OSAS are greatly influenced by the relatively small pharyngeal size in children.

Diagnosis

There have been numerous methods, techniques, and studies used to diagnose OSAS. The precise etiology remains uncertain, but OSAS is presumed to be caused by anatomic abnormalities, neuromuscular disturbances, or a combination of both. The oldest and most common method used to diagnose OSA is the history and physical examination. This has recently been supplemented by the use of flexible nasopharyngoscopy with or without the Müller maneuver to localize the level of obstruction. The Müller maneuver reportedly replicates obstructive events occurring during sleep. It involves introducing the fiberoptic nasopharyngoscope through the nasal cavity into the pharynx while the patient is sitting and supine. The tip of the scope is positioned at the lower oropharynx so the entire hypopharynx can be visualized. The patient is then instructed to close his mouth and vigorously inhale while the examiner occludes the nares. The degree of hypopharynx collapse is recorded as a percent of the entire hypopharyngeal cross-sectional area. The scope is then repositioned just cephalad and posterior to the free edge of the soft palate in the nasopharynx and again repeated and recorded. The literature reports the Müller maneuver to be between 33% and 87% accurate in predicting a good outcome (>50% reduction in AHI) from UPPP.

The initial history should focus on features supporting the presence of apnea and features suggesting the cause of

Chapter 18
Surgery of the Thyroid and Parathyroid Glands

GREGORY W. RANDOLPH

HISTORY

"The extirpation of the thyroid gland for goiter typifies better, perhaps better than any other operation, the supreme triumph of the surgeon's art." Halsted, 1920

Many misconceptions have punctuated our evolving understanding of thyroid and parathyroid function. Galen initially regarded the thyroid gland as a blood buffer to protect the brain from sudden increases in blood flow. Initially Graves' disease was interpreted as a cardiac illness, hypothyroidism as a neurologic and dermatologic disorder, and hyperparathyroidism as a bone disease. Early in the study of hyperparathyroidism, parathyroid gland enlargement was believed to be secondary to the underlying bone disease. In fact, in 1925, the European surgeon Mandel (the first to extract a parathyroid tumor in a patient with hyperparathyroidism) performed this procedure after his initial parathyroid tissue grafting procedure did not work. Even the relationship between postoperative cretinism and thyroidectomy in the pediatric patient was poorly understood initially. The Prussian otolaryngologist Felix Semon first suggested similarities between English myxedema patients and Swiss patients who had undergone thyroidectomy. In 1858, Billroth published his first series of 20 thyroidectomies, noting a 40% mortality rate. It was Theodore Kocher, whose meticulous technique during thyroidectomy allowed for the proliferation of thyroidectomy that, in turn, formed the foundation of the clinics of Lahey, Crile, and the Mayo brothers.

ANATOMY

The thyroid and parathyroid glands are endocrine glands located in the neck base. The normal adult thyroid gland weighs between 15 to 25 g and is composed of the two lateral nerves connected in the midline by an isthmus. The isthmus is attached to the trachea at the second to fourth tracheal rings by an anterior tracheal ligament, which is easily dissected. Laterally the thyroid lobes relate to the carotid sheath. Posteriorly the thyroid lobes relate to the paravertebral fascia and medially to the upper trachea and larynx. Ventrally, the thyroid is covered by the infrahyoid strap musculature. The main strap muscles of surgical consequence during thyroidectomy are the more medially placed sternohyoid and the somewhat more laterally placed sternothyroid. The thyroid is predominantly attached to the laryngotracheal complex by the posterolateral suspensory ligaments also known as the ligament of Berry. It is primarily the ligament of Berry that tethers the thyroid to the laryngotracheal complex, resulting in elevation of both with deglutition. Surrounding nodes in the central and lateral neck lack this synchronous movement. Each thyroid lobe is approximately 4 cm high, 1.5 cm wide, and 2 cm deep, although the exact size varies with patient size, sex, and functional status. The thyroid is associated with a rich intraglandular lymphatic network, which provides for intraglandular spread of papillary carcinoma. The central neck thyroid associated nodal groups include prelaryngeal (Delphian), pretracheal, paratracheal (recurrent laryngeal nerve chain), superior mediastinal, omohyoid associated, and internal jugular. In approximately one third of patients, the isthmus or the medial aspect of the left or right lobe forms a pyramidal lobe, which extends superiorly and represents a rudimentary thyroglossal duct cyst track remnant.

Berry's ligament can be considered as a condensation of the true thyroid capsule. There can be a varying amount of thyroid tissue infiltrating into the substance of the ligament. The greater the extent to which this occurs, the more the recurrent laryngeal nerve, as it passes under or through the ligament, will be brought into contact with thyroid tissue. The ligament of Berry is dense and well vascularized and derives its own separate branch from the inferior thyroid artery. This is the region of greatest difficulty in dissection of the recurrent laryngeal nerve. In 1935, Berlin reviewed the relationship between the recurrent laryngeal nerve, adjacent thyroid tissue, and ligament of Berry, with cadaver and surgical dissections. He found that in 30% of cases the recurrent laryngeal nerve traveled through the substance of the ligament of Berry, and in 10% of cases the recurrent laryngeal nerve actually penetrated thyroid gland parenchyma within the ligament of Berry. It is this set of anatomic concerns that prohibits capsular dissection as a method of preventing recurrent laryngeal injury.

The strap muscles, when elevated off the ventral surface of the thyroid, reveal loose areolar tissue, described as the perithyroid sheath. This interval can be associated with small bridging veins that can be easily cauterized. The inferior thyroid artery is a branch of the thyrocervical trunk and extends into the thyroidectomy field from the undersurface of the carotid artery. It extends medially with a small downward arching profile to ramify the thyroid lobe at the mid-lobar level. The inferior thyroid artery provides blood supply for the inferior parathyroid. The blood supply of the superior parathyroid is also frequently from the inferior thyroid artery. However, in approximately 40% to 50% of cases, the superior parathyroid is vascularized at least in part by the superior thyroid artery's posterior branch (Fig. 18–1). The thyroid ima artery is a separate midline inferior artery, which is present in 1.5% to 12% of cases and may arise from the innominate, carotid, or aortic arch directly. The superior thyroid vein travels with the superior thyroid artery and extends from the jugular to the thyroid superior pole. The middle thyroid vein travels without arterial complement and extends from the jugular vein to the mid-lobar level. The middle thyroid vein needs to be ligated to provide adequate lateral thyroid lobe exposure during thyroidectomy. The inferior thy-

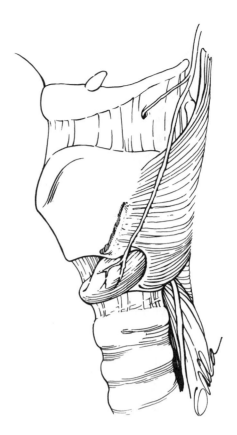

FIGURE 18-2. Side view of the larynx depicting the distal course of the recurrent laryngeal nerve in the tracheoesophageal groove. This nerve exits the thyroidectomy field by extending underneath the lowest edge of the inferior constrictor muscle. The external branch of the superior laryngeal nerve, also identified, and the superior polar region exposure are improved with sectioning of the superior portion of the sternothyroid muscle. (From Lee KJ, ed: Essential Otolaryngology, ed. 7. New York, McGraw-Hill, 1999; with permission.)

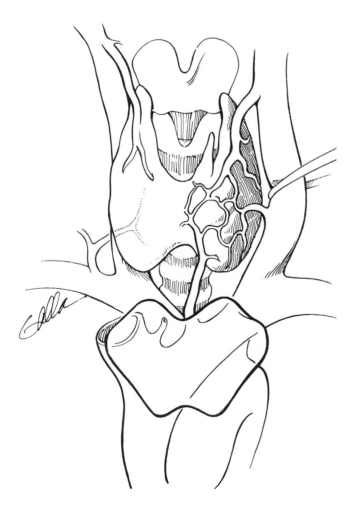

FIGURE 18-1. Right perithyroidal region depicts the arterial supply of the thyroid. On the left, the superior, middle, and inferior thyroid veins are shown. (From Lee KJ, ed: Essential Otolaryngology, ed. 7. New York, McGraw-Hill, 1999; with permission.)

roid veins also travel without arterial complement, arising from the internal jugular or brachiocephalic vein. These inferior veins can form an inferior venous plexus, termed the plexus thyroideus impar.

Both the external branch of the superior laryngeal nerve (SLN) and the recurrent laryngeal nerve (RLN) are at risk during thyroidectomy (Fig. 18–2). The SLN's internal branch brings general visceral afferents to the lower pharynx, supraglottic larynx and base of tongue, as well as special visceral afferents to epiglottic taste buds. The SLN's external branch brings branchial efferents to the cricothyroid muscle and inferior constrictor. The RLN contains branchial efferents to the inferior constrictor and all laryngeal intrinsics, except the cricothyroid muscle, as well as general visceral afferents from the larynx (vocal cords and below), upper esophagus, and trachea. These vagal branches also convey parasympathetics to the lower pharynx, larynx, trachea, and upper esophagus.

The right recurrent laryngeal nerve arises from the vagus as it crosses over the right subclavian and extends underneath the right subclavian, back up into the right thoracic and right thoracic inlet (Fig. 18–3). It extends at the level of the tracheoesophageal groove upward toward its laryngeal entry point. Owing to its more lateral entrance in the right thoracic inlet (compared with the left), it follows a secondary to changed neck positions or in recumbency. Some patients may have been erroneously diagnosed with asthma or obstructive sleep apnea. Melliere has shown that respiratory distress may occur acutely even in the setting of a chronic stabile goiter. The physical examination of such patients should focus on evaluation of respiratory status, identification of any laryngeal or tracheal deviation, or substernal extension. Pemberton's sign should be evaluated. A positive Pemberton's sign is the development of subjective respiratory discomfort or venous engorgement in the head and neck as a result of placing the arms above the head, which results in thoracic inlet obstruction in the setting of a large or substernal goiter. Patients with goiter should also have vocal cord mobility assessed. Thyroid hormone suppression is generally not effective for large goiters or multinodular goiters. Suppression is not possible if the patient's TSH is less than 1 mU/L. Aggressive thyroid hormone suppression is not possible in the elderly age group secondary to atrial arrhythmias. The reduction in size of a goiter in response to thyroxin suppression is unpredictable. Goiter size increase tends to recur once suppression is stopped. Surgery should be considered for all substernal goiters as the substernal component is unavailable for clinical monitoring through the physical examination or fine needle aspiration and may acutely enlarge secondary to hemorrhage within nodules of the substernal component.

Radionuclide scanning has been used in the past in the work-up of the thyroid nodule with the thought that if a nodule is cold it has lost differentiated function and may therefore represent a malignancy. However, almost 95% of all nodules when scanned are cold. It is true that the malignant nodules are cold, but the group of cold nodules is so large that the test is not helpful in identifying which nodules require surgery. It is true that nodules that are hot are infrequently malignant. Such testing, therefore, adds little in the work-up of a thyroid nodule and is not currently recommended.

Thyroid sonography can be very useful in the work-up of a thyroid nodule. Like radionuclide scanning, it does not provide information as to whether the nodule is malignant or benign, but it can provide accurate baseline information in terms of nodule measurement and may find contralateral nodules and surrounding lymphadenopathy. It is important to understand that the finding of cystic change within a nodule is not necessarily a sign that the nodule is benign. Sonography, although showing the intrathyroidal architecture with high resolution, does not provide adequate information regarding the relationship of the thyroid to the surrounding cervical viscera (trachea and esophagus) and does not provide clear information on the portion of the mass that extends substernally. These issues are best addressed with axial CT or MRI scanning. Sonography provides a clear-cut baseline before fine needle aspiration, suppression, or surgery to which the clinician will often refer. Sonography is also helpful to confirm the clinician's clinical examination.

Fine Needle Aspiration

Fine needle aspiration represents the central diagnostic test in the work-up of the thyroid nodule. It has decreased the number of patients operated on and increased the yield of carcinoma in surgical specimens. Fine needle aspiration accuracy relates to both the skill of the aspirator and the cytopathologist. During fine needle aspiration, significant time is taken in palpation and in stabilization of the nodule on adjacent structures or by tenting the nodule into a stable position relative to the skin. Fine needle aspiration is often performed with a 22- or 25-gauge 1.5-inch needle. A 10-mL syringe, with or without syringe holder, is used. The needle is inserted through the skin without suction applied. Once the needle tip is within the nodule, approximately 1 mL of suction is applied and the needle is oscillated within the nodule 10 to 20 times. This maneuver allows the passage of cellular material into the shaft of the needle. If bleeding occurs such that the hub of the needle or syringe fills with blood, the pass should be considered unlikely to yield adequate cellular material and should be repeated. Generally, about 3 to 6 passes are made. Once the aspirate is complete, suction is released and the needle is withdrawn. Pressure is placed over the region that has been aspirated for several minutes. The needle is taken off of the syringe, the syringe is filled with air, and the needle is placed back on the syringe. Air is used to expel the needle shaft contents onto a slide, which is smeared and quickly placed into alcohol fixative. Usually two slides can be made from each needle sample. The author believes that it is important to rinse the needle with cytologic fixative. This cytologic fixative can then be centrifuged, and a cellular pellet can be smeared, providing additional information. Lidocaine can be injected into the skin before aspiration. However, small nodules may be obscured by the effect of the lidocaine on the overlying skin. If a cyst is encountered, the cyst should be completely evacuated and then needle aspirate should be performed in the region of the collapsed cyst wall. It is the cellular material from this wall that provides for cytopathologic diagnosis. There appears to be no significant risk of skin carcinoma implantation of carcinoma with fine needle aspiration. The risk of such skin implantation does exist with larger-gauge needle sampling techniques.

Fine Needle Aspiration Cytopathologic Categories

Fine needle aspiration cytopathologic categories include (1) malignant, (2) suspicious (also described as indeterminate), (3) benign, and (4) nondiagnostic. The cytopathologic diagnosis of malignancy is usually quite accurate, with false-positive rates of only 1%. Cytopathologists are generally focusing on nuclear details when rendering a malignant diagnosis. The diagnosis of papillary carcinoma and anaplastic carcinoma are generally accurately made because of the unique nuclear features of these malignancies. Medullary carcinoma is often diagnosed through initial recognition of malignant nuclear changes present, which are not consistent with papillary follicular or anaplastic carcinoma. The diagnosis of medullary carcinoma can be obtained through calcitonin immunohistochemical staining. Thyroid lymphoma may be initially suggested by fine needle aspiration, but often additional tissue through open biopsy is required to confirm the diagnosis and subtype of lymphoma. Isthmectomy with or without tracheotomy is sometimes appropriate to obtain tissue to definitively diagnose thyroid lymphoma. The main difficulty in the diagnosis of malignancy with fine needle aspiration is in the differentiation of follicular adenoma from follicular carcinoma. This diagnosis hinges on a histologic finding of vascular invasion in pericapsular blood vessels. Fine needle aspiration then can only grade follicular lesions as to the degree of cellularity, presence of colloid, and degree of nuclear atypia. When a follicular lesion on fine needle aspiration is found to have large follicular profiles (macrofollicular arrays) and plentiful colloid with follicular cells arranged in sheets, it is believed to be a benign follicular lesion and is described as a macrofollicular lesion or colloid adenomatous nodule. When a follicular lesion aspirate shows small follicular profiles (microfollicular arrays) with a hypercellular aspirate and scant colloid, the lesion is described as a microfollicular aspirate. The risk of follicular carcinoma with such a follicular lesion ranges from 5% to 15% and increases with the nodule size. Fine needle aspirations that are quite hypercellular can also be described as embryonal, fetal, or trabecular and are also judged as suspicious follicular lesions with an underlying risk of follicular carcinoma. Hurthle cells are oxyphilic follicular cells with plentiful mitochondria. Hurthle cells may be present in a variety of different conditions, including multinodular goiter, Hashimoto's thyroiditis, Hurthle cell benign adenoma as well as Hurthle cell carcinoma. The Hurthle cell should be regarded as simply a variant of a follicular cell. The differentiation between benign Hurthle cell adenoma and Hurthle cell carcinoma is made by the same criteria used to differentiate follicular adenoma from follicular carcinoma; that is, by pericapsular vascular invasion. Thus, fine needle aspirations showing Hurthle cell predominance are read as Hurthle cell neoplasm, rule out Hurthle cell carcinoma, and are placed in the suspicious category.

False-positive aspirates (lesions that are benign but read as suspicious or malignant on fine needle aspiration) usually occur in the context of glands affected by Hashimoto's thyroiditis, Graves' disease or toxic nodules. These benign entities can often be diagnosed by checking TSH before fine needle aspiration. These disorders can result on fine needle aspiration in microfollicular arrays, lymphocytes, Hurthle cells, and cells with unusual nuclear features. Such nuclear features can be confused with those of papillary carcinoma.

For needle aspirates that are read as definitively benign, false-negative rates range from 1% to 6%. False-negatives primarily related to sampling errors occur with greater frequency with lesions smaller than 1 cm or greater than 3 cm. Because of this, it is reasonable to consider fine needle aspiration as a modality, which accurately diagnoses nodules within the size range of 1 to 3 cm. Beyond this size range, fine needle aspiration of thyroid lesions becomes less accurate. Because of the potential for false-negatives, when a patient is counseled regarding options in management of a thyroid lesion that is judged benign on fine needle aspiration, surgery should always be included as one possible management option. For patients with benign needle aspirates, treatment options should include (1) providing the patient with follow-up with repetitive examinations and sonograms in consideration for repeat aspiration; (2) suppressive therapy; and (3) surgery. Because errors may occur with fine needle aspiration, surgery should always be included in the list of options offered. This is especially true for nodules outside the 1- to 3-cm range in which fine needle aspiration is most accurate.

Nondiagnostic aspirates occur in about 15% of cases. Approximately 3% of these are ultimately diagnosed as malignant. If repeat aspiration is done, it is wise to consider sonogram guidance. Approximately 50% of cases, which are offered repeat aspiration, a cytologic diagnosis can ultimately be rendered.

For patients whose needle aspirations are described as suspicious or malignant, surgery is recommended, and this is typically hemithyroidectomy with frozen section with bilateral surgery if frozen section confirms malignancy. For patients with nondiagnostic fine needle aspirations, repeat aspiration is recommended. For those patients with multiple nondiagnostic aspirates, surgery can be offered.

Thyroid Hormone Suppression

Thyroid hormone has been shown to decrease the size of goiterous enlargement of the thyroid. Thyroid hormone suppressive therapy has been offered to control thyroid nodule growth. Control of thyroid nodule growth through suppressive therapy suggests it has an underlying benign nature, implying hormonal responsiveness. However, it is understood that thyroid malignancies contain TSH receptors and are controlled by suppressive therapy. This responsiveness to suppressive therapy is therefore certainly not specific before benign disease. Emerick showed that over 10% of patients who are ultimately diagnosed with follicular carcinoma had initially shown a decrease in size of the lesion on preoperative suppressive trials. It has also been found that growth on suppressive therapy is certainly not specific for malignancy; Rojeski found that only approximately 30% of nodules growing on suppressive therapy were malignant. Mazzaferri has noted that there are no randomized control trials that definitively show thyroid hormone suppression superior to placebo in the treatment of solitary colloid nodules. Suppressive therapy is associated with promotion of osteoporosis and the development of atrial arrhythmias in the elderly. Suppressive therapy also has no clear-cut, universally accepted criteria regarding duration, magnitude of TSH suppression, or success criteria. Suppressive therapy is generally avoided if TSH is less than 1 mU/L.

MANAGEMENT OF THE THYROID CYST

Almost one quarter of all thyroid nodules represent cysts. Cysts may be benign or malignant. Cyst formation may occur through accumulation of colloid or through hemorrhage within a solid nodule. Small cysts occasionally may be controlled through aspiration and post-aspiration suppressive therapy. Cysts that are greater than 3 to 4 cm in size generally recur after aspiration. Hemorrhagic cystic fluid and recurrence of cystic formation after initially successful aspiration raise the specter of malignancy. Such cysts, and in general cysts greater than 3 to 4cm in size, should be resected.

THYROID CANCER

There are approximately 14,000 new cases of thyroid carcinoma and just over 1,000 deaths from thyroid carcinoma each year. Papillary and follicular carcinomas with certain common features and overall favorable prognosis, yet distinct histologic and clinical characteristics, account for 30% of thyroid carcinoma. Medullary carcinoma of the thyroid derives from para-follicular C-cell (unlike papillary follicular, which derives from the follicular thyroid cell) and accounts for 5% of thyroid cancers. Anaplastic carcinoma, an undifferentiated carcinoma arising from follicular cellular elements with grave prognosis, and thyroid lymphoma, which is typically B-cell type and arises in the setting of autoimmune thyroiditis, account for the remaining cases of thyroid malignancy. Papillary carcinoma is characterized histologically by papillae formation consisting of neoplastic epithelium overlying a true fibrovascular stalk, unique nuclear features, and, in approximately 40% of cases, psammoma bodies, which represent laminated calcific densities believed to be the residua of necrotic calcified neoplastic cells. There are histologic variants of papillar carcinoma that have worse prognosis such as insular and tall cell carcinoma. However, the common follicular variant of papillary carcinoma in which follicular histologic features rather than papillary predominate follows a course consistent with typical papillary carcinoma. It is interesting to note that there is no benign neoplastic counterpart for papillary carcinoma of the thyroid.

Papillary carcinoma primary and nodal metastases may be primarily cystic. Papillary carcinoma is strongly lymphotrophic and spreads early on within the thyroid gland and to regional nodal beds. Approximately 30% of patients with papillary carcinoma of the thyroid will have regional nodal involvement at presentation. Distant metastasis, which occurs infrequently at presentation, most commonly affects lung and bone. Papillary carcinoma occurs more frequently in women than in men, with peak incidence in the third and fourth decades. In children, regional and distant metastasis is more common than in adults. Although advanced disease presentation is common in children, the overall prognosis is nonetheless favorable.

Approximately 20% of patients who are treated with low-dose radiation therapy subsequently develop thyroid nodules, with about 1.8% to 10% of patients subsequently developing papillary carcinoma. The vast majority of papillary carcinomas arise spontaneously. Latency periods between exposure to low-dose radiation therapy and subsequent thyroid malignancy range from 5 to 40 years. Individuals exposed to radiation through nuclear fallout including Hiroshima and, more recently, Chernobyl, have increased rates of papillary carcinoma with a shorter latency to development of cancer.

PAPILLARY CARCINOMA

Papillary carcinoma in the vast majority of cases is associated with a quite favorable prognosis. The unusually favorable course of papillary carcinoma can be understood when appreciating the rates at which papillary carcinomas are found in autopsy specimens and in the lack of clinical significance of microscopic disease. The numerous studies have shown that "occult" carcinomas are present in 5% to 36% of thyroid glands subject to serial section at autopsy in patients without a history of clinically apparent thyroid carcinoma. Microscopic papillary carcinoma is frequently present in the contralateral lobe (in up to 80% of patients) and ipsilateral neck nodes (in up to 50% to 80% of patients). Although frequently present microscopically, this disease in the contralateral lobe and ipsilateral neck is typically indolent and of little clinical significance. The development of clinically significant papillary carcinoma in an unresected contralateral lobe occurs only in about 5% of patients. The development of clinically significant nodal disease in a patient initially N0 occurs in only 4% to 9% of patients. The lack of clinical significance of microscopic neck disease was the impetus that lead to abandonment of prophylactic neck dissections performed for regional nodal microscopic disease in the 1960s and 1970s in patients presenting with N0 papillary carcinoma.

Most studies suggest that the presence of cervical lymph node metastasis has no significant prognostic implication in patients with papillary carcinoma of the thyroid. The presence of cervical lymph node metastasis may however increase the rate at which subsequent nodal disease develops.

Just over 10% of patients with papillary carcinoma recur after initial treatment. Recurrent disease may occur after many years of clinical stability. Even patients with known pulmonary metastasis may survive for decades. In patients initially thought to be free of disease after initial treatment, regional lymphatic metastasis occurs in 8% to 9%, thyroid bed (invasive) recurrence occurs in 5% to 6%, and distant metastasis (lung, bone) in 4% to 11%. Cervical nodal recurrences are most easily cured, but only 40% of thyroid bed recurrences and 15% of distant metastasis are cured. The development of thyroid bed recurrence or distant metastatic disease does worsen survival, although the development of regional nodal recurrence typically does not.

FOLLICULAR CARCINOMA

Follicular carcinoma of the thyroid is a well-differentiated thyroid malignancy with follicular differentiation. It is the identification of pericapsular vascular invasion that is the most reliable indication of follicular malignancy. Follicular carcinoma, unlike papillary carcinoma, arises as a unifocal thyroid lesion. It does not have papillary carcinoma's propensity for intraglandular or regional nodal spread. A recent review of bilateral thyroid resections for follicular carcinoma showed that the incidence of contralateral thyroid lobar disease for follicular carcinoma approaches zero. Follicular carcinoma also occurs more commonly in women but occurs in an older age group than papillary carcinoma, typically presenting in the sixth decade. Little is known regarding the etiology of follicular carcinoma, but it appears to occur more frequently in areas of iodine-deficient endemic goiter. It appears that follicular carcinoma probably does not arise from previously existing follicular adenomas. When follicular carcinoma is diagnosed, one must regard the possibility of distant metastatic disease, especially when considering that the histologic definition of follicular carcinoma involves vascular invasion at the level of the lesion's capsule. At presentation, the rate of distant metastasis for patients with follicular carcinoma is generally felt to be between 10% and 20%. For patients with follicular carcinoma judged to be free of disease after initial surgery, approximately 30% will recur, with 7% in regional nodes, 8% in thyroid bed, and 13% with distant metastasis. Only about 15% of patients with meta-static follicular carcinoma can be cured. The most important prognostic factor for follicular carcinoma relates to the degree of invasiveness of the primary. Insular and poorly differentiated forms of follicular carcinoma generally have poorer prognosis than follicular carcinoma.

Hurthle cell carcinoma is considered a subtype of follicular carcinoma. Its prognosis is somewhat worse than the stage equivalent follicular carcinoma in that its uptake of radioactive iodine is generally poor.

Patients with papillary and follicular carcinoma (well-differentiated thyroid carcinoma) have been grouped in a number of retrospective studies given their similarities regarding important prognostic features. A number of key prognostic variables allow us to segregate patients with well-differentiated thyroid carcinoma into a large low-risk group (approximately 90% of patients) and a small high-risk group (approximately 10% of patients). Mortality in the low-risk group is approximately 1% to 2%, whereas in the high-risk group, it is approximately 40% to 50%. The key elements of existing prognostic schema include age, degree of invasiveness/extra thyroidal extension, metastasis, sex, and size. Typically, for women less than 50 years of age and for men less than 40 years of age, prognosis is improved. Increased invasiveness increases the risk of local, regional, and distant recurrence and decreases survival. The presence of distant metastasis increases mortality, and men generally have a poorer prognosis than women. Patients with lesions larger than 5 cm have a worse prognosis than those with lesions smaller than 1.5 cm. Hay's scheme for papillary carcinoma is summarized by the pneumonic AGES for age, gender, extent, and size. Cady's prognostic schema for papillary and follicular carcinoma is summarized by the pneumonic AMES for age, metastasis, extent and size.

The extent of thyroidectomy has been a tremendously controversial issue. The studies that are currently available are all retrospective. Mazzaferri's recent large retrospective study with long-term follow-up on a large number of patients suggests that bilateral thyroid surgery improves survival and decreases recurrence. He recommends near total thyroidectomy for lesions greater than 1.5 cm, followed by radioactive iodine and T4 suppression. However, there are many retrospective studies showing no difference in survival between patients treated with hemithyroidectomy versus total thyroidectomy. Some studies also showed that recurrence is favorably affected by initial aggressive bilateral thyroid surgery, although others question the significance of extent of thyroidectomy on recurrence rate. The relationship of recurrence to distant metastasis and initial thyroid surgery is interesting. Grant found that, among patients recurring within the contralateral lobe after conservative thyroid, none died of recurrent disease. Rose found that the development in distant metastasis seemed unrelated to the development of recurrence within the contralateral lobe. Rossi noted that none of the deaths in the group of patients who recurred locally could have been prevented through the initial option of total thyroidecomy. Vickery noted no contralateral lobe recurrence in his series patients with conservative thyroid surgery. Recurrence in this series was typical nodal with no impact on long-term survival or distant with significant impact on long-term survival.

An argument that has been offered for total thyroidectomy in all cases is that it facilitates the use of thyroglobulin and radioactive iodine scanning and treatment in postoperative follow-up. The author has shown that, in patients treated with conservative thyroid surgery, low-dose I^{131} ablation results in TSH greater than 25 mU/L in 90% of patients and therefore allows for whole body scanning and thyroglobulin use as a marker. It is also to be noted in this discussion that total thyroidectomy, even in expert hands, results in significant thyroid bed radioactive iodine uptake in a substantial fraction of patients. Even in skilled hands, reports have ranged from 29% to 82% of patients undergoing total thyroidectomy had significant residual functional thyroid bed activity postoperatively. Although total thyroidectomy can be offered in selected centers of surgical experience, the bulk of the literature supports increased complication rates, mainly recurrent laryngeal nerve paralysis and permanent hypoparathyroidism with bilateral thyroid surgery.

A rational surgical plan, which blends aggressive oncologic resection and a commitment to not harm the patient, can be constructed for patients with well-differentiated thyroid carcinoma despite the divergent information in the literature. The basic concept relates to treating patients, depending on their prognostic risk grouping. Hay found that in low-risk group patients there was no difference in survival between unilateral or bilateral thyroid surgery. However, survival was improved in the high-risk group patients with the offering of bilateral surgery over unilateral thyroid surgery. However, in this high-risk group, total thyroidectomy offered no improved survival benefit above near total thyroidectomy. Surgery should then be undertaken with the primary intent of encompassing all gross disease in both thyroid and neck. Microscopic disease, although frequently present in the contralateral lobe and ipsilateral neck, is infrequently clinically manifest. Intraoperative palpation and preoperative sonography can help evaluate gross disease in the contralateral lobe. Most agree that bilateral thyroid surgery optimizes survival in patients in the high-risk group, but there is no decrement in survival with the offering of a near total thyroidectomy in this group of patients. Patients in the low-risk group with small intrathyroidal lesions are well treated with unilateral thyroid surgery if the contralateral lobe is negative on preoperative ultrasound and intraoperative palpation. The overriding philosophy is that gross disease should be resected; thus, patients without gross disease in the contralateral lobe in the low-risk group may be treated with conservative unilateral thyroid surgery. However, patients with gross airway invasion should be treated with segmental airway resection. In this respect, the extent of treatment is tailored to the level of risk. The degree of thyroid resection should also incorporate information on how the first side has gone, in terms of recurrent laryngeal nerve and parathyroid identification and preservation. If, after the first side of surgery, there are two parathyroids of good color and on good vascular pedicles with a recurrent laryngeal nerve that stimulates well electrically, contralateral thyroid surgery can be contemplated. If the first side has not gone well, contralateral thyroid surgery should be deferred or at least postponed.

The presence of cervical nodal disease in patients with well-differentiated thyroid carcinoma relates to recurrence rather than survival. Because of the tendency of papillary carcinoma to spread early on to regional nodal beds, the central and lateral necks should be inspected visually and through palpation intraoperatively. A systematic and compartmental neck dissection appears to reduce subsequent nodal recurrence when compared with "berry-picking" procedures. Extrathyroidal disease involving strap muscles or sternocleidomastoid should be managed with resection of the involved musculature. If the recurrent laryngeal nerve is involved with invasive disease and is preoperatively paralyzed, this nerve should be resected. If preoperative function is present, an attempt should be made to resect the disease with neural preservation, hopefully leaving only microscopic disease adjacent to the nerve to be treated with radioactive iodine. Disease that is adherent, but separable, from the airway, should be resected without airway resection. Disease that is grossly involving the airway should be treated with segmental airway resection and reconstruction.

Postoperatively, patients with well-differentiated thyroid cancer are treated with thyroid hormone suppression and considered for radioactive iodine ablation, scanning, and treatment. Such patients receive follow-up intermittently with physical examinations, sonography, chest films, and thyroglobulin measures and whole body iodine I^{131} scanning. Thyroglobulin is usually elevated after total thyroid ablation in patients with known metastatic disease and, along with whole body scanning, can be used to assess status of metastatic disease.

MEDULLARY CARCINOMA OF THE THYROID

Medullary carcinoma of the thyroid represents approximately 5% to 10% of all thyroid cancers and arises from the parafollicular C-cell, rather than the follicular parenchymal cell as for papillary and follicular carcinoma. Medullary carcinoma's behavior is one of role intermediate between well-differentiated thyroid cancer and anaplastic. Calcitonin, the hormonal product of C-cells and medullary cancer, is useful both in initial diagnosis and long-term tumor surveillance. Most medullary cancers represent sporadic neoplasms, typically presenting in the fourth decade as a unifocal lesion without associated endocrinopathy. About 25% of medullary carcinoma represents inherited disease. There are three specific forms of inherited medullary carcinoma. All are associated as an autosomal dominant trait, and all develop as a result of multifocal C-cell hyperplasia with gradual evolution of multifocal medullary carcinoma. MEN2A (multiple endocrine neoplasia 2A) typically presents in the third decade and is associated with pheochromocytoma and hyperparathyroidism. MEN2B usually presents in a younger age group (first or second decade) and is associated with pheochromocytoma and mucosal neuromata and Marfanoid habitus. Familial, non-MEN medullary typically presents in the fourth decade and has no associated endocrinopathies. All inherited forms of medullary carcinoma have been associated with RET oncogene point mutations. Although sporadically inherited forms appear to be easily recognizable discreet entities, approximately 30% of patients felt to be sporadic ultimately are diagnosed as inherited cases. Be-

cause of this, all patients with medullary carcinoma are recommended to have a total thyroidectomy.

Preoperatively, it is important to not only obtain calcitonin level but also to screen for parathyroid disease with a serum calcium and parathormone (PTH) and to screen for pheochromocytoma with a 24-hour urine collection for urinary catecholamines, vanillylmandelic acid (VMA), and metanephrines.

It is important to recognize that any patient with medullary carcinoma of the thyroid presenting with a palpable mass has a very high likelihood of having regional nodal involvement. Because of the tendency for early regional nodal involvement, neck dissection should virtually always accompany the total thyroidectomy. Recent work has emphasized the importance of having a low threshold for including not only central neck but also bilateral lateral neck dissections. During total thyroidectomy for medullary carcinoma, all four parathyroid glands must be explored. For MEN IIA, limited excision of only grossly enlarged glands results in a low rate of recurrence in patients with hyperparathyroidism.

Medullary carcinoma tends to metastasize early to cervical and mediastinal nodal beds and frequently recurs locally. Hematogenous metastases may occur ultimately to lung, liver, and bone.

LYMPHOMA

Thyroid lymphoma usually presents as a rapidly enlarging mass, often painless, in the elderly patient, often with a preceding history of hypothyroidism or Hashimoto's thyroiditis. Surgical treatment for lymphoma typically involves isthmectomy often combined with tracheotomy, depending on the status of the larynx. Treatment is with radiation therapy and chemotherapy.

ANAPLASTIC CARCINOMA

Anaplastic carcinoma is a rare and virulent malignancy arising from thyroid parenchyma. It typically presents in an older age group with a rapidly enlarging mass and typically with fixation to central neck structures, ipsilateral nodal disease, and sometimes vocal cord paralysis. It is important to differentiate anaplastic carcinoma, small cell type, from lymphoma. Surgical treatment is generally limited to isthmectomy for biopsy often combined with tracheotomy. It is important to obtain sufficient material to rule out lymphoma. Aggressive surgery generally has not been found to be effective. Treatment includes hyperfractionated external beam radiation combined with doxorubicin-based chemotherapy.

TECHNIQUE OF THYROIDECTOMY: SURGICAL ANATOMY

Thyroid surgical anatomy is revealed during thyroidectomy through attention to exposure, direct visualization of surrounding anatomy, and bloodless technique. Even minimal blood loss during thyroidectomy can stain parathyroidal planes and lead to difficulties in parathyroid recognition.

The author favors loupe magnification during thyroidectomy. Initial patient positioning helps to facilitate adequate neck base exposure. A thyroid inflatable bag or towel roll is placed under the shoulders with attention toward adequate head support. If nerve monitoring is anticipated, paralytic agents are avoided. The standard Kocher collar–type thyroid incision is made typically 1 to 2 fingerbreadths above the sternal notch in a normal skin crease. Generally, the lower the incision the more cosmetic the result. However, it is best in thin women to place the incision above the sternal notch if it is notably scaphoid. Access to lower and mid-lateral neck nodal groups can be obtained by simply extending the curvilinear incision in the skin crease laterally. If upper nodal groups are accessed, then an ascending limb is drawn. This ascending limb should be curved to prevent vertical scar banding. It is best to place this ascending limb as posteriorly as possible so that it is not apparent from front view. The subplatysmal flap is raised without uncovering strap musculature, leaving the anterior jugular vein and middle layer of deep cervical fascia down on the straps. Inferior subplatysmal flap is infrequently needed if incision is low. If strap musculature is exposed during flap elevation, the undersurface of the flap may scar to the strap musculature, leading to unsightly puckering of neck skin with deglutition postoperatively. The medial edge of the sternohyoid muscle is dissected bilaterally from the thyroid notch to sternum. As the sternohyoid is lifted ventrally, the medial edge of the underlying, more laterally set sternothyroid is identified. Both sternohyoid and sternothyroid are grasped and pulled ventrally. As this is done, the index finger pushes the thyroid down and medially to open the areolar tissue of the perithyroid sheath in the interval between the undersurface of the strap muscles and ventral surfaces of the thyroid lobe. There may be small bridging vessels here, which can be easily controlled with bipolar cautery. With invasive thyroid disease, the strap musculature may be fixed to the thyroid mass, and in this case, the affected strap musculature should be undissected on the ventral surface of the thyroid lobe and transected both above and below the involved segment. Aggressive or multiple fine needle aspiration attempts can lead to a mild scarring between the strap muscles and thyroid lobe. At this juncture, and before any true lateral dissection, it is the author's preference to identify the midline definitively, both above and below the thyroid isthmus. This allows for constant visual and palpable identification of the midline throughout the case, which is especially helpful in a setting of goiterous distortion of neck base anatomy. It is also an opportunity to dissect the prelaryngeal and pretracheal planes to examine and send for frozen section any suspicious adenopathy in these regions.

Lateral Thyroid Dissection

Once the midline and strap musculature is dissected, lateral to the thyroid region, it should be inspected. It is of critical importance that the lateral thyroid region be maximally exposed. This is obtained not only by lateral retraction of the strap muscle and, in some circumstances, the sternocleidomastoid muscle, but also by medial traction on the thyroid and laryngotracheal complex. Kocher referred to this as "me-

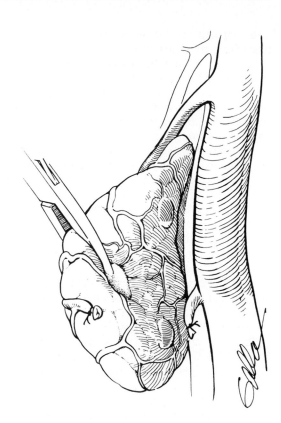

FIGURE 18–5. Division of the middle thyroid vein enhances the lateral thyroid region exposure. (From Lee KJ, ed: Essential Otolaryngology, ed. 7. New York, McGraw-Hill, 1999; with permission.)

dial dislocation of the goiter." This medial component to this medial traction is a significant component of adequate lateral thyroid region exposure. This maneuver typically presents the middle thyroid vein, which can then be dissected and tied (Fig. 18–5). Loss of control of the middle thyroid vein usually results in significant staining of the lateral thyroid region as it is a direct branch of the internal jugular vein. In those cases of goiterous enlargement, the strap muscle retraction does not provide for adequate lateral exposure, and the strap musculature can be incised superiorly to provide for preservation of inferiorly based innervation. If strap muscles are incised, they should then be clamped, tied, and retracted to make the most of the exposure that the incision has provided. It is of note that the lateral aspect of the strap muscles comes into very close proximity with the carotid sheath, specifically the jugular vein. As a result, it is important, to avoid injury to carotid sheath structures (carotid artery, vagus nerve, and internal jugular vein), that the lateral margin of the strap muscles be dissected with identification of carotid sheath structures before incision of strap musculature. In cases where strap musculature does not need to be incised, but the sternothyroid in its medially directed course toward the thyroid cartilage hoods the superior pole, the sternothyroid alone can be incised superiorly. This maneuver facilitates superior pole exposure to dissect the superior pole with full view of the external branch of the superior laryngeal nerve. At this juncture, it is reasonable to palpate the recurrent laryngeal nerve, paratracheal chain of nodes, and also the lateral neck jugular chain bilaterally.

Inferior Pole Inspection: Inferior Parathyroid Identification

There is a tendency at this juncture to move toward recurrent laryngeal nerve identification at the thoracic inlet. It is best to resist this temptation and instead inspect the inferior pole for the inferior parathyroid. The recurrent laryngeal nerve is best found more superiorly at approximately the mid-polar level. If it is found inferiorly and dissected superiorly, the surgeon puts at risk the lateral to medial oriented parathyroid blood supply. It is therefore best at this juncture to simply inspect the inferior pole of the thyroid to identify the inferior parathyroid, which is typically inferior or lateral to the inferior pole of the thyroid, usually resting in fat or thyrothymic horn. Because of the variability of inferior parathyroid position (more variable than the superior parathyroid owing to its longer embryologic migration course), the inferior parathyroid can not always be identified during routine thyroidectomy. If the inferior parathyroid can not be specifically identified, then the dissection of the thyroid's inferior pole should be performed with emphasis on reflecting all perithyroidal fat inferiorly with strict inferior pole thyroid capsule plane of dissection. This technique allows for preservation of the inferior parathyroid within the perithyroidal fat. The avoidance of dissection laterally, such as to find the recurrent laryngeal nerve at this juncture, helps to preserve the laterally oriented inferior parathyroid blood supply. Thus, even if the inferior parathyroid is not specifically identified, maneuvers facilitate its preservation and ongoing blood supply. With the inferior pole fully dissected, it can be drawn up and onto the trachea and the recurrent laryngeal nerve can be identified typically at a mid-polar level. At this level, the recurrent laryngeal nerve is crossing the inferior thyroid artery. If the inferior thyroid artery can be easily identified during the case, this helps to facilitate identification of the nerve. Also, by tracing out the inferior thyroid artery, clues can be obtained regarding the parathyroid location. It is best to do as little dissection of the inferior thyroid artery as possible to prevent injury to the tenuous distal branches supplying parathyroid tissue. Recurrent laryngeal nerve branching occurs in about one third of patients, with 90% of extralaryngeal branching occurring above the intersection of the nerve and inferior thyroid artery. Studies have shown that identification of the nerve during thyroidectomy results in a lower rate of injury during thyroidectomy than if the nerve is simply avoided through a "blind capsular dissection." Nerve stimulation can be used to facilitate nerve identification. Capsular dissection has been proposed as a method of avoiding and, therefore, not injuring, recurrently laryngeal nerve. However, the work of Berlin (1935) and, more recently, Wafae, suggests that in 10% to 20% of patients with recurrent laryngeal, nerve actually penetrate into thyroid tissue at the level of the ligament of Berry. In such circumstances, capsular dissection would lead to nerve transection. The recurrent laryngeal nerve is identified in its characteristic location in the tracheoesophageal groove, more laterally on the right than on the left, owing to variations in vascular mediastinal anatomy. On the right, should a nerve not be apparent on initial dissection, nonrecurrence should be considered. Goiterous enlargement of the thyroid can result in significant nerve displacement. The author has found that in about 15% of large cervical or substernal goiters, the nerve can be fixed or splayed on the surface of the thyroid in such a way that traction on the thyroid without nerve identification would lead to significant nerve injury. In these cases the recurrent laryngeal nerve should be searched through a superior approach by taking a superior pole down and finding the nerve at its laryngeal entry point. As the recurrent laryngeal nerve is dissected superiorly, it is dissected into the region described as the ligament of Berry. This is the area of most difficult dissection of the nerve. The nerve is typically deep to the ligament of Berry but can pass to within posterior components of the leaflet. Varying infiltration of thyroid tissue into the substance of the ligament of Berry brings thyroid tissue into close proximity to the nerve. In some cases, thyroid tissue may completely surround the nerve in this interval. The firmness of the ligament of Berry, its vascularity, and the proximity of thyroid tissue to the nerve make this area of dissection the most difficult. Extralaryngeal branching, if it is present, typically occurs at this level. The nerve should be identified at the base of the ligament and dissected through the ligament of Berry with attention toward resection of all adjacent thyroid tissue. If bleeding occurs in this area, it is typically controlled by gentle pressure for several moments. It is best not to indiscriminately clamp or cauterize aggressively in this region. If exposure is not good, there is a temptation to leave thyroid tissue here. Such thyroid tissue remains as a circular profile approximating the cut edge of the ligament of Berry and is responsible for thyroid bed uptake after "total thyroidectomy."

The author believes that the recurrent laryngeal nerve should be both visually and electrically identified through neural monitoring in all cases. The nerve has a characteristic caliber and wave-like profile. Usually there is a discreet vessel running along the back of the nerve. Electrical identification of the recurrent laryngeal nerve is analogous to electrical stimulation of the facial nerve during parotid surgery. The electrical identification reinforces its visual identification and provides the surgeon with a new functional dimension to surgical anatomy. Many methods have been used to electrically monitor the nerve during surgery. A simple method is to palpate the postcricoid region by placing the finger adjacent to the hypopharynx behind the cricoid and stimulating the nerve with any of a variety of nerve stimulators. This technique does not allow for passive monitoring and requires a finger to be placed behind the larynx whenever the nerve is tested. The author has used electrophysiologic monitoring of the recurrent laryngeal and vagal nerves in over 450 cases of thyroidectomy and parathyroidectomy at Massachusetts Eye and Ear Infirmary and has found that an endotracheal tube–based electromyographic system compares favorably with translaryngeal hook-wire vocal cord electromyographic monitoring and is reliable and safe. Electrophysiologic monitoring of the recurrent laryngeal nerve also allows for prediction of function postoperatively. It has been shown by several workers that recurrent laryngeal nerve surgical injury is often not recognized intraoperatively by the surgeon visually. Thus, in the majority of cases, the surgeon is unaware of recurrent laryngeal injury. It is this predictive value of electrophysiologic monitoring during thyroidectomy that is most important to the surgeon.

Once the recurrent laryngeal is dissected up into the ligament of Berry, exposure is further facilitated by then shifting to dissection of the superior pole. The superior pole region's exposure is optimized by transecting the sternothyroid muscle as it inserts into the thyroid cartilage. Lateral retraction on the superior pole and medial traction on the larynx help to open up this space. The external branch of the superior laryngeal nerve can be on or deep to the fascia of the inferior constrictor. Nerve stimulation of the external branch results in a discreet twitch of the cricothyroid muscle. Cernea has described the surgical anatomy of the external branch of the superior laryngeal nerve and has shown that in approximately 20% of cases, the nerve is intimately related with the superior pole capsule and vessels requiring wide exposure of this region to prevent injury to the external branch. Once the superior pole vessels are taken, the superior pole can be retracted down and medial, similar to the inferior pole where dissection has resulted in its upward and medial movement. At this point, the lobe is pedicled to the ligament of Berry, which can be dissected with full view of the recurrent laryngeal nerve as it relates to the ligament of Berry. Note that the superior parathyroid is typically identified in pericapsular fat, adjacent to the posterolateral aspect of the superior pole. It can be vascularized by the posterior branches of the superior thyroid artery, and care should be taken to preserve these branches as the superior pole is dissected. If the parathyroid turns completely black subsequent to dissection, its vascularity is very much in question. A biopsy should therefore be performed, and it should be minced into 1-mm cubes and placed into three separate muscular pockets in the ipsilateral SCM muscle marked with a clip, after frozen section confirms its parathyroid nature. It is of note that parathyroids may become ischemic without color change. Therefore, it is important to assess the vascular input to a gland. It is best to avoid dissection of the parathyroid from its surrounding fat and to leave undissected a span of tissue from the parathyroid directed out laterally to preserve incoming blood supply. If the parathyroid has not been dissected from surrounding fat, is of good color, and does have a laterally oriented undissected vascular pathway, it is reasonable to assume that it will function postoperatively. In those rare instances where initial lobectomy was not accompanied by adequate parathyroid identification and preservation and where contralateral thyroidectomy is necessary, consideration should be given to subtotal or near total technique on the contralateral side to avoid permanent hypoparathyroidism.

Once the thyroid lobe is fully mobilized, the isthmus can be transected after it is dissected off the front face of the trachea. A 2-0 running silk is placed on the isthmus stump. The specimen is sent to pathology after it is meticulously examined for possible resected parathyroids. Such resected parathyroids should undergo biopsy, and when confirmed as parathyroid, and then be re-implanted. As the isthmus is transected, a search for any pyramidal lobe is important. Contralateral thyroidectomy is then performed, depending on frozen section of the resected lobe. If no additional work is contemplated, anesthesia should supply several high-pressure ventilated breaths to identify any occult venous bleeding. The strap muscles are then approximated in the midline with attention to covering any exposed strap muscle to prevent scarring to the undersurface of the skin flap. The platysmal layer is then closed with 3-0 Vicryl, and the skin is closed with fine nylon suture. Drains are not typi-

cally necessary during thyroid surgery unless strap muscle division or a large goiter has been resected.

During surgery for goiter, patient positioning is very important. Generally, patients can be intubated in the standard way, but consideration should be given toward bronchoscopic-assisted transnasal intubation. Usually for large cervical goiters and substernal goiters, the recurrent laryngeal nerve can not be identified in the thoracic inlet. Some have recommended blind finger dissection of the goiter with mobilization without nerve identification. The author has found that about 15% of patients with large cervical or substernal goiters have fixation or splaying of the nerve on the surface of the goiter. These patients would have significant, and likely permanent, neural injury with blind finger mobilization of the goiter without prior nerve identification. Sinclair has noted a 17.5% incidence of vocal cord paralysis with this fingered dissection technique. The author recommends the superior approach to the nerve, identifying the nerve at its laryngeal entry point and then dissecting it retrograde off the surface of the goiter, before goiter delivery. Blood supply to substernal components of substernal goiters is almost always from the inferior thyroid artery and only rarely from the thyroid ima, subclavian, or internal mammary. Cysts within multinodular goiter can be decompressed with intraoperative fine needle aspiration. The author does not recommend morsalization of goiters, given the possibility of thyroid malignancy within the goiter and the potential for difficulty in hemostasis. The author has found that sternotomy is rarely needed, even with large cervical and substernal goiters. Total thyroidectomy is rarely necessary in these cases (Fig. 18–6). Even in the setting of significant tracheal compression and deviation, the author has not found tracheomalacia to be a problem postoperatively. What has previously been diagnosed as tracheomalacia may in fact have been undiagnosed bilateral vocal cord paralysis.

Should a nerve be transected during thyroidectomy, neurorrhaphy is best. Although laryngeal synkinesis will likely occur, ongoing motor tone will improve glottic function by providing for a less atrophic cord and a more normally positioned arytenoid. Should a nerve be clamped or ligated, it is best to simply free the nerve. Neurorrhaphy in this circumstance should not be performed.

Surgical Complications

Surgical complications involve neural injury (recurrent laryngeal nerve [RLN] and superior laryngeal nerve [SLN]), hypoparathyroidism, and a variety of nonspecific wound complications such as bleeding, infection, seroma, and keloid formation. Although significant hemorrhage is rare, airway obstruction may occur unless the wound is promptly opened.

Permanent recurrent laryngeal nerve paralysis is difficult to estimate after total thyroidectomy because many studies do not routinely involve postoperative laryngeal exams. Generally, expert rates are 1% to 2%, although many reports exist with significantly higher rates such as 6% to 7%, with rates as high as 23% being reported. Two recent reports document recurrent laryngeal nerve paralysis rates of approximately 10%. Martensson has shown that the incidence of RLN paralysis is higher with bilateral surgery, revision surgery, surgery for malignancy, or in patients brought back

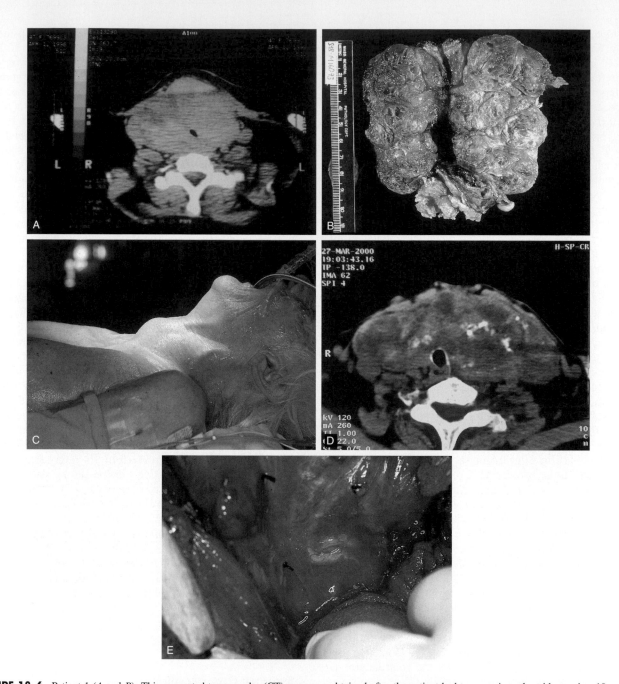

FIGURE 18-6. Patient 1 (*A* and *B*): This computed tomography (CT) scan was obtained after the patient had two previous thyroidectomies, 10 and 20 years before presentation. This surgery represented her third revision thyroidectomy. Preoperative diagnosis at an outside institution was asthma. The mass was benign. The recurrent laryngeal nerves were identified, and she had normal cord motion postoperatively. The trachea was compressed, but there was no evidence of tracheal malacia, and she did not require tracheotomy. Airway symptoms resolved postoperatively.

Patient 2 (*C, D,* and *E*): Elderly woman with a large multilobulated calcified cervical goiter. The recurrent laryngeal nerve was entrapped within layers of fascia adjacent to the lateral aspect of the left thyroid lobe (see the *white band* on the side of the goiter in *E*). Neural monitoring allowed identification and preservation of both recurrent laryngeal nerves with normal cord function postoperatively.

for bleeding. Sinclair noted a baseline rate of 1.1%, but a 17.5% incidence in surgery for substernal goiter. Superior laryngeal nerve external branch paralysis occurs in 0.4% to 3% of cases. The lack of cricothyroid muscle vocal cord tensing results in a loss of high vocal registers and in a cord which, on examination, is bowed lower than the normal contralateral cord. In such cases, the glottis is to be rotated toward the side of injury.

Postoperative transient hypoparathyroidism occurs in 17% to 40% of patients post–total thyroidectomy. In an American College of Surgery report reviewing over 24,000 thyroidectomies, Foster noted an average permanent hypoparathyroidism rate of 8%. Mazzaferri noted a 13% incidence of permanent hypoparathyroidism when total thyroidectomy was performed in the community setting. Calcium should be instituted if patients have a total calcium level of 7.5 or if patients develop symptoms. The first 24 to 48 hours are when the calcium level should be decreasing most rapidly. With significant hypocalcemia, intravenous therapy is warranted. Oral replenishment is typically initi-

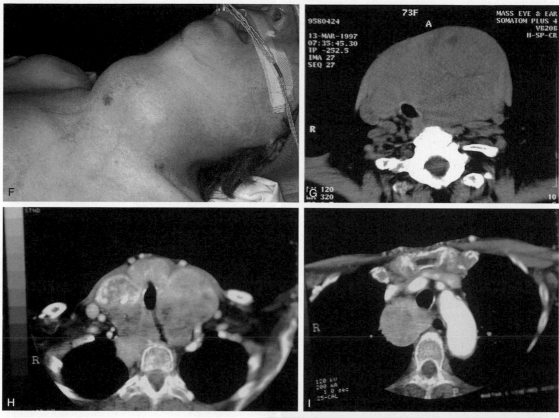

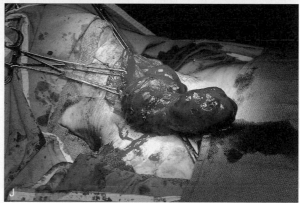

FIGURE 18-6. (*Continued*) Patient 3 (*F* and *G*): Large cervical goiter. Note redistribution of dermal veins secondary to jugular compression. The asymmetry of the goiter resulted in larynx rotation with the left recurrent laryngeal nerve entering into the side of the rotated larynx in the midline. The recurrently laryngeal nerves were identified and preserved with normal cord function postoperatively.

Patient 4 (*H, I,* and *J*): Patient with large cervical and substernal goiter. The mass was resected without sternal split transcervically with normal cord function postoperatively.

ated with 2 to 3 g of calcium carbonate divided three times a day with vitamin D, 1,25 dihydroxy cholecalciferol from 0.25 to 5 μg orally.

Parathyroid Surgery

Parathyroid hormone, the parathyroid gland's hormonal product, results in calcium serum elevation through increased gastrointestinal absorption, bone calcium mobilization, inhibition of renal calcium excretion, and stimulation of renal hydroxylase. The normal parathyroid glands are composed of chief cells as well as oncocytic cells and fat. Primary hyperparathyroidism involves the enlargement and hyperfunction of one or more parathyroid glands with ensuing hypercalcemia. Primary hyperparathyroidism is caused by single-gland enlargement in about 85% of cases and in four-gland hyperplasia in about 10% to 15% of cases. Double adenomas account for about 2% to 3% of cases. Carcinomatous degeneration of parathyroid tissue occurs rarely and accounts for 1% of cases with primary hyperparathyroidism. The differentiation between single-gland and four-gland disease is difficult in that the enlargement of parathyroids in four-gland disease can be very asymmetric. The diagnosis of single-gland adenoma versus four-gland hyperplasia incorporates both gross surgical and histologic information. If all four parathyroid glands are inspected and a single gland is enlarged, adenoma is suggested. The diagnosis of adenoma is confirmed, and four-gland hyperplasia ruled out if the adenoma is resected and the biopsy sample of a normal gland is a normal-appearing, non-hypercellular parathyroid gland.

Primary hyperparathyroidism is usually spontaneous but can occur in familial or MEN-associated syndromes. It occurs with increased frequency in patients with a history of low-dose external beam radiation therapy. Secondary hyperparathyroidism results from prolonged parathyroid

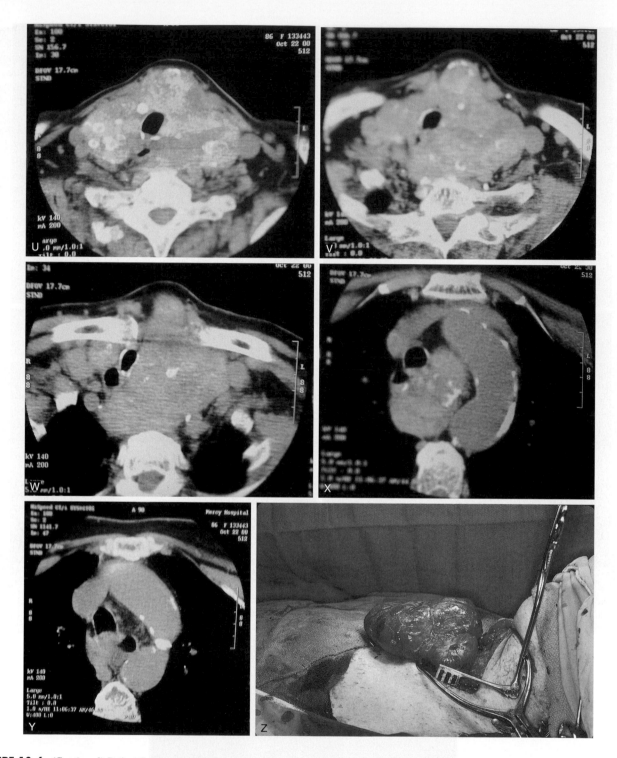

FIGURE 18–6. (*Continued*) Patient 7 (*U* to *Z*): Elderly woman with cervical goiter with significant left substernal extension to below the aortic arch down to the azygos vein. The mass was excised transcervically without sternal split, without change to preoperative vocal cord function.

lignancy, vitamin D and calcium excess intake, lithium and thiazide diuretics, immobilization, and benign familial hypocalciuric hypercalcemia. Benign familial hypocalciuric hypercalcemia can be easily confused with primary hyperparathyroidism as both calcium and PTH can be elevated in this autosomal dominant inherited disease characterized by excess renal calcium reabsorption leading to high serum calcium and low urine calcium levels. Urine 24-hour calcium levels should be less than 100 mg in a 24-hour sample in patients with benign familial hypocalciuric hypercalcemia.

In the past, patients would have presented primarily with the symptomatic sequela of long-term hypercalcemia, including "painful bones, kidney stones, abdominal groans, psychic moans and fatigue overtones." However, the majority of primary hyperparathyroidism today is detected on routine laboratory screening panels. Most endocrine surgeons and endocrinologists agree that patients who are symptomatic from hypercalcemia warrant surgical exploration. It is also generally agreed that patients who are young (less than 50 years of age) should be offered surgical exploration. The rationale for this offering is that studies have shown untreated hyperparathyroidism is associated with increased cardiovascular morbidity and that approximately 25% of patients who receive follow-up without surgery subsequently develop symptomatic hypercalcemia in long-term follow-up. Elderly patients who are asymptomatic have been a source of controversy. Recently it appears that bone density improvements after successful surgery argue toward consideration for surgery even in these elderly asymptomatic patients. The National Institute of Health consensus opinion has been developed regarding surgical exploration criteria for patients with hyperparathyroidism. Surgery is recommended according to this opinion in patients who (1) are symptomatic; (2) have calcium levels greater than 11.5; (3) are under 50 years of age; (4) have had a previous episode of life-threatening hypercalcemia; (5) are asymptomatic and over 50 years of age if there is evidence of (a) creatinine clearance decrease by 30% for age without other obvious cause; (b) urinary calcium greater than 400 mg/dL; or (c) if bone density is less than 2 standard deviations below the mean corrected for age, gender, and race.

During the preoperative evaluation, a history of radiation therapy, hypertension, or symptoms of pheochromocytoma should be elicited. A family history should also be taken for familial calcium, parathyroid conditions, or neck surgery of any type. Preoperative laboratory work, in addition to calcium, intact PTH, and phosphorus, should also include blood urea nitrogen, creatinine, albumin, and alkaline phosphatase, as well as a 24-hour urine for calcium and creatinine. Alkaline phosphatase may be elevated in patients with bone disease, which may result in prolonged hypocalcemia after successful surgery. Localization studies can be obtained to help guide the surgeon toward the presumptive adenoma (Fig. 18–7). Commonly used localization test modalities include ultrasonography, CT, MRI, and Sestamibi scanning. The author prefers the combination of sonography and Sestamibi scanning because this images the parathyroids from two different perspectives (structurally and functionally). Sonography is relatively expensive with sensitivities up to 80% to 90%. Sonography is very operator dependent and can miss lesions in areas of echo shadow typically behind the larynx or trachea or in the mediastinum. Sestamibi scanning has excellent sensitivity and specificity but can miss small adenoma and mediastinal disease and is poor in multigland disease. It appears to be more sensitive than sonography, MRI, or CT scanning.

Parathyroid Exploration

There is controversy regarding the minimum accepted surgery for parathyroid exploration. These arguments have been significantly affected by the introduction of localization testing and, recently, intraoperative PTH analysis. The author

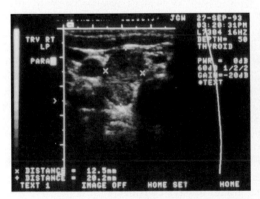
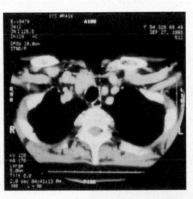
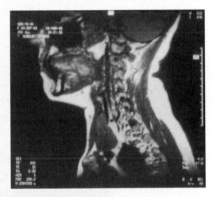
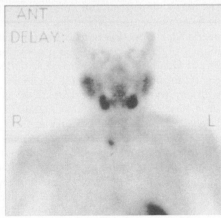
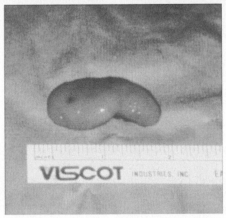

FIGURE 18–7. Parathyroid localization tests: parathyroid adenoma seen on sonogram, CT, MRI (top), and Sestamibi scanning (bottom). (From Lee KJ, ed: Essential Otolaryngology, ed. 7. New York, McGraw Hill, 1999; with permission.)

believes that the minimum effective surgery for patients with hyperparathyroidism is resection of the enlarged gland and identification and biopsy of a single normal-appearing gland. If the normal-gland biopsy comes back showing normal, nonhypercellular parathyroid, and intraoperative PTH falls within established criteria, surgery is complete and additional dissection is not necessary. In the past, before localization testing and intraoperative PTH, the gold standard was bilateral exploration and four-gland identification with resection of enlarged gland and biopsy of all remaining glands. Such approaches do result in increased rate of complications including hypoparathyroidism. It is important that if the degree of resection is reduced through the use of intraoperative PTH, very specific, safe criteria should be followed to optimize success.

In patients with four-gland hyperplasia, three and one-half–gland removal or four-gland resection with autotransplantation to forearm has been proposed. The exact type of four-gland hyperplasia should be considered when designing a surgical plan, as there is variability in aggressiveness within the various subtypes of four-gland hyperplasia. Milder forms of four-gland hyperplasia such as nonfamilial (sporadic) and MEN2A should be treated simply with resection of grossly enlarged glands. Such an approach has resulted in a low rate of hypercalcemic recurrence in these patients. However, in patients with more severe forms of four-gland hyperplasia such as familial hyperparathyroidism, secondary hyperparathyroidism, and MEN1-associated hyperparathyroidism, a more aggressive surgical approach including four-gland resection, bilateral thymectomy (given the incidence of supernumerary glands in these aggressive forms of hyperparathyroidism), and autotransplantation to forearm should be considered.

Parathyroid Surgical Anatomy

It is important to appreciate related embryology when attempting to identify parathyroid glands during exploration. Embryologic paths of descent and relationships to surrounding structures are essential. Individual normal parathyroid gland weighs between 35 to 40 mg and measures 5 × 3 × 1 mm. Parathyroid glands have a discreet encapsulated shape, which is beanlike or leaflike, often with a vascular strip down its midline. The parathyroid color has been described as yellow, tan, caramel, or mahogany. Adjacent fat, which the parathyroid is typically closely associated with, is softer, more amorphous, and a bright yellow by comparison. Adjacent thyroid tissue is redder and firmer. Lymph nodes are typically white to gray to red, firmer than parathyroids, and spherical to elliptical and often will have a slightly marbled surface. Thymic tissue, which is typically present as a finger of tissue that extends from the mediastinal thymus into the neck base to approximate the lower edge of the thyroid inferior pole, is typically a whitish-yellow color and has an encapsulated form. It is the movement of the parathyroids within the surgical field, within their surrounding fat, as discreet encapsulated structures with sharp margins that is the most helpful clue in their recognition. A strictly bloodless field needs to be maintained to appreciate these subtle characteristics. One should consider that most patients will

have four parathyroids. Approximately 5% to 13% of individuals will have more than four parathyroids.

The superior parathyroid descends from the fourth branchial pouch into its final adult orthotopic position, in close association with the lateral thyroid anlage c-cell complex. The variability of the superior parathyroid is less than that of the inferior parathyroid owing to its shorter migration. The superior parathyroid is typically located at the level of the cricothyroid cartilage articulation, approximately 1 cm above the intersection of the recurrent laryngeal nerve and inferior thyroid artery. In this location, the superior parathyroid is closely applied to the posterolateral surface of the thyroid's superior pole and often partially encased in fat. This parathyroid is located in a plane deep (dorsal) to the plane of the recurrent laryngeal nerve in the neck. The superior parathyroid is identified in this location as the layers of the perithyroidal sheath are dissected away from the thyroid in this region. The superior parathyroid tends, when ectopic, toward a retroesophageal posterior mediastinal location. The superior parathyroid is vascularized either directly by the inferior thyroid artery or, in approximately 45% of cases, either the superior thyroid artery or an anastomotic branch between the superior and inferior thyroid artery systems.

The inferior parathyroid arises from the third branchial pouch migrating closely with the developing thymus. It enjoys a greater varying adult position owing to this longer embryologic path relative to the superior parathyroid gland. The inferior parathyroid is typically within 1 cm inferior or lateral to the inferior pole of the thyroid. In such locations, the inferior parathyroid is closely associated with thyrothymic fat. When ectopic, the inferior parathyroid can, through incomplete migration, occur much higher in the neck, at the level of the hyoid bone or carotid bifurcation. In such upper neck locations, such undescended inferior parathyroids are usually associated with thymic remnants. The inferior parathyroid is located superficial (ventral) to the recurrent laryngeal nerve. The inferior thyroid artery provides blood supply to the inferior parathyroid.

Parathyroid exploration starts initially as with preparation for thyroidectomy. Given localization testing information and intraoperative PTH, more limited incisions have been considered in some cases of parathyroid exploration. However, one should always consider, in preoperative discussions with patients and in framing out the initial incision, the potential for multigland disease and the need for full, bilateral neck exploration. Localization tests dictate the initial region to be dissected. When a normal-appearing parathyroid is identified, it is important to dissect this tissue sufficiently to rule out an attached adenoma. This must be done with an eye toward prevention of devascularization. Akerstrom has noted a positional symmetry of the superior glands in 80% of cases and inferior glands in 70% of cases. All glands that are identified should be marked with a titanium clip. It is important that normal glands are identified and undergo biopsy but are never removed. It is important not to rupture an enlarged gland as one proceeds in its dissection because neoplastic parathyroid cells will seed the wound and lead to multifocal recurrence, which can be difficult to manage. Once an enlarged gland is identified, a search is performed for an ipsilateral normal-size gland. The ipsilateral normal-size gland can undergo biopsy at its nonhilar distal tip. If this confirms normal parathyroid tissue and the adenoma shows an enlarged hypercellular gland, the diagnosis of adenoma is reasonably correct. If intraoperative PTH falls appropriately, the diagnosis is confirmed and additional dissection is unwarranted. Should multiple enlarged glands be found, treatment should include consideration for removal of enlarged glands versus three and one-half–gland resection or four-gland resection with autotransplantation depending on the exact subtype of multiglandular disease. When enlarged, parathyroid glands can migrate. This is especially true for the superior parathyroid glands, which can descend posteriorly in a retroesophageal location along prevertebral fascia to the posterior mediastinum. Inferior glands can migrate to some degree as well, typically into the anterior mediastinal thymus. Should three normal glands be identified during dissection, a targeted exploration for the missing gland should be performed. Intrathyroidal parathyroids occur in 0.5% to 3% of cases. Rather than empirically offering thyroid lobectomy, it is best to perform a thyroidotomy to access the intrathyroidal lesion. Preoperative ultrasound becomes useful when considering intrathyroidal parathyroid adenoma. It is also possible to manipulate the thyroid lobe and generate a PTH spike intraoperatively to confirm the need for thyroidotomy.

Complications of Parathyroid Surgery

Parathyroid surgery, in experienced hands, is quite successful, with persistent hypercalcemia occurring in only approximately 5% of patients. There is a higher failure rate for patients with multigland disease, ranging from 10% to 50%. Reasons for failure of parathyroid exploration include (1) failure to find an adenomatous gland; (2) failure to recognize multigland disease (either second adenoma or four-gland hyperplasia); (3) failure to identify a supernumerary gland; (4) regrowth of an adenoma from an unresected stump; (5) unrecognized parathyroid carcinoma; and (6) incorrect diagnosis (eg, benign familial hypocalciuric hypercalcemia). Most studies that examine patients with missed adenomas find that the adenomas are within the neck. Excessive dissection during parathyroid surgery can lead to permanent hypoparathyroidism, which occurs rarely in patients with adenomas but in about 10% to 30% of cases of multigland disease or secondary hyperparathyroidism.